G000135200

From S
to Citizens

The Integration of Immigrant Communities in Britain, Ireland and Colonial America, 1550–1750

From Strangers to Citizens

The Integration of Immigrant
Communities in Britain, Ireland and
Colonial America, 1550–1750

Edited by

Randolph Vigne and
Charles Littleton

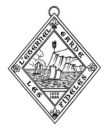

The Huguenot Society
of Great Britain and Ireland

sussex
ACADEMIC
PRESS

BRIGHTON • PORTLAND

2 4 6 8 10 9 7 5 3 1

First published 2001 in Great Britain by
THE HUGUENOT SOCIETY OF GREAT BRITAIN AND IRELAND
The Huguenot Library, University College, Gower Street, London WC1E 6BT
and
SUSSEX ACADEMIC PRESS
PO Box 2950
Brighton BN2 5SP

and in the United States of America by
THE HUGUENOT SOCIETY OF GREAT BRITAIN AND IRELAND
and
SUSSEX ACADEMIC PRESS
5824 N.E. Hassalo St.
Portland, Oregon 97213-3644

British Library Cataloguing in Publication Data
A CIP catalogue record for this book is available from the British Library.

Library of Congress Cataloging-in-Publication Data
From strangers to citizens : the integration of immigrant communities in Britain, Ireland, and colonial America, 1550–1750 / edited by Randolph Vigne and Charles Littleton.
p. cm.
Proceedings of a conference convened in London on 5–7 April 2001 by the Huguenot Society of Great Britain and Ireland.
Includes bibliographical references and index.
ISBN 1–902210–85–9 (hc : alk. paper) — ISBN 1–902210–86–7 (pbk. : alk. paper)
1. Great Britain—Ethnic relations—History—Congresses. 2. Great Britain—Emigration and immigration—History—Congresses. 3. North America—Emigration and immigration—History—Congresses. 4. Great Britain—Colonies—North America—History—Congresses. 5. Ireland—Emigration and immigration—History—Congresses. 6. North America—Ethnic relations—History—Congresses. 7. Immigrants—Great Britain—History—Congresses. 8. Immigrants—North America—History—Congresses. 9. Ireland—Ethnic relations—History—Congresses. 10. Immigrants—Ireland—History—Congresses. 11. Huguenots—Congresses. I. Vigne, Randolph. II. Littleton, Charles. III. Huguenot Society of Great Britain and Ireland.
DA125.A1 F76 2001
304.8'41'00903—dc21   2001042007

Typeset and designed by G&G Editorial, Brighton
Printed by Bookcraft, Midsomer Norton, Bath
This book is printed on acid-free paper.

Contents

———————

———————

CONTENTS

CONTENTS

CONTENTS

Illustrations

---

*The Huguenot Society of Great Britain and Ireland and Sussex Academic Press grate-
fully acknowledge permission to reproduce copyright material, as detailed below.*

*Colour plates appear after page 296. Page numbers of black and white illustrations in
the text are denoted by square brackets.*

Acknowledgements

Sincere thanks are due to the very large number of institutions and individuals who helped bring about the conference which this book perpetuates in print, and to the smaller circle concerned with its publication. First, the wholehearted personal endorsement of HRH The Prince of Wales, of both conference and book, was deeply appreciated and attracted that of many others. A valuable contribution was made by Mrs Kathryn Michael, whose support in fund-raising and planning before and administration during and after the conference was invaluable, as was her hard work and assiduity in assembling the illustrations for the book and raising the funds to meet these extra costs. Other Huguenot Society colleagues concerned and helpful with both projects were the Hon. Treasurer, Martin Harcourt Williams, the Hon. Secretary, Mary Bayliss, the Society's President in 1998–2001, Paul Minet and the Librarian, Stephen Massil. With Paul Minet, whose start-up funding for the conference was matched by that of the Johannes a Lasco Library, Emden, must be linked Professor Walter Schulz, who also both urged the publication of this book in this form at the conference itself and made available the further injection of funds from his institution which brought it about. The Huguenot Society is indebted also to the Scouloudi Foundation for a most welcome grant towards production costs. The Marc Fitch Fund contributed generously to the funding needed for the colour-plate section. Our co-publishers, Sussex Academic Press, in the person of Anthony Grahame, the editorial director, expressed support for the conference from the start and has proved a worthy colleague since.

Other institutions who expressed their confidence in the conference through generous support (and we regret having space only for the institutions and not for the individuals with whom we worked) were the Huguenot Society itself, the British Academy, the Dutch Church of London and the French Huguenot Church of London Charitable Trust. Other organizations to whom we owe thanks for funding in cash or kind are: Cazenove & Co, the German Historical Institute, the Paul Mellon Centre for the Study of British Art, the Peter Minet Trust, the Royal Historical Society, the Spitalfields Centre, the William and Mary History of Toleration Committee, and, by no means least, the Worshipful Companies of Carpenters and Drapers, as well as of Fanmakers, Goldsmiths, Mercers and Weavers.

The members of the committee (of which the editors were, respectively, chairman* and secretary*) who organized the conference were: Mrs M. Bayliss, A. Bienfait, Dr A. Fahrmeier, G .A. Forrest,* Prof. M. Greengrass, Dr R. D. Gwynn, C. Knook, A. Lawes, D. Levesque, Dr L.B. Luu, Mrs K. Michael, Prof. J. Miller (acting chairman on several occasions),* Dr S. Nishikawa, Dr S. Parissien,* E. Samuel, Dr A. Spicer,* Mrs H. Termeulen, Dr B. van Ruymbeke and Prof. R. Whelan.

Bodies who collaborated in varying ways and degrees were the French Protestant Church of London, the Jewish Historical Society of England, the Public Record Office, the Institute of Historical Research, the Commission de l'Histoire de l'Eglise Wallonne (Leiden) and the Spanish and Portuguese Jews' Congregation.

Before and during the conference itself, and in running its parallel events, much service was performed by members of the Dutch Church of London, outstandingly Mrs Henny Termeulen, and of the Huguenot Society, of whom we have space here to single out only Lady Monson and Mrs Barbara Julien. Others who contributed their time and energy to the many events were Susie Symes of the Spitalfields Centre, Aidan Lawes of the Public Record Office, Edgar Samuel at Bevis Marks synagogue, David Titterington, the Dutch Church organist, Gareth Harris of the Spitalfields Historic Buildings Trust, Max and Isabelle Engammare at the French Church of London, Soho Square, and the Clerks and staffs of the Carpenters' and Drapers' Companies whose halls were so generously made available to us. The last should be first: The Bishop of London, the Right Reverend Richard Chartres, who opened the conference so fittingly, both as successor to Bishop Grindal, who followed Johannes a Lasco as Superintendent of the stranger churches, and as an honorary fellow of the Huguenot Society.

Those who chaired conference panels were, in addition to members of the committee starred above: Dr Ian Archer, Dr Toby Barnard, Dr Raingard Esser, Dr David Feldman, Mr Graham Gibbs, Dr Philippa Glanville, Prof. Joyce Goodfriend, Dr Robin Howells, Prof. Michael Hunter, Dr R.C. Nash, Prof. Kenneth Parker, Ms Margaret Pelling, Prof. Giorgio Vola, Prof. Peter Wende and Dr David Wykes.

We thank all those who gave papers and who attended and participated from the floor or between sessions. The former, led by the keynote speakers, Prof. Hugh Trevor-Roper, Prof. Patrick Collinson, Dr Robin Gwynn and Prof. Christoph Strohm, made the conference the success it was and produced the contents of this book. The latter made up the unexpectedly large numbers which confirmed our committee's belief in the relevance of our theme, to historians and the public — and thus the value of publishing the proceedings as a whole.

THE EDITORS

Abbreviations

Add.	Additional
BL	British Library
Bodl.	Bodleian Library, Oxford
CLRO	Corporation of London Record Office
CSP	Calendar of State Papers
CSPC	Calendar of State Papers, Colonial
CSPD	Calendar of State Papers, Domestic
CSPF	Calendar of State Papers, Foreign
DNB	Dictionary of National Biography
FCL	Library of the French Protestant Church of London, Soho Square
GL	Guildhall Library
HMC	Historical Manuscripts Commission
HSP	Huguenot Society Proceedings
HSQS	Huguenot Society Publications (Quarto Series), *see below*
LPL	Lambeth Palace Library
NS	New Series
PCC	Prerogative Court of Canterbury
PRO	Public Record Office
SP	State Papers
SPD	State Papers Domestic
SPF	State Papers Foreign
STC	Short-title Catalogue (Pollard and Redgrave and/or Wing)
TJHSE	Transactions of the Jewish Historical Society of England

HUGUENOT SOCIETY PUBLICATIONS (QUARTO SERIES)

The following titles in the series 'Publications of the Huguenot Society of London', 1887–1985, and 'of Great Britain and Ireland', 1985– (the 'Quarto Series') are referred to in endnotes.

1   W. J. C. Moens (ed.), *The Walloons and their church at Norwich: their history and registers. 1565–1832* (1887).
2   A. C. Chamier (ed.), *Les actes des colloques des Eglises françaises et des synodes des Eglises étrangères refugiées en Angleterre, 1581–1654* (1890).

3 W. Minet and W. C. Waller (eds.), *Transcript of the registers of the Protestant church at Guisnes from 1668 to 1685* (1891).

5 R. Hovenden (ed.), *The registers of the Walloon or strangers' church in Canterbury*, Part 1 (1891), Part 2 (1894), Part 3 (1898).

7 J. J. Digges La Touche (ed.), *Registers of the French conformed churches of St Patrick and St Mary, Dublin* (1893).

8 W. Page (ed.), *Letters of denization and acts of naturalization for aliens in England, 1509–1603* (1893).

9 R. E. G. Kirk and E. F. Kirk (eds.), *Returns of aliens dwelling in the city and suburbs of London from the reign of Henry VIII to that of James I*, Part I, 1525–1571 (1900), Part II, 1571–1597 (1902), Part III, 1598–1625, Additions, 1522–1595 (1907), Index (1908).

11 W. Minet and W. C. Waller (eds.), *Registers of the church known as La Patente in Spittlefields from 1689 to 1785* (1898).

12 W. J. C. Moens (ed.), *Register of baptisms in the Dutch church at Colchester from 1645 to 1728* (1905).

15 F. W. Cross, *History of the Walloon and Huguenot church at Canterbury* (1898).

17 H. Peet (ed.), *Register of baptisms of the French Protestant refugees settled at Thorney, Cambridgeshire, 1654–1727* (1903).

18 W. A. Shaw (ed.), *Letters of denization and acts of naturalization for aliens in England and Ireland, 1603–1700* (1911).

19 T. P. LeFanu (ed.), *Registers of the French Church of Portarlington, Ireland* (1908).

21 W. Minet and S. Minet (eds.), *Livre des tesmoignages de l'église de Threadneedle Street, 1669–1789* (1909).

22 W. Minet and S. Minet (eds.), *Livre des conversions et des reconoissances faites à l'église françoise de la Savoye* (1914).

26 W. Minet and S. Minet (eds.), *Registres des églises de la Savoye, de Spring Gardens et des Grecs, 1684–1900* (1922).

27 W. A. Shaw (ed.), *Letters of denization and acts of naturalization for aliens in England and Ireland 1701–1800* (1923).

38 E. Johnston (ed.), *Actes du consistoire de l'église française de Threadneedle Street, Londres*, Vol. I, 1560–1565 (1937).

43, 44 F. Gardy, *Correspondance de Jaques Serces*, Vol. I, 1720–1748 (1952), Vol. II, 1749–1761 (1956).

49 A. P. Hands and I. Scouloudi, *French Protestant refugees relieved through the Threadneedle Street church, London, 1681–1687* (1971).

50 R. Smith, *The archives of the French Protestant Church of London. A handlist* (1972).

51 R. Smith, *Records of the Royal Bounty and connected funds, the Burn Donation, and the Savoy Church in the Huguenot Library, University College, London. A handlist* (1974).

52, 53 C. F. A. Marmoy, *The French Protestant Hospital: extracts from the archives of 'La Providence' relating to inmates and applications for admission 1718–1957 and to recipients of and applications for the Coqueau charity 1745–1901*, Vol. I, Introduction, Entries A–K; Vol. II, L–Z, Appendices (1977).

54 R. D. Gwynn (ed.), *A calendar of the letter books of the French Church of London from the Civil War to the Restoration* (1979).

55 C. F. A. Marmoy (ed.), *The case book of 'La Maison de Charité de Spittlefields'* *1739–41* (1981).
56 I. E. Gray, *Huguenot manuscripts: a descriptive catalogue of the remaining manuscripts in the Huguenot Library* (1983).
57 I. Scouloudi, *Returns of strangers in the metropolis, 1593, 1627, 1635. 1639: a study of an active minority* (1985).
58 R. D. Gwynn, *Minutes of the consistory of the French Church of London, Threadneedle Street, 1679–1692* (1994).
59 O. Boersma and A. J. Jelsma (eds.), *Unity in multiformity: the minutes of the coetus of London, 1575, and the consistory minutes of the Italian Church of London, 1570–1591* (1997).

CONVENTIONS

Where dates are provided, 1 January is taken to be the first day of the year. Dates from contemporary sources which take 25 March as the beginning of the year are adjusted to reflect modern dating practice.

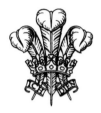

ST. JAMES'S PALACE

'From Strangers to Citizens' marks the 450th anniversary of the charter granted by King Edward VI to give immigrants and refugees – 'strangers' – the right to hold Reformed services in their own places of worship in England. It is a thought-provoking anniversary, and I am delighted both that the Huguenot Society have chosen to draw attention to it in this way, and that they have been kind enough to make the connection back to my Family by inviting me to be Patron of the conference.

Even those of us who rejoice in the multicultural character of today's United Kingdom often forget that this character – and our tradition of tolerance, of which the British can be proud – are not new phenomena. It helps to be reminded that today's waves of refugees are only the latest of many; our understanding of contemporary opportunities and challenges, in this area as in so many others, can be enormously enhanced by a better grasp of our own history. A walk through Spitalfields, past weaver's house, synagogue and Bangladeshi grocer's, is a good start. This conference will probe much more deeply, and its main themes – the integration of immigrant groups, the ways in which they maintained their own distinctive identities, their experiences in Britain, Ireland and the colonies, and the contributions which they made to their host societies – are all subjects of both historical *and* contemporary interest.

So I should like to send my very best wishes for a stimulating and enjoyable discussion to all involved in 'From Strangers to Citizens'. I am sad that I cannot join you, but I much look forward to reading your conclusions. I want, too, to congratulate in particular the organisers and co-sponsors on arranging such a worthwhile and fascinating event.

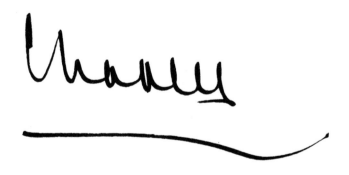

The Johannes a Lasco Library, Emden

In grateful acknowledgement of the support given to the 'From Strangers to Citizens' conference and towards the publication of this book by the Johannes a Lasco Bibliothek, Emden, we present the following statement by that institution's Director.

The Johannes a Lasco Library, Emden: towards the achievement of a self-supporting library

WALTER SCHULZ

In the 16th century, at the time of the Reformation, the two most important places with foreign Protestant communities were London and Emden. In both places, first in Emden and later, from 1550 to 1553, in London, the Polish nobleman John a Lasco was the superintendent of these small but well-educated and skilled groups of exiles. At Emden, the Dutch refugees were integrated into the Emden Reformed Church, because the Dutch and Low German languages were closely related. The French- and English-speaking refugees built up their own communities. Approximately 8000 to 10,000 refugees had settled in Emden by the mid-16h century. When the harbour of Antwerp was closed in the early 1560s, Emden gained European importance for some years. Even though Emden had no university, the Reformed Church became a training centre for Reformed preachers who were prepared for their work in the new Reformed communities in the occupied Dutch area. Emden also advanced during this period towards becoming an important place of book printing. Classical authors of Reformed literature (John Calvin, Heinrich Bullinger, Ulrich Zwingli; John a Lasco, Marnix van St Aldegonde and others) had their works published in Emden for the Dutch, and in part for the English, market. In 1571, the first synod of Dutch Reformed Christians took place in Emden. This led to the constitution of the Dutch Reformed Church. So the 'Grand Church' in Emden helped to give birth to Reformed Protestantism, especially in Holland, but also in the larger area of north-western Europe. In Germany, Reformed Christians are a minority today, as they are in Poland, where John a Lasco, during the last years of life, also founded the Polish Reformed Church.

The Polish humanist John a Lasco, a nephew of the Primate of Poland and a student of Erasmus of Rotterdam, whose library he purchased, found his way to Protestantism, and also to Emden, through the Dutchman Albert Hardenberg. John a Lasco was the only Superintendent (bishop) of East Frisia for the Protestant Church from 1542 to 1549. He also represented Reformed Protestantism in its human-istic tradition and had an important influence on the structural and organizational questions within the reformed churches. A Lasco's influence was international as well as interconfessional. He had political and religious contacts throughout Europe. His great achievements had an impact on the East Frisian, Dutch, English and Polish church history.

The 'Grand Church' in Emden, consecrated to Cosmas and Damian in the Middle Ages, was destroyed in December 1943, along with almost the whole old town centre of Emden. Only the eastern choir with three wings remained, later on a monument against war in the new post-war town of Emden.

The library project and its architecture

During the period from 1992 to 1995, 15.6 million DM was spent on the project. Finance was provided by three sources: 5.2 million DM by the Reformed Church (Synod of the Reformed Churches of Bavaria and Northwest Germany), 5.2 million DM by the Foundation of Lower Saxony – up to now the largest donation they have granted to any project – and 2.6 million DM each by the state of Lower Saxony and by the city of Emden. Built on a foundation measuring 1020 square meters (30m x 34m) the library has about 3000 square meters of usable floor space and encloses a space of 13,000 cubic metres.

'A graceful though mighty house, full of character' said someone in noting the tension between the old brick ruins and the modern construction. The architectural design was guided by the following principles: a reconstructive project to restore the late-Gothic sacred character did not seem appropriate due to the fact that the building was planned for use as a library. The modern design makes as much use as possible of the existing historic ruins.

One library — three functions

The main objective of our project was, of course, to build a library, although we use it in different ways and for quite different events.

(1) *A research centre and library*: The library has approximately 100,000 titles, nearly 10,000 of which were printed before 1800, mostly in the 16th and early 17th centuries. We started only some years ago to set up a modern library function and organization. Having a valuable book collection does not mean the same as having a library.

Up to 1990 the library had an acquisition budget of only 10,000 DM. In recent years we have spent some hundreds of thousands of DM every year on recent publications. A PICA-LBS computer system had been planned from the beginning. Since October 1991, and all the time during the building project, the library has been connected to the system of the University of Groningen. Today we have a PICA-system within the Göttingen Association of Libraries (GBV), and in co-operation with the University of Applied Sciences in Emden. A CD-ROM network and a microfilm/microfiche reader/printer is also available. With the digital camera we have started to digitize the 16th-century book collection of Albert Hardenberg, a friend of John a Lasco. We receive financial support from the Deutsche Forschungsgemeinschaft and the state of Lower Saxony. With financial support of the EU (Interreg-program), we have started to set up a database and online publishing project for the World Alliance of the Reformed Churches (www.reformed-online.net).

(2) *A conference centre*: An important aspect of our project was not only to have a library in the traditional sense, but to use it as the basis of a research centre. The open central nave of the former ruins is an attractive place for meetings. While the library was opened as early as November 1995, we could start with a conference programme only in the spring of 1998. We have our own symposia, mostly in the wider field of Reformed Protestantism or history. Besides this we also host conferences for other organizations. Up to now we have held many conferences and meetings. An advisory board oversees the policies and projects of the library: the members are recognized in the field of theology or history and come from Berlin, Oxford, Zurich, Groningen, Apeldoorn, Münster, Hannover and Munich. The chair is Professor Christoph Strohm, University of Bochum.

(3) *An open library*: As our conference facilities are very attractive, we offer them for hire to a wider public. And it is not only conferences with an academic background that are possible, but also concerts, receptions, exhibitions of the museum of modern art and banquets. All this then takes place in a library, surrounded by books. The former German foreign minister Hans Dietrich Genscher opened the exhibition of the Russian paintings of Henri Nannen, a famous German journalist and art collector. All the important exhibitions of the art museum attract many people to the library. The memorial ceremony for Henri Nannen, sponsor of the museum, who died in October 1996, also took place in the library, as well as synodal conferences of the Reformed Church. Receptions of firms such as Phillips-Petrol, Statoil, Daimler-Chrysler, Volkswagen, Commerzbank and many others were important steps to our achieving in a few years a widespread reputation as a unique conference hall. In February this year, we held a congress hosted by Volkswagen with some 600 participants, intended to encourage young people to become entrepreneurs . In June 2000 the German chancellor Schroeder opened a conference about the importance and future of the German maritime industry. Other events are booked for 2001, such as the official inauguration of activities by 'Brot für die Welt', an important Protestant organization for development aid in Germany. This event will be broadcast on television. All of this takes place in a church library: it is an open library in every way. These past and forthcoming events might be regarded as strange or even as disturbing burdens on the core work of librarianship and research. They also entail much work and require great efforts from all staff. On the other hand, wide public acceptance of the church library has been gained by this policy, an achievement that cannot be taken for granted nowadays . So the open-library concept opens our library doors to the public.

The library foundation

In 1993 the former book collection of the Reformed community was reorganized as a foundation under German civil law. This was a very important step and paved the way for a positive development. The presiding committee of the foundation is made up of representatives of the Reformed Church, the city of Emden, the University of Groningen, the European Leuenberg Community of Protestant Churches and the World Alliance of Reformed Churches at Geneva.

Our operation costs have to be paid from the rent received for the property of the foundation, and that is approximately 1.2 million DM per year. Whenever we need more, whatever it may be for, we have to get it as a support from the state or the Deutsche Forschungsgemeinschaft, the office of unemployment benefits, the EU, or private foundations. And we do need more.

The main objective for the future of the foundation is very clear: to exploit all possibilities to increase the assets in order to reach our goal: a totally self-supporting library foundation.

Introduction

————————

In 1550 King Edward VI granted Protestants fleeing to England across the Channel a charter allowing them to worship in their own churches according to their own rites, independently of the authority of the Church of England. Their first superintendent was one such stranger, the Polish baron known to the English as John a Lasco. The relationship of the new, post-Reformation wave of immigrants with their host country raised many issues which have affected the thinking of the English-speaking world ever since.

On 5–7 April 2000 the Huguenot Society of Great Britain and Ireland, with the support of a number of other historical societies and institutions, convened a conference to mark this 450th anniversary. Its aim was to examine the immigrants over the first two centuries after Edward VI's charter, specifically regarding integration into their host societies in Britain, Ireland and the north American colonies. Close to 300 academics and members of the public from all five continents gathered to share the results of their research.

The conference was held in the Dutch Church of London, which traces its origin back to the charter of 1550 and still stands on the site in the City of London of the Augustinian priory which was given to the strangers for their use by Edward VI. Considering the royal origins of the church, we were very pleased that HRH The Prince of Wales graciously acted as Patron for the conference. It was opened by the Rt Revd Richard Chartres, Bishop of London, whose predecessor Edmund Grindal had succeeded A Lasco as superintendent with the accession of Elizabeth I.

This volume stands as a record of the proceedings of those three days. Of the 58 papers originally presented at the conference all but one, delivered extempore, are provided here. They deal with a wide range of topics and chronological periods, employ differing approaches, and come from both well-established scholars and from post-graduates presenting the first fruits of their researches. The very richness and variety of themes and approaches indicate the continuing vitality of research on this topic. The strength of some aspects and relative sparsity of others demonstrate the sort of work that still needs to be done. Individual case studies of immigrants and their adaptation to, and influence on, English and Irish life (especially in Parts III and IV) accompany general discussions of immigrant groups in general and their long histories in England (Part V). Similarly wide is the chronological and geographical scope of the papers, as again are the ethnic and religious groups they discuss.

A resumé of the unifying principle of each section, and the themes covered, may prove useful to the reader.

Part I covers the foundation and early years of the stranger churches in the 1550s and '60s. The papers in this section stress the influence in England of a group of Continental Protestant intellectuals and theologians – Jean Véron, Johannes a Lasco, Nicolas des Gallars, Jacopo Aconcio. Part II continues to emphasize the primacy of the strangers' religion, both to themselves and to their hosts, with examinations of the relations between strangers and natives during the struggles of the 'Protestant International' in the late 16th and early 17th centuries. This section also introduces us to aspects of the stranger communities in the towns of East Anglia and the Fens further north, often neglected in favour of the London communities.

With Part III we move from a chronological to a thematic focus, by looking at the work of stranger artists and craftsmen and its influence on the development of British art. This set of essays, surveying Gheeraerts to Roubiliac, David Willaume the gold-smith to Peter Le Keux the silkweaving master, suggests how much of British art in this period was executed or inspired by Continental immigrants. The papers in Part IV examine the strangers' intellectual contribution to Britain. The influence was again significant, as can be seen by the fact that out of the six papers in this section which deal specifically with individuals, four of them concern men who were elected Fellows of the Royal Society – Henri Justel, Jean Chardin, Jean-Théophile Desaguliers and Emanuel Mendes da Costa.

The paper on Mendes da Costa reminds us that there were immigrants other than the Protestants of north-western Europe, and this is the larger theme of Part V, where the papers examine the presence in Britain and Ireland of those settlers and visitors who came from less familiar regions in Asia and Africa and were not even Christian, let alone Protestant. Having such a mosaic of peoples from different cultures was more a feature of the developing British colonies in the Americas, and the non-British settlers in those colonies provide the focus of Part VI. There the contributors draw our attention to the importance of Dutch, Huguenot, German and Jewish settlers to religious and social developments in the British American colonies.

Parts VII–IX deal with the period of increased immigration to Britain from Europe in the late 17th and early 18th centuries. Part VII looks at various aspects of this Huguenot immigration of the late 17th century – relations with the Church of England; among neighbours and in the streets and workshops of London; and with their former king, Louis XIV, whose power they tried to diminish both through the sword and pen. Part VIII moves to Ireland, where a substantial Huguenot immigration was encouraged and effected, not least to shore up Protestant power there. Many of these papers directly address the issues of integration, with close studies of the Huguenot communities in Portarlington and Dublin, for instance, which highlight their differences from similar communities in England. Part IX takes us up to the mid-18th century and introduces another immigrant group that was growing in increasing numbers during this period – the Germans, whether they be the 'poor Palatines' of 1709 or the many Hanoverians who came over with the new dynasty. The final paper deals again with integration by showing the subtle shifts in naming practices found among second- and third-generation Huguenot immigrants.

The innumerable ways in which immigrants, in the early modern period and ever since, have added to British national life is emphasized by HRH The Prince of Wales, the patron of the conference, in his open letter to the delegates, which is reproduced in this volume. We believe that the papers here presented confirm his statements and take them into further realms. We hope that they will add to public awareness and debate on the role of immigration in British, Irish and North American society, in the past, present and future.

THE EDITORS

Part I

The foundation of the stranger churches and their early years

The Netherlandish presence in England before the coming of the stranger churches, 1480–1560

RAYMOND FAGEL

———————

'An important milestone': that is how Andrew Pettegree described the founding of the stranger churches in the summer of 1550. Nonetheless, he reminded his readers that 1550 was not the start of something completely new. 'On the contrary', he said, 'foreign merchants and workmen had been making their homes in the city [London] for several centuries, and were an established part of the London scene'. The importance of studying this pre-history can also be defended by another quote from the same author: 'It was indeed extremely important for the first generation of foreign Protestant refugees that they were able to join a well-established and settled foreign community in the city, and many of these foreign residents of an earlier generation would give the foreign churches sturdy support in their first difficult years'.[1]

The immigrants I am interested in came from the Low Countries, the Netherlands, which corresponded more or less with the present countries of Holland, Belgium and Luxembourg, as well as the northern part of France. I shall refer to the Netherlands as they existed during the reign of the Emperor Charles V around 1548, when the Burgundian Circle gained a considerable degree of independence from the German Empire. The period I wish to examine is that *between* the late Middle Ages and 1560; that is to say, between the last decades of the 15th century and the early years of the stranger churches. In this way I wish to combine the many studies on immigrants in medieval England with those on the Protestant communities of the second half of the 16th century and onwards. What can we say about the Netherlandish presence in England between 1480 and 1560?

The answer to this very general question depends on two enormous and, at the same time, completely interrelated problems. First, is it possible to separate the Netherlanders from the other immigrants, and secondly, what sources do we possess for this period? At the same time, I shall try to compare my answers to the situation in the late 15th century, referring for the most part to the book on the alien communities of London by J. L. Bolton, and to the situation around 1550, using the book by Andrew Pettegree on the foreign Protestant communities in 16th-century London.[2]

The sources

There seem to exist three important quantitative sources for the history of the immigrants during the early Tudor period. First of all, there is at the local level the registers of those purchasing the freedom of a city. Laura Hunt Yungblut has collected some information from these sources in her book on the aliens in Elizabethan England. Her conclusion is that aliens rarely bought the liberty of a city before Elizabeth's reign and that there were probably very few strangers in the cities at this time, in any case. Between 1500 and 1558 there were nine aliens registered in Colchester and 16 in Norwich between the 1380s and 1558. Using our second source, the subsidy rolls, she further tells us that there were only 15 aliens to be found in the York subsidies between 1524 and 1549.[3]

The subsidy rolls, however, do not always indicate low numbers of aliens present in England, although in this case we are mostly referring to London. Bolton's edition of the 1483–4 London subsidy rolls and the ones edited as 'returns of aliens' by the Huguenot Society, show the existence of thousands of aliens. Bolton listed 1,595 aliens in the city, while the returns from 1523 onwards also showed large numbers of aliens. The subsidies, however, are not a very informative source. In 1483–4, 1,307 aliens are described as Theotonicus, or Theotonica, meaning Germans, and in the later subsidies they were mostly just called strangers or aliens, although we do find some nationalities such as Frenchman, Gallus, Doch or Ducheman or Teutonicus.

At this point we can draw two preliminary conclusions: firstly, that the immigrants were mostly to be found in London, and secondly, that they consisted of a large and unidentified mass of aliens, whose names we know, but whose origin generally remains a mystery, giving us little information on the specific presence of the Netherlanders. In order to continue, we need the third type of source, also published by the Huguenot Society: the letters of denization and acts of naturalization for aliens in England, 1509–1603.[4] This source has both advantages and disadvantages. On the one hand, when compared to the subsidies, it refers only to a small percentage of the immigrants, those who required denization or naturalization in order to protect their residence in England. These petitioners were probably fairly integrated, either by marriage or by long residence, and they belonged to the more advantaged levels of society. Another disadvantage is the fact that the number of applications does not relate directly to the number of immigrants, but rather to the necessity of petitioning. This means that it was during periods of trouble that we find most of the immigrants; for example, when there were difficult international relations between the English Crown and the immigrant's country of origin, or when there was a negative general sentiment towards strangers in England, as resulted perhaps from a downturn in the economic situation. This means that it is impossible to use the numbers of denizations and naturalizations as a direct correlation to the number of immigrants coming to England. On the other hand, the advantage of this source is that the information is sometimes more detailed than in the subsidies. This makes it possible for us to study the importance of London and the Netherlandish presence there in more depth.

The Netherlandish presence and the origin of the immigrants

As was the case with the other sources, most of the immigrants are also listed here under a general description. The Netherlanders are to be found under the following descriptions: 'from under the dominion of the Emperor', 'under the rule of the Emperor', 'under the jurisdiction of the Emperor' or 'under the obedience of the Emperor'. As most of the information used dates between 1519 and 1555, 'the Emperor' almost always refers to Charles V. Under these descriptions we find some 640 persons registered between 1521 and 1560, with no one at all in the period between 1509 and 1520. They form more than 70 per cent of those labelled 'Central Europe' by William Page in 1893. Three separate years seem to have been the most important for these immigrants from the empire of Charles V; the years 1535, 1541 and 1544 together saw more than 400 denizations and naturalizations granted. Only the year 1551, with 67, comes close to these numbers, but this almost completely relates to one specific group under Vallerand Poullain which went to Glastonbury. The reasons for the large number of petitions in 1535, 1541 and 1544 are explained in the volume's introduction by William Page.

When we compare the numbers with those between 1560 and 1580 we can put everything into perspective. In this case I am using the numbers given by Page for all petitioners from 'Central Europe'. We find the decade 1561–70 to be clearly the central period. Eight hundred letters of denization and acts of naturalization were granted during this decade, with the year 1562 accounting for more than 460. The pre-1560 period never reached such heights; however, when we compare, for example, the period 1541–50 with the period 1571–80, the numbers are almost equal, totalling just below five hundred in each decade.

Table 1.1 Letters of denization and acts of naturalization of subjects of the Emperor (described as dominion, rule, jurisdiction, or obedience)

Period	Subjects of the Emperor
1509–20	–
1521–30	11
1531–40	143
1541–50	98
1551–60	90
Total	642

Source: Page, *Letters of denization*.

But how do we determine from the categories 'Central Europeans' and 'subjects of the Emperor' just how many were Netherlanders? The only way to achieve this is to use those acts and letters where the description of 'subject of the Emperor' is combined with a more specific geographical reference, such as the country, region or city of origin. References to what I call 'the Netherlanders' are clearly dominant, but they were far from the only nationality included under that description. There are many references to places within the German Empire, and even a few individual subjects of the Emperor coming from Italy, the Basque country or Aragon. Important regions of origin are also the Bishoprics of Liège and Cologne, and the Duchy of Cleves, this last probably being related at least in part to the marriage between Anne of Cleves and Henry VIII. Liège and Cologne are difficult descriptions to deal with, as part of the Netherlandish territories of the Emperor belonged ecclesiastically to these bishoprics, whose remaining territories were situated outside the Netherlands. The fact that both bishoprics also often appear without any accompanying description related to 'the Emperor' makes it tempting to see here the separation between territories within the dominions of the Emperor and outside. The fact that many Netherlandish territories also appear without a reference to the Emperor makes this idea useless. Cologne, Liège and Cleves seem to have been considered as under the Emperor's influence, without taking into account strict juridical differences. An argument could be made to include these territories during the 16th century within the history of the Netherlands. As I have shown, there are also regions and places in the Netherlands which do not include a reference to the Emperor in their descriptions in the acts and letters. In conclusion, we might say that such a reference to the Emperor almost always relates to a place of origin within the Netherlands or in the regions adjacent to its territory, but that there are also some examples of places of origin other than within the vast dominions of Charles V.

When we look more closely at the regions and cities within the Netherlands we can get an even clearer picture of who these immigrants were. The first conclusion is obvious: Brabant and, including within Brabant the city of Antwerp, is the most frequently mentioned origin. To a somewhat lesser degree we find Gelderland, Flanders and Holland, in this order, but close to each other in frequency of mention. The number of immigrants produced by the other regions together could be compared to one of these last regions. This shows again clearly which were the core provinces of the Netherlands, although it is surprising to find Gelderland at this level, ahead of Flanders and Holland. Two elements might help to explain this: that perhaps Anne of Cleves brought some Geldersmen with her, but more importantly, that Gelderland was the last to join the territories of the Emperor and was therefore possibly mentioned separately more often than the others. Whatever the reason, I think it remains an interesting fact that cannot be ignored completely. We must also consider the influence of the almost continuous warfare in Gelderland during the first half of the 16th century. Unfortunately, the history of Gelderland has never received as much attention as the history of the other central regions that were to form the core of the later national states of Belgium and Holland.

Another point worth mentioning is that, apart from Antwerp which was mentioned eleven times, most cities are only listed sporadically; in the province of Holland, Haarlem is mentioned three times, and Delft twice, while Bruges in Flanders is also mentioned twice. Another remarkable feature is that, whereas the immigrants from Brabant appear to have come from the larger cities, the Flemish petitioners often came from smaller villages. An anachronistic comparison setting the number of immigrants coming from the provinces that were to become the Dutch Republic against those from the later Spanish Netherlands would show that close to 55 per cent came from the future Dutch Republic.

Table 1.2 Geographic origin of the Netherlanders as mentioned in denizations and naturalizations, 1509–60

Region	NR	%	SE	%	Total	%
Brabant	21	22	21	34	42	27
Gelderland	26	27	5	8	31	20
Flanders	18	19	10	16	28	18
Holland	15	16	11	18	26	17
Artois	3	3	5	8	8	5
Utrecht	2	2	6	9	8	5
Zeeland	4	4	1	2	5	3
Friesland	2	2	2	3	4	3
Hainault	2	2	–	–	2	1
Tournai	2	2	–	–	2	1
Total:	95	100	61	100	156	100

Source: Page, *Letters of denization*.
Notes: NR: No reference to the Emperor; SE: mentioned as subject of the Emperor.[5]

It is difficult to find comparable information on the origin of the other Netherlanders living in England. Bolton returns to the much-used and detailed information from the 1436 subsidy roll, when the subjects of the Duke of Burgundy had to ask for letters of protection.[6] At that time the majority came from Holland and Brabant, with Flanders and Zeeland rather far behind. Of course we have to remember that large parts of the Netherlands were not yet part of the territory of the Duke. The only conclusion that can be drawn is that Holland was more predominant in 1436 than in the period of the denizations, and that Brabant remained very important throughout. At the city level, the year 1436 is also totally different when compared to the denizations. Antwerp played only a minor role, having the same number as Hoogstraten, Schoonhoven and Diest. The most frequently mentioned is Haarlem with 26 letters, followed by Den Bosch, Middelburg, Gouda, Bruges and Dordrecht, all having between 10 and 13 letters.

Table 1.3 Geographic origin of the Netherlanders in England. Comparison between the 1436 Letters of Protection and the denizations and naturalizations, 1509–60

Region	1436	%	Den./Nat.	%
Holland	170	29.6	26	14
Brabant	114	19.8	42	22
Flanders	49	8.5	28	15
Zeeland	39	6.8	5	2.5
Gelderland	39	6.8	31	16
Utrecht	23	4.0	8	4
Liège	21	3.6	23	12
Cologne	15	2.6	27	14
Total	484	100	190	100

Sources: Bolton, *Alien communities*; Page, *Letters of denization*.

The second problem referred to at the beginning of this paper is the domination of London over all other regions and cities as the residence of aliens. To address this problem, I have looked at those petitioners who are identifiable as Netherlanders or subjects of the Emperor, and of whom we know both their professions and their place of residence. The non-London group is estimated to have numbered approximately 30 per cent of the immigrants living in London, Southwark and Westminster. This does indeed point to a clear London domination, but it still means that almost one-third did not live in London. Compared to the very marginal numbers given by Yungblut, this new information could lead to a re-evaluation of the rest of England as a home of aliens. The concentration on London sources and London research, which involves looking at a large group of aliens living close together, stands out against the enormous task of gathering information about strangers from all over England, one by one. These non-London immigrants worked in cities such as Oxford, Cambridge, Plymouth, Canterbury, Salisbury and Colchester, as well as places like South Molton in Devon and Bridport in Dorset. There were also a few brewers working in Calais which of course was an English town until 1558.

Professions

This same group of petitioners, whose professions we know, but whose origins are often vague, makes it possible to study the ways in which the Netherlanders and other subjects of the Emperor earned their living in England. The three most frequently mentioned professions indicate that they were mostly occupied with clothing the English; for example, 36 per cent of the aliens were shoemakers, cordwainers and tailors, although aliens practised many other professions as well. Perhaps the best way of presenting these results is to compare them with the numbers and divisions given by Bolton for the late 15th century and with those by Pettegree for the members of the Dutch Church in its early years.

Table 1.4 Professions of early members of the Dutch Church in London, compared to professions in the denizations and naturalizations, 1509–60

Professions	Pettegree	%	Den./Nat.	%
Shoemakers and cobblers[7]	50	19	50	25
Tailors	45	17	23.5	12
Woodwork craftsmen[8]	37	14	21	11
Metalworkers[9]	30	11	10	5
Weavers[10]	17	7	2	1
Hat and glovemakers	16	6	4	2
Printing tradesmen	15	6	3.5	2
Basket makers	8	3	6	3
Glassmakers	6	2	5	3
Rest	36	14	71	36
Total	260	100	196	100

Source: Pettegree, *Foreign Protestant communties*, 82; Page, *Letters of denization*. Categories from Pettegree.

Pettegree was not very complete, as his book was not an economic study, but we can use his categories for a rough comparison. Trades involving the production of shoes and clothing were also dominant within the Dutch Church, and the percentages for this between the two groups are almost equal. More than 35 per cent of the church members were dedicated to these professions and the same is true for the petitioners for denizations and naturalizations. The most remarkable differences are to be found with the metal workers, the weavers and the printing tradesmen. In the church, they accounted for almost one fourth of the total, while among the petitioners they make up under 10 per cent. This difference might be explained by the distinction that Pettegree makes when discussing the relation between profession and Protestantism. In his opinion, the new religious ideas were primarily attractive to two groups of craftsmen, those working in highly skilled professions, such as the goldsmiths, and those working with innovative technology, such as the book trade and the weavers.[11] The attraction of Protestantism and the resulting refugee movement did change the labour structure of the immigrant community in England. It seems that the old immigrant colony of brewers, for example (7 per cent of the denizations and naturalizations), did not join the Dutch Church in the same numbers, as was also the case with the London joiners of alien origin.

Table 1.5   Professions of the Germans in London in 1484, as compared to professions in the denizations and naturalizations, 1509–60

Categories	1484	%	Den./Nat.	%
Cloth /Clothing production	110	31	48	24.5
Leather/ Leather working	60	17.5	51	26
Metal working	42	12	13	6.5
Brewing	34	9.5	22	11
Victualling	3	1	1	0.5
Craftsmen	14	4	11(12).5	6
Merchants	20	6	1	0.5
Building	9	2.5	14	7
Miscellaneous	64	18	33.5	17
Total	356	100	196	100

Sources: Bolton, *The alien communities*, 134–8; Page, *Letters of denization*. Categories from Bolton.

The other comparison can be made with the London 'Germans', as they are called in the book by Bolton, as they appear in the 1484 subsidies. The first difference is the size of the group of merchants in 1484. This may have been caused by the fact that they did not need to petition for denizenship or naturalization in the same numbers as did the other immigrants. Other differences are less easy to explain, such as the predominance of metal workers (mostly goldsmiths) in 1484, and of building workers, in the denizations and naturalizations. But we must not forget that the subsidy concerned London and all 'Germans', not only those from the Netherlands and the dominions of the Emperor. Were there relatively more goldsmiths from further away in the German Empire, or were there more in the city of London?

Even more striking than the differences are the common general features, such as the importance of craftsmen and brewers, and even more so the predominance of two sectors: clothing and leather workers. Cloth and leather working accounted for half of the strangers, both in 1484 and in the denizations and naturalizations. The smaller categories used by Pettegree showed that more than 35 per cent were shoemakers, cobblers and tailors, this being the case for both members of the Dutch Church as well as for the petitioners between 1509 and 1560. This general characteristic seems to have originated in the 15th century and survived the whole period leading up to the formation of the Dutch Church.

When we look more closely at specific trades, there are more differences to be found. Within the category of cloth and clothing production, weavers and hatters were much more important in 1484 than later on, whereas in the category of leather and leather working, the predominance of cobblers in 1484 gave way to that of shoemakers and cordwainers among the denizations. Although the differences may be partly explained by a changing vocabulary, it might be interesting to look more closely at these changes. The presence of weavers in 1484 fits in very well with the weavers mentioned by Pettegree in the Dutch Church. The denizations and naturalizations almost completely lack reference to members of this profession. The question is whether or not their absence during the first half of the 16th century reflected reality, or if it can be explained by the fact that weavers did not need denizenship and naturalization in order to protect their presence in England.

Marriage and duration of residence before petition

The information given in some of the years in the letters of denization and the acts of naturalization makes it possible to study two other factors regarding the residence of the Netherlanders in England, particularly those during the important years of 1541 and 1544. The first element is the duration of their stay before applying for their papers. In 1541, almost all immigrants from, as it was called in the sources, 'the dominions of the Emperor', mentioned their years of residence in England; this amounted to about two hundred persons. Three years later, a new wave of petitioners, about one hundred, also mentioned quite consciously the duration of their stay in England. Most of the new denizens had resided in England between eight and 32 years. In 1541, however, we also find a group of approximately thirty long-established immigrants who had resided in the country between 32 and 64 years. Three years later there were only a few of these very ancient petitioners. It seems that they had almost all grasped their opportunity in 1541.

Another way of looking at these numbers is to calculate the strangers' years of arrival. When we consider both years together, we can oversee the results of the immigration to England between 1477 and 1541. Approximately 10 per cent of the immigrants were said to have arrived before or during the early years of Charles V (1477–1509), as well as roughly 60 per cent during the period more or less comparable to the years of the regency of Margaret of Austria (1509–28), which leaves approximately 30 per cent for the years between 1529 and 1541. The years around 1500 and then again around 1520 seem in particular to have resulted in relatively large numbers; however, as the petitioners were likely to have given round figures such as 10, 20 and 30, it is difficult to draw more solid conclusions.

The last point to consider is the marital status of the group of immigrants from the dominions of the Emperor who petitioned in 1541 and 1544. Being married to an Englishwoman seems to have been the most common status. This was the case in more than 60 per cent of the new denizens in 1541, that is, 112 persons. The bachelors formed only a small minority, with a mere 15 per cent in 1541 listed as unmarried. The more limited information for 1544 shows the same tendencies: those married to an Englishwoman numbered 19, with only one of the total of 35 listed as unmarried.

Conclusions and intentions

The letters of denization and the acts of naturalization between 1509 and 1560 can help us to understand better this rarely studied period of the alien presence in England and to combine the knowledge of the medievalists with that of the specialists on the Protestant churches and early modern immigration. We shall probably never be able conclusively to separate the Netherlanders from the other inhabitants of the German Empire, or from other subjects of the Emperor, but it appears that they made up the majority of the group as a whole, especially when the Bishoprics of Liège and Cologne and the Duchy of Cleves are included. The number of petitioners in the 1540s was even larger than in the 1570s, thereby making immigrants an important issue even before the coming of the refugees.[12] Brabant and Antwerp seem to have been the most frequent areas of origin within the Netherlandish colony, but even more surprising was the influential position of newcomers from Gelderland.

The professions of the new denizens reflect above all the continuity in the crafts related to cloth and clothing, leather and leather working. Although the noted changes may have been partly the cause of the special character of my sources, there is something to be said for the change of the Netherlandish labour structure which came about as a result of the arrival of Protestant refugees, mostly from Flanders and the southern provinces. The evidence regarding marital status and length of residence show that we are dealing here with a very well-integrated group of aliens.

I began by quoting Andrew Pettegree on the importance of the old residents for the new refugees and their new churches. I believe that this point does not require any additional comment. However, what happened to the old immigrant group as a result of the coming of the refugees? This question does not seem to have been posed very often.[13] As only a small percentage of refugees entered into the stranger churches, what must have happened to all the others? This Netherlandish presence, both before and after 1550, can be further studied at several additional levels: their presence within the trades and guilds, in fraternities, and at the court of the English kings. A last element consists in studying the regulations from central and local authorities. We have now reached a fitting place to embark on discussing the years after the foundation of the stranger churches.

NOTES

1 A. Pettegree, *Foreign Protestant communities in sixteenth-century London* (Oxford, 1986), 9.
2 J. L. Bolton (ed.), *The alien communities of London in the fifteenth century: the Subsidy Rolls of 1440 and 1483–4* (Stamford, 1998); Pettegree, *Foreign Protestant communities*.
3 L. Hunt Yungblut, *Strangers settled here amongst us: policies, perceptions and the presence of aliens in Elizabethan England* (London, 1996), 10–13.
4 HSQS 8.
5 As some places have not been identified, the calculations are not complete.
6 M. R. Thielemans, *Bourgogne et Angleterre: relations politiques et économiques entre les*

Pays-Bas et l'Angleterre 1435–1476 (Brussels, 1966), 283–306.

7   Under the Denizations and Naturalizations this category also includes cordwainers.

8   Woodwork craftsmen as defined by Pettegree are: joiners, boxmakers and coopers. Under Den./Nat. they are: joiners, carpenters and coopers.

9   Pettegree mentions 10 cutlers and 12 goldsmiths among this group. Under Den./Nat. this group includes goldsmiths, smiths, goldbeater and farrier.

10   Under Den./Nat. this group consists of one corse-weaver and one fuller.

11   Pettegree, 105, 107–8.

12   The importance of denization and naturalization of members of the Netherlandish community in England was greater than that of naturalization of Netherlanders in France during the reign of Francis I. R. P. Fagel, 'Les hommes des Pays-Bas et le roi de France: gens des Pays-Bas en France à la Renaissance, 1480–1560', *Revue du Nord* (forthcoming).

13   A Ph.D. study of the aliens in London after 1550, not focusing on the stranger churches, is Lien Bich Luu, 'Skills and innovations: a study of the stranger working community in London, 1550–1600' (University of London Ph.D. thesis, 1997).

2

Bringing Reformed theology to England's 'rude and symple people': Jean Véron, minister and author outside the stranger church community

CARRIE E. EULER

Jean Véron was among the earliest French Protestant refugees in England. His letters of denization in July 1544 state that he had been in the country for over eight years, indicating his arrival in England in or around 1536.[1] He remained in England until his death in 1563. During the reign of Edward VI, he did not join the French stranger congregation in London, but became a priest in the Church of England and served as the rector of St Alphage in Cripplegate. He was imprisoned during the reign of Mary I, but not executed. He went on to hold several clerical positions in London during Elizabeth I's reign, including vicar of St Martin's in Ludgate and a prebendary of St Paul's, and he preached at least once in front of the Queen at Whitehall.[2] Throughout Edward's and Elizabeth's reigns, Véron also produced many religious publications, including translations of Continental literature and writings of his own. During the reign of Edward VI, he was responsible for the publication of two tracts by Huldrych Zwingli, the leader of the Reformation in Zürich;[3] three by Zwingli's successor Heinrich Bullinger;[4] two treatises of his own against the Mass;[5] a compilation of Patristic opinions on the Lord's Supper;[6] and one non-religious publication, a tri-lingual French-Latin-English dictionary.[7] In 1561–2, he published a series of dialogues in which Philalethes (who symbolized the lover of truth) leads Albion (England gone astray under Catholicism) back to the Protestant teachings on predestination, purgatory, free will, justification by works, invocation of the saints, and clerical celibacy.[8] His goal in all of these publications was to bring the word of God to the 'rude and symple people', those unskilled in Latin, ignorant of Reformed doctrine, and thus most susceptible to error.

Despite this prolific career, Véron has been neglected by historians. The only studies of him are two outdated articles. The first, written by Baron F. de Schickler in 1890, presents a summary of the facts of his life and career and a brief evaluation of his writings.[9] The second, a very short piece written by Philippe Denis in the early 1970s, suggests that Véron is worthy of further study as a writer who 'vulgarized' Continental theology for English readers.[10] However, no further study from Denis or any other scholar ever emerged. Instead, references to Véron that have appeared in monographs by English Reformation scholars consistently lack context and knowledge of Véron's background or career. The result is that they are often misleading or incorrect.[11]

The study of Véron's career is important because it offers insight into the processes of evangelization in England and the relationship between the English and Continental Reformations, and it does so at a level different from that of most previous studies. Véron was not directly involved with the universities, with other foreign Protestant divines in England, or with Archbishop Cranmer. His position as a parish minister in London brought him closer to the English people than were many of Cranmer's elite circle. Nevertheless, as a translator of Zwingli and Bullinger, he was aware of the intricacies of Continental theology and its potential value for the Reformation in England.

This essay focuses on two aspects of Véron's career. First, it examines his integration into the English community. Véron's involvement in the English evangelical movement is an example of the international character of the Reformation under Edward VI and the atmosphere in which the Stranger Churches were founded. Evidence reveals that neither Véron nor his English colleagues thought his stranger status was significant; what was more important was that he was a fellow brother in Christ and a servant of the Reformation. Second, this essay briefly investigates Véron's theology and the role his writings played in the evangelization of England. It demonstrates that negative attacks on various Catholic and radical Protestant beliefs, such as those found in his writings, formed an important part of the formation of Protestant orthodoxy in England, and that his interest in the writings of Zwingli and Bullinger over Calvin is an example of the importance of Zürich theology for the Reformation under Edward VI.

I

In his article, Philippe Denis asserted that Véron 'shared the life of Englishmen'. 'He was', Denis continued, 'for all practical purposes an Englishman, although his contemporaries continued to call him "a Frenchman".'[12] To the contrary, Véron's actions and words indicate that he thought of himself as neither French nor English, but as a true Christian, teacher, and preacher to the 'rude and symple people' of England. His English colleagues, moreover, accepted him as such and never referred to him as a Frenchman.

Véron does not seem to have had much contact with other foreigners. The only evidence about his life during the reign of Henry VIII is his letters of denization which state that in 1544 he was a teacher of gentlemen's children.[13] During this time, he was probably working on his one non-religious publication, a version of the French humanist Robert Etienne's French and Latin dictionary, complete with Véron's own English entries added for every word. Véron dedicated this work to the youth of England, with the hope of facilitating the reading and understanding of 'good letters' among English students.[14]

During Edward's reign, Véron did not join the French 'Stranger Church', but instead was ordained as a priest in the Church of England in August 1551. His name does not appear in the extensive collections of correspondence between English and Continental evangelicals, and there is no evidence that he had contact with other foreign divines in England, such as Martin Bucer or Peter Martyr Vermigli. Rather, he seems to have become acquainted with some of the better-known English evangelicals in London. Nicholas Ridley, then Bishop of London, ordained Véron in 1551. When Véron did not flee England after Mary's accession, he was arrested along with John Bradford, John Rogers, and Thomas Becon in connection with a riot at St Paul's in August 1553.[15] During Elizabeth's reign, he preached several times at St Paul's and once in front of the Queen at Whitehall. Thus, in many ways, Véron did share the life of native English evangelicals.

Véron's own words confirm his belief that his stranger status was unimportant. The titles of nine of his 16 publications refer to him as 'John Veron, Senonois', most likely a reference to his birth in Sens, France. Yet, he only refers directly to his French origins twice in all his writings, and in both of these instances, he argues that it should not hinder his ability to communicate his message to the reader. In the introduction to *The godly saiyngs of the old auncient faithful fathers,* a compilation of views of the Church Fathers on the sacrament of Communion produced by Véron in 1550, he suggested that his readers might need more than average patience in dealing with his crude English. He explained 'Because I was in Fraunce . . . born & brought up, & not in . . . English . . . learned and taught: do I earnestlye, now you al that in England do dwell, and professe Christ . . . desyre and pray, to take in good worth, [what] I have here wroughte & set furthe'.[16] In a dedication to Elizabeth I in 1561, he reiterated the notion that true Christians will appreciate his message, regardless of his foreign background. He wrote:

> Some . . . wyll mervaile and wonder, that I beyng but a pore stra[n]ger, dwellinge here wythin your graces dominion, dare be so bold to dedicate any maner of booke unto your maiestye . . . But they shall, I truste, cease from marvailing when they shall both call to remembraunce thys saying of Paul: there is neyther Jewe nor Grecian, ther is neyther bond nor free, there is neyther man nor womanne: for, [they] are all one in CHRIST JESUS.[17]

Véron's choice of dedicatees also reveals his integration into English society and his concern for the spread of the Gospel to the English people. Like most writers and translators, Véron dedicated nearly all of his publications to powerful individuals. The list of his dedicatees includes Protector Somerset, King Edward VI, Queen Elizabeth, Robert Dudley and Nicholas Bacon. These dedications were not just bids for patronage, however. Véron understood the importance of godly magistracy for the spread of the true faith among the ignorant. Thus, he urged Sir John Gates of Essex to protect the simple people by driving out all the Anabaptists and other heretics from the region.[18] He asked Queen Elizabeth to accept his gift of a book defending pre-destination, because he hoped it would 'passe forth, through your highnes name & permissyon, into the handes of your unfained and faithfull subiectes'.[19] Véron did, however, dedicate one book to a commoner, his dialogue defending clerical marriage. We know the man only by the Véron's description: 'Master George Balford, Leather Sealer, Citizen of London'. This man seems to have done Véron a favour in the past. Addressing Balford at the end of the dedication, he wrote 'althoughe I haue not seen you this great while yet I am not vnmindeful of you, nor of the gentle kyndenes, that [you] haue shewed to m[y] warde at all tymes'.[20]

Two references we have to Véron from other contemporary sources indicate that English evangelicals accepted him as one of their own and believed his efforts to bring the Word of God to the English people were worthwhile. In his *Acts and Monuments*, John Foxe included a letter from Nicholas Ridley to John Bradford, when the two were in separate prisons in 1555. 'It should do us much comfort', Ridley wrote, 'if we might have knowledge of the state of the rest of our most dearly beloved, which in this troublesome time do stand in Christ's cause, and in the defence of the truth thereof . . . We long to hear of father Crome, Dr Sands, master Saunders, Veron, Beacon, Rogers, etc'.[21] Upon his death in 1563, John Awdelie wrote a poetic epitaph for Véron. I quote here an excerpt from Awdelie's tribute.

> From pasture unto pasture he dyd thee bryng to feede,
> And never ceased to make thee from fayth to fayth proceede.
> There restes no more for you hys paynes now to requite,
> But so to walke as he you taught, and speake of hym the ryght.
> And thou, O England, now, to ende and mone wyth th[ose],
> Lament thou mayst also wyth us, a woorkeman thus to l[ose].[22]

Neither of these two references to Véron mentions his French origins. In fact, though Véron continued to attach the title 'Senonois' to his name, the only person to refer to his being French was the diarist Henry Machyn, who was, for some unknown reason, hostile towards Véron. Machyn mentions Véron by name 16 times in his diary, and once simply as the unnamed vicar of St Martin's of Ludgate. In seven of these 17 citations, he refers to Véron as a Frenchman.[23] In two, he relates how after a sermon of Véron's, the congregation sang 'the tune of Geneva', the implication being that the singing of foreign songs was a result of the foreign origins of the minister.[24] The most interesting references, however, are two which describe two men, one of whom was Machyn himself, having to do public penance at St Paul's for slandering Véron. Specifically, Machyn was punished for passing on a rumour that Véron was 'taken with a wench'.[25]

We cannot know for certain the reason for Machyn's hostility to Véron, if Véron was truly keeping a mistress, or if the 'wench' was simply a wife. The editor of Machyn's diary states that Machyn sympathized with the Catholic religion, and it is likely that his animosity had roots in these religious differences. Regardless, it is interesting that the only man to refer to Véron as a Frenchman was an enemy, certainly an enemy of Véron's and possibly an enemy of the Reformation.

This completes our picture of Véron's integration into the English community, one that is full of contradictions. He was a man who cared more about being a Protestant than being French or English, but never stopped calling himself 'Senonois'. He was acquainted with powerful English evangelicals, yet he presided at many funerals of London citizens and dedicated one book to a London artisan. He earned the love and respect of his colleagues in the ministry, but was slandered by others. His life and career are, therefore, examples of the international character of the English Reformation in the mid-Tudor period and the penetration of international influences down to the level of the common citizen, but also of the tensions that could arise between strangers and native Englishmen.

II

The second part of this essay deals with Véron's theology. All of his religious works possess a negative orientation; that is, their main goal was to prove false the arguments of some heretical sect or group. His three translations of Bullinger were all from one long dialogue against the Anabaptists that Bullinger wrote in 1531. The two translations of works by Zwingli both focused on how to tell true preachers of God from false prophets, and true interpretations of Scripture from erroneous ones; the main targets in these works were Catholics. The Mass itself was the victim of Véron's attack in a short book of his own composition, entitled *The V. abhominable blasphemies co[n]teined in the masse*. In his compilation of Patristic views on the sacrament of Communion, Véron's objective was to prove erroneous both those who 'attrybute to muche to the holy sacramentes', (in other words, Catholics) and those who 'of a lyghtnes and inconstancie ... attribute to little vntoo them' (presumably radical sacramentarians).[26] In another small book, *Certayne litel treaties, setforth by John Veron Senonoys, for the erudition and learnyng, of the symple & ignorant peopell*, he attacked the Mass, but also a group he called Anthropomorphists, who believed that God has human features and limbs.[27]

Finally, five of Véron's six Elizabethan dialogues took on particular aspects of Catholic belief: justification by works, free will, purgatory, saint worship, and clerical celibacy. In the title of the sixth dialogue, that on predestination, Véron claimed he wrote it not against Papists, but as 'an answer made to all the vain and blasphemous obiections that the Epicures and Anabaptistes of our time canne make'.[28] In the dedication of this work to Queen Elizabeth, however, Véron substituted 'papists' for 'Epicures'. He wrote that his goal in this and all his other publications was

> to advaunce and set foorth gods glorye and to arme his church and faythfull congregation againste all maner of heretics and abhominable erroures both of the papistes and of the Anabaptistes, and of all other sectaryes, that do now moleste and trouble the Godlye quyetnesse and peace of the church.[29]

The negative approach of Véron's work was common in early modern religious polemic. It is a reminder of just how much definitions of Protestant orthodoxy depended on arguments against Catholics on one side of the religious spectrum and Anabaptists on the other. For example, anti-Anabaptism was a driving force behind England's first confession of faith. Two of the Forty-Two Articles, those confirming original sin and denying the communality of goods, state directly the intention of refuting the opinions of the Anabaptists. Eight more, including those commending infant baptism and affirming the value of Old Testament moral codes, address issues stemming from Anabaptism. Moreover, articles on justification by faith, grace, and predestination simultaneously refute both Catholic and Anabaptist doctrine.[30]

Nearly all of these points are found in Véron's translations of Bullinger's dialogue against the Anabaptists. In translating these pieces, Véron was not only protecting the 'rude and symple people' of England against Anabaptist heresy, but also presenting them with important elements of Swiss Reformed doctrine. Véron seemed particularly concerned with impressing upon his audience the importance of secular and religious obedience. In the introduction to the translation of Bullinger's chapters on civil authority, Véron draws an analogy between Anabaptists and the rebels who took part in the uprisings in East Anglia in 1549.[31] For Véron, as for Bullinger, resistance to the king was itself a heretical act, a crime against God equal to proclaiming false doctrine. By associating the rebels with Anabaptism, even though there were very few Anabaptists in England and none involved with the rebellions, Véron made the connection between rebellion and heresy clearer. By suggesting that Anabaptists were a threat to the stability of England, he hoped to inspire fear and horror in his audience, so that his and Bullinger's simultaneous arguments for Reformed doctrine and for secular obedience would prove all the more powerful and persuasive.

The Anabaptist dialogues are just one example of how Véron employed Zürich theology towards the evangelization of England. Véron's choice to translate Zwingli and Bullinger instead of Calvin attests to the need for historians to revise their assumption that Calvin was always the dominant Continental theologian in the English Reformation. During the first half of the century, Zürich's influence was equally strong, if not stronger, than Geneva's. As we saw with Véron's Anabaptist dialogues, one reason that Bullinger's theology was especially appealing to evangelicals in England was because it placed religious authority in the hands of the magistrates, a situation applicable to England under the royal supremacy. Moreover, Véron was only one among many English translators to produce works by Zwingli and Bullinger. From the beginning of the Reformation until the death of Edward VI, nine separate titles by Bullinger were published in English, in addition to four by Zwingli. This is similar to 11 titles by Luther and 11 by Calvin. Even in the 1560s, when Calvin's influence in England was on the rise, Véron's dialogues were more concerned with refuting Catholic practice than with asserting Genevan theology.[32]

Three important points should be drawn from this study of Jean Véron. The first is the openness of the English evangelical community in London during the reign of Edward VI, an openness that fostered the founding of the Stranger Churches. Second is the importance of Continental influences on the English Reformation during this period, not only in the upper echelons of Cranmer's church and Edward VI's government, but also at the parish level. And third, these Continental influences, even when coming from the pen of a Frenchman, were not necessarily Calvinist.

NOTES

1   HSQS 8, 246; HSQS 10, pt. 1, 82.
2   These and other facts about Véron's career are found in George Hennessy (ed.), *Novum repertorium ecclesiasticarum parochiale londinense* (London, 1898), 38, 86, 125, 293, 383; and Henry Machyn, *The diary of Henry Machyn,* ed. J. G. Nichols (Camden Society vol. 42, 1848), 211–12, 214, 228, 248, 257, 263, 265, 271–3, 284. John Strype also mentions Véron several times in his *oeuvre,* but since Strype took most of his material from Machyn, I do not cite him separately.
3   Huldrych Zwingli, *A short pathwaye to the ryghte and true understanding of the holye & sacred Scriptures* (Worcester, 1550) [STC 26141]; idem, *The ymage of bothe Pastoures* (London, 1550) [STC 26142].
4   Heinrich Bullinger, *An holsome antidotus or counterpoysen, agaynst the pestylent heresye and secte of the Anabaptistses newly translated out of lati[n] into Englysh by John Veron,*

Senonoys (London, 1548) [*STC* 4059]; *idem, A most necessary & frutefull Dialogue, betwene y[e] seditious Libertin or rebel Anabaptist, & the true obedient christia[n]... well translated out of Latyn into Englisshe, by jho[n] Veron Senonoys* (Worcester, 1551), [*STC* 4068]; *idem, A moste sure and strong defence of the baptisme of children, against ye pestiferous secte of the Anabaptystes... nowe translated out of Laten into Englysh by Jhon Veron Senonoys* (Worcester, 1551) [*STC* 4069].

5   Jean Véron, *Certayne litel treaties setforth by John Veron Senonoys, for the erudition and learnyng, of the symple & ignorant peopell* (London, 1548), [*STC* 24676]; *idem, The V. abhominable blasphemies co(n)teined in the masse, with a short a(n)swere to them, that saie, we ronne before the kyng and his counsayle* (London, 1548), [*STC* 24679].

6   *Idem, The godly saiyngs of the old auncient faithful fathers vpon the sacrament of the bodye and bloude of Chryste* (Worcester, 1550), [*STC* 24682].

7   Robert Etienne and Jean Véron, *Dictionariolum puerorum, tribus linguis Latina, Anglica & Gallica conscriptum* (London, 1552), [*STC* 10555]. This went through two more editions during the Elizabethan period, after Véron's death. See *STC* 24677, 24678.

8   Jean Véron, *A fruteful treatise of predestination* (London, 1561), [*STC* 24680]; *idem, The huntynge of purgatorye to death* (London, 1561), [*STC* 24683]; *idem, A moste necessary treatise of free will* (London, 1561), [*STC* 24684]; *idem, The over throw of the iustification of workes* (London, 1561), [*STC* 24685]; *idem, A stronge battery against the idolatrous inuocation of the dead saintes* (London, 1562), [*STC* 24686]; *idem, A stronge defence of the maryage of pryestes* (London, 1562?), [*STC* 24687]. Hereafter, I will refer to Véron's publications by their *STC* numbers only. All of these dialogues appear to be original except for the one on purgatory. Though he used his own names for the interlocutors and added some original material, Véron lifted the majority of *The huntynge of purgatorye* from two dialogues by Pierre Viret in his *Disputations chrétiennes* (Geneva, 1544): 'L'Alcumie du Purgatoire' (also published as 'La Cosmographie infernale') and 'Le Purgatoire'. For a different 16th-century English translation, see *The Christian disputations, by Master Peter Viret*, trans. John Brooke (London, 1579).

9   F. de Schickler, 'Le réfugié Jean Véron, collaborateur des réformateurs anglais, 1548–1562', *Bulletin de la Société de l'Histoire du Protestantisme français* 39 (1890), 437–46.

10 Philippe Denis, 'Jean Véron: the first known French Protestant in England', *HSP* 22 (1970–6), 257–63.

11 Susan Brigden, *London and the Reformation* (Oxford, 1989), 459; Irvin B. Horst, *The radical brethren: Anabaptism and the English Reformation to 1558* (Nieuwkoop, 1972), 106–7.

12 Denis, 258.

13 See n. 1 above.

14 *STC* 10555, preface.

15 In addition to sources cited in n. 2, see also David Loades, *The reign of Mary Tudor: politics, government, and religion in England, 1553–1558* (New York, 1979), 151–2.

16 *STC* 24682, sig. A2v.

17 *STC* 24681, preface.

18 *STC* 4068, sig. C2v-C3r.

19 *STC* 24681, preface.

20 *STC* 24687, preface.

21 John Foxe, *The acts and monuments*, ed. Stephen Reed Cattley (London, 1838), vol. 7, 124.

22 John Awdelie, excerpt from 'An Epitaphe upon the Death of Mayster John Viron, Preacher', in *Select poetry... of the reign of Queen Elizabeth*, ed. E. Farr (Cambridge, 1845), vol. 2, 540. A fragment of a 16th-century edition of this poem exists in the Huntington Library, San Marino, California, shelf-mark 18264.

23 Machyn, *Diary*, 214, 248–9, 257, 263, 265, 272–3, 284.

24 *Ibid.*, 228.

25 *Ibid.*, 271–3.

26 *STC* 24679, preface.

27 Véron argued here against literal interpretations of the Bible; for example, taking a reference to God's 'hands' or 'eyes' to mean that the deity actually possessed these features. Véron made no indication, however, as to whether he was targeting an actual sect called 'Anthropomorphists' or simply all radical Christians who interpreted the Bible literally.

28 *STC* 24680, title.

29 *STC* 24681, sig. E8v.

30 *Articles agreed vpon by the Bishoppes . . . for the auoiding of controuersie in opinions* (London, 1553) [*STC* 10034].

31 *STC* 4068, sig. A2r-C3v.

32 I would argue that Véron's use of Pierre Viret's dialogues against purgatory in his own (see n. 8) is not indicative of Genevan or Calvinist theological influence, but of Véron's identification with Viret's ironic and vituperative literary style.

3

Discipline and integration: Jan Laski's Church Order for the London Strangers' Church

Christoph Strohm

On 24 July 1550, Jan Laski, a Polish baron, was nominated by King Edward VI to be superintendent of the 'Strangers' Church' in London, which brought together the French, the Dutch-German, and the Italian congregations.[1] At the same time, the King guaranteed an annual payment of £100 from his own coffers, and a royal decree assigned to the stranger churches the former monastery of the Austin Friars (Augustinian order), a 13th-century church in the centre of London. The decision to assign this important, centrally-sited building to the stranger churches was astonishing. Not less surprising were the extensive powers granted by the King to the superintendent and the four pastors who were his assistants. The stranger churches did not come under the jurisdiction of the Bishop of London, and were permitted to order their affairs very much as they pleased.[2]

With the Strangers' Church, Jan Laski was faced with a double problem of integration. In the first place, it was necessary to integrate the exile congregations into the changes which were being brought about in the English Church as a result of the Reformation and the consequent formation of the national Church. Secondly, Laski needed to address the problem that the congregations under his authority drew together people from very different national, cultural and ecclesiastical contexts, whose understandings of the teaching and order of the Church varied accordingly. But before I consider the tasks of integration facing Laski in more detail, I wish to discuss the background to the surprising fact that an exile like Jan Laski could find himself in such a privileged situation at all.

Laski's life and background

Jan Laski (Johannes a Lasco) was born in 1499 in Lask, a small town west of Lodz in Poland.[3] From 1510 to 1531 his father's brother was Archbishop of Gnesen and Primate of Poland; he also served as Chancellor to King Sigismund I. Laski's education was supported by his uncle, who intended it to fit him to serve in the highest echelons of the Polish Church. The young Jan Laski studied in Bologna (1515–18) and Padua (1518–19). He was deeply influenced by a period spent at the University of Basle during 1525–6. Here he lived together with Erasmus of Rotterdam in the house of Froben, the printer, and learned Greek and Hebrew from Conrad Pellikan. Ordained in his teens and already holding significant benefices in the Polish Church, Laski was appointed in his twenties to still higher offices. As a humanist and student of Erasmus, he was open to reform in the Church, while at the same time being a strong opponent of Martin Luther.

Political events in Hungary brought an important change in Laski's life. In the late 1520s his brother Jaroslaw supported the efforts of Johann Zápolya, a Transylvanian count, to be elected King of Hungary, fighting with Zápolya and joining with him in a treaty with the Turks against the Habsburgs. In the course of these campaigns, Jaroslaw Laski entrusted his brother Jan with diplomatic missions. The failure of these endeavours brought financial and political ruin to the Laski family, and neither upon the death of his uncle in 1531 nor later was Jan Laski able to succeed to a Polish see, as had been planned.

In 1537, Laski met the reformer Philip Melanchthon. However, Laski's break with the Roman Catholic Church did not become obvious until 1540, when he married the daughter of a burgher in Louvain, where he had gone to continue his studies. As a consequence he was forced to flee to Emden, where he lived for some time as a private householder before being appointed as the first superintendent of East Frisia in 1542. In Emden, Laski followed the example of the Prince Archbishop of Cologne, Hermann von Wied, who, with the help of Melanchthon, Martin Bucer, and Laski's old friend Albert Hardenberg, sought to introduce a moderate reform into his diocese. The apparently irreconcilable tensions within the East Frisian Church meant that Laski's work there often seemed close to failure; the many Anabaptists who had fled from the Netherlands were especially hard to integrate. With the defeat of the Protestants in the Schmalkadic War (1546/7) and the imposition of the Augsburg Interim by the Emperor in 1548, Laski's position in East Frisia became untenable.

The relationship of the Strangers' Church to the English Church

Laski was one of the first reformers to be invited by Archbishop Thomas Cranmer to come to England after the death of Henry VIII. His name is already found on a list of desirable visitors drawn up in 1547.[4] Cranmer reiterated the invitation in July 1548, but Laski was not able to respond immediately. Cranmer was keen to encourage leading Protestants to come to England, not only in an attempt to further the Reformation in England after the death of Henry VIII, but also because the Council of Trent and the consequent intensification of the Counter-Reformation had convinced him of the necessity of a pan-European Protestant council. After the reverses suffered by the Protestant cause in Continental Europe as a result of the Schmalkadic War, Cranmer believed that the Church in England had a particular role to play. After the failure of the attempts at reformation in Cologne and the Emperor's demand that Hermann von Wied should resign his Archbishopric,

Cranmer directed his attention to Laski. Cranmer had followed the progress of von Wied's reform of Cologne's *Erzstift* in the years 1542 to 1546 with close attention, for this was the first attempt by a Prince-Bishop of the German empire to introduce a moderate Reformation. The Reformation in Cologne was moderate in that it left the ecclesiastical structures of the old Church largely intact. For example, the Prince-Bishop should remain. The theological basis of the Reformation in Cologne, Melanchthon's and Bucer's *Einfältiges Bedenken* of 1543,[5] was one of the most important influences upon Cranmer's Reformation, and in particular on the Book of Common Prayer. Once the Archbishop of Cologne was no longer available as a Protestant leader and could not initiate a Protestant council in opposition to the Council of Trent, Cranmer saw himself as entrusted with this task.

Laski was intended to help achieve this aim. Cranmer saw Laski, who was in close contact with Hermann von Wied and his theological advisers Martin Bucer and, in particular, Albert von Hardenberg, as a colleague and ally of the Archbishop of Cologne. He knew Laski as a member of the Polish high nobility and nephew of the Primate of Poland, and viewed Laski's role as 'reforming bishop' in East Frisia as the continuation of a tradition established by von Wied. And so, during his six months' stay in England from 18 September 1548 until the middle of March 1549, Laski lived initially in Cranmer's palace at Lambeth, moving later to Windsor, but remaining in close contact with Cranmer during his entire visit. On his return from England, Laski left Emden immediately for East Prussia, where he entered political negotiations with Duke Albrecht.[6]

Laski returned to England on 13 May 1550. He was received with open arms and continued to enjoy the hospitality of Cranmer, whom he referred to as his 'patron and father'.[7] The Polish baron, now appointed by the King as superintendent of the London Strangers' Church, was far from being a simple exile. Cranmer hoped that Laski would offer advice and support in the Reformation of the English Church, and, given his origins, his political and diplomatic contacts, and his episcopal role as the organizer of the Reformation in East Frisia, he seemed eminently qualified to do so. His contacts were also intended to be put to use in organizing a Protestant general council. Moreover, Laski's work as superintendent of the Strangers' Church served to integrate these extremely heterogeneous groups. The moderate Reformation of England's Church was not to be endangered by the multiplicity of heterodox opinions which could be found amongst the Protestant exiles. Finally, Cranmer intended that the stranger churches should serve as role models for the Reformation in England as a whole. The stranger churches offered a precisely defined field for experiment which made possible the stringent realization of Reformation principles in a way which seemed impossible in the wider church.

The integration of the London Strangers' Church into the developing English Church was not uncomplicated. Conflict soon broke out with Nicholas Ridley, Bishop of London, who was unwilling to accept Laski's refusal to use English liturgy and ceremonial in his congregations. Laski's use of his own Eucharistic rites was a particular bone of contention. In the controversy about the retention of vestments in episcopal consecrations, Laski sided with John Hooper and quarrelled with Cranmer. Cranmer, himself influenced by Erasmus, had clearly overestimated the extent of common ground shared by himself and the Erasmian Laski, and was incensed by Laski's lack of willingness to compromise. Hooper's concessions did much to soothe

the controversy, but Cranmer's and Laski's relationship had not recovered by the time the latter fled England on the accession of Mary Tudor to the throne in 1553.

A programme of integration through church discipline

On his appointment in 1550, Laski immediately took energetic steps to build up Protestant congregations amongst the exiles. He sought to give the Strangers' Church a common character through a statement of faith composed by himself and four other pastors appointed by the King. Every member of the Strangers' Church was required to sign this text, the so-called *Confessio Londinensis*, printed in 1551.[8] Laski was particularly concerned with the necessity of compiling a common church order. The *Forma ac ratio tota ecclesiastici Ministerii*, first printed in 1555, offers a detailed description of the offices of the church, their duties and responsibilities, and of the orders for church services.[9] In reality, this church order was valid only in the Dutch-German part of the church which as a whole gathered together 3000–4000 exiles,[10] and the French-Walloon congregation oriented itself along the lines of the *Ordonnances ecclésiastiques* of Calvin's Geneva.[11]

Laski's *Forma ac ratio* for the London church centres on the *disciplina ecclesiastica*, to which more than a fifth of the text is devoted.[12] For Laski, the *disciplina ecclesiastica* is the decisive means of integration within the congregation. The establishment of a common *disciplina ecclesiastica* is necessary firstly in order to create a common identity amongst the exiles, who lived in different parts of London and who were using, or drawing on, very different doctrines, rites and liturgies. Moreover, a consistently applied *disciplina ecclesiastica*, in the sense of a unifying commitment to mutual support, could have a positive stabilizing effect on the rootless exiles and their community and thus be a significant aid to survival.[13]

While superintendent in East Frisia, Laski had already become convinced that the establishment of a *disciplina ecclesiastica* represented the means for the internal integration of a congregation. The background to this recognition was both his particular ethical interest as a student of Erasmus and the necessity of dealing with the Anabaptists and other representatives of the left wing of the Reformation. Their rigorous practice of church discipline had led Laski to see a connection between a failure in *disciplina ecclesiastica* and the spread of Anabaptists and other sects. In a letter to his friend Albert Hardenberg of 26 July 1544, he emphasized that the key problem of the integration of the Anabaptists and the struggle against the sects could not be solved as long as no convincing *disciplina* had been introduced into the Church as a whole.[14] In his opinion, the 'Epicureans in their own ranks', that is, the burghers of Emden whose increasing wealth made them unwilling to submit to a strict church discipline, must share the blame for the expansion of the sects.[15]

Because of his humanist interest in ethics, *disciplina ecclesiastica* was already the central element of the thought of the Erasmian Laski. This tendency was further strengthened by the fact that his work as superintendent of the East Frisian Church was shaped by the need to integrate the Anabaptists and other groups of the radical Reformation into the Protestant Church. It is against this background that in the London church order Laski further developed his understanding of *disciplina ecclesiastica* as the decisive means for maintaining the *unity* and *community* of the church.

This is the particular characteristic of Laski's understanding of *disciplina ecclesiastica* in comparison to that of other reformers.

In accordance with biblical foundations and with the reformers Oecolampadius, Bucer and Calvin, Laski defines *disciplina ecclesiastica* as 'a particular certain way of gradually coming to a mutual observance of Christian admonitions from the Word of God amongst all the brothers in the Church of Christ, so that both the whole body and its individual members may be held in their office for as long as that is possible. [. . .]'[16] *Disciplina ecclesiastica* thus forms the decisive means by which the *community*, a gift of Christ, central to Laski's theory of the Church, is realized (or in the theological sense more accurately, actualized) and maintained.[17] Moreover, *disciplina ecclesiastica* is itself community put into practice.[18]

For Laski, the most important aspect of *disciplina ecclesiastica* is the consummation and maintenance of the community of the body of Christ, constituted through the *lex caritatis*. This takes place in opposition to the abuse of *disciplina ecclesiastica* by the Anabaptists. 'Firstly, it must be sprung from true Christian love and from a pure and loving heart; not from the zeal to convict one's brother, but to win him; not from a wish for personal glorification, but for the building up of the whole church. Then we must be certain that that for which a brother is admonished offends . . . against our faith and our love. [. . .] Finally, we must apply Christian restraint and intelligence in our admonishments of this kind. Surely, if the reason why a brother is to be admonished be uncertain, it can be exposed through loving questioning.'[19]

Further, Laski discusses the case that incriminating behaviour may endanger the entire body: 'The law of love itself requires that the good of the whole body or of a number of members in one and the same body be regarded as more important than that of one member and that it is therefore better (as Christ himself taught) that the body itself together with all the remaining members should be saved, if it is disabled by one member or another, than that the whole body together with all its members should be dissipated.'[20]

Laski's discussion of a number of punishments – often taken to be the central focus of the English translation of *disciplina ecclesiastica* as 'Church discipline' – is marginal and for extreme cases. Even when Laski does turn to a detailed discussion of excommunication, in the sense of temporary exclusion from the congregation, in detail, he pays a great deal of attention to the measures which can be taken to reinstate the offender into the community.[21] He is not interested in matching certain punitive measures to certain offences. The deciding factor is whether the person whose exclusion or acceptance is under discussion is prepared to submit to *disciplina ecclesiastica* by attending to the admonishments of the brothers; that is, whether he or she is ready to reopen the damaged or broken channels of communication and thus to enable *communio* to be reinstated.[22] Laski emphasizes that excommunication is the result, not of particular sins or offences, but of the disdaining of admonishments – and thus of the community – by those affected.

It is clear that this model could quickly be converted into a system of force and punishment, and indeed it was. However, it is impossible to miss Laski's attempts to oppose the legalistic and loveless practice of church discipline which he had encountered in East Frisian Anabaptist circles by his wish to define *disciplina ecclesiastica* entirely in terms of the Church's *communio*, shaped by *lex caritatis*.[23] The unique nature of Laski's understanding of *disciplina ecclesiastica* is most clear on this point.[24]

Kirchenordnung/Wie die
vnter dem

Christlichen

König auß Engelland/
Edward dem VI.in der Statt
Londen/in der Niderlendischen Ge-
meine Christi/Durch Kön. Maiest. man-
dat geordnet vnd gehalten worden/mit
der Kirchendiener vnd Eltesten
bewilligung/

Durch

Herrn Johann von Las-
co/Freiherren in Polen/Su-
perintendenten derselbigen Kirchen
in Engelland in Lateinischer sprach weit-
leufftiger beschrieben/Aber durch Mar-
tinum Micronium in eine kurtze Sum
verfasset/Vnd jetzund
verdeutschet.

Gedruckt in der Churfürstlichen
Statt Heidelberg/Durch Jo-
hannem Mayer.

1 5 6 5.

Neither Bucer nor Calvin – besides Oecolampadius, the two most important influences on Laski's interest in church order – take *communio* shaped by *lex caritatis* as the background to *disciplina ecclesiastica* in this way. Moreover, and in contrast to Calvin, Laski does not see church discipline as a prerequisite for the participation in Holy Communion.[25] Church discipline does not serve as a cleansing in preparation for Holy Communion. Rather, it is the expression and fulfilment of the gift of *communio* through the Eucharist.[26]

The key role of the *disciplina ecclesiastica* in the *community* of the church is directly linked to its significance for the *unity* of the church. Final agreement about questions of doctrine or outward ceremonies is not necessary for the unity of the church,[27] for this unity comes into being in the form of the lived community arising from the practice of *disciplina ecclesiastica*.[28] Laski here shows himself to be influenced by the heritage of his teacher, Erasmus.[29] Laski praised Erasmus's *Liber de sarcienda ecclesiae concordia*[30] of 1533 very highly;[31] in the 1550s he was to react to Gnesiolutheran attacks on his Eucharistic theology by quoting Erasmus's warning that the Lutheran tyranny would prove to be even worse than that of the Papists.[32] From the beginning, Laski's reforming impulses were characterized by his attempts to preserve, or restore, the community of the church from all possible party differences.[33] Particular examples of this, besides his work towards integrating the Anabaptists and the establishment of a doctrinal consensus with the followers of Luther in East Frisia, can be found in his attempts to negotiate a settlement in the Eucharistic controversy of the 1550s,[34] and his work towards bringing about unification of the divided Protestant movements in Poland during the final years of his life.[35]

Conclusion

Laski's understanding of *disciplina ecclesiastica*, developed in London at the beginning of the 1550s, is one of the most detailed presentations of Protestant *disciplina ecclesiastica* to be found in the 16th century. Its particular focus on the unity and community of the Church – to the extent that *disciplina ecclesiastica*, the binding relationship between church members in the form of encouragement and admonition, forms a decisive means for the realization of the community of the church – has a number of roots: the inheritance of Erasmus; the attempts to integrate the Anabaptists into the church in East Frisia; the influence of Oecolampadius, Bucer, and Calvin; and the particular situation of the Strangers' Church in London, for whose life a settled community was necessary.

Laski's programme of 'integration through *disciplina ecclesiastica*' could be realized at least within the Dutch-German part of the Strangers' Church. Moreover, the integration of the Strangers' Church into the changes brought about by the Reformation in the English Church, although not free of conflict, was nevertheless successful. Through his church order, Laski was able to bring together the culturally and ecclesiastically heterogeneous groups of exiles who fled to England from Continental Europe, to meld them into a disciplined unity and to prevent the spread of anti-Trinitarian and other false doctrines. Despite the conflicts between Laski and Ridley about the independence of the Strangers' Church and between Laski and Cranmer over the question of the retention of Roman ceremony, the Strangers' Church was able to function for some years as a field of experiment and as a role model to encourage what was, on the whole, a rather cautious Reformation within the English Church.[36]

NOTES

1 Johannes a Lasco, *Opera tam edita quam inedita*, ed. Abraham Kuyper, 2 vols. (Amsterdam/The Hague, 1866) (hereafter: *K I* and *K II*), vol. 2, 279–83. With thanks to Charlotte Methuen for her translation of this text.

2 Compare Dirk W. Rodgers, *John à Lasco in England* (New York, 1994) (American University Studies, Series VII: Theology and Religion 168), 28f.

3 For Laski's biography, see Oskar Bartel, *Jan Laski*, trans. by Arnold Starke (Berlin, 1981); Menno Smid, 'Laski, Jan (1499–1560)', in *TRE* 20 (Berlin/New York, 1990), 448–51.

4 Laski to A. Hardenberg, 11 October 1547: *K II*, 611; for what follows, see Diarmaid MacCulloch, 'The importance of Jan Laski in the English Reformation', in Christoph Strohm (ed.), *Johannes a Lasco (1499–1560). Polnischer Baron, Humanist und europäischer Reformator. Beiträge zum internationalen Symposium in der Johannes a Lasco Bibliothek Emden* (Tübingen, 2000) (Spätmittelalter und Reformation, NR 14), 315–45; Rodgers, *John à Lasco*.

5 Hermann von Wied, 'Einfaltings Bedencken' in Christoph Strohm/Thomas G. Wilhelmi (eds.) with Stephen E. Buckwalter, *Schriften zur Kölner Reformation* (Gütersloh, 1999) (Martin Bucers Deutsche Schriften, Band 11:1), 163–429. It was translated into English: 'A simple and religious consultation' (London, 1547; London, 1548).

6 Laski wished to discover whether the accession to the throne of King Zygmunt August would offer him any chance to return to Poland and work for the Reformation there. In his support he carried a letter from Edward VI to Zygmunt August, which included the request that Laski be allowed to return to his homeland. (see Bartel, 127f.).

7 Laski to Cranmer, August 1551: *K II*, 657.

8 *Compendium doctrinae de vera unicaque Dei et Christi Ecclesia, eiusque fide et confessione pura: in qua Peregrinorum Ecclesia Londini instituta est, autoritate atque assensu Sacrae Maiestatis Regiae* (1551), in *K II*, 287–339.

9 Johannes a Lasco, *Forma ac ratio tota ecclesiastici Ministerii, in peregrinorum, potissimum vero Germanorum Ecclesia: instituta Londini in Anglia, per Pietissimum Principem Angliae etc. Regem EDVARDVM, eius nominis Sextu: Anno post Christum natum 1550. Addito ad calcem libelli Priuilegio suae Maiestatis*, in *K II*, 1–283. For a discussion of the content of the *Forma ac ratio* and of the situation in which it was compiled, see Otto Naunin, 'Die Kirchenordnungen des Johannes Laski', in *DZKR* 19 (1909), 197–236, 348–54; Ulrich Falkenroth, 'Gestalt und Wesen der Kirche bei Johannes a Lasco' (unpublished Ph.D. thesis, Göttingen, 1957), 20–121; Anneliese Sprengler-Ruppenthal, *Mysterium und Riten nach der Londoner Kirchenordnung der Niederländer (ca. 1550 bis 1566)* (Cologne/Graz, 1967); Bartel, 140–7; Rodgers, 51–79. The title is probably inspired by a work of Johannes Oecolampadius, in which he describes the reformed order for baptism and eucharist and the rules pertaining to exclusion from the church recently introduced in Basle: Oecolampadius, *Form und gestalt wie der kinder tauff Des herren Nachtmal und der Krancken heymsüchung jetz zü Basel von etlichen Predicanten gehalten werden* (1526) (Ernst Staehelin, *Oekolampad-Bibliographie* (Nieuwkoop, 1963), no. 135). Laski valued Oecolampadius's work highly and studied it carefully.

10 The size of the congregation has been so estimated by Andrew Pettegree, *Foreign Protestant communities in sixteenth-century London* (Oxford, 1986), 77f.; and compare also his 'The foreign population of London in 1549', in *HSP* 24 (1984), 141–6. In 1522/3, the Dutch-German congregation probably had approximately 1400 members (see Rodgers, 41). There

was also a French-Walloon congregation and Italian congregation. Naunin, 196, refers (misleadingly) only to French-Walloon and German congregations.

11 On the tense relationship between the French-Walloon and the Dutch-German congregations, see Rodgers, 39f., 48.

12 *K II*, 170–226.

13 The exclusively positive interpretation (to modern ears somewhat problematic) of concepts associated with order or discipline can be better understood against the background of the fate of exiles who experienced their age as a time of radical change and upheaval. For Laski, the term *disciplina* refers primarily to the kind of order which allows peace and growth. See, for instance, *K II*, 61f.: 'Sed ordinem retinendum esse publicarum Eleemosynarum in Ecclesia iuxta Apostolicam ordinationem, ut veris pauperibus Ecclesiae prospiciatur cum Ecclesiae aedificatione.' Compare also *K II*, 64 ('publicae alioqui tranquillitatis atque ordinis politici retinendi in Ecclesia custodem'); on the relationship between crisis and order in the later 16th century, see Christoph Strohm, *Ethik im frühen Calvinismus. Humanistische Einflüsse, philosophische, juristische und theologische Argumentationen sowie mentalitätsgeschichtliche Aspekte am Beispiel des Calvin-Schülers Lambertus Danaeus* (Berlin/New York, 1996) (AKG 65), 540–652, especially 542–6.

14 Hardenberg refused Laski's repeated suggestion that he should be called to Emden or to East Frisia (see, for example *K II*, 576) on principle because of his distaste for the ' furiae anabaptistorum' which reigned there. Hardenberg went as far as to refer to the area as ' the most miserable nursery of all evil, in which there are as many heresies, sects, and schisms as there are heads'. See Wim Janse, *Albert Hardenberg als Theologe. Profil eines Bucer-Schülers* (Leiden/New York, 1994) (SHCT 57), 351f. (with sources).

15 'Meditamur nunc quandam disciplinam in nostra hac Ecclesia, cui omnes fere hactenus manibus, quod dicitur, ac pedibus restiterunt, qui me adiuvare potissimum debebant. Dicebam, nunquam fore, ut sectis careamus, si, dum in alios severi sumus, in vitiis interim ipsi nobis indulgeamus. Quae cum inter nos regnarent, statuendum etiam nobis esse discrimen in nostra Ecclesia, dum ita in alios severi sumus, inter eos, qui sese ad resipiscentiam volunt componere, et qui Dei Ecclesiam eiusque disciplinam contemnunt.– Breviter, post multos clamores id tandem effeci, ut nobis ministris adiuncti sint quatuor cives, viri alioquin graves, et, quantum iudicare possumus, pietatis studiosi, qui a tota Ecclesia potestatem nobiscum habeant in mores civium inquirendi, admonendi quenquam sui offici, et ad extremum etiam nomine totius Ecclesiae excommunicandi nobiscum, si quos admonitionum nostrarum contemptores haberemus': *K II*, 574f. In the London Church Order, Laski emphasized that a 'legitimate restoration of the churches and of religion' seemed to him unthinkable without regaining a legitimate application of *disciplina ecclesiastica*, particularly for office-holders: *K II*, 223f.

16 'Disciplina Ecclesiastica est certa quaedam e scripturis petita ratio observandi gradatim Christianas admonitiones ex verbo Dei inter fratres invicem omnes in Ecclesia Christi, ut et corpus universum singulaque illius membra in suo officio, quoad eius fieri potest, contineantur, – et, si qui in illa deprehendantur obstinati admonitionum istiusmodi contemptores, ut Satanae ad extremum per excommunicationem tradantur, si quo modo per talem pudefactionem et caro in illis interire, quod ad affectus illius attinet, et spiritus ita demum revocari ad resipiscentiam ac proinde servari etiam possit': *K II*, 170.

17 For the meaning of 'communio' in Laski's early theology, see 'Epitome doctrinae' (1544), in *K I*, 568–70; and compare Falkenroth, 129f., 154 ('his understanding of community is fundamental throughout'); on the key role of 'communio' in Laski's eucharistic theology, see Cornel A. Zwierlein, 'Der reformierte Erasmianer Johannes a Lasco und die Herausbildung seiner Abendmahlslehre 1544–1552', in Strohm (ed.), *Johannes a Lasco*, 35–99, esp. 65–96.

18 'Deinde usu legitimae excommunicationis conservatur Ecclesia in suo officio, discit sollicita

esse pro salute membrorum suorum, docetur quam res sit invisa Deo planeque intolerabilis admonitionum Ecclesiasticarum contemptus, coadunatur indies magis ac magis per quotidianas invicem ex verbo coadunatur indies magis ac magis per quotidianas invicem ex verbo Dei inter sese admonitiones ac consolationes atque assiduis istiusmodi exercitiis in unanimi semper consensu confirmatur': *K II*, 200.

19 'Diximus eas admonitiones, quae ita gradatim observari debeant, oportere esse Christianas, ut intelligamus tria nobis peculiariter observanda esse in illarum usu. Primum, ut ex mera charitate Christiana candidoque et amanti pectore proficiscantur, non equidem traducendi, sed lucrifaciendi fratris studio, neque item ad nostri ipsorum ostentationem, sed ad Ecclesiae totius aedificationem. Deinde, ut nobis certe constet, id, de quo frater aliquis sit admonendus, pugnare omnino cum verbi Divini doctrina facereque contra fidem nostram aut charitatem. Alioqui hypocriticum est potius, quam Christianum, ea redarguere velle, quae cum doctrina verbi Dei consistere simul possunt. Postremo, ut modestiam ac prudentiam Christianam in nostris istiusmodi admonitionibus adhibeamus. Nempe ut, si res incerta sit, de qua frater aliquis debeat admoneri, amanti aliqua sciscitatione duntaxat temperetur. Si vero res plane sit certa, ut rursum videamus, multisne iam sit cognita nec ne, multosne secum item aut totam forte etiam Ecclesiam ita involvat, ut in discrimen aliquod induci possit. Si enim res multis iam est cognita multosque secum periculo alicui involvit, plures sane adhiberi possunt in prima etiam admonitione. Si vero ad totam alioqui Ecclesiam eiusve ministerium pertineat, ut ad Seniores Ecclesiae protinus deferatur, quibus sane curam et gubernandae et conservandae Ecclesiae demandatam esse constat. Christi enim doctrina de solo fratre primum omnium privatim admonendo ad eos duntaxat pertinet, qui unum duntaxat aliquem, non autem simul multos, nedum totam Ecclesiam aut offenderunt aut in discrimen aliquod induxerunt': *K II*, 171f. See also *K II*, 177f.: 'Quae autem plebis totius ac singulorum membrorum in Ecclesia officia ad mutuam fratrum invicem omnium societatem pertinent, in hoc imprimis consistere videntur: 1. Ut quisque in Ecclesia totius simul corporis Ecclesiae imprimis, deinde vero singulorum ipsius membrorum inter sese, quoad eius fieri potest, pacem concordiam atque unitatem sub verbi divini obedientia observet custodiat promoveat ac tueatur pro sua virili neque illam, quod in ipso est, scindi quoquo modo perturbarive sinat.'

20 'Et lex ipsa charitatis hoc postulat, ut totius corporis pluriumve adeo membrorum etiam in uno eodemque corpore maior sane, quam unius duntaxat membri, ratio habeatur, et, quemadmodum Christus ipsemet docet, praestat, corpus ipsum, cum reliquorum membrorum compage servari, uno aut altero membro mutilatum, quam ut propter unum membrum corpus totum eiusque compages dissipentur': *K II*, 172. Laski often emphasizes that a brother may be excommunicated only with the clear agreement and support of the whole congregation, and not simply as the result of a decision taken by the superintendent or the preachers and elders (see *K II*, 187–9, 195, 199).

21 *K II*, 196, 203, 208–22. Compare also *K II*, 199: 'Exponit Ecclesiastes, excommunicationis usum non solum non pugnare cum lege charitatis Christianae, sed gravissime etiam violari legem charitatis in Ecclesia Christi, si legitimus excommunicationis usus non observetur.'

22 *K II*, 194. See also *K II*, 196–8: '1. Exponit Ecclesiastes, quid sit et quid in se complectatur, quamque vim obtineat ipsa excommunicatio. Docet esse Christi Domini institutionem ad retundendum in eius Ecclesia comtemptum legitimarum omnium admonitionum ordinatam, quae nos etiam nostrae invicem omnium aliorum pro aliis curae ac sollicitudinis admoneat, qui nos unius in Christo corporis membra esse profitemur. [. . .] 2. Docet Ecclesiastes, non tam equidem crimina ipsa atque flagitia, quantumvis gravia, quam comtemptum potius rebellem ac praefractum, excommunicationis remedio ab Ecclesia Christi arceri. Nullum enim tam esse atrox facinus ac flagitium, quod Ecclesia ferre non debeat, cum et ipsa sit omni infirmitatis genere circumdata, praeter obstinatum rebellem ac praefractum contemptum admonitionum ex verbo Dei.' Compare further *K II*, 200f., 204,

208, 213–16, 220f. For Erasmus's sharp criticism of those who destroy the unity of the Church, see his 'Liber de sarcienda ecclesiae concordia', in *Desiderii Erasmi Roterodami Opera omnia emendatiora et auctiora*, ed. Joannes Clericus, 10 vols. (Leiden, 1703–6; reprinted Hildesheim 1961/2), vol. 5, 498B; see also note 30 below.

23 See Naunin, 217: 'This view of church discipline, unified and circumspect as it is, has a strong element of social awareness. Its fundamental principle is pastoral love, which must not, however, be allowed to compromise the well-being of the church. As far as possible, it seeks to take care of the sinful brother, in order to save him if at all possible.'

24 That this is a particular characteristic of Laski's thought can be seen from the fact that precisely this point is not so obvious in the shorter versions of the London Church Order which appear in Dutch and High German in Micron's *Ordinancien* (1554/65). The translation of *disciplina ecclesiastica* as 'christliche Straffe' ('Christian punishment') sets a significantly different accent (see particularly Emil Sehling (ed.), *Die evangelischen Kirchenordnungen des XVI. Jahrhunderts* (Leipzig, 1902–13 and Tübingen, 1955–), vol. 7/II,1, 638–43.

25 *Disciplina ecclesiastica* is discussed after the section on the Eucharist in Laski's *Forma ac ratio*: *K II*, 114–69, 170–228.

26 'Unde perspicuum est etiam, usum legitimum disciplinae Ecclesiasticae ad Sacramentorum ministerium omnino pertinere, quod illam finis ille praecipuus omnium Sacramentorum complecti manifeste videtur. Etenim qui sibi Ecclesiae gubernationem concreditam habent, sive per verbi et sacramentorum, sive per gladii ministerium, facile intelligunt esse id debiti officiique sui, ut peccandi licentiam iuxta suum utrique ministerium coerceant; atque huius sui se officii commonefieri sentiunt proculdubio, siquidem signa Sacramentorum renovationis nostrae signa esse, vere et ex animo credunt; et qui id secum non reputant circa usum Sacramentorum, adeoque et nihil huius ad se pertinere arbitrantur, hi equidem communionis nostrae cum Christo mysterium, aut nondum intelligunt, aut, si intellectum negligunt, rei proculdubio fiunt corporis et sanguinis Christi in usu Sacramentorum, tum quod mysterium ipsorum non diiudicent, ut debent, tum quod mysticum Christi corpus, Ecclesiam inquam, incuria negligentiaque sua dedecorant, dum illud, laxatis omnis disciplinae habenis, variis flagitiorum generibus pollui contaminarique patiuntur': *K I*, 166.

27 Like Erasmus, Laski understands only a consensus about fundamental truths to be necessary. In the Eucharistic controversy he attempts to avoid being tied down to any one of the opposing views. His *Epitome doctrinae* of 1544, which was never published, consciously leaves open the main point of controversy, the question of Christ's presence in the eucharistic elements. See also Laski to A. Hardenberg, 30 September 1546: 'Ita ego pacem cum omnibus habeo, quantum in me est, quod quidem ad coenae dignitatem attinet, quandoquidem idem cum omnibus coenae mysterium agnosco, nempe communionem corporis et sanguinis Christi. Sed sunt quibus hoc non satisfaciat, hos ego permitto iudicare quod velint: interim illos pro fratribus habeo, si id patiantur. Certe do operam, ne a me quoquomodo laedantur' (*K II*, 609).

28 Laski to K. Pellikan, 31 August 1544: 'Ecclesiae vestrae de tanto doctrinae consensu gratulor. Caeremoniarum eandem formam non magnopere requiro, ne rursum ad novum aliquem Pharisaismum posteri nostri anxia caeremoniarum observatione delabantur. Quin potius concordem aliquam illarum varietatem retineri mallem, ut homines intelligant Religionem non caeremoniarum una atque eadem facie, sed studio pietatis constare. Ego hic nullas certas caeremoniarum leges praescribo, quas equidem pro temporum ratione mutari oportere semper puto. Illud tantum ago, ut abolita superstitione, et impietate Papistica, puras minimeque operosas caerimonias habeamus. Caenam alii stando, alii ad mensas accumbendo sumant, alii in azymo, alii in cibario pane, ut constet sua libertati ratio. Sed doctrinae consensum modis omnibus urgemus et de disciplina instituenda cogitamus.' (*K II*, 584). See also the fragment of a letter from Laski to an unknown recipient: *K II*, 765.

29 On Laski's attempts to bring about unity in the Church, see K. Eduard Jordt Jørgensen, *Ökumenische Bestrebungen unter den polnischen Protestanten bis zum Jahre 1645* (Copenhagen, 1942); Herwart Vorländer, 'Der ökumenische Grundzug im Denken und Wirken des Johannes a Lasco', in *ZKG* 80 (1969), 50–60; for the Erasmian heritage in these attempts, see the (admittedly not very analytical and apparently somewhat haphazard) comments in Oskar Bartel, 'Johannes a Lasco und Erasmus von Rotterdam', in *LuJ* 32 (1965), 48–66, 63–5. Later conflicts with followers of Luther did not show this irenical side of Laski's work. This is not a negation of the argument for Erasmus's influence, but suggests that Laski retreated from it in the course of developing his own theology.

30 Printed in Erasmus von Rotterdam, *Opera*, vol. 5, 469–506. The work is briefly summarized by Cornelis Augustijn, *Erasmus von Rotterdam. Leben–Werk–Wirkung. Aus dem Holländischen übersetzt. von Marga E. Baumer* (München, 1986), 159–61. In 1534, Wolfgang Capito published a German translation of this work under the title 'Von der Kirchen lieblicher Vereinigung' in Strasbourg. For its wide reception, especially by Reformation theologians such as Bucer, see Robert Stupperich, *Der Humanismus und die Wiedervereinigung der Konfessionen* (Leipzig, 1936) (*SVRG* 160), 27–52, especially 27–32.

31 'Libellus suus de ecclesiae concordia, postquam mihi perlatus est, tantum arrisit animo meo, ut numquam ab initio operis fuerim crediturus; utinam sint qui ipsius secuti consilium positis dissidiorum studiis ac moderata utriusque vehementi sane illa nimiaque fortassis pertinaci sua omnia terendi constantia id agant potiusque in hoc totis viribus incumbant, ut – postquam utrique negare non possumus nos non carere vitiis – utrique alter in alteris simus mitiores, alterius onera tanto facilius feramus quanto magis perspicuum est non deesse in utrisque. Quod summus ille nostrum omnium Nomothetes sit olim vehementer desideraturus, sistemur [. . .] illic omnes etiam [. . .] quorum partes erant luxata corporis mystici membra suis locis restituere potius quam resecare ac angularis illius lapidis calce divulsum hunc magna ex parte jam parietem connectere potius quam deturbare': Laski to Jodocus Decius, 5 June 1534, in Hermann Dalton (ed.), *Lasciana nebst den ältesten evangelischen Synodalprotokollen Polens 1555–1561* (Berlin, 1898, reprinted Nieuwkoop, 1973) (Beiträge zur Geschichte der evangelischen Kirche in Rußland 3), 175f.

32 'Colloquia nulla admittunt legitima, sed nos ad academias suas ablegant, haud aliter quam papistae Lutetiam Lovaniumve aut Coloniam provocare solent; denique ita rem gerunt ut mihi Lutheropapistica tribunalia instituere velle videantur, planeque ego videam, verum esse quod ab Erasmo olim Roterodamo pluries me audisse memini: nempe fore, si Lutherani isti rerum potiantur, ut multo graviorem sub illis quam sub plerisque papistis tyrannidem sustinere cogamur. Sed sic est mundi ingenium': Laski to J. Calvin, 13 March 1554, in Dalton, *Lasciana*, 336. See also the criticism of H. Bullinger for his strong language against Luther: Laski to H. Bullinger, 25 August 1545, in *K II*, 595.

33 'Ad tollendum doctrinae dissidium pacificandasque Ecclesias ita sum affectus et fui semper, ut nulli hac in parte sim cessurus, sed sic, ut veritas obtineat, non autem obscuretur aut dissimuletur quoquo modo in hominum gratiam': Laski to A. Hardenberg, 28 March 1554, in *K II*, 699). Laski's concern about the unity of the Church goes so far that he changes the classical definition of the *notae ecclesiae*. The third characteristic, besides faith and public confession, is 'age and uninterrupted existence': 'Huius porro Ecclesiae tres notas Spiritus Sanctus nobis indicavit, quibus ab aliis simulatis Ecclesiis discerni facile possit: vetustatem illius cum perpetua duratione, fidem eius praeterea, et publicam professionem' (*Londoner Katechismus* (1551), in *K II*, 296; and compare *K II*, 300).

34 For a summary of Calvin's, Melanchthon's and Laski's attempts at unity, see Wilhelm H. Neuser, 'Dogma und Bekenntnis der Reformation: von Zwingli und Calvin bis zur Synode von Westminster', in Carl Andresen (ed.), *Handbuch der Dogmen- und Theologiegeschichte*, vol. 2: *Die Lehrentwicklung im Rahmen der Konfessionalität* (Göttingen, 1980; Studienausg. 1988), 279–81.

35 See Jørgensen, *Ökumenische Bestrebungen*; Bartel, 242–89; George H. Williams, 'The Polish-Lithuanian Calvinism during the "Superintendency" of John Laski, 1556–1560', in Brian A. Gerrish (ed.), *Reformatio perennis: essays on Calvin and the Reformation in honor of Ford Lewis Battles* (Pittsburgh, PA, 1981), 129–58.

36 For the influence of the *Forma ac ratio* in England, see Rodgers, 79f.

4

Nicolas des Gallars and the Genevan connection of the stranger churches

Jeannine E. Olson

Although I started out as a student of Tudor and Stuart England, most of my scholarly research has been in Geneva, where I work in the archives of the 16th century when John Calvin and his successor, Theodore Beza, led a religious Reformation that spread throughout Europe to the British Isles. In this paper, though, I will bridge the distance between Geneva and England in the person especially of Nicolas des Gallars, pastor of Geneva, who came to London in 1560 to be pastor of the church for French refugees or the 'Strangers' Church'. I shall start with a few words about the origins of the stranger churches before considering des Gallars's role there in 1560–3.

The formation of the Strangers' Church

Foreigners had been residing in Britain for economic reasons long before the religious Reformation of the 16th century, but with the advent of the Reformation, the nature of the foreign community in England began to change as religious refugees, escaping persecution on the Continent of Europe, joined those who had come seeking economic opportunity. England became more attractive as a land of refuge upon the death of Henry VIII in 1547 and the accession of Edward VI. Once in England, the foreign communities desired churches of their own, with services in their own language, and soon congregations were forming even before ministers were called and churches were formally recognized. This was a typical pattern for Reformed churches (churches reformed on the Swiss model), many of which sprang up spontaneously on the Continent as well. First the congregation formed, and then the pastor was found.[1]

It was not a foregone conclusion that the strangers' wish for a church of their own in London would be fulfilled, however. There was opposition to an independent church with its own style of service and church organization in the middle of the capital. But as Henry VIII was dead, Thomas Cranmer, the Archbishop of Canterbury, was able to move ahead with his own projects. In 1548, when the Interim of Augsburg prohibited Protestant worship in the Empire, Cranmer invited Protestant leaders from Europe to England and allowed them to worship in Canterbury.[2] Pierre Alexandre arrived in 1548, for instance. He was an ex-Carmelite monk and had been preacher at the court of Mary of Hungary, sister of the Emperor Charles V and Governor of the Low Countries.[3] Cranmer procured for Alexandre a prebend at Canterbury, and Alexandre became one of Cranmer's principal secretaries.[4] Another of these Continental reformers who came to England was John à Lasco, a distinguished Polish noble and cleric, a convert to Protestantism and superintendent of the churches in the region of Emden in East Friesland.[5] He was a leading force behind government recognition of the Strangers' Church in England and stayed close to Cranmer at Lambeth in 1550.[6]

Even before John à Lasco arrived, the stranger community approached the government for the use of buildings for worship in the spring of 1550. Recorded in King Edward's journal on 29 June 1550 is the grant to the strangers of the church of the Augustinian (or Austin) friars in London, the largest friary church in England. The priory itself had been dissolved some 12 years previously. On 24 July a charter confirmed the recently-arrived Lasco as superintendent of the Strangers' Church and named the Church's first ministers.[7] The church of Austin Friars was intended for all strangers but ended up in the use of the Dutch alone, who agreed to share with the French congregation the rent and repairs for the former hospital of St Anthony in Threadneedle Street. Thus the Strangers' Church, though one in the original charter, consisted of two congregations: one Dutch-speaking and the other French-speaking.

Even before the Strangers' Church had possession of the buildings, it was organized on a Reformed or Genevan model, with supervisory elders and deacons for church finances and for the care of the poor. Once established in Austin Friars, the Dutch wrote a church order.[8] For the French congregation, two small 1552 liturgies in French have been discovered. There are few documents for these first few years of its existence.[9] Lasco's hope was that the Strangers' Church would be a model that the English Church could emulate, but soon that experiment was over. With the death of Edward in 1553 and the accession to the throne of his Catholic older sister, Mary, the French and Dutch Churches were shut. Mary's government encouraged the foreign theologians and ministers to leave the country. Many complied. On 17 September 1553 Lasco and 165 members of the Dutch and French congregations filled two ships to capacity and sailed for the Continent. Others escaped through other means, including Pierre Alexandre, secretary to Cranmer.[10] Other members of the stranger congregation remained in England and escaped the fires of Smithfield either because they conformed to the Church under Mary or because they were not noticed.

The restoration of the stranger churches under Elizabeth I

Upon the accession of Elizabeth I, Protestants moved back to England from abroad with hopes aroused for what the Church of England under her might become. Some of those who returned were the strangers, and they wanted the Strangers' Church to be reconstituted. Former church members tended to think, of course, in terms of what the Strangers' Church had been before, that is, a Church that was independent of outside control. This was not to be under Elizabeth. In high circles in England there was favour for a reborn Strangers' Church but less enthusiasm for its independent status. Perhaps John à Lasco's open criticism of practices in the Church of England while he was superintendent of the Strangers' Church from 1550–3 had turned powerful individuals against it, for he had found fault with the prescribed vestments, with the 1549 prayer book, and with the practice of kneeling to receive Communion, which was retained in the second prayer book of 1552.[11] Perhaps Elizabeth's desire to have a church which she clearly controlled, ruling through her bishops, made an independent church impossible under the new regime. At any rate, Jan Utenhove, a powerful elder from the earlier Dutch congregation, agitated for a reconstitution of the Strangers' Church. What he received was a Strangers' Church under the Bishop of London. Fortunately for the strangers, that bishop was to be Edmund Grindal.[12]

The reconstituted Strangers' Church was to be not one church but two: Dutch and French. In much the same manner as Jan Utenhove worked on behalf of the Dutch, Pierre Alexandre would work on behalf of the French congregation, and Bishop Grindal himself took an interest. In addition, William Cecil appeared to look favourably on the stranger churches, perhaps in large part, as Andrew Pettegree has suggested, because Cecil realized the advantages of welcoming foreigners, who had skills that the English did not have, to the English economy. Not only would this help with the balance of trade, as fewer luxury goods would have to be imported, but it would also foster domestic industry in England.[13]

Just as the Dutch got their church, so did the French. It is on that French congregation that this paper will focus. One of the first steps in reconstituting a church, of course, is organization. This the stranger churches did, on a Reformed model. For the French, the community could provide elders and deacons, but who would they have as a pastor? On 18 March 1560 elders and deacons in the French community wrote to John Calvin and his colleagues asking for a pastor from Geneva, even suggesting several men by name 'a Viret, a Théodore de Bèze, a Nicolas des Gallars, a Macar, a Colonges . . . '. The ministers and elders of the Dutch Church signed the letter, too, and Bishop Grindal himself added his own name and several sentences on behalf of the petition of the French Church for a pastor, adding a request for prayers for the state of 'our Churches not yet sufficiently constituted according to our desire', an interesting comment as Bishop Grindal may have been referring to the Church of England, 'not yet sufficiently constituted according to our desire', as well as to the stranger churches.[14]

Calvin and the Venerable Company of Pastors of Geneva, which consisted of all the pastors of the city and of the outlying towns under Genevan jurisdiction, were familiar with requests for pastors, as such requests had been coming in for several years. The years 1560–1, during which time this letter arrived, was a period during which, according to Robert M. Kingdon, the Calvinist Reformation was at its peak, not only in Geneva itself but in other countries. In France, for instance, Protestantism was spreading rapidly. Within Geneva, Calvin's career was at its height, the Libertines,[15] or Perrinist opposition, having been defeated half a decade before, in 1555, and a definitive edition of Calvin's *Institutes of the Christian Religion* just coming off the press.[16] As Reformed congregations formed in France and elsewhere, many looked to Geneva for a pastor. Geneva was coming to be viewed as the capital of French Protestantism and a source of personnel. But continuing to supply pastors was difficult for the Venerable Company.[17] The Geneva Academy had recently been formed, with Théodore Beza at its head, in 1559, essentially to train pastors; but there were still not enough adequately trained men available.[18]

It was a tribute to the importance of the post in London, that the Venerable Company, after some indecision and with the approval of the Genevan city council, chose a member of the Venerable Company of Pastors of Geneva and a close friend of Calvin, Nicolas des Gallars, to take up this London post:

> Friday, 3 May 1560. Spectable Nicolas des Gallars, minister, came to thank messieurs [the city councilors of Geneva] and said goodbye in order to go to England . . . being accompanied by two who came. . . . One prayed God to bless them on their voyage and, notably, to make prosper the churches there and . . . to serve to his glory and to our joy and consolation.[19]

Nicolas des Gallars, Seigneur de Saules, was probably from Paris or the surrounding area, although it has not been possible to find his baptismal records or extensive information on his family. The civil records of Paris burned in the 19th century and have been only partially reconstituted. There is almost nothing extant, but according to *La France Protestante*, des Gallars was born about 1520, was well educated, and came to Geneva c.1543–4 'to learn theology at the lessons of Calvin of whom all his life he was a faithful disciple'.[20] Des Gallars married in Geneva and started a large family.

Des Gallars was perhaps just over ten years younger than Calvin, who had been born in 1509, and I believe this played a role in their relationship. Although des Gallars became a pastor of Geneva, he also assisted Calvin with his publications, copying Calvin's lectures and readying them for publication. Des Gallars had publications of his own, too, but Emile Doumergue calls des Gallars a secretary of Calvin, for des Gallars was almost serving the role of a private Latin secretary to Calvin for a time.[21]

The age difference between the two men had other ramifications as well. If it is true that des Gallars was about 23 or 24 years old when he came to Geneva, it must have been shortly after he had completed his education – or perhaps he considered himself still in the process of being educated. It is important to what happened in England that almost all of Nicolas des Gallars's adult life up to the point at which he came to London was spent in Geneva under the tutelage of Calvin. When des Gallars arrived in London he had had almost no other experience than that of Geneva. He had been sent once to an outlying village in 1553 but was still a member of the Company of Pastors of Geneva as were the other outlying pastors. Des Gallars had also been sent to Paris in 1557, but he was too well known there to stay in safety, especially after the incident of the rue St Jacques, when Parisians who had gathered in a private home for Protestant services had been overheard singing Psalms and had been raided by the authorities. Des Gallars returned from Paris to Geneva in less than six months.[22]

Unlike some of Calvin's other friends from whom Calvin had become disaffected, des Gallars appears to have been a loyal and admiring disciple. The letter from Calvin in 1560 when he designated des Gallars as pastor of the Strangers' Church in London indicates that it may have been difficult to persuade des Gallars to leave Geneva and difficult for Calvin to part with him.[23] No doubt it was equally difficult for des Gallars to come. He was about 40 years of age when he uprooted himself, and he left his family behind in Geneva as did many of the missionary pastors sent out from Geneva. When he arrived in England in June 1560, he immediately had troubles to deal with, not the least of which was that during the time between the French Church's initial request for a Genevan pastor and des Gallars's arrival, Pierre Alexandre had increasingly taken the role of leader of and preacher to the French refugees, and was loath to give up this role. Alexandre even offered to serve the community without pay. There were members of the congregation who were sympathetic to Alexandre. It was with the backing of Bishop Grindal that Nicolas des Gallars was able to persevere and to assume leadership of the community, but it is noteworthy that Grindal refused to allow an election to let the congregation decide between the two men.[24] During this time, des Gallars corresponded in Latin with Calvin, expressing anxieties about the situation. Calvin encouraged des Gallars and kept him informed of news on des Gallars's wife and children.

Some have claimed that des Gallars managed the French congregation with excessive strictness or even intolerance. This is reflected, for instance, in his attitude toward the French who had stayed in London during the reign of Queen Mary and had compromised their beliefs. It was not until December 1560 that the church order was written, the elders and deacons chosen, and the first Communion celebrated, in part because all those who had attended Catholic ceremonies under Mary had had to recant and repent individually of what they had done.[25]

Des Gallars may well have been strict on this point, but he would not have viewed himself as overly severe, for des Gallars had just come from a city and a mentor, John Calvin, who condemned Nicodemism, that is, camouflaging one's Reformed convictions for the sake of expediency by participating in Roman Catholic religious practices, just as Nicodemus in the New Testament had come to Jesus at night under the cover of darkness so as not to be seen (John 3:1–21).[26] In des Gallars's eyes, the French who had remained in England under Mary and conformed to her Church were in need of repentance and reacceptance before being allowed to participate in the Lord's Supper. It should be no surprise, given des Gallars's Genevan background, that the new church order he composed for the French strangers in London, and his own attitudes, reflected the views of the Genevan Church toward discipline and Nicodemism.

Fortunately for our pursuit of information on the minister, these first few years of the French Church's existence after it was reconstituted under Queen Elizabeth I are well-documented. There is not only the church order of the French Church itself, published by John Day,[27] and the correspondence between Calvin and des Gallars, already mentioned, but the letters of Bishop Grindal and of Nicolas Throckmorton, English ambassador to France, who corresponded with des Gallars and with others about des Gallars when the Genevan minister became a delegate to the 1561 Colloquy of Poissy.[28]

Des Gallars received an invitation to the important Colloquy of Poissy, which was held in the summer of 1561 outside Paris in an attempt to reconcile Catholics and Protestants and to avoid war in France, then under the rule of Catherine de Medici, regent for her son Charles IX, and under the chancellorship of Michel de l'Hôpital, who was conciliatory towards the Huguenots. The English took such an interest in the Colloquy at Poissy that des Gallars's account of it was translated into English and published in London.[29] Unfortunately for his wife and children, who had come to England in 1561, des Gallars left them for the Colloquy in France for several months.

As for other records, besides his correspondence with Calvin, for the period of des Gallars's ministry in London (1560–3), we have the minutes of the consistory of the French Church. These minutes were published by the Huguenot Society of London in 1937,[30] approximately sixty years before the first minutes of the consistory of the Church of Geneva were published in 1996.[31] This is a phenomenal accomplishment for the Huguenot Society of London, although some of the credit must go to an elder in the French Church of London, Anthoine Poncel or Antoine du Ponchel, the consistory scribe, to whose legible handwriting we owe part of the credit for the early publication of the consistory registers of London.

These minutes reveal a consistory that resembles that of Geneva in many respects, but which was, of necessity, different. The consistory of Geneva was composed of all of the pastors of Geneva, whose numbers during the peak of Calvin's career almost equalled the 12 members called elders who were selected from Geneva's governing councils.[32] The consistory of the French Church of London, in contrast, was composed of the church's pastor or pastors and of elders elected from the congregation itself. There was no governmental representation on the French Church consistory. Sometimes the deacons from the congregation, in charge of congregational poor relief, were invited to attend.

The consistory of Geneva, founded by the Genevan Ecclesiastical Ordinances of 1541,[33] functioned like a church court, sitting weekly to hear breaches in conduct by church members. The consistory of the French Church of London also had the function of governing church members' conduct, but, in addition, the consistory also had to run the church itself. In Geneva, financial decisions about the church were in the hands of the Genevan city council and the pastors were paid by the city, but in London, it was the consistory and the deacons who controlled the pastor's salary. It was the consistory, for instance, that agreed to make it possible for des Gallars's wife and several of their small children to join him in London in January 1561.[34]

Other than these structural differences, the atmosphere and underlying attitude of the consistory of the French Church of London is similar to that of the consistory of Geneva. There was the same practice of summoning people before the assembled pastors and elders and there admonishing them for their infractions of the Ten Commandments, or simply for their inability to get along with each other. The consistory of London, as well as that of Geneva, consulted witnesses, elicited confessions from people, demanded contrition, and admitted or rejected people from the Lord's Supper.

Des Gallars was willing to accept other previous practices of the early Strangers' Church, but the 'discipline' was central to des Gallars's view of the church, and by that he meant 'discipline' similar to that of Geneva, for that is what he had known. By 'discipline' the Reformed tradition meant both the way in which a church was organized, that is, its 'discipline' or church order, and the church's attempt to insist that members adhere as much as possible to the Ten Commandments. Thus Reformed church consistories inquired into marital irregularities, blasphemy, lack of attendance at services, scandalous dress or behaviour (such as dancing), mistreatment of servants by masters, dissent in marriages and among friends, broken financial commitments, and quarrelling. Each member of the congregation was supposed to be reconciled with all the others before he or she could partake of the Lord's Supper, and contrition, often insisted upon, was open and verbal, either before the consistory itself or before the congregation as a whole. The consistory controlled who could go to Communion, and who was to be barred. Anyone who has read early modern Reformed consistory minutes cannot help but be impressed by the Reformed churches' insistence on proper human conduct and responsibility towards one's peers, compared to the flabbiness of church discipline today.

Now all this is not new to the French Church under des Gallars. In the early 1550s in the Strangers' Church under John à Lasco, discipline and a structure of church government with pastors, elders, and deacons existed. These offices are a part of the Reformed tradition, but some would say that the discipline under des Gallars and his successors was stricter than it had been before. Some would say the discipline was stricter because of the influence of Geneva, or, one is tempted to say, because of the influence of Geneva as it was transmitted by des Gallars as the leader of the French Church of London.

When we look at Geneva in the 1560s, the discipline of the church and of the city was evolving over the years and in some ways was becoming stricter – although when one is discussing the regulation of human behaviour, there are always frustrations and limitations to what one can do. For instance, in Geneva by the 1560s adulterers were no longer merely jailed, banished, or admonished for their misconduct. If a man and woman were married to other partners and had sexual intercourse with each other they were both to be put to death. However, if the woman was married and the man was not married, only she was to be put to death, unless the man was a servant, in which case, he was to be put to death, too. But if only the man was married and the woman was not married, they both got off with only being imprisoned on bread and water for twelve days.[35] Despite the double standard, the penalties were becoming harsher for adultery in Geneva for both sexes. Discipline is characteristic of these early Reformed communities, and stricter discipline in the 1560s was perhaps in step with the times and with the nature of institutions in general, which tend to solidify and to become more structured over time.

Des Gallars stayed only three years in London. He claimed that the weather of England was bad for him and Grindal seconded this view in a letter to Calvin. But there might have been other factors involved in his desire to leave England, such as better opportunities abroad or difficulties with the English language, about which matter we read nothing in des Gallars's correspondence. In addition, des Gallars's wife and several of his children died while in England.[36] After des Gallars' departure in June 1563, the French Church of London continued to favour pastors with connections to him or to Geneva, and he maintained some contact with the church and England. For instance, des Gallars dedicated his 1569 commentary on the church father, Irenaeus, to Bishop Grindal.[37]

In 1563 des Gallars went back to the Continent, to Geneva, first, and then on to Orléans, headquarters of the Protestant cause during the first War of Religion in France. There des Gallars served as pastor and professor in the newly constituted Reformed faculty of theology until he and the other Reformed pastors fled Orléans in 1568. He considered escaping to England, but after stopping at the French estate of Renée of France, he retired to Geneva until he was called in 1571 by Jeanne d'Albret, Queen of Navarre, to her court in Navarre, which straddles the Pyrenees between France and Spain. He remarried there in the city Pau, for his contract of marriage with Françoise de Contades is dated 7 March 1572.[38] He was professor at the Reformed Academy in Lescar, and he died shortly before 14 August 1581, as evidenced by a receipt of that date to Daniel des Gallars, his son and heir, settling Nicolas des Gallars's will.[39] That receipt and the marriage contract were discovered in October 1999 when

I was doing research in Pau. They are important because historians had long been somewhat uncertain about Nicolas des Gallars's date of death. With these discoveries we need be uncertain no more.

NOTES

1 For information on the foreign community in England prior to the foundation of the Strangers' Church see Andrew Pettegree, *Foreign Protestant communities in 16th-century London* (Oxford, 1986), 9–25.

2 Francis Cross, *History of the Walloon and Huguenot Church at Canterbury*, HSQS 15, 3–5.

3 The footnotes to Nicolas des Gallars's 7 March 1563 letter to John Calvin in the Sarrau collection are an excellent concise source on Pierre Alexandre: *Les lettres à Jean Calvin de la collection Sarrau*, ed. Rodolphe Peter and Jean Rott (Paris, 1972), 82 n9–84 n11.

4 *Ibid.*, 83; Diarmaid MacCulloch, *Thomas Cranmer: a life* (New Haven, 1996), 395.

5 For material on John à Lasco in English see Basil Hall, *John à Lasco, 1499–1560: a Pole in Reformation England* (London, 1971) and *The Oxford Encyclopedia of the Reformation*, 'Laski, Jan'. Note that *The Oxford Encyclopedia* mentions only the one visit of John à Lasco to England, that of 1548, and gives the impression that his appointment as superintendent of the Strangers' Church was earlier than 1550, whereas John à Lasco left England early in 1549 and went back to his position in Emden. He then returned to England in May 1550 when Emden could no longer resist the imposition of the Interim. Pettegree, 30–31.

6 Pettegree, 31.

7 For the charter see J. Lindeboom, *Austin Friars: history of the Dutch Reformed Church in London, 1550–1950* (The Hague, 1950), 198–203.

8 The church order was completed in 1551 but not published until 1554 after the dissolution of the church. Martin Micron, *De christlicke ordinancien* (Emden, 1554) [*STC* 16571a]. In January 1551 the church's confession of faith was published, the *Compendium doctrinae de vera unicaque Dei et Christi ecclesia* (London, 1551) [*STC* 15263], also in *Joannis a Lasco opera tam edita quam inedita*, ed. A. Kuyper (Amsterdam, 1866), vol. 2, 285–339. Lasco's longer explanation of the customs and liturgy of the church was not published until 1555, the *Forma ac ratio tota ecclesiastici minsterii, in peregrinorum, potissimum vero Germanorum ecclesia: instituta Londini* (Frankfurt, 1555). [*STC* 16571], also in *Lasco opera*, vol. 2, 1–283. A year later a French translation was published at Emden, *Toute la forme et maniere du ministere ecclesiastique en l'eglise des estrangers, dressée a Londres* (Emden, 1556) [*STC* 16574.]

9 *La forme des prieres ecclesiastiques. Avec la maniere d'administrer les sacramens* (London, 1552) [*STC* 16572.3]; *Doctrine de la penitence publique* (London, 1552) [*STC* 16572.7].

10 Andrew Pettegree, 'The stranger community in Marian London', in *Marian Protestantism: six studies* (Aldershot, 1996), 41–5.

11 Pettegree, *Foreign Protestant communities*, 40–43, 74–6.

12 Fernand de Schickler, *Les Eglises du refuge en Angleterre* (Paris, 1892), vol. 1, 84–5.

13 Pettegree, *Foreign Protestant communities*, 139.

14 Grindal's sentence reads: 'Nostrarum ecclesiarum statum nondum satis ex animi nostri sententia constitutarum tuis et caeterorum fratrum precibus commendo': Letter 3170, 'Ecclesia Belgica Londinensis Calvino et Collegis', in *Joannis Calvini opera quae supersunt omnia*, eds. Gulielmus Baum, Eduardus Cunitz, Eduardus Reuss [hereafter *CO*], vol. 17 (Brunswick, 1877), cols. 29–32. In French, Grindal's comment reads: 'Je recommande à vos prières et à celles de tous les autres frères l'état de nos Eglises, non encore suffisamment constituées selon notre gré'. There is a French translation of this letter in the appendix of

de Schickler, *Les Eglises du refuge*, vol. 3, 44–7 ('No. IX. Lettre de l'Eglise française de Londres à celle de Genève. L'Eglise française de Londres à Calvin et à ses collègues, les très fidèles pasteurs de l'Eglise de Genève').

15 *Encyclopedia of the Reformation*, Jeannine Olson, 'Libertines'.

16 Robert M. Kingdon, *Adultery and divorce in Calvin's Geneva* (Cambridge, MA, 1995), 118–19.

17 For the story of the dispatching of pastors from Geneva to serve churches in France see Robert M. Kingdon, *Geneva and the coming of the Wars of Religion in France, 1555–1563* (Geneva, 1970).

18 *Encyclopedia of the Reformation*, Jeannine Olson, 'Geneva Academy'.

19 Archives d'Etat de Genève [hereafter AEG], Reg. Con., vol. 56, 1560–2, fo. 35: 'Vendredi 3 de May 1560 en Conseil . . . [in margin] Spectable Nicolas des Galars ministre est venu remercier messieurs et prendre conge pour sen allee en angleterre . . . . estant accompagne de deux qui le sont venu . . . son a pris dieu les benir en leur voiage et notamment de faire prosperer les eglises de par de la et . . . servir a sa gloire et a notre joie et consolation.

20 'Des Gallars . . . s'être rendu de bonne heure à Genève pour apprendre la théologie aux leçons de Calvin dont il fut toute sa vie un disciple fidèle': Eugène and Emile Haag, *La France Protestante* (2nd edn., Paris, 1886), 'Des Gallars (Nicolas)'. There is an earlier article on des Gallars in the first edition of E. and E. Haag, *La France Protestante ou vies des Protestants français* (1st edn., Paris, 1852), 'Des Gallars (Nicolas)'.

21 Emile Doumergue, *Jean Calvin: les hommes et les choses de son temps*, vol. 3: *La ville, la maison et la rue de Calvin* (Geneva, 1969, reprint of original published Lausanne, 1899–1927), 597–605.

22 Peter and Rott, *Les lettres à Jean Calvin*, 81 n1.

23 *CO*, vol. 18, letter 3201, 'Calvinus Ecclesiae Flandricae Londinensi', col. 90. There is an English translation of this letter 'To the Bishop of London' in *Letters of John Calvin selected from the Bonnet Edition with an introductory biographical sketch* (Aylesbury, 1980), 226–8.

24 Pettegree, *Foreign Protestant communities*, 151–4.

25 *Ibid.*, 125, 155.

26 *Encyclopedia of the Reformation*, 'Nicodemism'.

27 Nicolas des Gallars, *Forma politae ecclesiasticae, nuper institutae Londini in coetu Gallorum* (London, 1561). [*STC* 6774.5].

28 On Throckmorton, see A. L. Rowse, *Ralegh and the Throckmortons* (London, 1962).

29 Nicolas des Gallars, *A True Report of All the Doynges at the Assembly Concernyng Matters of Religion, Lately Holden at Poyssy in Fraunce. Written in Latine by Mayster Nicolas Gallasius, Minister of the Frenche Churche in London, and Then Present, One of the Disputers in the Same, Translated into English, by J. D., 1561* (London, 1561) [*STC* 6776]

30 HSQS 38.

31 *Registres du consistoire de Genève au temps de Calvin*, vol. 1: *1542–1544*, eds. Thomas Lambert and Isabella Watt (Geneva, 1996).

32 Kingdon, *Adultery and divorce*, 14.

33 'Ordonnances ecclésiastiques', in *Registres de la Compagnie des Pasteurs de Genève au temps de Calvin*, vol. 1: *1546–1553*, ed. Jean-François Bergier (Geneva, 1964), 6–7, 11–13. For an English translation see 'Draft Ecclesiastical Ordinances', in *Calvin: theological treatises*, ed. J. K. S. Reid (Philadelphia, 1954), 58–72.

34 On 9 January 1561, Nicolas des Gallars, brought the subject up with the consistory of the French Church in London: 'Ledyt Jour monsieur de solle proposoit touchant pour faire venire sa femme scavoir sy la debvoit faire venire par france ou par lalemaigne et pria la compagnie de y aviser lequel chemin seroit le plus comodde et plus expedient'. 'Mardy 21 dudyt au Consistoire, monsieur de Solles proposy present les diacres pour avoir conseil par

quel chemin il pourroit faire venire sa femme, scavoir est par la france ou par Lalemaigne, et quel moyen pour Lamener sur quoy Ladvis des freres fut de la faire venire par la france estoit le plus court et le plus expedient et le meilleur marchiet, et pour brief expedition fut arreste dy envoier dycy homme expres pour la conduire surquoy nicolas binet nostre diacre se presenty de faire la paine volentiers, sy on le trouvoit suffisant pour cela, . . . en le Remercyant grandement de telle offre sy liberale le priant que il se prepary de se metre a chemin dycy a xv jours ou trois sepmaines sy luy est posible et que sil troeuve bon daller a cheval leglise luy permet dachapter quelque petit cheval pour faire ledyt voiage' The deacon Nicolas Binet was given twenty-four ecus for the trip. HSQS 38, 24, 26, 31.

35   Only in 1566, two years after John Calvin's death, did Geneva have an official law that punished adultery with death. However, already by 1560–1 there were several cases of adultery punished with death in Geneva. Kingdon, *Adultery and divorce*, 116–18.

36   *CO*, vol. 20, letter 3969, 'Grindallus Calvino', London, June 1563, cols. 43–5.

37   See the letter of six pages from Nicolas des Gallars to Edmund Grindal ending with 'Genevae pridi Cal. Februarii, M. D. LXIX' in *Divi Irenaei, Graeci scriptoris eruditissimi, Episcopi Lugdunensis, libri quinque adversus portentosas haereses Valentini & aliorum, accuratius quàm antehae emendati, additis Graecis quae reperiri petuerunt: opera & diligentia Nicolai Gallasii, S. Theologiae professoris: una cum eiusdem annotationibus* (Geneva?, 1570).

38   Archives Départementales des Basses-Pyrénées, Registre E. 2001, 1570–73, fos. 274v-5v: 7 March 1572, contract of marriage between Nicolas des Gallars, minister, and Françoise de Contades.

39   Archives Départementales des Basses-Pyrénées, Registre E. 2003, 1579–81, fos. 353v-4: 14 August 1581, 'Quittance de 200 écus par Jean de Chorinit, capitaine de la garde de Catherine de Navarre, à Daniel Des Galas, fils and héritier de de Saulle, ministre, pour legs fait par ce dernier'.

5

Acontius's plea for tolerance

AART DE GROOT

Shortly after his arrival in England, the Italian stranger Jacopo Aconcio (Jacobus Acontius), an engineer and writer, became a naturalized resident of 16th-century London.[1] In 1559, after a precarious life, the hunted exile – 'propter evangelicae veritatis professionem extorris' – had finally found a safe haven in England, where he spent the rest of his years. Almost nothing is known about his youth and his education. Born in Trent around 1500, he had grown to become a real 'Renaissance man' and had obtained high positions in the service of some Italian prelates. After his conversion to the Protestant faith he had fled to Switzerland in 1557, where he came in contact with the most influential leaders of the so-called Radical Reformation. But within two years he had crossed the Channel. In England, Acontius's technical abilities and skill had received due appreciation. On 27 February 1560 the Queen granted him an annuity of £60 and on 8 October 1561 he was granted naturalization.[2]

Appreciated and accepted as an engineer, Acontius remained an outsider in his religious and theological opinions, and he frequented the Dutch Church in Austin Friars.[3] At that time, this community was divided into two parties, for and against its minister Adriaen van Haemstede.[4] The discord was caused by Haemstede's unorthodox thought and his behaviour towards a group of Anabaptist refugees, whom he refused to condemn as dangerous heretics. Because of his friendly overtures to those Anabaptists, Haemstede was thought to endanger the reputation of the community. In the end he had to leave the fray and was excommunicated on 17 November 1560, and again in August 1562.[5] Acontius still gave his friend unqualified support, even after Haemstede's banishment. Twice he wrote to the Bishop of London, Edmund Grindal, the Superintendent of the Dutch Church and other refugee churches, in order to pursue the *status quaestionis* and to defend Haemstede's position. His letters had no success: Acontius himself was also condemned. Disappointed, he applied for membership of the Italian Church. He died around 1567.

It is not because of his career as an engineer that Acontius earned a reputation in Europe in his own day and afterwards. It was his book *De Stratagematis Satanae libri octo*, edited in Basel in 1565, that established his fame.[6] The book – immediately translated into French, and later also into other European languages – was a passionate appeal for tolerance within the Church and outside it. Its title occurs in every work about the history of tolerance and ecumenism, and it is this book, *The Stratagems of*

Satan, to which I would like to call your attention on this occasion, for it was in the divided congregation of the Dutch Church at Austin Friars, in whose building our conference is being held, that Acontius found his motivation to write about Satan's stratagems.

In neither the book's preface nor its eight chapters are the names of Haemstede or other *dramatis personae* in the conflict of the Dutch Church mentioned. Acontius preferred writing in a general way to expressing himself in concrete terms.[7] Anybody who tries to imagine the situations described in the book will be confronted with events and scenes which were typical of 16th-century Europe: everywhere people are engaged in furious discussions about questions concerning Christian faith and ethics; there are rumours, trickery and complicated manoeuvres; prelates and kings are invested with authority over life and death; cocksure theologians impose their own interpretations of the Bible upon laymen; church members are frequently excommunicated; there is a constant danger that spiritual life will be overruled by selfishness and that the power of empty traditions will be unmasked. Yet unmistakably some elements of the description point to the specific conditions of the Dutch exile community.[8]

In commenting on Acontius's book, one might be inclined to leave aside all those details of an all-too-human tragedy and to concentrate instead on its main themes: tolerance for the heretic, unity of the churches, open-mindedness in listening to God's voice. But in taking this approach, it would appear to us as if Acontius had been composing a sort of manual for tolerance. According to Jordan's wording, 'his treatise was cool, calm, detached and philosophical'.[9]

In my view, however, *Satan's Stratagems* is a loose composition. Its chapters are full of repetitions and Acontius's remarks about Satan's strategy and stratagems are spread out over the different chapters. The author himself had to admit his short-comings in style and the inadequacy of his arguments, which he ascribed to lack of time.[10] But more importantly, Acontius was in no way 'detached and philosophical' in his writing. He was reacting to specific events, and first of all, his book is meant as a charge against the misuse of power by people of authority and reputation, especially in the church.[11]

In his recently published essay about the historiography of tolerance, H. A. Oberman argued that we should not stick to 'the grand saga of tolerance with its traditional stages marked by Erasmus, Castellio and Locke', but 'replace a timeless, immutable and therefore ahistorical principle of rationality with actual historical situations and specific events'.[12] It is one of the merits of Jelsma's biography of Haemstede to put the origins of *The Stratagems of Satan* in its historical context, namely the trial against Haemstede.[13] Many pages of the proceedings of the consistory of the Dutch Church in London are devoted to the so-called 'causa Haemstedii'.[14] I will not go into the further details of this moving story, which is indeed a well-known chapter in the history of the Dutch Church. Yet, following in Jelsma's tracks, I would like to place the book of Acontius even more firmly within the framework of the London exile churches of those days. Therefore we need to analyse the text precisely.

Observing the madness of the world on his wanderings in Italy, Switzerland and France, Acontius was extremely concerned about the constant deterioration of Christian brotherhood. His conviction was that it was Satan himself who was trying to defend his throne against God's Kingdom and to catch men and women in his snares. He felt compelled to study all those sad and alarming developments more thoroughly. Now the tragic 'causa Haemstedii' appeared to him to be the culmination and crystallization point of Satan's stratagems, recapitulating all his experiences under one theme.

We know that in the 16th century it was still common belief that Satan was the cause of every evil.[15] Satan really existed in Acontius's view.[16] His book confronts us with Satan's stratagems[17] in the world as well as in our own heart, within the Church and outside it.[18] The writer unfolds a remarkable psychological insight in depicting the various instruments Satan produces to reach his goals.[19] The question confronts us: How to resist?

Not only do we need a firm belief in God, in Christ's redemption, we must also be prepared to obey God's Spirit. 'Put on the whole armour of God' (Ephesians 6) is not only the theme of the concluding chapter, but of many passages throughout the book. In writing so, Acontius is addressing himself to the individual reader. God's Spirit speaks to us individually. The Christian, who believes that God's Word is sealed in Holy Scripture – 'divina oracula quae sacris sunt literis consignata' (Koehler, 55:24) – has to listen to the voice of God, who is still speaking to his children in our own day: 'Consulendus est optimus magister spiritus' (Koehler, 178:8). It is a remarkable spiritualistic feature of the book, which did not please all its readers.[20] In Acontius's opinion the willingness to hear the voice of the living God precedes Bible reading.[21]

It was this belief that may have led Acontius, the newly arrived Italian refugee, who presumably did not even understand Dutch, to the Dutch Church of London. For this church had the so-called 'prophecy', an unique institution in the Protestant world of the 16th century.[22] We learn about this particular institution through the instructions John a Lasco formulated in his church order for the stranger communities (1555).[23] Once a week a meeting had to be held in order to give the church members the opportunity to put questions to their ministers, especially concerning the sermons. It was agreed that a committee composed of members of the consistory and other respected members of the congregation should first approve the questions, so that the talks could be kept within bounds, without Satan's interference.[24] The proceedings of the Dutch consistory offer us an insight not only into how questions could be put, but also how new questions arose, caused by prophecies which were given by its members.[25] Let us look at an example.

Without doubt, Acontius had witnessed the notorious Justus Velsius proclaim his eccentric ideas about justification and utter his criticism on the Reformed sermons during one of these prophecy gatherings. Immediately afterwards it was agreed that everything necessary should be done in order to avoid a repeat of such a scandal in the city.[26]

New conflicts arose after the installation of Godfried van Wingen, the successor to Haemstede, mainly because of his ideas concerning baptism and godparents. Again Bishop Grindal was asked to intervene in the matter. In September 1564 Grindal and other ecclesiastical authorities issued a decree underwriting the authority of the minister and elders and their order relating to baptism, a sort of *formula pacificationis*. The peace, however, did not last very long. The main point of the discussions was the authority that should be given to the consistory.[27]

The 'prophecies', a sensational experiment to activate the layman's participation in the spiritual policy of the whole congregation, were ended on 8 February 1571 — partly because of the 'many unedifying proposals and questions' they produced and partly because the sessions brought more 'devastation and discord' than 'godly lessons'.[28]

We can understand that important factors in the failure of the 'prophecies' were psychological ones, like the tensions that already existed between ministry and laity throughout the Reformed churches. Furthermore, the heavy emphasis on the Bible as the sole source of revelation did not further speaking freely. Besides that, there was the threat of Anabaptist and other sectarian groups infiltrating the sessions. Nevertheless, Acontius himself was deeply convinced that the New Testament prescripts on prophecy in the church assembly (1 Corinthians xiv, 1 Thessalonians v) were to be followed for the present, as in the Apostolic age.[29]

Many passages in *The Stratagems of Satan* dealing with the rules of good debate and discussion seem to indicate that the author himself liked a good debate. Most likely he had wished to participate in prophesying too. I do not know whether he made a sharp distinction between prophecy and discussion in general, but I am sure that Acontius was accustomed to putting questions to the ministry, penetrating questions without doubt, at every opportunity.

At the very least Acontius was convinced that the theologians felt they had a monopoly of wisdom. The unwillingness of the Dutch consistory to make concessions in the Haemstede cause, not to mention the inflexibility with which the Bishop handled it, made Acontius very sensitive about the layman's participation in church affairs (Koehler, 101:10–103:39).

On one occasion Acontius became very angry – as may be seen at a particular point in *The Stratagems of Satan* – about a clergyman who claimed, with an air of arrogance, that the parishioners could not have said one intelligent word about the Gospel without learning it first from the clergy (Koehler, 130:5ff., 19ff.). Ministers had obviously become little popes. They were the ones who decreed the doctrine.

Acontius made a considerable effort to put forward a better procedure for the prophecy-gatherings. A large problem arose when somebody would be allowed to speak as a prophet or to reveal a heaven-sent message, only to have an equally inspired church member set forth a conflicting prophecy. A similar problem arose concerning the various confessions of faith, all of which claimed obligatory force. In the Protestant churches there were already too many conflicts and consequently the many confessions of faith in the Protestant world do not do any good, Acontius argued (Koehler, 180:6–14).[30] Afraid as he was of endless disputes and mutual hatred – in all that discord Satan is on the look-out, even in London itself! – Acontius constantly repeated his message: let us together look for mutual love and unity. What really matters is a common understanding of the main points of our faith. Acontius then offered a practical proposal to restrain the confusion and quarrels: let us agree to stop discussing fundamental Christian truths, and at the same time let us leave each other free to disagree in all other points. So in Book 7 of *The Stratagems* he summed up the main points of his 'confession', a very short statement, later known as the *Symbolum Acontianum* (Koehler, 186:35–187:35), in order to oppose Satan's efforts to spread discord between the Christians in their churches as well as in their prophecy meetings (Koehler, 183:24; 189:35ff.). His proposal for the short *symbolum* has been typically placed at the centre of his treatment of prophecy.

In the following centuries, this text assumed a life of its own. Some treat it as a precursor of a rationalistic minimum programme of Christian tenets, as propagated in the era of the Enlightenment.[31] Acontius in effect designed a sort of *Wesen des Christentums*, according to others.[32]

Certainly, the clear and rational way in which Acontius deduced the main themes of Christian faith did make a profound impression on his many readers. But should we, with Collinson, circumscribe Acontius's method: 'Reason in its free interpretation of the Scripture is the sole judge'?[33] In my opinion, here 'reason' (*ratio*) acquires the meaning given to it by the rationalistic philosophers of the following century, indicating the instrument of human knowledge. In *The Stratagems of Satan*, however, *ratio* primarily means 'a way of arguing or debating' (e.g. Koehler, 10:23ff.; 17:20ff.).[34] The first English translation (1651) has 'reasons' for '*ratio*'. O'Malley (1940) translates it as 'reasoning' and that is in accordance with the purpose of the book as a whole.

A clever and trained debater, as Acontius was, – his letter to Bishop Grindal is a fine example of his style[35] – he did not, on the other hand, like it when he was silenced. He felt he should not be troubled with such trivialities. The rules of debate are to be formulated lucidly and carefully, but in no way narrow-mindedly. Mutual trust and confidence is of primary importance. The purpose of every discussion must be to edify the church in love to the honour of God. One should not annoy the church by repeating the same questions ('perpetuo obtundere', Koehler, 192:17ff.).

This brings me to the much discussed question, whether or not Acontius was an anti-Trinitarian. His orthodoxy was disputed from the very beginning.[36] Rather surprisingly, some modern historians even call upon the verdict of 17th-century Calvinists to find in favour of Acontius's heresy.[37] Acontius himself never said one word that could justify such accusations. That is indeed only to be expected, for he knew, what the consequences would be. In view of the rules we find in his book on Satan's stratagems, the main reason for his silence about this most controversial topic must have been his fear of provoking discord. Under the circumstances of those days one could not expect a meaningful, objective exchange of ideas. At least that was Acontius's conviction on the basis of his experiences within the exile churches in London. Anti-trinitarian or not, Acontius's spirit was free from dogmatism, and independent of ecclesiastical authority.

To sum up, Acontius's book on the stratagems of Satan may be called a plea for tolerance. At the same time and even more purposefully, it is a protest against all oppression and an attempt to win for the Christian a place of personal freedom against church tyranny.

NOTES

1   For his life and writings see the bibliography in A. Gordon Kinder, *Alumbrados of the kingdom of Toledo* (Baden Baden, 1994), 55–117; W. K. Jordan, *The development of religious toleration in England from the beginning of the English Reformation to the death of Queen Elizabeth* (London, 1932), 304–17.

2   HSQS 8.

3   About the history of the Dutch Church in London in the 16th century: J. Lindeboom, *Austin Friars* (The Hague, 1950); Andrew Pettegree, *Foreign Protestant communities in sixteenth-century London* (Oxford, 1986); Owe Boersma, *Vluchtig voorbeeld: de Nederlandse, Franse en Italiaanse vluchtelingenkerken in Londen, 1568–1585* (Kampen, 1994).

4   A. J. Jelsma, *Adriaan van Haemstede en zijn Martelaarsboek* (The Hague, 1970).

5   Patrick Collinson, *Archbishop Grindal 1519–1583: the struggle for a Reformed Church* (London, 1979), 136ff.

6   I refer to the edition of W. Koehler: Jacobus Acontius, *Satanae Stratagematum libri octo*, ed. Walter Koehler (Munich, 1927) [hereafter Koehler in the notes and text]. The Latin text has also been edited by G. Radetti: Giacomo Aconcio, *Stratagematum Satanae libri VIII*, ed. Giorgio Radetti, Edizione nazionale dei classici delpensiero italiano, 7 (Florence, 1946).

7   Nominibus peperci, res ipsas tantum, in quibus latere laqueos intelligerem, persequutus sum (Koehler, Praefatio, 2:16–18).

8   See the very realistic painting of the closed character of the exile community, full of suspicion and backbiting in Koehler, 113. See also Ole Peter Grell, 'Exile and Tolerance', in Ole Peter Grell (ed.), *Tolerance and intolerance in the European Reformation* (Cambridge, 1996), 164–81.

9   Jordan, 363.

10 'Quasi abortum' (Koehler, Praefatio, 4).

11 Koehler, Praefatio, 2:7–14. See also E. R. Briggs, 'An apostle of the incomplete Reformation: Jacopo Aconcio (1500–1567)', *HSP* 22 (1970– 6), 488ff.

12 Heiko A. Oberman, 'The travail of tolerance: containing chaos in early modern Europe' in Grell (ed.), *Tolerance and intolerance*, 29, 17.

13 Jelsma, *Adriaan van Haemstede*, esp. 206–28; see also C. D. O'Malley, *Jacopo Acontio*, Uomini e Dottrine 2 (Rome, 1955), 56–65.

14 A. A. van Schelven (ed.), *Kerkeraads-protocollen der Nederduitsche vluchtelingen-kerk te Londen 1560–1563*, Werken uitgegeven door het Historisch Genootschap III/43 (Amsterdam, 1921), 445–66.

15 Jeffrey Burton Russell, *Mephistopheles: the Devil in the modern world* (Ithaca, 1986), 30; Auke Jelsma, 'The Devil and Protestantism' in Auke Jelsma, *Frontiers of the Reformation: dissidence and orthodoxy in sixteenth-century Europe* (Aldershot, 1998), 25–39.

16 The only place where Russell refers to Acontius is in his discussion of growing scepticism about the existence of the Devil, without giving any evidence for his claim that Acontius doubted the reality of the Devil.

17 The Greek word *stratagema* ('stratagem', 'trick', 'ruse') does not occur in the Greek New Testament. The classical story of Satan's ultimate 'stratagem' is in Genesis iii.

18 Typical of the atmosphere in the London stranger churches are the letters and writings of their Superintendent John a Lasco, who often hints at Satan's activities: Joannes a Lasco, *Opera tam edita quam inedita*, ed. A. Kuyper, vol. 2 (Amsterdam, 1866), 350, 352, 647, 674, 690, 706. See. also the church order of the French Church composed by Nicolas des Gallars (1561), in Boersma, *Vluchtig voorbeeld*, 271.

19 Jelsma, *Frontiers*, 101.

20 In the Dutch translation by Jean de la Haye, the Reformed pastor of the Hague (1611), De la Haye translated 'testimonium divinae vocia' as 'testimony of God's Word': Jacobus Acontius, *VIII. Boecken van de arglistigheden des Satans*, trans. Johannes de la Haye (Amsterdam, 1660), 55. On Acontius's spiritualism, see Erich Hassinger, *Studien zu Jacobus Acontius*, Abhandlungen zur Mittleren und Neueren Geschichte 76 (Berlin-Grunewald, 1934), 84ff.: 'seinem Spiritualismus fehlt alles Enthusiastische'.

21 Hassinger, 84ff. characterizes Acontius as a biblicist.

22 On the prophecy in 16th century Protestantism, see G. H. Williams, *The Radical Reformation* (3rd edn., Kirksville, MO, 1992), 518–21; Philippe Denis, 'La prophétie dans les églises de la réforme', *Revue d'histoire ecclésiastique* 72 (1977), 289–316.

23 Johannes a Lasco, *Forma ac ratio tota ecclesiastici ministerii, in peregrinorum, potissimum vero Germanorum Ecclessia* (Frankfort am Main, 1555), reprinted in A. Lasco, *Opera*, ed.

Kuyper. vol. 2, 101–5. The Dutch version is in Marten Micron, *De Christlicke ordonancien der Nederlantscher ghemeinten te Londen* (1554), ed. W. F. Dankbaar (The Hague, 1956), ch. 12, 71–3.

24 'Want daer syn over al veel twistighe, herdtneckinghe, curioese ende opgheblasen menschen, doer de welcke de Duyvel allesins soucken soude, de Ghemeinte te beroeren ende te schoeren': Micron, 72.

25 A. J. Jelsma, O. Boersma (eds.), *Acta van het consistorie van de Nederlandse gemeente te London 1569–1585*, Rijks Geschiedkundige Publicatiën, kleine serie 76 (The Hague, 1993), in voce 'profetie'.

26 Van Schelven, *Kerkeraads-protocollen*, 478–81.

27 Collinson, 141ff.

28 Jelsma and Boersma, *Acta*, 167ff.

29 Williams, 1204, on Acontius's defence of 'prophecy' (according to the so-called *lex sedentium*), although he does not mention the existing practice of prophecy in the London stranger churches of the 1550s introduced by John a Lasco. Nor does Hassinger give attention to the London prophecy-gatherings in connection with Acontius's support for prophecy: Hassinger, 84ff. I believe that Acontius would not have acknowledged the Dutch prophecy-meetings as fully apostolic because of the controlling role of the church authorities (Koehler, 101:28ff.; 192:8ff.).

30 Certainly in the Dutch Church, after being reinstated in 1559, there must have been much discussion about the controversies with the Lutheran authorities during the peregrinations of A Lasco and his congregation during the mid-1550s. See Grell, 'Exile and tolerance'.

31 Briggs, 494.

32 Walter Koehler, 'Geistesahnen des Johannes [*sic*] Acontius', *Festgabe von Fachgenossen und Freunden Karl Müller zum siebzigsten Geburtstagdargebracht* (Tübingen, 1922), 199ff.

33 Collinson, 136. Collinson gave this interpretation of Acontius's reasoning on the basis of Jordan, 362: 'Acontius extolled reason and free inquiry as the solutions for the evils which beset the Church'. In his interpretation of the use of 'reason' Jordan is referring to the wording of the French edition, 57, where the Latin edition uses *argumenta* (Koehler, 42:29), without justifying his terminology

34 Hassinger, 88, 96, doubts whether Acontius could be treated as a rationalist thinker. Williams, 521, calls Acontius an Evangelical rationalist.

35 'Epistola apologetica ad Grindal, episcopum Londinensem, 1564' in Koehler, 235:7–242:32.

36 Acontius's contacts with the Spanish Church in London harmed his reputation: Boersma, *Vluchtig voorbeeld*, 33.

37 Delio Cantimori, *Italienische Haeretiker der Spätrenaissance,* trans. Werner Kaegi (Basel. 1949), 319: 'Man darf nicht leichthin das Urteil revidieren wollen, das die Häupter jener Kirchen (= der lutherischen und calvinistischen Kirchen) gefällt haben . . . Gallasius und die Häupterdes kirchlichen Lebens in England standen in unmittelbarem Kontakt mit Calvin; wenn sie Acontius zu den Täufern und andern Häretikern zählten, können wir von diesem Urteil nicht absehen.' Cantimori distances himself from Hassinger's treatment of Acontius's orthodoxy.

Part II

The strangers and their churches in the late 16th and early 17th centuries

6

Europe in Britain: Protestant strangers and the English Reformation

PATRICK COLLINSON

In 1555 Jan Laski told the king of his native Poland: 'Nous pensions, en effet, qu'encouragé par cet exemple les Eglises Anglais elle mêmes seraient unanimes dans tout le royaume a revenir au culte apostolique dans toute sa pureté.' Here, neatly encapsulated, was the idea of the stranger churches in England, and especially in London, serving as a kind of ecclesiastical Trojan horse for the intrusion of a 'sincere' and 'pure', rather than a merely political and moderated, Reformation. With Mary on the throne, Laski was speaking in the past tense, giving expression to what might have been as he made his way back to Poland via Denmark, Emden and Frankfurt.[1]

But with Mary's half-sister Elizabeth presiding over yet another reversal of the state religion, John Calvin linked the despatch of his distinguished colleague Nicolas des Gallars to take charge of the resuscitated French Church in London with renewed anxiety about the direction and pace of the English Reformation. 'Je déplore vivement que les Eglises de tout le royaume ne soient pas organisées comme tous les gens de bien le désireraient et avaient esperé a l'origine.'[2] Bishop Edmund Grindal of London, appointed under the new dispensation to Laski's old office of Superintendent of the stranger churches, echoed these concerns, asking Geneva to pray for 'the state of our churches', 'non encore suffisament constituées selon notre gré'.[3] At Grindal's invitation, des Gallars preached twice a week in Latin, presumably for the benefit of his London clergy, and three years later, Grindal assured Calvin that des Gallars had been 'of great use both to myself and our churches'. 'Master Gallasius, who brings you this letter, can give you the best information of the state of our kingdom and church'.[4]

The imposition of a bishop as their superintendent modified the status of the stranger churches as a *corpus corporatum et politicum* and might appear, on the face of it, to have placed restrictions on their freedom. But under the new arrangements the consistories were free to function, and there was no question of imposing French or Dutch translations of the Book of Common Prayer, something which would not be attempted before the 1630s. In effect, the strangers were exempt from the terms and requirements of the Act of Uniformity. Calvin had assured des Gallars that in Grindal he had 'un fidèle et sincère protecteur de votre liberté.'[5]

When Grindal instructed his clergy not to admit foreigners to Communion unless they brought the written consent of their own ministers, the clerk of the French consistory noted: 'Acte de levesque remarquable'.[6] 'Acte remarquable' or not, it was repeated 50 years later when the Dutch Church asked Archbishop George Abbot to take steps to prevent members of their congregation who were defying its discipline, 'sundry licentious persons', from taking Communion in the parishes in which they lived. Bishop John King of London duly ordered that none of his clergy should receive such persons, and he frankly acknowledged a fundamental difference between the stranger churches and his own parishes, referring to such as avoided censure in their own churches by transferring themselves to 'another congregation where happily ['haply'] noe such censure is used'. That was as much as to admit that the Church of England lacked rigorous, Reformed discipline.[7] The freethinking Jacobus Acontius had already drawn embarrassing attention to this anomaly when he pointed out to Grindal that whereas a heretic like himself was not permitted to communicate in the stranger churches, he was not only allowed but actually compelled to attend his parish church, and that he spoke not only for himself but for many who were dissidents not in respect of one doctrine but of the whole orthodox package.[8]

On the other hand, there is no evidence that any Englishman was ever prevented from or presented in court for taking Communion in the French Church, and the record shows that several did, including, in 1568, the Earl of Leicester, the clerk noting that this was a first for any 'seigneur notable d'Angleterre'.[9]

It is clear that far from using his office to impose an episcopalian 'Anglicanism', Grindal, much like the 'quasi-episcopal' Laski,[10] hoped that the churches of foreign Protestants would exercise an exemplary and progressive influence in countering conservative elements in the English Church (as well as radical 'Anabaptist' tendencies among the strangers themselves). Amongst these conservatives was a person who could never be named, the Supreme Governor, Queen Elizabeth herself, whose commitment to the godly cause was to be lauded in public but doubted in private. Perhaps that was one of the problems which des Gallars was to discuss with Calvin by word of mouth.

The migrant churches of Western Europe in the 1550s and 1560s were everywhere catalysts of religious polarization and the beginnings of confessionalization. The hostile reaction of local Lutheran leaders to the presence in north German cities of congregations who in doctrine were sacramentarian and in discipline proto-Reformed (or Laskian), together with the reaction to those reactions of, especially, Calvin, helped to precipitate the definitive divorce of the Evangelical and Reformed (or 'Calvinist', a neologism of that moment) tendencies and traditions. Emigration for religious reasons was therefore a force making for more clearly defined religious identities.[11]

But in England the story was different. The presence of foreign Protestants who adopted early forms of Reformed worship and discipline had a limited defining impact on the polity of the Church of England, while it served to exacerbate a somewhat contradictory religious situation: the marriage of Reformed doctrine to a liturgy still shaped by the old faith; and a structure and government which was hierarchical and tempered with the Erastianism of the royal supremacy. This was a reformed but not properly Reformed church, without ministerial parity, elders, consistories or mechanisms for congregational participation in decision-making and discipline.

The fifth-column role played by the stranger churches in the strategy of the more extreme Edwardian Protestants to remedy these defects and deficiences, the in some ways destabilizing alliance of Bishop John Hooper with Martin Micron and Jan Utenhove, together with the signal importance of Laski's liturgical and constitutional experiments, have always been acknowledged by historians both of the Edwardian Reformation and of the refugee communities themselves.[12] The continuing influence of the foreign churches on the Elizabethan ecclesiastical scene was rescued from relative neglect in my 1963 lecture to the Huguenot Society, 'The Elizabethan Puritans and the foreign Reformed churches in London'.[13] But we may ask for how long the role of the stranger churches as model churches lasted, or, to alter the question slightly, in what ways it may have changed with the passage of time.

The argument will be one not only of relations but of ratios, and also of generations. The Elizabethan Protestants, and especially the early Elizabethan Protestants, who were actively involved, as co-religionists and brethren, with the foreign congregations, were virtually in a congregational situation themselves. By a parliamentary-cum-ecclesiastical fiction, all English men and women were deemed to be members of what in liturgy and doctrine was now a Protestant Church and were legally bound to participate in its services. In the caustic judgment of a radical separatist, 'all this people, with all these manners, were in one day, with the blast of Queen Elizabeth's trumpet, of ignorant papists and gross idolaters, made faithfull Christianes and true professors'.[14]

The reality, of course, was very different. The Edwardian Protestants, even when they were in some ways in a politically more advantageous situation than obtained under Elizabeth, thought of themselves as a small embattled minority,[15] and this was existentially the case, even in London, in the early years of Elizabeth's reign. Those who had formed a gathered, secret congregation in Mary's reign, which, as we n now know, had ordained at least one minister, retained their semi-separatist identity.[16] Religiously, they merged with the general mass of London's population as readily as oil mixes with water. So much is clear from developments in 1567, when the imposition of 'popish' clerical vestments on the London parish clergy drove these 'gospellers' back into the conventicles, deliberately reviving the Marian underground experience and apparently using the Genevan form of prayer.[17] It is clear from John Knox's letters of 1559–60 to a veteran of the Geneva congregation, the wealthy merchant's wife Anne Locke, that back in England the Genevans kept themselves somewhat apart, and in Mrs Locke's case perhaps wholly apart, since in one of his letters Knox approved her principled absence from parochial assemblies.[18]

From Brett Usher, we are learning more about the enterprising and concerted activities of such members of this loose grouping as the seriously rich Culverwell family. These city magnates were not involved, so far as we know, with Separatist conventicling. But their financial operations were, if not sectarian, distinctly partisan, and they included the relief of Protestants of other nations, both overseas and in England.[19] When Richard Culverwell wrote his will in December 1584, he bequeathed a gold chain which he had been 'frankly' given by the Queen of Navarre, together with other jewels of great value, recalling her 'honourable zeale' for the 'furtherance and defence of the Ghospell and suche as sincerely professed the same'.[20] It sounds as if Culverwell and his friends were acting as international pawnbrokers, and that Jeanne d'Albret's jewels were pledges against sustenance in money or kind. In 1559 Knox had hoped that some of these same syndicates might be willing to bail out the financially strapped Lords of the Congregation, and so save the day for the Reformation in Scotland, but also, he suggested, in England itself. Mrs Locke reported that this was thought to be a state responsibility which ought not to be, as it were, privatized.[21] However, David Trim has uncovered the tip of a large iceberg in telling us about the assistance given by private persons, especially military persons, to the international Protestant Cause.[22]

In the cameo which I use to open my 1963 lecture, the multi-national funeral in London of the Scottish minister James Lawson, which happened in October 1584, we see the procession of 'gentlemen, honest burgesses, famous and godlie matrons', 'manie godlie brethren, ministers and citicens', numbering about 500 persons, said to be an unusually large turnout.[23] But this was roughly the same number as the suspected heretics briefly arrested in London 45 years earlier, and it represents less than one per cent of the population of the city.[24] By 1584, such people were often nicknamed 'Puritans'. One might say that when most people became, after a fashion, Protestants, real Protestants became Puritans.

In other words, the ratio of godly, fully committed English Protestants to their fellow Reformed Protestants of other nations in the core membership of the stranger churches was roughly equal. And the English Puritans will have regarded the godly strangers as 'brethren' in a sense that conformist, conventional English church-goers were not.

Forty or fifty years on, the situation had changed. In London, the alteration was more fundamental and structural than the succession, as bishop-superintendents, of Edwin Sandys, who was friendly, John Aylmer, who appears to have taken little or no interest, and, soon, Richard Bancroft, who was downright hostile to all forms of what he called 'the pretended holy discipline'. The relation was also affected by the progressive indigenization of the strangers, as they evolved into established language communities and sub-cultures on the English and London scene. But most relevant to the changed relationship was the altered ratio. So-called Puritanism was now more widespread and diffuse, so that soon, not least in London, it became something like the mainstream of English religious life, its ideological infrastructure, whether articulated or not, Calvinist.[25] In these circumstances, the stranger churches, *qua* churches, were now more distinctly alien and 'other'. That is to state a paradox, since, as Andrew Pettegree has shown, the economic and social integration of individual immigrants, certainly in London, was steadily advancing.[26]

As for the provincial centres, there is no evidence that the strangers contributed very much to the local Protestant cause. Take Norwich and Canterbury, cities with very substantial immigrant populations. In Norway a Dutch and Walloon community which was planted in 1565 with the arrival of some 300 migrants had swelled by 1570 to 4000, something like a third of the population.[27] Yet the most recent history of the Reformation in Norwich finds it necessary to refer to the foreigners in only a couple of paragraphs. Apparently they had little or nothing to do with Muriel McClendon's subject, called, in her sub-title, *The emergence of Protestantism in Tudor Norwich*.[28] Other sources not consulted by Dr McClendon might perhaps have told a different story, and it may be significant that many strangers were clustered in the vicinity of St Andrews, the godliest of all Norwich parishes.[29] However, pending further research, it remains striking that it has proved possible to tell the story of how the second city in the kingdom became Protestant without reference to the strangers in its midst.

The archives I consulted in the course of writing the history of Canterbury Cathedral between 1540 and 1600[30] suggested that unless one was advised from other sources, one would never have guessed that here too foreign migrants made up about a third of the population.[31] In the depositions given in evidence by hundreds of witnesses, a cross-section of Canterbury society – in cases involving marriage, inheritance, defamation – Walloon names are conspicuous by their absence. Endogamy within communities which for generations remained legally alien, outside the freedom of the city, was probably persistent. Nigel Goose told us that in Colchester there was little intermarriage before the later years of the century.[32] In 1581 the consistory of the Canterbury church censured a female member who was intending to marry an Englishman while already contracted to another; and generally, the consistory regarded intermarriage as contrary to ecclesiastical discipline, while English sponsors very rarely appeared at Walloon baptisms.[33] In 1574 Archbishop Parker had expressed surprise and disappointment that the consistory of the Dutch Church in London should have excommunicated a woman in their congregation only for having married an Englishman, 'and that you should thus wish to keep yourselves apart.'[34]

Relations between natives and migrants in these two towns were not necessarily hostile. 'Ambivalent', a term preferred by Charles Littleton, might be a better word. Both Norwich and Canterbury knew on what side their bread was buttered, and that the presence of foreign skills had halted and even reversed a process of economic and demographic contraction. Landlords with property to rent were certainly in favour of the immigrants. Almost the only occasion that McClendon has to mention the Dutch in Norwich is in the context of an abortive Catholic conspiracy in 1570, which planned to rally the common people to 'beat the strangers out of the city'. This is certainly evidence that the strangers were significant symbols of a Protestant regime which the conspirators hoped to eradicate. But there is no evidence that this call met with any popular resonance.[35]

When, two generations later, Archbishop Laud took steps to destroy the independent existence of the foreign Protestant congregations in Maidstone, Sandwich and Canterbury, one might have expected the approval of xenophobic local elements, resentful of the strangers. But Canterbury in 1630 was not Dover in 2000. There was some ecclesiastical opposition to the Canterbury Walloons in the Cathedral precincts, as well there might have been, since every Sunday morning a congregation of as many as 2000 raised the roof of the crypt with psalms which, according to one cleric, made 'very harsh and untuneable discords' right underneath the choir. But the fact is that even the Dean and Chapter made no attempt to evict the Walloons, while the Mayor and Commonalty of Canterbury were among those who petitioned Laud to relax his demands.[36]

To sum up this part of my argument. By the early 17th century, we are looking, religiously speaking, at what the sociologists, in a very convenient, elastic sort of word, call 'routinization'.

Let us go back to the 1560s and 1570s, reminding ourselves of some details of a period of interactive solidarity of the stranger churches in London with elements in the English Church eager for 'further reformation'. This was the time of international Calvinism *par excellence*, when the radical London preacher and publicist Thomas Wilcox could ask 'is a reformation good for France? and can it be evyl for England? Is discipline meete for Scotland? and is it unprofitable for this Realm?';[37] and when the Scottish Presbyterian John Davidson could tell Wilcox's fellow agitator John Field that he had received on consecutive days letters from Field in London and from La

Rochelle. 'It is no small comfort, brother, . . . to brethren of one natione to understand the state of the brethren in other nationes.'[38]

There are two aspects of this solidarity which deserve attention: imitation of the exemplary model, and cross membership. Let us take first cross membership, participation by English Protestants in the worship and life of the London stranger churches. Not all adherents, or even members, of the various stranger churches were of the appropriate and designated nation or language. In the 1560s an actual minority of the members of the Italian congregation, an extreme case, were Italian by birth. The majority were Dutch, in 1568 numbering at least 63. The Italian Church also had some English adherents who, Roger Ascham tell us, simply wanted to brush up their Italian. But we may well suspect a more serious motivation in the case of William Winthrop, uncle of the future Governor of Massachusetts, John Winthrop, and an elder of the congregation. In 1570 three of the six elders of this church were English: in addition to Winthrop, Michael Blount and Bartholomew Warner.[39]

It is well known that John Bodley, an elder of the English congregation in Geneva, printer of the Geneva Bible and the father of the founder of the Bodleian Library, was an elder of the London French church for more than 20 years. In July 1560 three returned English exiles had helped to preside over the first election of officers in the French congregation.[40] The Dutch Church also numbered among its officers for a time an English elder and an English deacon, although they had Dutch connections. The English Genevans seem to have attended the French Church with some regularity, the clerk of the consistory noting that this was allowable, 'a cause qui sont unis de foy avec nous'.[41] Occasional attenders included William Whittingham, translator of the Geneva Bible (whose wife was French-speaking), William Fuller, another office-bearer in Geneva, the diplomat Henry Killigrew and his wife Catherine, sister-in-law of Lord Burghley and Sir Nicholas Bacon, 'et plusieurs aultres englois'.[42] By 1581 some London clergy were complaining to Convocation that 'manie citizens' were deserting their parish churches in favour of the Dutch and French congregations.[43] In 1569 a Dutch minister proposed that the monthly meetings of the inter-congregational coetus should be attended 'si commodum videbitur' by one or other of the 'precipuis anglicarium ecclesiarum ministris'.[44]

A context for these fragments of evidence is provided by what had been happening across the Channel in 1562 and 1563: English intervention on the side of the Huguenots in the first War of Religion. The Earl of Warwick, Leicester's brother, was commander of the English forces at Le Havre ('Newhaven'). His man of business, secretary to the Council of War, was Thomas Wood, a former Geneva elder. Among the preachers in Newhaven garrison were William Whittingham and William Kethe, Genevan veterans both. And it was hoped to recruit none other than Knox's closest friend, Christopher Goodman, whose political views made him *persona non grata* with the Queen but who was patronized by the Dudleys. Killigrew was at Newhaven as a military volunteer, which put his life in danger when he was wounded and captured, but not before he had written to his brother-in-law Cecil, describing how he and 'a great many Christian soldiers' had participated in a Reformed Communion service. 'You will think me over holy for a soldier.'[45] In short, the Newhaven camp, with its godly discipline and Reformed worship, was a Cave of Adullam for frustrated English Calvinists. However, it rather spoils the atmosphere of ecumenicity to have to report that as the pressure built up on the hard-pressed garrison, the Privy Council recommended driving the French, mostly good Calvinists 'of the religion', right out of Le Havre, lock, stock and barrel.[46]

Back in England, and at a ministerial level, there was practical collegiality among the French pastors and the Puritan clergy, whose correspondence with Geneva and Zurich was regularly routed through the French congregation. In 1572 'nos Freres les Ministres Anglois' used the same intermediaries to communicate with the Synod held in Nimes.[47] Presently this Anglo-French solidarity was strengthened by the arrival in England as refugees from the St Bartholomew Massacre of no fewer than 60 French pastors, who immediately attracted an exceptional response from what we may call the card-carrying English godly. Whittingham, now dean of Durham, sent £10, a charitable donation equivalent to some thousands today.[48]

There is no lack of evidence that as the Elizabethan Puritan movement gathered momentum, from the 1560s through to the 1580s, the stranger churches were admired and even envied as examples of everything which the Elizabethan Church was not. In 1600 an elderly London minister wrote retrospectively of the foreigners who 'never dyd receive our Booke of Common Prayers', and who enjoyed congregational discipline and the free election of their officers.[49] In 1572 an abortive Parliamentary bill 'concerning rites and ceremonies' proposed that the bishops should be empowered to license their clergy to use forms of worship divergent from the Prayer Book, provided they were the forms in use in the French and Dutch Churches, the bill itself noting that there were freely available in print, 'and therefore wilful ignorance not to knowe it.'[50] An anonymous Puritan manifesto makes it clear that such orders were not considered foreign at all but part of a common heritage of Reformed worship and discipline in which English Protestants were fully participant. It spoke of 'the liturgie used by our country men persecuted in Queen Maries tyme, and now used in Fraunce, Scotland, Flanders, and others for the profession of the Gospell within this Citye and by others abroade at Geneva and els where.'[51]

The response from time to time of the Elizabethan authorities was predictable. In October 1573 the Queen fired a warning shot across the bows of the French and Dutch Churches in a couple of stiff letters from the Privy Council. We accept, they said, that there has always been a legitimate diversity of rites and ceremonies among Christians, and we approve of what you do insofar as it conforms to the practice of the countries from which you come. But do not even think of stirring up religious dissension in this Church. The Queen would rather banish the whole lot of you out of her kingdom, 'exigere vos omnes', 'wt haer rijke drisen', than have it disturbed by the ingratitude of guests welcomed in the name of piety. And above all do not admit dissident Englishmen to your Communions. The Dutch said that of course they would do nothing of the kind. The reply of the French is not preserved. It took a little time for the dust to settle, after that.[52] When, early in James I's reign, the French minister de la Fontaine paid his respects to the new Bishop of London, Richard Vaughan, Vaughan spoke warmly of the memory and legacy of Laski, but rather pointedly said that he hoped that the stranger churches would not pour oil on the fires of domestic discord but would rather do their best to extinguish them.

That did not need to be said. The stranger churches and their liturgies and discipline were no longer a distinct source of inspiration for a Puritan case which had now gone cool on Presbyterianism, and nor did they pose a threat to Anglicans. Meanwhile, neither the English state nor the Church threatened the stranger churches, until

William Laud began his unprecedented but ultimately abortive attack on their liberties in the early 1630s. To state what is almost a paradox in the context of a volume called 'From Strangers to Citizens', with the passing of what one may call the Genevan generation, the churches were now more and not less foreign and 'other'. La Fontaine's response to Bishop Vaughan was to say that the French were well aware that strangers ought not to interfere in matters which were none of their concern: 'peregrinos qui rebus alienis nequaquam nos immiscere debeamus'.[53]

Not that English Protestantism now pulled back, tortoise-like, into is own insular shell. It would be easy to make that mistake, and it has been made, by those who have misunderstood the rhetoric of English exceptionalism, the theme of England the 'elect nation'. It is true that one preacher declared (and his sermon could be paralleled a hundred times over) that England was 'Gods Signet, Gods Jewel, . . . the one Nation, almost, that doth openly and solely professe the true Religion of God!' But note the 'almost'. The whole point of such rhetoric was to complain that England had treated God's mercy towards her with shameful contempt.[54] Just as it was a great credit to Protestant England that it gave sustenance and shelter to the godly of other nations, so it was a particular cause of shame when England failed in those obligations. That was the whole point of the poet Milton's boast about England's 'precedence of teaching other nations how to live'.[55] Protestant nationalism and internationalism were two sides of the same coin.

But in an earlier essay I suggested that 'there was more of fantasy and nostalgia in "the Protestant Cause" than substance, given the reluctance of the monarchy to identify with it.' So far as there was substance, it was financial and voluntary. The international Protestant Cause was, in modern terminology, a Non-Governmental Organization, and no doubt the seamless unity of the Protestant cause throughout Europe was most apparent to the more prodigiously religious membership of the English Church, 'the godly', and it was the purse-strings of the godly which were most readily loosened.[56]

These were the critical moments in the godly, voluntary and almost sectarian response to the international cause: the Massacre of St Bartholomew, the defence of Geneva in the early 1580s, and again in 1590 and 1603, and the relief of the Calvinists of the Rhenish Palatinate in the 1620s. In 1583, the fundraising agent for the Genevan government, Jean Maillet, met with the *classis* of the London presbyterian ministers, eight of them, with Walter Travers in the chair. But he was advised that it would be too risky to work through these unauthorized channels, and that he should deal with the bishops, who, indeed, proved helpful.[57] Much charitable funding was generated in the preaching fasts which were a conspicuous feature of English Calvinist culture, exact counterparts of the *jeunes* ordered by the *coetus* of the stranger churches on no fewer than 30 occasions in the 23 years covered by its minutes.[58]

The English contribution to the Palatine relief fund far outstripped the help given by the established Calvinist churches in Switzerland, France and the Netherlands, as the Palatine ministers were prepared to testify to 'the whole sympathizing Christian world'. But while there was a very substantial governmental input to the fund, with money raised, according to Royal letters patent, in every parish in England, this would probably not have happened without the political pressure applied by the godly great and good, while a significant share of the response was explicitly or implicitly voluntary. William Laud, as Bishop of London, was put in charge of the first official collection, but it was obvious that it was not Laud's idea to have one. The Palatine refugees did their homework, discovered that there were more than 8700 parishes in England, and doubted whether the money raised represented a sufficient or truly national response. Some of the first aid had been organized by such leading puritan divines in London as John Davenport, Richard Sibbes and William Gouge. So almost conspiratorial did these fund-raising activities appear to the suspicious ecclesiastical authorities that the London ministers were prosecuted in the Court of High Commission. Further funds were raised by the puritan mafia in provincial towns, and especially through the effort of John White, the famous patriarch of Dorchester, who took four Palatine asylum seekers into his own household.[59]

This large subject has been explored, so far as the Dutch Church and its connections are concerned, by Ole Grell. Grell has uncovered the central role of the officers of Austin Friars in forwarding the moneys collected in England and liaising with the relief committees in Germany, none of whose members spoke any English. Their accounts detail the enormous sums of money involved, counting the Royal collections, a total of £12,510; which takes no account of the funds raised and spent on Palatine refugees in England itself. We may compare the money raised for flood relief in Mozambique in 2000, when this country, as in the 1620s, was more generous than any other: £20 million from the government, £16 million from private and voluntary sources, a total of £36 million, or say £36,000 in 17th-century money; but from a nation ten times more populous than 17th-century England and a thousand-fold richer.[60]

Europe in Britain? The story of the stranger churches between the mid-16th and mid-17th centuries is one of complex interaction, some otherness and some together-ness. Some of this was predictable, other aspects transcendental.

NOTES

1   Laski's words appeared in the dedication to King Sigismund of his *Forma ac ratio*, and are quoted (translated) in *Actes du consistoire de l'église française de Threadneedle Street, Londres* vol. 1: *1560–5*, ed. Elsie Johnston, HSQS 38, xiiin. See Andrew Pettegree, *Foreign Protestant communities in sixteenth-century London* (Oxford, 1986), 30–5; Diarmaid MacCulloch, 'The importance of Jan Laski in the English Reformation', in Christoph Strohm (ed.), *Johannes a Lasco: Polnischer Baron, Humanist und europäischer Reformator* (Emden, 2000), 315–45; Basil Hall, *John à Lasco, 1499–1560: a Pole in Reformation England*, Friends of Dr Williams's Library 25th Lecture (London, 1971).

2   Baron F. de Schickler, *Les églises du réfuge en Angleterre* (Paris, 1892), vol. 3, 45, quoting and translating from *Joannis Calvini opera selecta*, ed. E. Cunitz and G. Baum (Munich, 1926), vol. 18, no. 3199, cols. 87–8.

3   Schickler, vol. 3., 46–7.

4   *The Zurich letters*, ed. Hastings Robinson, The Parker Society, 2nd series (Cambridge, 1845), 96.

5   Calvin to des Gallars, June 1560: Schickler, vol. 1, 85–6.

6   *Actes du consistoire*, xxvi, 108

7   *Ecclesiae Londino-Batavae archivum*, ed. J. H. Hessels, vol. 3 (Cambridge, 1897), 1225–8, 1260–2.

8   *Ibid.*, vol. 2 (Cambridge, 1889), 224–34.

9   Bochetel de la Forest to King Charles IX, 25 March 1568: PRO, Baschet Transcripts 31/3/26, fo. 207. I owe this reference to Professor Wallace MacCaffrey.

10 MacCulloch, 324.

11 Andrew Pettegree, 'The London exile community and the second sacramentarian contro-versy, 1553–1560', in his *Marian Protestantism: six studies* (Aldershot, 1996), 55–85 (chap. 3).

12 Pettegree, *Foreign Protestant communities*, 46–76; Diarmaid MacCulloch, *Thomas Cranmer: a life* (New Haven, 1996), 477–80; MacCulloch, 'Importance of Jan Laski', 327–33.

13 Patrick Collinson, 'The Elizabethan Puritans and the foreign Reformed churches in London', *HSP* 20 (1964), 528–55, reprinted in Collinson, *Godly people: essays on English Protestantism and Puritanism* (London, 1983), 245–72.

14 *The writings of Henry Barrow, 1587–1590*, ed. Leland H. Carlson, Elizabethan Nonconformist Texts 3 (London, 1962), 283.

15 Catherine Davies, '"Poor persecuted little flock" or "Commonwealth of Christians": Edwardian Protestant concepts of the Church', in Peter Lake and Maria Dowling (eds.), *Protestantism and the national Church in sixteenth-century England* (London, 1987), 78–102.

16 Brett Usher, '"In a time of persecution": new light on the secret Protestant congregation in Marian London', in David Loades (ed.), *John Foxe and the English Reformation* (Aldershot, 1997), 233–51.

17 'An examination of certayne Londoners before the Commissioners', in *A parte of a register* (Middelburg, 1593), 23–36, reprinted in *The remains of Edmund Grindal*, ed. W. Nicholson, Parker Society (Cambridge, 1843), 210–16.

18 Patrick Collinson, 'John Knox, the Church of England and the women of England', in Roger Mason (ed.), *John Knox and the British Reformations* (Aldershot, 1998), 91–2.

19 Brett Usher, 'Backing Protestantism: the London godly, the Exchequer and the Foxe Circle', in David Loades (ed.), *John Foxe: an historical perspective* (Aldershot, 1999), 105–34.

20 Collinson, *Godly people*, 271–2.

21 Collinson, 'John Knox', 85–6.

22 David Trim, 'Protestant refugees in Elizabethan England and confessional conflict in France and the Netherlands, 1562–c.1610', elsewhere in this volume.

23 Collinson, *Godly people*, 245–6.

24 Susan Brigden, *London and the Reformation* (Oxford, 1989), 320–1.

25 Patrick Collinson, *The religion of Protestants: the Church and English society, 1559–1625* (Oxford, 1982), *passim*.

26 Pettegree, *Foreign Protestant communities*, 296–309.

27 HSQS 1, 17–20, 25–35.

28 Muriel McClendon, *The quiet Reformation: magistrates and the emergence of Protestantism in Tudor Norwich* (Stanford, 1999), 211–12, 224–5.

29 I owe this point to an oral communication by Professor Ralph Houlbrooke. See also Moens, 21–4.

30 Patrick Collinson, 'The Protestant cathedral, 1541–1660' in Patrick Collinson, Nigel Ramsay and Margaret Sparks (eds.), *A history of Canterbury Cathedral* (Oxford, 1995), 154–203.

31 HSQS 15.

32 Nigel Goose, 'The Dutch in Colchester in the 16th and 17th centuries: opposition and integration', elsewhere in this volume.

33 Cross, 31–2.

34 *Ecclesiae Londino-Batavae*, vol. 3, 266.

35 McClendon, 224–5.

36 Ole Peter Grell, 'The struggle for survival: Archbishop Laud and the foreign congrega-

tions', in Grell, *Dutch Calvinists in early Stuart London: the Dutch Church in Austin Friars, 1603–1642* (Leiden, 1989), 224–48 (chap. 6); Collinson, 'The Protestant cathedral', 192–3.

37 'An admonition to the Parliament', in *Puritan manifestos: a study of the origin of the Puritan revolt*, ed. W. H. Frere and C. E. Douglas (London, 1907; reprinted, 1954), 19.

38 Collinson, *Godly people*, 249.

39 HSQS 59, 21–30, 133. For Winthrop's involvement with the strangers, see Collinson, *Godly people*, 268–9; and for the context, Francis Bremer, 'William Winthrop and religious reform in London, 1529–1582'. *London Journal* 24:2 (1999), 1–17.

40 Collinson, *Godly people*, 267–8.

41 *Ibid.*, 263–4.

42 *Ibid.*, 262.

43 *Ibid.*, 264–5.

44 *Ecclesiae Londino-Batavae*, vol. 3, 311–14. It is not clear whether the minister, George Wybo, meant by 'precipuis . . . ministris' the English bishops or such leading Presbyterian Puritans as Walter Travers or John Field.

45 Wallace T. MacCaffrey, 'The Newhaven expedition, 1562–1563,' *The Historical Journal* 40 (1997), 1–21; Christopher P. Croly, 'Religion and English foreign policy, 1558–1564' (unpublished Ph.D. thesis, Cambridge University, 2000), chaps 5 and 6, esp. 213–14; Patrick Collinson, 'Letters of Thomas Wood, Puritan, 1566–1577', in Collinson, *Godly people*, 47–9; 'The Life of Mr William Whittingham', ed. M. A. E. Green, *Camden Miscellany* vol. 6 (London, 1870); Amos C. Miller, *Sir Henry Killigrew: Elizabethan soldier and diplomat* (Leicester, 1963), 74–92, esp. 82.

46 Croly, 235.

47 Pettegree, *Foreign Protestant communities*, 273; Collinson, *Godly people*, 259.

48 Collinson, *Godly people*, 269–70.

49 Notebook of Thomas Earl, Rector of St Mildred's, Bread Street: Cambridge University Library, MS Mm.1.29, fos. 1–2.

50 Collinson, *Godly people*, 261. John Field's copy of the *Forma politiae ecclesiasticae* of Nicolas des Gallars survives in BL, Add. MS 48096 (Yelverton 150), where it is bound with the minutes of the Italian Church: *Unity in multiformity*, 111–32.

51 *The seconde parte of a register*, ed. Albert Peel (Cambridge, 1915), vol. 1, 165.

52 *Ecclesiae Londino-Batavae*, vol. 2, 456–62, 482–5.

53 John Strype, *Annals of the Reformation*, 4 vols. (Oxford, 1824; reprinted New York, 1966), vol. 4, 551.

54 William Whateley of Banbury, quoted in Patrick Collinson, 'Biblical rhetoric: the English nation and national sentiment in the prophetic mode'. in Claire McEachern and Debora Shuger (eds.), *Religion and culture in Renaissance England* (Cambridge, 1997), 29.

55 Patrick Collinson, *The birthpangs of Protestant England: religious and cultural change in the sixteenth and seventeenth centuries* (Basingstoke, 1988), 5, 17.

56 Patrick Collinson, 'England and international Calvinism, 1558–1640', in Menna Prestwich (ed.), *International Calvinism, 1541–1715* (Oxford, 1985), 203–10.

57 *Ibid.*, 205–6.

58 *Ibid.*, 204; *Unity in multiformity*, 58–110 *passim*.

59 Collinson, 'England and international Calvinism', 207–10.

60 Ole Peter Grell, 'The collections for the Palatinate', in Grell, *Dutch Calvinists*, 176–223 (chap. 5).

7

Protestant refugees in Elizabethan England and confessional conflict in France and the Netherlands, 1562–c.1610

D. J. B. TRIM

This paper briefly explores the ways by which different communities in Elizabethan England supported militant Protestants in France and the Netherlands, from the start of the first 'guerre de religion' until the conclusion of the Twelve Years' Truce. This essay stresses that the 'stranger churches' of Elizabethan England played an active *military* role in the wars of religion in their homelands, but also emphasizes that they generally did so jointly, together with native Englishmen. Aid to the Continent from Elizabethan England is often portrayed as coming *either* from stranger churches, *or* from sympathetic English nobles, such as the Earl of Leicester. In fact, while the indigenous population generally took the leading role in helping Continental co-religionists, 'stranger' Protestant refugees were an integral part of 'English' efforts to resist papal tyranny in Europe. This essay also argues that the co-operative nature of this support given to French and Dutch Protestants helped to integrate immigrants into English society. In 'transcending traditional xenophobia' in England, 'religious solidarity' was a factor of great importance,[1] but it owed as much to shared endeavour as to shared doctrine.

Combined action was the order of the day from the very beginning. The relatively large force of English 'volunteers' who went to Normandy in the first War of Religion (1562) co-operated closely with Huguenot exiles as well as with the local Protestant forces.[2] During the third civil war in France (1568–70) the Protestants received much assistance from England – assistance that was the fruit of co-ordinated action between English and French. The emphasis at this time was not on supplying troops: a few exiles did return home to fight, but as individuals; the only *units* were entirely English. However, considerable quantities of arms and other 'matériel' were supplied thanks to the efforts of many people on both sides of the Channel. Two exiles, Odet de Coligny, *quondam* Cardinal de Châtillon, and the Vidame de Chartres were of particular importance because they were crucial links between, on the one hand, Condé,

Navarre and the other Huguenot leaders in France, and on the other, their English sympathizers in the city of London, in the country and at court – men such as Nicholas and Richard Culverwell, successful merchants from a godly London family; or Sir Arthur Champernowne, Vice-Admiral of Devon, whose nephew Henry was a trusted lieutenant of the Prince of Condé and whose son Gawain married a daughter of the comte de Montgommery, a leading Huguenot commander.[3] Montgommery had emigrated to England in 1559 and though he returned to France, his family stayed as refugees in England from 1563 until after the Comte was captured and executed in 1574. They were admitted to Communion at the French church in Southampton in 1575, and in many ways became integrated into English society, though the children eventually returned to live in France.[4]

During the 1566 rebellion in the Netherlands, in which returned exiles are known to have played an important role, the involvement of Englishmen is often overlooked.[5] Two English merchants participated in the Calvinist movement at Bergen-op-Zoom, one of them even serving as a member of the consistory. In Antwerp, Englishmen as well as émigrés were among the iconoclasts who 'cleansed' the city's churches in August 1566. One was executed at the order of the Prince of Orange for theft and sacrilege, whilst another, the ardently anti-Catholic Thomas Churchyard, was chosen by the mob as one of their captains due to his military experience.[6] From 1567, a number of Englishmen fought with the *bosgeuzen* (or Wood Beggars), whose guerrilla war in the *Westkwartier* of Flanders was co-ordinated by the Dutch churches in Sandwich, Norwich and London and seems to have been funded jointly by those churches and by sympathetic English merchants.[7] Between 1568 and 1572 the Dutch *watergeuzen* (or Sea Beggars) *and* the Huguenot corsairs of La Rochelle recruited not only from Dutch and French exiles in England, but from native Englishmen, with whom they also co-operated intimately in equipping their enterprises.[8] The commander of the King of Navarre's fleet, Jean de Sores, was a member of the French church of Southampton and, in the words of G. D. Ramsay, this 'international camaraderie . . . made possible . . . the setting-forth of ships, whether as privateers or pirates, with crews of mixed nationalities'.[9]

It was, however, from 1572 that co-operative military activity really took off, stimulated by the beginning of the *opstand* in the Netherlands and the horrific St Bartholomew's Day Massacre in France. The Comte de Montgommery led an expeditionary force of English (and Welshmen) as well as Huguenot refugees to La Rochelle, helping it to survive the great royal siege of 1573. After peace was concluded, this multi-national force went to the Netherlands to aid the Dutch rebels.[10] At the beginning of the fifth war of religion in early 1574, Montgommery led another expedition (to be his last), this time to Normandy. His force was made up of his followers from France, of English soldiers and probably of men from both the French and Dutch exile communities in England, and it was funded partly by English supporters and partly by the French congregation in Southampton.[11]

Meanwhile, in the Netherlands in 1572, the year of the *opstand*, it is well known that, from the storming of Den Brielle by Lumey de La Marck on 1 April, the rebellious Dutch towns bombarded England, particularly the stranger churches, with appeals for military assistance.[12] These appeals met with a positive response: soldiers and supplies crossed the North Sea in April and May. In the fullness of time, Thomas Morgan and Sir Humphrey Gilbert led a large number of Anglo-Welsh 'volunteers' to Flushing in

June and July: because of its size and the complicity of the Elizabethan regime in its dispatch, their force has overshadowed all other English succour to the rebels. The standard historical accounts of these events, though essentially accurate, are nevertheless somewhat misleading. First, they portray the early assistance sent from England as being supplied solely by the stranger churches; second, they indicate that the only significant English intervention in the Netherlands at this time was that led by Morgan and Gilbert; and third, they depict the support of the refugee communities as distinct from that of English captains and grandees.[13]

Let us take these points in order. The strangers undoubtedly made an important contribution to the war effort across the narrow seas. By the end of April, the French Church of London had raised £300, the Austin Friars congregation £200, and the two churches had jointly bought enough arms for 1700 men; while Lumey in Den Brielle had received volunteers from London and Sandwich.[14] In May, the fund-raising efforts continued in London, where the French Church recruited 200 men who were sent to Flushing, while the Norwich church raised 125 soldiers at the behest of an agent of the Prince of Orange, who led the men to Ter Veere.[15] Just half a dozen Dutch families in Ipswich sent six of their men to Den Brielle, having equipped three of them and raised an extra £15, whilst the Dutch Church in Colchester raised and shipped over to Flushing nearly 40 soldiers.[16] The support of the exile congregations was not restricted to April and May. In June, although more than 25 of the members of the Dutch Church in Norwich who had gone to Flushing in May had already been slain, over a hundred more Dutch and French exiles, raised at a cost of £160 to the Dutch Church, crossed the North Sea.[17] By the end of 1572, Austin Friars, as a church, had raised £1400 and sent to Flushing 200 fully equipped soldiers, while wealthier members of the church, acting as individuals, had sent another fifty men to Holland and Zeeland. Even the small community at Maidstone had raised £13.[18]

However, it is not clear that those 250 men raised by the members of the Dutch Church of London, for example, nor any of the other troops raised by the various refugee communities, were recruited only from immigrants. Thus we come to the second point. Native English military assistance to the Dutch rebels was not restricted to Morgan's and Gilbert's force – it was more common and widespread. Reports from Spanish diplomatic agents in London, the correspondence of émigré congregations, and the records of officers of the English companies in Zeeland, all alike indicate that many Englishmen, including discrete units, were among the ranks of the troops raised by the stranger churches.[19] English soldiers had already played as significant a role as had returned refugees during the fighting in April and May. Englishmen (as well as Huguenot exiles) served in de La Marck's own company at the storming of Den Brielle and his force also included at least one distinct English foot-band.[20] The appeal of the magistrates and captains of Flushing to all the Dutch churches in England on 26 April 1572 for men and money is well known[21]; it is less well known that some three hundred English soldiers had already disembarked at Flushing two days earlier.[22] De La Marck received three more foot-bands, raised in England from the indigenous population, as reinforcements in May.[23] When Louis of Nassau captured Mons in that same month there were a number of English volunteers in his force, including some in his own guard; they served in the campaign in Hainault throughout the summer and remained with him until the bitter end in the autumn.[24]

Nor were the men of Humphrey Gilbert's well-known force the only English troops to arrive in the Low Countries after summer had come. Edward Chester, son of Sir William Chester (a former Lord Mayor of London and a notable patron of godly ministers), led to Ter Veere a force raised probably partly independently of Gilbert, though Chester later linked up with the main English body.[25] At around the same time that Gilbert's brigade left England for Flushing, a unique battalion arrived in Den Brielle. Commanded by a Dutchman and possible refugee, Jan van Tryer, it was extraordinary and of special interest to students of integration of immigrant communities, because of the composition of its rank and file. Generally, Englishmen served in Dutch units only as isolated individuals, while the nominally English bands *were* made up almost entirely of English and Welshmen, rather than Continentals. However, van Tryer's unit comprised 163 Dutch and Walloons, all of them returning refugees, plus 179 English and Welsh volunteers – all fighting together under the same captain.[26]

This last example leads us to the third point: the co-operative nature of the military and financial aid delivered to the Dutch rebels from Elizabeth's realm. Just as the soldiers supplied by foreign congregations were not necessarily refugees, not all the money collected by the stranger churches came from exiles. As Professor Collinson has shown, the stranger churches included Englishmen in their membership, while other native members of the population regularly co-operated with the churches' leadership or contributed to the strangers' fund-raising enterprises.[27] How was the cash raised in Threadneedle Street and Austin Friars, the Cinque Ports and East Anglia actually delivered to Flushing, Den Brielle and Enkhuizen? Most of it was transferred as bills of exchange by the English merchant Ferdinand Pointz, who also arranged the transportation of the bulk of the arms and munitions. However, he simply took a leading role at this time. Later, in the autumn of 1572, he raised jointly with a merchant from Flushing the extraordinary sum of £20,000 to buy and transport to Holland munitions, powder, beer, biscuit, salt meat and corn.[28] In early 1573 he was a member of a consortium of English and Dutch merchants who arranged the sale in England of goods captured by Zeeland privateers, with the profits used to provide 'victuals . . . stores' and 'payment' to the English companies still in Flushing.[29]

Thus, I do not seek to denigrate the efforts of the émigrés; but it needs to be understood that the supply of men, money, or arms and armour was generally the action not of *either* English *or* exiles, but of both, frequently acting together. The rising in Holland and Zeeland in spring and summer 1572 was only the beginning of joint action between the stranger churches and a variety of English mercenaries and merchants. The revolt was soon confined to those two rebellious provinces and the English government tried to distance itself from what appeared to be a lost cause, 'preferring an uncertain peace to uncertain wars'.[30] As a result, the stranger churches took on a new importance. William of Orange and his supporters bombarded all the stranger churches with appeals for help from the end of 1572 throughout 1573. He several times had cause to reproach them for their lack of zeal in assisting their brothers in the Netherlands, but though they were not always able to provide what the Prince asked (or as much as he asked), they were still, in relative terms, quite supportive, furnishing money (in particular) and men (albeit to a lesser degree) for the forces already in the Netherlands.[31] They served as a valuable source of information for the Dutch rebels about developments in England[32] and they must also have been an invaluable line of communication to the English sympathizers whose support, as Philip II of Spain recognized, was crucial to the rebel cause.[33]

In addition to Pointz, other English merchants also played an important role in supplying the rebels, shipping lead and gunpowder to de La Marck in Brielle in 1572–3, for example.[34] In the mid-1570s, another London merchant, Thomas Pullison (who lived in the London parish of St Antholin's, then known as a hotbed of Puritanism) actually took over the States of Holland's debts to Colonel Edward Chester in order that his men should be paid and fed and so keep fighting.[35] Two fellow parishioners at another radical parish, St Mary Aldermanbury in Cripplegate, were Elizabeth's famous Puritan Secretary of State, Sir Francis Walsingham, who also worshipped at the French Church at Threadneedle Street, and an affluent 'godly' merchant, Thomas Myddelton, who was additionally a member of the Dutch Church at Austin Friars. Myddelton began his career as an apprentice to Ferdinand Pointz, for whom he was factor at Flushing in 1578. By 1582, he was in business for himself at Antwerp; his brother William fought as a mercenary under the celebrated Sir John Norreys and Thomas Morgan (who returned to the Netherlands in 1578) and it is therefore not surprising that Myddelton advanced cash to Morgan and to Henry Norreys (Sir John's younger brother) for their personal mercenary bands.[36]

In 1583, the 4000 Anglo-Welsh troops then in the Low Countries still relied to a great extent on initiatives of English merchants, due to the financial situation of the States-General; but some supplies of 'beer, bread and other victuals, besides much merchandise, as shoes and such other', probably came from the stranger churches of Sandwich and Dover.[37] In sum, the craftsmen and merchants of the Dutch and French communities in south-east England did make a major contribution to the Calvinist war effort on the Continent, but as part of a much wider network of merchants, English and émigré alike, who took on considerable financial commitments, with poor chance of profits.

Even when the war effort was taken over by the English crown in 1585 the Austin Friars congregation raised £1072 to help equip troops in the Earl of Leicester's expeditionary force.[38] Furthermore, exiles continued to serve alongside English and Welshmen, including those raised through the efforts of private sympathizers. The numbers of troops in Leicester's army were equalled by volunteers in the pay of the States-General. These companies, though mostly English, included at least one company under 'a Wallowne Captayne', made up of men of the stranger communities of Norwich, Colchester and elsewhere in East Anglia.[39] Francis Castilion, one of the Earl of Leicester's officers in the Netherlands in 1586, was a member of the Italian immigrant community, the son of Gian Batista Castiglione, Elizabeth's Italian tutor.[40] In 1588, the stranger churches raised 500 men to reinforce the Queen's garrison in Bergen-op-Zoom.[41] Later, in the 1590s, the four sons of the Dutch statesman, Adolf van Meetkerke (whose support for the Earl of Leicester had resulted in his family being exiled to England in the late 1580s), all led companies or regiments of the English army. In 1602 the Dutch congregations of London, Norwich, Sandwich, Rye, Winchelsea, Maidstone and Dover were targeted by the recruiting parties of Sir Francis Vere, raising troops to succour the garrison of besieged Ostend.[42]

Under the circumstances it is unsurprising that, though there were mixed feelings in England generally about the economic consequences of immigration,[43] Englishmen who had participated in Europe's wars of religion were normally positive about those with whom they had fought shoulder to shoulder, literally as well as metaphorically. It is notable that the muster-master of Norwich allowed Dutch strangers to serve in its trained bands.[44] This was probably due at least partly to their knowledge of gunpowder technology,[45] but it still indicates that soldiers were accepting of 'strangers'. Among the intimate friends of Robert Devereux, 2nd Earl of Essex, was Gabriel de Montgommery, younger son of the comte de Montgommery, who spent his youth in exile in England after his father's death in 1574 and who may have had an Englishwoman as his first wife.[46] Baldwin van Meetkerke, second son of Adolf van Meetkerke, was a client of the Earl's, by whom he was knighted at Cadiz in 1596, and at this time several of the other, indigenous, soldiers and diplomats in Essex's circle were friends of the well-known Dutch historian Emmanuel van Meteren, who lived much of his life in London.[47]

So greatly was English soldiers' xenophobia diminished that trans-ethnic marriages became relatively common. In 1591, Sir Thomas Bodley, the friend of a number of members of the exile communities in London, as his father had been before him, wrote to Lord Burghley that about 40 English soldiers had married Dutch wives; and the municipal archive of Leiden, an English garrison town, preserves records of many marriages between English soldiers and townswomen in the 1590s and early 17th century.[48] Lust is, of course, a more obvious motivation for ordinary soldiers stationed abroad to marry local females than pluralist acceptance of foreigners, but it was also the officers and gentlemen in the English units who contracted such alliances. Some were probably motivated by money, but others are known to have married for love. In 1588, Sir William Browne, Lieutenant-Governor of Flushing, married a Huguenot exile.[49] L'Estrange Mordant, later a captain in Ireland and a baronet, married the daughter of a former citizen of Antwerp (his family themselves exiles in the Dutch Republic) around 1600.[50] From 1590 into the early 1600s, four colonels (Sir Callisthenics Brooke, Sir Edward Conway, Sir Thomas Knollys and Sir John Ogle), a lieutenant-colonel (Thomas Holles) and at least two captains (Thomas Pointz – a cousin of Ferdinand Pointz – and Captain Randolf) all married Dutch women. Conway even named a daughter after Den Brielle in Holland, where she was born while her father was governor. Ogle went further, naming three daughters after the cities in the Netherlands where they were born and, though his wife and children settled in England, they were never naturalized. Thomas Pointz's family settled permanently in the Netherlands; and Holles's son grew up to speak 'French and Dutch . . . better than English'.[51]

John McGurk, in examining the marriages of Irish soldiers settled in the Spanish Netherlands to local women, rightly warns of the danger that 'highly selective evidence' will 'lead to . . . exaggerated conclusion[s] about assimilation'.[52] However, the marriages just cited arguably represented more than simply the normal adjustment to local conditions that takes place whenever soldiers are garrisoned in a foreign country. A number of marriages that took place across national and linguistic borders were not to locals, but to women from Dutch immigrant families in England. In 1607, for example, Lieutenant John Braddedge married a Flemish woman who had emigrated to England and settled in Lambeth with her husband. Sir Edward Conway's foreign wife, similarly, came from a Ghentish family that had fled to London, where her first marriage had been to John West, a grocer.[53] At least one member of the aristocratic Cromwell family, many of whom fought in the Netherlands, married an émigré Dutch woman.[54] Similar marriages were also made by the rank-and-file. For example, at Leiden in 1603, Thomas Smith wed Jannetgen Swyetijn of Colchester. Also at

Leiden in 1603, William Segar married Sara Meeuwels of Sandwich; when Segar died in 1607, Sara re-married another English soldier, Giles Hall, and in the same year Oliver Augustine of Gloucester married Cathelijne Douwes of Sandwich, also at Leiden.[55]

The inculturation of English soldiers by foreign service can also be seen in the experience of Sir Thomas Morgan – the same man who fought at Flushing in 1572 and received financial aid from Thomas Myddelton. In 1589, Morgan eloped with a daughter of Jan van Merode, Marquis of Bergen. The Marquis and, more particularly, his wife were not happy at having as a son-in-law a grizzled Welsh veteran closer to their age than their daughter's. In the end, it was Morgan's Dutch friends, including some on the Council of State, who intervened to mend fences between Morgan and his mother-in-law. Later, the son born to this union (named in honour of Maurice of Nassau) also married a Dutch noblewoman.[56] Thomas himself, when writing to a Continental confidant, used English, French and Dutch: all in the one letter.[57]

This is indicative of how mutual participation in confessional conflicts on the Continent could integrate indigenes and immigrants. Whatever their language, they were all fighting for the reformed faith, for the Holy Scriptures, which taught them 'There is neither Jew nor Greek, neither slave nor free . . . for you are all one in Christ Jesus.'[58] Sir Arthur Champernowne reflected this in the year of crisis, 1572, writing to the queen:

> Of one side your highnes may see Flushing, the Flemmyngs, and germans in good labor, on the other side, Rochell and the persequted frenchemen, at hard point, . . . we be made up with them in one band together . . . with them to stande in strength . . .[59]

This sense of being part of a common cause – 'la cause commune' – was not felt by all English people, but was felt especially strongly by those who were committed to the Protestant cause and they applied it not only to Protestants in foreign countries but to foreign Protestants who had emigrated to England. In the words of one English military writer at the end of the century, 'this noble and most mighty nation of Englishmen . . . are always most loving . . . & ready to cherish & protect strangers'.[60] A few years later, William Bradshaw took such sentiments to their logical conclusion in an oft-quoted passage: members of the stranger churches, 'being all the same household of faith that we are . . . are not aptly called forreyne . . . [A]ll members of the Church, in what country so ever they be, are not . . . accounted Forreyners one to another, because they are all Citizens of heaven'.[61]

I conclude with a last example of how confessional conflict helped to integrate refugees into English society. Adolf van Meetkerke's four eldest sons were all born in the Netherlands, but each served in English units during the war against Spain, fighting in the Low Countries, in Portugal and in Spain itself; two lost their lives in the Queen's service. Were they Dutch? Were they 'strangers'? In virtually all contemporary English narratives they are clearly regarded as English. Sharing the burden of confessional conflict helped to engender a sense of unity; that shared burden and the shared experiences that resulted made English and refugee alike better appreciate each others' qualities and helped to break down barriers. It was one way by which strangers became citizens.

NOTES

1   Patrick Collinson, *The birthpangs of Protestant England: religious and cultural change in the sixteenth and seventeenth centuries* (Basingstoke, 1988), 16.

2   See D. J. B. Trim, 'The "foundation-stone of the British army"? The Normandy campaign of 1562', *Journal of the Society for Army Historical Research* 77 (1999), 71–87; Amos C. Miller, *Sir Henry Killigrew: Elizabethan soldier and diplomat* (Leicester, 1963), 75–8, 84–5; *CSPF, Elizabeth I*, vol. 5, 66 (no. 130).

3   D. J. B. Trim, 'The "secret war" of Elizabeth I: England and the Huguenots during the early Wars of Religion', in *HSP* 27:2 (1999), 189–99, esp. 190–3 and the sources cited at 198–9. See *DNB*, vol. 5, 288; Patrick Collinson, 'The Elizabethan Puritans and the foreign reformed churches in London', *HSP* 20 (1964), 554–5; Brett Usher, 'The silent community: early Puritans and the patronage of the arts,' in Diana Wood (ed.), *The Church and the arts*, Studies in Church History 28 (Oxford, 1991), 287–302; Anthony Emery, *Dartington Hall* (Oxford, 1970), 73–80.

4   Andrew Spicer, *The French-speaking Reformed community and their church in Southampton 1567–c.1620*, Huguenot Society New Series 3 (London, 1997), 133; G. E. C *et al.*, *The complete peerage* (rev. ed., 13 vols. in 12, London, 1910–59), vol. 9, 138; Bibliothèque Nationale, Paris [hereafter BN], Fonds Clairambault MS 1907, fos. 132–3.

5   Andrew Pettegree, 'The exile churches during the *wonderjaar*', in J. van den Berg and P. G. Hoftijzer (eds.), *Church, change and revolution: transactions of the fourth Anglo-Dutch Church history colloquium*, Publications of the Sir Thomas Browne Institute [hereafter PTBI], NS 12 (Leiden, 1991), 82, 84.

6   Randal Starkey and George Kyghtley to William Cecil, June 1568: *Relations politiques des Pays-Bas et de l'Angleterre, sous le règne de Philippe II*, ed. Kervyn de Lettenhove [hereafter KL], (11 vols., Brussels, 1882–1900), vol. 5, 108 (no. 1690); G. D. Ramsay, *The Queen's merchants and the Revolt of the Netherlands* (Manchester, 1986), 48; Thomas Churchyard, *A lamentable and pitifull description of the wofull warres in Flaunders* (London, 1578), 22–34; *idem, A pleasant discourse of court and wars with a replication to them both* (London, 1596; repr., 1816), sig. A2v.

7   M. F. Backhouse (ed.), 'Dokumenten betreffende de godsdiensttroebelen in het Westkwartier: Jan Comerlynck en tien zijner gezellen voor de Ieperse vierschaer 1568–69', *Handelingen van de Koninklijke Commissie voor Geschiedenis* 138 (1972), 138, 191, 268, 293–97, 335–6, 344; *idem*, 'Guerrilla war and banditry in the sixteenth century: the Wood Beggars in the Westkwartier of Flanders (1567–68)', *Archiv für Reformationsgeshichte* 74 (1983), 234–40, 247–9; Andrew Pettegree, *Foreign Protestant communities in sixteenth-century England* (Oxford, 1986), 252–3; *idem*, 'Exile churches', 84–5, 95–6.

8   Richard Clough to Thomas Gresham, 28 Sept. 1567: KL, vol. 5, 15 (no. 1622); Guzmán de Silva (Spanish Ambassador in London until Sept. 1568) to Elizabeth I, 14 July 1568: BL, Galba MS C iii, fo. 233; Guerau de Spes (Spanish Ambassador in London from Sept. 1568), Memorandum, March 1569: KL, vol. 5, 320 (no. 1860); Louis of Nassau to Earl of Leicester, 17 Oct. 1569: BL, Galba MS C iii, fo. 306; de Spes to Duke of Alba, 23 June 1570 and to Cecil, 27 July 1570: KL, vol. 5, 669 (no. 2078), 681 (no. 2088); J. C. A. de Meij, *De watergeuzen en de Nederlanden 1568–1572*, Verhandelingen der Koninklijke Nederlandse Akademie van Wetenschapen, NS 77:2 /Werken uitgeven door de Commissie voor Zeegeschiedenis, vol. 14 (Amsterdam, 1972), 37–42, 169, 313–16; *Niuewe Nederlandsch biografisch woordenboek*, ed. P. C. Molhuysen *et al.* (10 vols., Leiden, 1911–37), vol. 8, cols. 71, 365, 977, 1254; M. J. French, 'Privateering and the Revolt of the Netherlands: the *watergeuzen* or Sea Beggars in Portsmouth, Gosport and the Isle of Wight 1570–1', *Proceedings of the Hampshire Field Club and Archaeological Society* 47 (1991), 171–80 (I

am grateful to Alastair Duke for calling this article to my attention); M. Delafosse, 'Les corsaires protestantes à La Rochelle (1570–1577)', *Bibliothèque de l'école des Chartes* 121 (1963), 191, 215; Spicer, 131–7.

9   Jean de Pablo, 'L'armée de mer huguenote pendant la troisième guerre de religion', *Archiv für Reformationsgeschichte* 47 (1956), 65–6, 74–6; Spicer, 133–4; Ramsay, 86.

10 BN, MS Français 20787, fo. 5; Roger Williams, *The actions of the Lowe Countries*, in *The works of Roger Williams*, ed. John X. Evans (Oxford, 1972), 138, 241n.; Sigismond di Cavalli (Venetian Ambassador to France) to the Signory, 27 May and 12 July 1573: *Calendar of state papers... in the archives and collections of Venice*, vol. 7 (London, 1890), 488–9 (nos. 550–1); [Fogaça] to Alba, 9 June 1573: *Calendar of letters and state papers... in the archives of Simancas* [hereafter *CSPSpan.*], vol. 2 (London, 1894), 470–1 (no. 386).

11 James W. Thompson, *The Wars of Religion in France 1559–1576* (Chicago, 1909), 472–3, 484–5; William Drury to Earl of Rutland, 31 March 1574: *HMC, Duke of Rutland MSS*, vol. 1 (London, 1888), 101; anon. newsletter, 5 May 1574: Universiteitsbibliotheek Leiden, MS Vulc. 104/13; Spicer, 132.

12 Community of Flushing to Elizabeth I, 20 April 1572: KL, vol. 6, 4391 (no. 2391); to the Dutch Churches of England, 26 April 1572: J. H. Hessels (ed.), *Ecclesiæ Londino-Batavæ archivum* (4 vols. in 3, Cambridge, 1887–97), vol. 2, 397–9 (no. 112); Magistrates of Flushing to Elizabeth I and Lord Burghley, May 1572: KL, vols. 6, 410 (nos. 2406–7); Diedrich Sonoy (Minister of Enkhuizen) to the Dutch Church of London, 4 and 10 July 1572: Hessels, vol. 2, 420–5 (nos. 119–20) (the latter letter refers to letters to the refugee communities of King's Lynn and Norwich which have not survived); Pettegree, *Foreign Protestant communities*, 253–5.

13 E.g. Ramsay, 176; Conyers Read, *Lord Burghley and Queen Elizabeth* (New York, 1960), 73; Geoffrey Parker, *Spain and the Netherlands, 1559–1659* (London, 1979), 212.

14 François de Sweveghem to Alba, 23 April 1572: KL, vol. 6, 395 (no. 2393); anon. report from the Netherlands, 30 April 1572: KL, vol. 6, 403 (no. 2398).

15 Antonio de Guaras to Alba, 12 May 1572: *CSPSpan.*, vol. 2, 390 (no. 327); anon. report from the Netherlands, 24 May 1572: KL, vol. 6, 412 (no. 2408); Herman Moded to the Dutch Church of London, 29 May 1572: Hessels, vol. 3:i, 166–7 (no. 195).

16 Dutch community of Ipswich to Dutch Church of London, 11 and 14 May 1572: Hessels, vol. 2, 403–4 (no. 114), 408–9 (no. 116); Dutch community of Colchester to Dutch Church of London, 12 May 1572: *ibid.*, 405–6 (no. 115).

17 Herman Moded to the Dutch community of London, 5 June 1572: Hessels, vol. 3:i, 168 (no. 197).

18 Hessels, vol. 2, 438–42 (no. 123).

19 See de Sweveghem to Alba, 23 April 1572: KL, vol. 6, 395 (no. 2393); Dutch community of Colchester to the Dutch Church of London, 12 May 1572: Hessels, vol. 2, 405 (no. 115); de Guaras to Alba, 18 May, and [Antonio Fogaça] to Alba, 22 July 1572: *CSPSpan.*, vol. 2, 391 (no. 329), 397 (no. 339); Thomas Morgan to Burghley, 16 June 1572: KL, vol. 6, 426 (no. 2414), referring to 'Englyshe men in bandes *and skateryd amonge others*' (emphasis mine); and see also Williams, 108 – 'the *Count's deputies* had sent him [the] three *English* companies', that reinforced Den Brielle in May 1572 (emphasis mine).

20 BL, Lansdowne MS 1204, fos. 114, 121v, 123; Churchyard, *Lamentable and pitifull description*, 51–2; Williams, 104.

21 Printed in Hessels, vol. 2, 399 (no. 112).

22 Claude de Mondoucet (French Ambassador in Brussels) to Charles IX, 27 April 1572, BN, MS Fr. 16127, fo. 39.

23 Williams, 108.

24 Francis Walsingham to Burghley, 21 May [1572], in *The compleat ambassador...*, ed. D. Digges (London, 1655), 202; Williams, 83–4, 87; Mondoucet to Charles IX, 4 Jan. 1573:

BN, MS Fr. 16127, fo. 126v; Thomas Churchyard, *A generall rehearsall of warres* (London, 1579), sigs. K2v-K4, and *Lamentable and pitifull description*, 51, 54; P. J. Blok (ed.), *Correspondentie van en betreffende Lodewijk van Nassau en andere onuitgegeven documenten*, Werken van het Historisch Genootshcap te Utrecht, NS 47 (Utrecht, 1887), 102.

25 KL, vol. 6, 440 (no. 2425); Devereux Papers, MS II, fo. 9. The Devereux Papers are cited by permission of the Marquess of Bath, Longleat House, Warminster, Wiltshire.

26 Algemeen Rijksarchief, The Hague [hereafter ARA], Collectie Ortell 73 (unfoliated); Williams, 108.

27 Patrick Collinson, 'John Field and Elizabethan Puritanism,' in S. T. Bindoff, J. Hurstfield and C. H. Williams (eds.), *Elizabethan government and society: essays presented to Sir John Neale* (London, 1961), 141; *idem*, 'Elizabethan Puritans and the foreign reformed churches', 528–55; and 'England and international Calvinism, 1558–1640', in Menna Prestwich (ed.), *International Calvinism 1541–1715* (Oxford, 1985), 204–9, 211–12.

28 De Guaras to Alba, 24 May 1572: *CSPSpan.*, vol. 2, 391, 394 (no. 330); [Fogaça] to Alba, 17 and 18 Nov. 1572: *ibid.*, 441 (no. 365), 447 (no. 368).

29 [Fogaça] to Alba, 16 Feb. 1573: *ibid.*, 464–65 (no. 380).

30 Daniel Rogers to Abraham Ortell, 20 Oct. 1572: Hessels, vol. 1, 101 (no. 42).

31 Jan van der Beke to the Dutch community of London, 29 Dec. 1572: Hessels, vol. 3:i, 186–7 (no. 215); Antonio de Guaras to Alba, 16 Feb. 1573: *CSPSpan.*, vol. 2, 463 (no. 379); William of Orange to the Dutch Churches in England, 26 Feb. 1573: Hessels, vol. 2, 447–53 (no. 125); and to the Dutch communities of Norwich, Thetford and Ipswich, 27 Feb. 1573: M. Gachard (ed.), *Correspondance de Guillaume le taciturne, Prince d'Orange*, vol. 3 (Brussels, 1851), 73–4 (no. 534); the Magistrates of Flushing to the Dutch community of London, 7 April 1573: Hessels, vol. 3: i, 215 (no. 238); the Magistrates of Veere to the Dutch Church of London, 7 June 1573: *ibid.*, 230 (no. 254); the Dutch community of Sandwich to the Dutch community of London, 18 June 1573: *ibid.*, 231 (no. 255); the Dutch Church of Norwich to the Dutch Church of London, 27 June 1573: *ibid.*, 232–3 (no. 257); William of Orange to the Dutch, French and Italian Churches of London, 13 Dec. 1573: *ibid.*, vol. 2, 472–5 (no. 129); and to the Dutch Church of London, 29 Dec. 1573: *ibid.*, 490–2 (no. 132). (These refer to military-related activity; the numerous cases of charitable assistance to communities in the Netherlands are excluded).

32 E.g. William of Orange to Elizabeth I, 31 March 1574: KL, vol. 7, 97 (no. 2710).

33 Parker, 35.

34 'Rekening van Maerten Ruychaver, Thesaurier in het Noorder-Kwartier, 1572/1573', ed. N. J. M. Dresch, *Bijdragen en mededeelingen van het historisch genootschap* 49 (1928), 98–9.

35 R. G. Lang (ed.), *Two Tudor subsidy assessment rolls for the City of London: 1541 and 1582*, London Record Society Publications 29 (London, 1993), 199 (I owe this reference to Brett Usher); Pullison to Joachim Ortell, 12 May and 16 June 1576: ARA, Collectie Ortell 54, unfoliated.

36 A. H. Dodd, 'Mr Myddelton the merchant of Tower Street', in *Elizabethan government and society*, 250–1, 254, 263; Collinson, 'England and international Calvinism', 211; *HMC, 2nd Report* (London, 1874; repr., Liechtenstein, 1979), 73.

37 J. Jernegan to Walsingham, 3 August (n.s.) 1583: *CSPF, Elizabeth I*, vol. 18, 36 (no. 43).

38 Ole Peter Grell, *Dutch Calvinists in early Stuart London*, PTBI, NS 11 (Leiden, 1989), 28–9.

39 Sir Robert Jermyn to William Davison, 25 Aug. 1585: Bodl., MS Tanner 78, fo. 73.

40 Simon Adams, 'A Puritan Crusade? The composition of the Earl of Leicester's expedition to the Netherlands, 1585–1586', in *The Dutch in crisis, 1585–1588: people and politics in Leicester's time* (Leiden, 1988), 23; *idem* (ed.), *Household accounts and disbursement books of Robert Dudley, Earl of Leicester, 1558–1561, 1584–1586*, Camden Miscellany, 5th ser., vol. 6 (Cambridge, 1995), 196 (n. 414).

41   R. B. Wernham, *After the Armada: Elizabethan England and the struggle for Western Europe 1588–1595* (Oxford, 1984), 36.

42   Privy Council to Lord Cobham and the Mayors of London and Norwich, 7 April 1602: *Acts of the Privy Council*, NS, vol. 32 (London, 1907), 487, 'for the leavying of voluntaries out of the Dutch congregations in the several places' – Cobham was Lord Warden of the Cinque Ports, which of course included Sandwich, Rye and Winchelsea.

43   Grell, 7; Nigel Goose, 'The "Dutch" in Colchester: the economic influence of an immigrant community in the sixteenth and seventeenth centuries', *Immigrants and Minorities* 1 (1981), 265–71.

44   I am obliged to Mark Fissel for this information, which derives from his work in the Norwich archives.

45   Compare Goose, 269.

46   Walter Bourchier Devereux (ed.), *Lives and letters of the Devereux, Earls of Essex, in the reigns of Elizabeth, James I, and Charles I 1540–1646*, vol. 2 (London, 1853), 478, 485, 491; Devereux Papers, MS I, fo. 28; BN, Fonds Clairambault 1907, fo. 133.

47   PRO, SP 12/259, fo. 179 (I owe this reference to Paul Hammer); van Meteren's *album amicorum*, Bodleian Library, MS Douce 68, fo. 42v. On van Meteren's circle, mostly comprising other Dutchmen resident in London, see J. A. van Dorsten, ' "I. C. O.": the rediscovery of a modest Dutchman in London', in J. van den Berg and Alastair Hamilton (eds.), *The Anglo-Dutch renaissance: seven essays*, PTBI, NS 10 (Leiden, 1988), 8–20.

48   Alice Clare Carter, 'Marriage counselling in the early seventeenth century: England and the Netherlands compared', in Jan van Dorsten (ed.), *Ten studies in Anglo-Dutch relations*, PTBI, general series 5 (Leiden, 1974), 94, citing Bodley to Burghley, PRO, SP 84/41, fo. 152. The registers of betrothals, marriages, citizenship, and court sentences held in the *gemeentearchief* of Leiden are printed in Johanna W. Tammel *et al.* (eds.), *The Pilgrims and other people from the British Isles in Leiden: 1576–1640* (Isle of Man, 1989).

49   Browne to Walsingham: *CSPF, Elizabeth I*, vol. 21, iv, 37.

50   G. E. Cokayne (ed.), *The complete baronetage* (Exeter, 1900–06), 61–2.

51   John Chamberlain to Dudley Carleton, 28 Feb. 1603: *The letters of John Chamberlain*, ed. N. E. McClure, Memoirs of the American Philosophical Society 12, 2 vols. (Philadelphia, 1939), vol. 1, 187 (no. 61); Cokayne, *Complete peerage*, vol. 3, 400; *DNB*, vol. 8, 1275, vol. 14, 934–5; H. F. K. van Nierop, *Van ridders tot regenten: de Hollandse adel in de zestiende en de eerste helft van de zeventiende eeuw* (2nd edn., Amsterdam, 1990), 82; Gervase Holles, *Memorials of the Holles family 1493–1656*, ed. A. C. Wood, Camden Miscellany, 3rd ser., vol. 55 (London, 1937), 84–5 at 85; Koninklijke Bibliotheek, The Hague, *handschriften*, lias 132.G.27; ARA Collectie Aanwinsten 1098, fo. 82; *HMC, De L'Isle and Dudley MSS*, vol. 2 (London, 1936), 520.

52   J. McGurk, 'Wild Geese: the Irish in European armies (sixteenth to eighteenth centuries)', in Patrick O'Sullivan (ed.), *The Irish world wide: history, heritage, identity*, vol. 1: *Patterns of migration* (Leicester, 1992), 40.

53   A. L. Rowse, *Simon Forman: sex and society in Shakespeare's age* (London, 1974), 52; Cokayne, *Complete peerage*, vol. 3, 400.

54   Robert Parker Sorlien, ed. *The diary of John Manningham of the Middle Temple 1602–1603* (Hanover, NH, 1976), 86.

55   Tammel, 32, 241, 245.

56   Van Nierop, 82–4; Morgan to Christian Huygens, 27 April 1589: ARA, Collectie Aanwinsten 593; Carter, 94; R. B. Wernham (ed.), *List and analysis of State Papers, Foreign Series, Elizabeth I*, vol. 6 (London, 1993), 101 (no. 79).

57   ARA, Collectie Aanwinsten 593. Morgan was not unique among English soldiers in Dutch pay, for though the Veres conducted all their correspondence with their Dutch paymasters in French, at least two other mercenary officers, Captain Edmund Bishop and Anthony

Slingsby also wrote in Dutch. See Bishop to William Davison, 15 April 1578: PRO, SP 83/6, fo. 19; and Slingsby's petition to the States General, 1606: ARA, Archief van Johan van Oldenbarnevelt, no. 2979.

58   Galatians 3:28.

59   8 Oct. 1572: BL, Lansdowne MS 15, fo. 199v.

60   George Silver, *Paradoxes of defense* (London, 1599) – online edition available at URL <http://www.pbm.com/~lindahl/paradoxes.html>.

61   William Bradshaw, *A myld and just defence of certeyne arguments* ... (1606), quoted by Collinson in 'England and international Calvinism', 213 and in *Birthpangs of Protestant England*, 16, and by Alastair Duke, 'Perspectives on European Calvinism', in Alastair Duke, Gilliam Lewis and Andrew Pettegree (eds.), *Calvinism in Europe, 1540–1620* (Cambridge, 1994), 1.

8

Fictitious shoemakers, agitated weavers and the limits of popular xenophobia in Elizabethan London

Joseph P. Ward

Historians of European immigrant communities in early modern England often remark on the inherent xenophobia of the English and especially of non-elite Londoners. Anne Oakley suggests that in Canterbury relations between natives and aliens were generally good, unlike 'in London where Londoners were frequently admonished for calling the strangers rude names in the streets'.[1] Ole Peter Grell finds that Queen Elizabeth periodically collected information about the size of the alien population in London in order to alleviate 'escalating xenophobia', and that the Privy Council tried to act discreetly in such matters 'to prevent general xenophobia and individual troublemakers within the host population from taking action against the immigrants'.[2] Laura Hunt Yungblut reports that among 'the central difficulties' the Elizabethan government faced when developing its policies towards immigrants was 'the fact that the English had a reputation for xenophobia'. Although she maintains that the 'twin traditions of asylum and xenophobia existed side by side', she also asserts that 'popular sentiment' was hostile to aliens because 'according to extant sources, the English, especially Londoners, actively disliked' immigrants, and notes in her conclusion that the 'unusually large number of aliens in London and other southeastern towns brought the legendary English xenophobia to the surface on many occasions'.[3]

Despite such scholarly consensus, it is worth considering how little we actually know about popular attitudes towards Continental immigrants. The evidence supporting a broadly based xenophobia consists largely of examinations of disturbances such as the Evil May Day riots in 1517, petitions from English trade guilds and other economic interest groups to the Crown asking that the immigrants not infringe upon the trading rights of natives, and plays and other literary sources that display the strangers in an unflattering light. Alongside these may be placed other evidence of a similar nature indicating that popular sentiment could view the aliens, and the societies in which they originated, far more positively. To probe further into early modern Londoners' opinions of strangers, this essay will analyse the relationship between native and alien artisans in the final years of Queen Elizabeth's reign as portrayed in two quite different texts. The first is one of the better known comedies of the era, Thomas Dekker's *The Shoemaker's Holiday*, which was first performed in London in 1599. The play has a happy ending only because it assumes cordial relations between native and alien shoemakers. However, because it is difficult to determine the extent to which a popular literary work offers an accurate portrayal of social relations during the time of its production, the discussion will then shift to a letter that several weavers sent to the elders of the French Church in London in 1595. The letter indicates that the native weavers seemed always ready to complain about aliens taking advantage of their hospitality, but that this concern came with the corollary that if the strangers would play by the economic rules laid down for them, then the Londoners would treat them kindly. Read together in this way, these two texts suggest that, rather than being inherently hostile to European immigrants, Elizabethan London artisans could have embraced them.[4]

The Shoemaker's Holiday

Literary historians have in recent years been quite interested in the topic of English national identity in the Renaissance. According to Richard Helgerson, England was coming into its own as a 'nation' in the later part of the 16th century, a development that manifested itself in a wide range of cultural productions.[5] In the theatre, Janette Dillon maintains that the representation of aliens on the English stage at the end of the 16th century demonstrated that the 'particular threat they posed was double-edged: they fought England abroad, but they also threatened jobs, housing and safety in England'. It was in response to such threats that the trade guilds of London treated the aliens with, at best, ambivalence for the 'paternalism of the London companies . . . was one side of a parochialism that sought to protect a narrowly defined community of residents by identifying its difference from those others who threatened its coherence'.[6]

For the purpose of understanding how late 16th-century English people – and especially London artisans – may have viewed aliens, one of the most compelling texts is Thomas Dekker's *The Shoemaker's Holiday*.[7] Literary and social historians have recognized it as one of the most sophisticated theatrical representations of London's artisanal world.[8] Set in the era of the 15th-century wars with France, the plot accelerates when Rowland Lacy, the heir to the Earl of Lincoln, deserts his continental regiment and returns to London disguised as the Dutch shoemaker Hans Meulter to be nearer to his true love Rose, the daughter of Lord Mayor Sir Roger Oatley. Lacy's choice of a craft is explained to the audience in an earlier conversation between Lincoln and the mayor in which the Earl mentions that Lacy was such a spendthrift that on his way to Italy as part of his grand tour he ran out of money before he had passed through Germany and was forced by necessity to work for a shoemaker [I, 16–30].

At first glance, Hans seems very much a standard alien character on the stage, but the others greet him in an unconventional manner. When he first appears, Hans is singing a Dutch song about a drunken man from Gelderland, a scene that doubtless elicited laughter from the audience. His song soon leads to Hans being offered a job as a journeyman shoemaker in the shop of Simon Eyre. Contrary to our expectations about the attitudes of English artisans towards aliens, Hans's job is secured not as a result of Eyre's desire to exploit his skill but rather at the behest of Eyre's foreman Hodge and his journeyman Firk. When Firk first glimpses Hans, he tells Eyre:

> Master, for my life, yonder's a brother of the Gentle Craft! If he bear not Saint Hugh's bones, I'll forfeit my bones. He's some uplandish workman. Hire him, good master, that I may learn some gibble-gabble. 'Twill make us work the faster. [IV, 48–52]

But the master dismisses the suggestion with the words:

> Peace, Firk. A hard world; let him pass, let him vanish. We have journeymen enough. Peace, my fine Firk. [IV, 53–54]

Soon Hodge enters the conversation, imploring Eyre that:

> 'Fore God, a proper man and, I warrant, a fine workman. Master farewell . . . If such a man as he cannot find work, Hodge is not for you. [IV, 63–65]

After further entreaties from Firk – including his own threat to leave the shop – Eyre relents and takes Hans into his employment [IV, 68–111].

This is a complicated exchange. It is unclear how seriously Dekker assumed his audience would take the pleadings of Hodge and Firk. They certainly participate in the ribaldry and mocking that typifies English attitudes towards the appearance of aliens on the stage, and yet they also seem to put their own economic positions at risk. Firk's references to Hans's language as 'gibble-gabble' indicates clearly that he recognizes Hans as an alien.[9] But it is perhaps more telling here that Firk's initial response to seeing Hans – or, perhaps, to hearing him sing – is to identify him as a 'brother of the Gentle Craft', reminiscent of the way that members of London's trade guilds commonly referred to one another.[10] By having Firk's first impression of Hans indicate the willingness of a London artisan to embrace a stranger as a 'brother', Dekker – who may have had Dutch parents himself – suggests an openness to aliens that is at odds with the common assumption of historians and literary critics that xenophobia was widespread among Elizabethan London artisans.[11]

The subsequent unfolding of the plot of Dekker's play buttresses this point, for Hans's position as an alien and his employment in Eyre's shop lead to the dramatic turns that produce the play's happy ending. Hans's connections in the Dutch community bring him wind of an opportunity to enrich his master. Discovering from a Dutch ship's captain that he has a full load of precious commodities waiting to dock in London, Hans, Firk, and Hodge help Eyre disguise himself as an alderman so that he may appear to have the necessary credit with which to buy the ship's cargo, which he subsequently sells at huge profit [VII].[12] The money he gains from his fraudulent transaction enables Eyre to launch a political career that culminates in his elevation to the mayoralty. At the end of the play, and after Lacy removes his disguise, Lord Mayor Eyre has an audience with the King in which he persuades him to forgive Lacy's disloyalty during the French war and to bless the marriage of Lacy and his beloved Rose [XXI]. Dekker's London audience may have found this plausible as well as amusing, especially because the records of London's trade guilds contain ample evidence of freemen employing a wide array of deceitful and sharp practices in the marketplace.[13] At the same time, showing a legendary lord mayor like Eyre resorting to such a connivance is at odds with the Elizabethan trend of commemorating famous citizens.[14]

Dekker's depiction of Eyre's rise to wealth and power also departs somewhat from that offered in the prose fiction writer Thomas Deloney's *The Gentle Craft, Part I* (1597), a popular work recounting the heroic and romantic adventures of shoemakers throughout history, which is considered the main source for Dekker's plot. In Deloney's version of the story, a French shoemaker living with Eyre asks him to help the ship's captain find someone to purchase the cargo, whereupon Eyre and his wife concoct the scheme involving the disguise. In Dekker's play, the ship's captain first informs Hans of the opportunity to enrich his master and then Hans turns to Firk and Hodge to convince Eyre to take advantage of the opportunity. This emphasizes the camaraderie and trust between the English and alien shoemakers that facilitate Eyre's rise to wealth and fame and, eventually, the audience with the King.[15]

In short, *The Shoemaker's Holiday* is a play that spins the stock dramatic characterization of aliens in a positive way. Not only do Dekker's fictional artisans welcome the Dutch stranger into their shop, but they then come to rely on him for the information required to make their crafty plot work. The result is happiness all round: Eyre is lord mayor, while Lacy secures the love of Rose. Notably absent from this fictitious portrayal of London artisans is the xenophobia and parochialism that historians and literary critics often have ascribed to them. The problem remains, however, to determine the extent to which a play like *The Shoemaker's Holiday* may have reflected attitudes maintained by Elizabethan artisans.

Strangers and citizens in the Weavers' Company

The Elizabethan government encouraged the immigration of skilled artisans from the Continent in order to bolster English industry. Pointing to the French Wars of Religion and the Dutch Revolt as evidence that Protestants were being persecuted on the Continent, the government adopted measures to encourage Dutch and French religious refugees to settle in England. Although the new immigrants occupied many trades, in the towns of the south-east they seemed to have a particularly noticeable influence in the textile industry. According to a list of strangers' trades in greater London from 1593, the production of cloth, including silk, was by far the largest single occupation, with just over 500 aliens employed.[16] Subsequently, London's governors worried that such large numbers of aliens might provoke a hostile reaction from the native population in the metropolis during a time of pronounced social stress that had been marked by, among other things, the unusual occurrence of food riots in June 1595. According to Ian Archer, the aldermen 'feared that the tense situation in the city might lead to further riots against the aliens, tapping a rich vein of popular xenophobia'.[17]

A letter from members of the Weavers' Company to the elders of the French Church of London in June 1595 reveals an attitude towards the aliens that is more complex than the agitation of that year may at first glance suggest. The letter appeals to the elders to encourage members of their congregation to obey the regulations governing their participation in the metropolitan economy, but it is also filled with the language of Christian brotherhood, suggesting that many London artisans could have imagined living harmoniously with the strangers. In their letter, the freemen maintain that 'The liberty which they [the aliens] have amongst us is not small nor lightly so regarded, for they are suffered, and we are content therewith . . . to keep houses and servants, to come into our City to fetch and carry their work, to buy and sell in as ample a manner as any freeman amongst us, and yet they are not satisfied'.[18] As a result of the aliens' violation of the rules governing their activities, they gain unfair advantages over native weavers, driving them out of work. The freemen continue, 'To be brief, they live not like strangers of another country, nor like obedient subjects to the laws and customs of this land nor like Christian brethren, nor like friends, nor like good neighbours'.[19] The native weavers make it clear that they are content to have the aliens in their midst if they would follow the rules of their trade, saying to the elders of the French Church: 'if you allege that strangers ought to be cherished and well entreated, we know it, and grant it, so far forth as their doings stand with the benefit of the commonwealth, so long as their life may not be our death, not their welfare our woe, so long, say we, we will nourish and tender their estates'. 'But', they suggest in an ominous tone, 'we must need count it more than common ingratitude that they, like the viper, should seek to destroy their nourishers'.[20]

To drive this point further, the freemen undertake an exercise in comparative jurisprudence. Noting that during Queen Mary's reign they found 'that in the well-governed city of Geneva, where the persecuted Englishmen fled thither, and that the Governor and the rest of the States of the city seeing the multitude of strangers daily to increase made a decree that no stranger should buy any victuals in the market before the clock had struck ten; and that the citizens were first served the like care they had'. They also report that 'the like was in many other cities in Germany, very carefully also do many cities in France and Flanders maintain their privileges, which we speak to their commendations, for as good men had never purchased privileges, as to suffer every one to infringe it'.[21] By taking this comparative approach, the native weavers not only impress upon the French Church elders the essential fairness of their position but also criticize their own governors, including the Queen. 'If it be alleged that our Queen favours strangers', they assert, 'we grant it is true, but she will favour them no further than may stand with the good estate of her loving subjects'. Having surveyed their attitudes towards the aliens, the weavers then adopt a decidedly moderate tone with their closing, in which they insist that 'we have written these our letters unto you, hoping you will use persuasions of love and agreement between them [the aliens] and us, whereby God will be well pleased, and both we and they shall the better prosper'.[22]

This letter requires anyone to pause before generalizing about the xenophobia of London artisans in 1595. This sort of letter is inherently difficult to interpret, for we have few means by which to reconstruct its context in order to gauge either the sincerity of its language or the extent to which its arguments reflect the sentiments of London artisans generally. The limited literacy rates of the time and the polished quality of its argument suggest that it was unlikely the sole work of artisan weavers.[23] Indeed, the author of *The Gentle Craft*, Thomas Deloney, who was also a silk weaver, signed the letter himself and was among those subsequently arrested for presenting the letter to the elders of the French Church.[24] Even if the letter does not express the opinions of all those who felt themselves threatened economically by the presence of aliens in London in 1595, it certainly suggests that there were London freemen who were aggrieved by the activities of many aliens in the metropolis and yet could still imagine finding a way to live alongside them peacefully. Or, to put it in the form of a rhetorical question, what sort of xenophobe would construct a letter that both extends a welcome to those aliens who would follow the rules of their trade and criticizes Queen Elizabeth for not sufficiently defending her subjects' economic interests?

Members of the London Weavers' Company were also aware that their economic positions were being undermined by the behaviour of their fellow citizens. Some of the aliens who migrated to London in the late 16th and early 17th centuries became integral parts of the metropolitan economy. Rather than trying to block this development, the Weavers' Company sought to manage it by creating new levels of company membership that enabled aliens to find employment in the shops of citizens.[25] By offering employment to a stranger, a master weaver may not have been expressing his great affection for the alien, but neither can it be assumed that the offer of employment was a manifestation of hostility. The weavers arrested in 1595 subsequently alleged that officers of the Weavers' Company ignored the regulations governing the employment of aliens in London.[26] As time passed, the company's officers gradually replaced the aliens as the primary targets of the poorer freemen's complaints. An anonymous, undated report kept among the Weavers' Company papers from the early 17th century mentions 'sundry evil minded freemen' who 'not respecting their oaths of the general good' of the City had 'for some profit to themselves, or of other sinister respects' agreed to have apprentices bound to work with themselves and then turned them over to work with 'strangers and foreigners'. These disputes culminated in the disenfranchisement of the company's beadle.[27] The co-operation of native and alien weavers in an effort to circumvent the regulations governing the weaving trade in London – reminiscent of the co-operation between Hans, Firk, and Hodge in Dekker's play – suggests that some London artisans saw it to their advantage to have immigrants in their midst.

When read alongside *The Shoemaker's Holiday*, the records of the Weavers' Company demonstrate that there were limits to the popularity of xenophobia among London's artisans. The sources discussed above clearly indicate that, in certain circumstances, the aliens could have felt welcome in London. They each suggest the possibility that natives and aliens could have belonged to a common family: the play articulates an international brotherhood of shoemakers while the weavers' text alludes to an international brotherhood of Protestants. They each further assume that some London citizens were willing to employ and to trade with the strangers. While this may not constitute xenophilia, it is something far short of xenophobia.

Historians therefore should avoid leaping to the conclusion that xenophobia was an essential characteristic of life in early modern London. There surely was, at times, considerable antipathy towards aliens among some Londoners, but even in the highly competitive economic environment of the late 16th century there was also sympathy among the non-elite for their plight as religious refugees. If, as the weavers' letter to the elders of the French Church suggests, they wanted aliens in London treated the same way the English were treated in Geneva, that would indicate their adherence to an international standard for charity and economic fair play rather than a deeply rooted aversion to all strangers. Although we cannot be certain that Dekker wrote his play in response to the criticisms sometimes directed at alien artisans in the metropolis of his day, it certainly can be viewed as an appeal by one Londoner to his audience to consider the happiness that could result from native artisans embracing their alien craft brethren.

NOTES

1 Anne M. Oakley, 'The Canterbury Walloon congregation from Elizabeth I to Laud', in Irene Scouloudi (ed.), *Huguenots in Britain and their French background, 1550–1800* (London, Totowa, NJ, 1987), 67.

2 Ole Peter Grell, *Calvinist exiles in Tudor and Stuart England* (Aldershot, 1996), 2–3.

3 Laura Hunt Yungblut, *Strangers settled here amongst us: policy, perceptions and the presence of aliens in Elizabethan England* (London, 1996), 2–3, 9, 115.

4 Throughout this essay, the aliens being discussed are immigrants from Europe who sought to settle in England. For Elizabethan attitudes towards non-European aliens, see Emily C. Bartels, *Spectacles of strangeness: imperialism, alienation, and Marlowe* (Philadelphia, 1993) and, more generally, Ivo Kamps and Jyotsna G. Singh (eds.), *Travel knowledge: European 'discoveries' in the early modern period* (New York, 2000).

5 Richard Helgerson, *Forms of nationhood: the Elizabethan writing of England* (Chicago, 1992). More recent discussions include Andrew Hadfield, 'From English to British literature: John Lyly's *Euphues* and Edmund Spenser's *The Faerie Queen*', in Brendan Bradshaw and Peter Roberts (eds.), *British consciousness and identity: the making of Britain, 1533–1707* (Cambridge, 1998), 140–58 and Willy Maley, 'The British problem in three tracts on Ireland by Spenser, Bacon and Milton', in *ibid.*, 159–84.

6 Janette Dillon, *Language and stage in medieval and Renaissance England* (Cambridge, 1998), 175–6.

7 All parenthetical references are to Thomas Dekker, *The Shoemaker's Holiday*, ed. R. L. Smallwood and Stanley Wells (Manchester, 1979).

8 David Bevington, 'Theatre as holiday', in David L. Smith, Richard Strier, and David Bevington (eds.), *The theatrical city: London's culture, theatre, and literature, 1576–1649* (Cambridge, 1995), 101–16; Paul Seaver, 'The artisanal world'', in *ibid.*, 87–100; Lawrence Manley, *Literature and culture in early modern London* (Cambridge, 1995), esp. 441–3.

9 George Evans Light, 'All hopped up: beer, cultivated national identity, and Anglo-Dutch relations, 1524–1625', *Journal x*, 2:2 (Spring 1998), 167.

10 For examples, see Ian W. Archer, *The pursuit of stability: social relations in Elizabethan London* (Cambridge, 1991), 116 and Joseph Ward, *Metropolitan communities: trade guilds, identity, and change in early modern London* (Stanford, 1997), 66.

11 Julia Gasper, *The dragon and the dove: the plays of Thomas Dekker* (Oxford, 1990), 18–20.

12 Gasper, 31–2 demonstrates that Dekker meant his audience to understand that Eyre was not an alderman when he donned the alderman's robe in order to convince the ship's captain he had sufficient credit to purchase the cargo.

13 Ward, *Metropolitan communities*, 46–57.

14 Ian W. Archer, *The history of the Haberdashers' Company* (Chichester, 1991), 74 and Joseph Ward, 'Godliness, commemoration, and community: the management of provincial schools by London trade guilds', in Muriel C. McClendon, Joseph Ward and Michael MacDonald (eds.), *Protestant identities: religion, society, and self-fashioning in post-Reformation England* (Stanford, 1999), 141–4.

15 Merritt E. Lawlis, *The novels of Thomas Deloney* (Bloomington, 1961), 142–5, 361; Smallwood and Wells (eds.), *The Shoemaker's Holiday*, 20–1.

16 Robin Gwynn, *Huguenot heritage: the history and contribution of the Huguenots in Britain* (London, 1985), 60–4; Irene Scouloudi, 'The Stranger community in the metropolis 1558–1640', in Scouloudi (ed.), *Huguenots in Britain*, 43–8; Bernard Cottret, *The*

Huguenots in England: immigration and settlement c. 1550–1700 (Cambridge, 1991), 54–65.

17 Archer, *Pursuit of Stability*, 1.

18 GL, MS 4647 (Weavers' Company Ordinance Book), 126. The spelling and capitalization is modernized from the original manuscript consulted by the author. Another transcript of this letter is printed in Frances Consitt, *The London Weavers' Company*, vol. 1 (Oxford, 1933), 312–16.

19 GL, MS 4647, 126–7.

20 *Ibid.*, 131.

21 *Ibid.*, 132.

22 *Ibid.*, 134.

23 For the drafting of petitions for London artisans see Ward, *Metropolitan Communities*, 75–83.

24 Consitt, *The London Weavers' Company*, 146–7 and Lawlis (ed.), *Novels of Thomas Deloney*, xxvii.

25 Alfred Plummer, *The London Weavers' Company 1600–1970* (London, 1972), 16–17; Charles G. D. Littleton, 'Geneva on Threadneedle Street: the French Church of London and its congregation, 1560–1625' (unpublished Ph.D. thesis, University of Michigan, 1996), 49–68, 166–90.

26 GL, MS 4647, 138.

27 *Ibid.*, 364.

9

The Dutch in Colchester in the 16th and 17th centuries: opposition and integration

Nigel Goose

Late in 1561 the Corporation of Colchester agreed that Benjamin Clere, one of the bailiffs, should treat with the Privy Council for the taking in of Dutch refugees.[1] Dutch settlers arrived in 1565, via Sandwich in Kent, numbering 55 people in 11 households. Their numbers grew slowly at first, producing an alien community of 185 by 1571, of whom 177 were Dutch. Two years later this had more than doubled to 431, no doubt a product of the economic dislocation that afflicted the Low Countries in the early 1570s, but the real influx was yet to come, for by 1586 a total of 1,291 Dutch settlers were present in the town. As in late 16th-century London, some individuals returned home, some new settlers arrived, and it is impossible to trace detailed fluctuations in the size of the community over time. Nevertheless, a return of 1616 records 1,271, another of 1622 lists 1,535, whilst the average number of baptisms in the Dutch church during the mid-17th century, on a conservative estimate, suggests a total population of around 1,500.[2]

These numbers take on more significance in the context of the size of the settlement they joined. London would have swallowed them up, but not so Colchester. Unfortunately Colchester is as bereft of useful demographic data as almost any early modern town, and therefore estimates of its population are particularly tenuous. Nevertheless, a list of 'inhabitants swearing fealty' to the Crown of 1534 suggests a total in the region of 3700. By the 1570s, the baptism data surviving for six of the 16 parishes suggests a total of *circa* 4200, excluding the Dutch settlers, whilst a similar calculation for the 1620s indicates that considerable growth had been achieved, producing a total of *circa* 9600, again excluding the Dutch.[3] In the very early years, therefore, the Dutch community was little more than a makeweight to the indigenous population, but within ten years there was approximately one immigrant to every ten native English. Ten years later the situation had been transformed, for by the mid-1580s, although the indigenous population was now growing steadily too, the Dutch formed over 20 per cent of the town's population, and thus there was one immigrant for every four native English residents. As a proportion of the total, as the town expanded in the later 16th and early 17th century, their significance declined, but still by the 1620s some 14 per cent of the town's population were Dutch. They congregated most heavily in the parish of St Peter where the Dutch Bay Hall was established, but were found in at least eight other parishes.[4] Through from the 1580s, therefore, the Dutch settlers constituted a significant section of the town's population, a section that in the context of a town of up to 11,000 inhabitants must have been highly visible, and inevitably influential in many different ways.

How did they fit in? It is impossible to discuss the question of integration of immigrant communities without also discussing the question of opposition to them, its provenance, its nature, its extent and its implications. Here we must grasp a somewhat controversial nettle, and consider the nature of the reaction they provoked.

There are good reasons to expect that the Dutch would have been warmly welcomed, and equally good reasons to expect difficulties. Dutch settlers were by no means new to the town in the 1560s. In the Exchequer lay subsidies of 1524–5, as many as 103 of the 996 individuals named in either one or both of the returns were distinguished as aliens. Most were of modest means, but a few were relatively wealthy, including James Godfrey, beerbrewer, of St Leonard's parish, born in the Gelderland, assessed on £63 in goods in 1524 and £50 in 1525, or Anthony Jacob of the same parish, assessed on £30 in goods in 1524 and £24 in 1525.[5] A list of inhabitants 'sworn in the tithing of the king' at the Law Hundred held in 1521 includes 38 aliens out of a total of 445, whilst a smaller number, many clearly of Low Countries origins, are identified in the 1534 list.[6] This is unsurprising, given geographical proximity, the existence of direct trading links and the fact that the German Hanseatic merchants trading to Colchester in the 15th century often made use of Dutch ships.[7] Indeed, Dutchmen can be found entering the freedom of the town in the 15th and the early 16th centuries. Anthony Jacob again, born at Flushing, was admitted as a burgess in 1513 for the standard fine of 20s, as were Roger Godfrey and Richard Shelbury in 1519, whilst six were admitted in the 1550s.[8] Richard Shelbury appears amongst the town officers in 1533–4 as a keybearer, but only briefly, for the court roll records that he was excused office on payment of a 40s fine.[9] Wynken Greenrice, born in Gelderland and admitted in 1538, was to rise to prominence in the 1550s as a councillor, holding the onerous office of chamberlain in the year 1557/8.[10] So Dutch residents were familiar in the town, it had long been considered appropriate for them to enjoy the privileges that the freedom conveyed, and it was by no means unknown for them to achieve considerable economic, and even occasionally political, success.

The settlers who arrived in the 1560s, of course, were Protestant refugees, 'banished for godes word' as the original invitation reads.[11] Colchester had long been a centre of Lollardy, but despite evidence of notable schismatism the leading townsmen were cautious and ambivalent in their early response to the Reformation.[12] Nevertheless, following the Elizabethan settlement there is evidence of greater enthusiasm for the Reformed church, symbolized by the appointment of a town preacher in 1561, 'to the increase of God's glory and maintenance of his word', reinforced the year following by an order that 'every week upon the Friday when the common preacher shall make any sermon there shall be of every household within the town one person at the least at the same sermon as well for their edifying as for good example and comfort of the preacher'.[13] This clearly helped to bridge any potential religious gulf between the indigenous population, or at least its leadership, and the Dutch. In religious terms, therefore, the Dutch were most acceptable, and the establishment of their church in the town was unproblematic.

We must also remember that the Dutch, far from being unwelcome refugees, were *invited* to settle in Colchester. The economy of Colchester towards the middle of the 16th century was in the process of readjustment. Cloth production had long been central to the town's economy, employing 30 per cent of the occupied male population in the early 16th century, but by mid-century this had fallen to just 18 per cent, and lack of employment found expression in a threatened uprising in 1566.[14] Compulsory rating for poor relief was introduced in 1557, besides voluntary collections at sermons in 1561, and a new hospital was erected in the early 1570s.[15] Eastern coastal trade was expanding in the early 16th century and Colchester may have shared in this, while more intensive regulation of internal trade in the 1550s and 1560s might also indicate expansion here too. The 1550s saw a substantial increase in the number of burgesses purchasing the freedom, though interestingly only 16 per cent of those admitted between 1550 and 1570 were textile workers.[16] Perhaps like Norwich, as its textile industry waned, the town was reorienting towards greater reliance on its trading role.[17] All of this notwithstanding, declining cloth production was bound to exacerbate unemployment and poverty, for the industry was highly labour intensive, and the Corporation had little doubt that the introduction of the Dutch settlers would bring economic benefits.[18]

This was the key point that was returned to time and again: the Dutch brought economic benefits through the introduction of the lighter, cheaper cloths known collectively as the 'new draperies', and provided employment for the poor. Indeed, when a group of settlers transplanted from Colchester to Halstead by an order of 1576 returned to the town, Halstead petitioned Walsingham for their return to continue their baymaking, claiming that their departure had impoverished the neighbourhood, and eight similar petitions were issued from surrounding parishes.[19] In Colchester itself, in 1580 Nicholas Chalyner and Robert Lewis, preachers, along with Robert Searle and Robert Monke, wrote to Walsingham in defence of the Dutch, emphasizing their civility, honesty and godly behaviour, but also the advantages to the town in terms of the employment created.[20] In 1603 a letter written on behalf of the Dutch congregation to Sir Thomas Lucas emphasized the benefits produced by bringing new manufactures to the town.[21] In 1607 the bailiffs wrote to the Earl of Salisbury in support of a petition from the Dutch merchants objecting to the proposed imposition of a double subsidy on the new draperies, arguing that this would lead them to leave off their trade, 'and many poor people will be very much distressed for want of work, which now they have by reason of that trade'.[22] The Letters Patent to the Dutch community in Colchester issued by James I in 1612 also stressed 'how beneficial the strangers of the Dutch congregation had been and were unto the said town, as well as in replenishing and beautifying it, as for their trades which they daily use there, setting on work many of his poor people and subjects both within the said town and in other towns and places thereabouts . . . '.[23]

These benefits were undeniable. On the back of the new draperies, the Colchester cloth industry experienced a remarkable revival, until by the early 17th century the textile industry accounted for as much as 37 per cent of the occupied male population of the town, whilst the leading occupation was that of baymaker.[24] Evidence from fines paid to the Dutch Bay Hall for faulty workmanship suggest production continued to grow in the 17th century, reaching a peak in the 1680s.[25] Overseas trade also expanded considerably, based largely upon the growing volume of new drapery exports to the Low Countries, whilst imports also grew and diversified.[26] There is no doubt that, despite short term setbacks, the Colchester economy prospered in the later 16th and 17th centuries, permitting the substantial growth in population noted above. This is why the Dutch were granted substantial economic privileges and authority in the town, and why, in the face of all complaints, they were given fair hearing, were protected, and had their privileges upheld.

But it was inevitable too that there would be difficulties. The sheer scale of the influx in the 1570s and early 1580s must be appreciated, roughly an additional 1,000 residents in a town that previously had only housed some 4,000. This was an enormous proportional increase by any standards, suggesting there must have been at least some spare capacity in the town for it to be able to cope. It is hardly surprising that this created problems and generated fears amongst some of the indigenous population, and the first of a string of complaints issued in 1575 concerned the increase in levels of rent that their numbers caused.[27] The sheer pressure of numbers by 1580 led the Corporation to issue an order against further increase, and required the removal of all who were not members of the Dutch congregation or had arrived within the past fortnight. No more were to be admitted without written consent of the aldermen and bailiffs, for 'there are a great number of strangers inhabiting within this town pre-supposed more than the town can well sustain and bear'.[28] This was a similar situation to that at Sandwich, a smaller town still that was almost overwhelmed by the scale of immigration in the 1570s, leading to much more drastic action to reduce the number of settlers.[29] Still, at Colchester, even on this occasion voices were raised on their behalf, and no wholesale expulsion resulted.

This was by no means the last time complaint was voiced against the Dutch, but it was the last occasion upon which there was any suggestion of expulsion. In times of economic difficulty the Dutch provided useful scapegoats, particularly for the poorer residents of the town, whilst the growing confidence of the indigenous population as they absorbed the skills learned from the Dutch and established their own regulatory organizations inevitably led to competition. But while both the Corporation and the Privy Council listened to these complaints, they acted with an even-handedness that left their privileges essentially intact: for example in 1631 when it was ordered that the Dutch were to be allowed to continue to search and seal bays and says at the Dutch Bay Hall, but not new textile stuffs, which were to be searched and sealed at the English hall.[30] Furthermore, it is undoubtedly true that the influx of strangers to Colchester helped fuel the fires of inflation, as rents and food prices steadily rose into the 17th century.[31]

But it was not only the Dutch strangers that exacerbated the inflationary trends of the period: this was due to population growth generally and internal migration as much as from overseas. Time and again *English* strangers were targeted by the authorities: injunctions against incomers – particularly poor incomers – abound in the Corporation records, as do injunctions against craftsmen practising without serving proper apprenticeships or purchasing the freedom, unlicensed trading, forestalling and regrating, and trading outside the official town markets.[32] Amongst the complaints issued against the Dutch in 1631, it was suggested that they bought up bays and says by agreement without bringing them to the public market, and also bought commodities in inns and other private places.[33] But this is a theme that finds an echo in corporation records up and down the country in this period, the vast majority of which had no experience at all of foreign settlements.[34]

It would be a gross injustice, therefore, to characterize the English reaction to the Dutch as xenophobic. Time and again their privileges were upheld, and they were defended from the unfair criticism that occasionally arose from small sections of the population. In the complaints levelled at them, there was no overarching distaste for foreigners, merely a concern that they played by the rules laid down and observed the same regulations that were imposed upon the indigenous population, both long term residents and new migrants from the English countryside.

Full integration of the Dutch community was a long process, operating on many levels. Economic integration came quickly, as the establishment of the Dutch as over-seers and regulators of production of the new draperies was the very essence of their settlement. Although not their sole economic activity, and they quickly also estab-lished themselves as market gardeners and later as tailors, cardmakers, and furniture makers amongst other occupations, this was the fundamental contribution that wedded them to the Colchester economy. There is no doubt that, despite the occasional complaint that they kept their secrets to themselves, their skills were quickly disseminated through the town's population. From 1579 apprentice in-dentures are regularly recorded in the town's Court Rolls and Books, and Dutch baymakers feature almost immediately amongst the masters taking apprentices: for example, Richard Bassana in 1584; William Strickson in 1585 and 1586; and Hugh de Lobell in 1585, 1590, 1594 and 1598, de Lobell having been admitted to the freedom in 1582. He was not alone in this: William Grewynkhoff was admitted in 1590 to sell aquavita and other 'waters', soap and candles.[35]

The Dutch also established themselves quickly in overseas trade, being charged 14s 6d per exported shortcloth from 1604 compared to the 6s 8d paid by English merchants.[36] Trade with Holland, particularly Rotterdam, quickly became central to the town, and if Colchester merchants rarely became substantial operators in their own right, Dutch factors resident in Colchester were active on behalf of more substantial merchants based in London, or in Holland and Zeeland.[37] In 1605 strangers paid £350 10s customs on the double and single bays they exported from Colchester, a figure well over half the average amount paid by all merchants in 1608, 1611 and 1613.[38] Economic success quickly followed, and Dutch settlers were soon to feature amongst the wealthier members of Colchester society. As early as 1630 Francis Pollard, saymaker, bequeathed over £520 in cash legacies, whilst eight years later Francis Hockee left £660 in cash to his children. Later in the century more substantial bequests still were being made by members of the congregation.[39]

Political assimilation was to follow, but far more slowly. A small step in this direc-tion was made by granting the freedom to some members of the congregation, and it was not long before second generation Dutch were following suit, such as Samuel De Hame, loommaker, born in Colchester, admitted for the rather large sum of £4 in 1618.[40] A steady flow of Dutch burgesses followed, including James Dehame in 1630, Simon Drybutter in 1631, later assessed at £80 towards the fine imposed by Fairfax after the siege of Colchester in 1648, Jacob Burkin in 1642 who paid £400 after the siege, Isaac Degrave in 1660 and John Debart in 1669.[41] It was not essential for the Dutch to become freemen, for an annual payment of £60 covered their collective 'foreign fines',[42] but becoming a free burgess did, at least in theory, give greater economic freedom besides a small degree of political purchase. It is equally clear, however, that purchasing the freedom was by no means necessary to economic success: Charles Tayspill, assessed in 1648 at the huge sum of £485, had gained the freedom in 1642, but George Tayspill, assessed at £500, does not appear to have done so, and nor had Francis Tayspill, assessed at £250.[43]

The proportion of the stranger community purchasing the freedom is unknown, but it does appear that involvement in borough politics remained marginal to their interests until the 18th century. A complete examination has been made of the membership of the corporation of Colchester in the 137 years between 1576 and 1713 which, across this period, comprised either two bailiffs or (from 1635) a mayor, 8–12 aldermen and generally 32 subordinate officers (rising to 36 in the early 18th century), the latter constituting two tiers of the common council.[44] Wynken Grenerice, 'cordiner', was listed in 1571 as a denizen resident in Colchester for about 46 years, and continued to serve the town, as a common councillor on the first tier of the council, from 1577 until 1585 when he died.[45] His will shows little sign of his Dutch origins: he held several tenements in Colchester, a house and lands at Ardleigh, was brother-in-law to George Northey, common preacher of the town, and left £5 to the poor.[46] For the next Dutch representative on the council we have to wait until October 1599 when Hugh de Lobell appears on the first tier of the common council, serving for five years through to September 1604, an unusually short term.[47] When he drew his will in 1621, aged about 72, his continued attachment to the Dutch congregation is reflected in a bequest of £2 to the Dutch poor, and through mention of Jonas Proost, minister of the congregation.[48] After de Lobell, there is no sign of Dutch representation on the Corporation for over 50 years. Indeed, the appearance of the next representative, Andrew Fromanteel in 1659, coincided with the issue of a new charter, serious parliamentary interference in the town's government, and a shake out of all of those deemed to have neglected their duties. Fromanteel became an assistant in July 1659, the first tier of the common council, but was quickly elevated to alderman by January 1660.[49] In January 1660 also Francis Pollard appears as a common councillor, only to disappear again after 29 July 1662, another year in which there was a considerable shake up of the Corporation's membership.[50] Pollard was a man of considerable wealth: in 1670 he left cash bequests in excess of £1,300, lands in Fordham and West Bergholt, £5 to the poor of St James and £3 to the Dutch poor.[51] Andrew Fromanteel junior appears as a common councillor in August 1663, graduating to the position of assistant by August 1667, just two months before his father was elected mayor. After his term of office as mayor, Andrew Fromanteel senior remained an alderman until his death in 1672/3, whilst his son was never promoted above the level of assistant, a position he held until 1684, three years before his death, and another year of political controversy in the town and considerable turnover amongst the Corporation.[52]

No further Dutch representative can be found until the turn of the century, and it is only then, almost 140 years after their original settlement, that they begin to appear more regularly. The Tayspill family had long been prominent in the town, and were amongst the wealthiest inhabitants. John Tayspill the elder bequeathed cash legacies in excess of £2200 in 1657, besides a number of tenements in St Botolph's; George Tayspill in 1666 also left £2200, plus another £1000 if his wife was to bear a child within eight months.[53] But it was not until August 1703 that Michael Tayspill junior and

Benjamin Tayspill were elected to the common council, Michael being quickly elevated to the position of assistant in the following year. Thomas Benne joined them in 1704, immediately rising from common councillor to assistant, whilst Jacob Valender also became a councillor in that year. Other Dutch names to shortly appear include Charles De Boys in 1706, and Peter and John Hendrikx in 1708 and 1709.[54] For the appearance of Isaac Rebow, Sir Isaac from 1693, we have to wait until 1714, for although he was MP for the town in 1694, he held no office until 20 years later when he was rushed through in one day from common councillor to alderman, graduating to mayor in 1716.[55]

Political assimilation, therefore, was remarkably slow. The Dutch, occasional exceptions notwithstanding, appear to have shown little interest in participating in local government until well over a century after their arrival. It was not only in terms of office holding that this appears to be true. When the first contested parliamentary election was held in Colchester in 1654, the names of all 200 who voted are recorded in the town's Assembly Book. Of these, a mere 14 names can be identified as Dutch, just 7 per cent, only half of what one might expect given the size of the Dutch Community, and excluding many wealthy members of the Congregation.[56] Perhaps it was only as the Congregation itself waned in the later 17th century, indicated by the declining numbers of baptisms in the Dutch Church, that they turned to alternative hierarchies of power and influence, or perhaps it was a product of their decreasing ability to control the bay trade, resulting eventually in the closure of the Dutch Bay Hall in 1728.[57] The rise of Whig and Tory factions within the town may also have been influential, allied to the considerable extension of the franchise that this rivalry produced.[58] Another possibility, of course, is that the Dutch had more sense than to waste their energies on local politics, preferring to get on with the much more important business of making money, an undertaking at which they were remarkably successful – arguably in itself both cause and effect of their failure to be distracted by involvement in local government.

Finally we can turn to demographic integration. Despite the considerable comings and goings amongst the Dutch in the later 16th century, there is little doubt that they intended to settle. The earlier listings reveal a mixed community, comprising family men, their wives, children and occasionally servants too, many in their 30s and 40s.[59] The 1573 list includes 208 men and their wives, 200 children and 23 servants.[60] This was a community on the move and in the making, a fact further underlined by the rapidity with which their numbers increased. Hence of the 1,291 strangers listed in 1586, whilst 176 are identified as 'children born out of the realm' as many as 504 are listed as 'children born in the realm'.[61] Likewise in 1622, of the 1,535 strangers just 234 are described as 'householders, aliens', 379 as 'householders inborn of Dutch parents', 798 as 'children born here' and 124 as 'men and maidservants born here'.[62] The Dutch had come to settle, and by the 1640s they were producing children at the rate of over 48 on average per year.[63]

Whilst the Dutch community were contributing to the natural growth of Colchester's population, they also shared in another aspect of the urban demographic experience: the relationship between migration, poverty and mortality. Although Colchester appears to have achieved a small natural surplus of baptisms over burials across the later 16th and early 17th centuries as a whole, some parishes suffered more unfavourable demographic conditions.[64] One of these was St Botolph, where a natural deficit rather than a surplus was the common experience, and plague impacted with frequency and ferocity. The Hearth Tax of 1674 shows that St Botolph contained more than its share of poorer inhabitants, a fact endorsed by the Corporation's instruction that All Saints parish should contribute towards the relief of its poor.[65] During the 1620s and 1630s the St Botolph parish register, quite unusually, identifies the poor that were buried here, and frequently also identifies children, widows and the Dutch, as well as many occupations.[66] 'Poor weavers' – the predominant Dutch occupation according to the listing of 1622 – feature very prominently, whilst the register amply testifies to the high level of child mortality experienced in this parish, affecting both Dutch and English alike. In periods of crisis mortality, notably the plague outbreak that racked up mortality levels in 1625–6, the Dutch feature particularly prominently. In 1616 roughly half the Dutch population lived in St Peter's, which would mean that the level of concentration in others parishes in the town was far less than the 14 per cent calculated for the town as a whole in 1622. Nevertheless, taking the period from January 1625 to December 1626 inclusive, over 13 per cent of burials in St Botolph were burials of Dutch inhabitants.

More interesting still, in the peak months of mortality from September to December 1626, the Dutch constituted 23 per cent of the total number buried. It is possible that these high levels of mortality amongst both children and the Dutch may reflect a greater vulnerability to plague and other diseases produced by a shorter opportunity to acquire immunity, and this may have been an experience they shared with recent migrants from the English countryside. What is certain, however, is that whilst the Dutch baymakers and merchants waxed rich in circumstances propitious for economic growth, the Dutch community contained its share of poor just as did the English, and their demographic experience, particularly their vulnerability to plague, was of a kind with that of the native poor.

A more welcome form of demographic integration for the Dutch was inter-marriage. In the early years this may have been frowned upon: when Abraham de Horne married an English woman, apparently the first of the Dutch congregation so to do, it was said that his fellow countrymen were almost prepared to disown him.[67] But attitudes and hence practices changed over time, and the surnames of Dutchmen's daughters mentioned in extant wills provide a useful benchmark. Of 35 married daughters identified in wills proved before 1660 only five appear to have married outside their own community; but of 34 identified between 1660 and 1700 as many as 12 did so.[68] Marital integration thus proceeded slowly, but wills reflect predominantly the experience of the relatively wealthy, where one might expect to find a higher degree of endogamy than amongst the poor.

Many examples can be found of the continuing strength of the bonds within the Dutch community: for example, the will of John Rebow, father of Sir Isaac, proved 1699, bequeathed £100 to the poor of the Dutch congregation but just £10 to the poor of St Mary at the Walls where he lived. He also names the Dutchman Abraham Hedgethorne his executor, and mentions the Dutchman Abraham Langley as his book-keeper, whilst his sister-in-law, Sarah Tayspill, was a member of another prom-inent Dutch family, as was the occupant of one of his tenements and near neighbour Charles Tayspill.[69] Other wills show greater signs of integration: in 1687 Andrew Fromanteel left £5 to the Dutch congregation, but also £5 each to the parishes of St Martin and St Nicholas for the use of their poor, whilst at least one of his three executors, Thomas Reuse, gentleman, was English.[70] Reuse (or Ruse) in turn, when he wrote his will in 1688, named the Englishman William Mott of Colchester, esquire, as one executor but the Dutchman John Rebow of Colchester, merchant, as another.[71] If by this time there are distinct signs of demographic and social integration amongst the will-leaving population, one might expect it to have proceeded further lower down the social scale, where potential marriage partners were more numerous and the protection of assets cannot have been such an important consideration.

Integration, therefore, can be viewed from a range of perspectives. It is a multi-layered process, not monolithic and all-embracing. Depending upon which aspect of the process one examines, the depth and the speed of integration of any immigrant community is likely to vary considerably: in the case of the Dutch in Colchester, in some respects it was extremely rapid, in others remarkably slow. Economic integration proceeded with great speed, and was the essential feature of the Dutch presence from their own and the host community's point of view, both very sensibly operating according to the principle of enlightened self-interest, and each benefiting accordingly from the level of tolerance that that principle required. The more formal aspects of economic integration were not essential to this: acquiring the freedom of the town was not necessary to Dutch economic success, and accepting the authority of the Dutch Bay Hall as a separate hierarchy of authority was good for the reputation and hence prosperity of the town as a whole. The Dutch were, however, expected to operate according to accepted standards, their privileges notwithstanding, and were required to conform to the basic economic regulations that bound all who worked and traded in the town; in this respect, they were being treated no differently from any other inhabitant.

Demographic integration can be viewed on three levels. First, it is clear the Dutch came to settle, to set up homes and to raise children. Second, they quickly came to share the demographic experiences of the native population, perhaps particularly the strong association that existed between poverty and plague. Third, demographic integration via intermarriage came more slowly, and – for the will-leaving stratum of the population at least – appears to have become common only towards the latter part of the 17th century. Political integration was slowest of all, and the paucity of Dutch representatives on the Corporation of the town throughout the 17th century, despite their notable economic success, is quite startling. It was not until the early 18th century that this was to change, some 140 years after their original settlement, when we can begin to identify a real sea change, a change that can be detected too in the waning significance of the Dutch church as a place to baptize children, in greater social integration between the Dutch and native elite, and shortly too in the demise of both the Dutch Bay Hall and the Dutch church. As the Dutch finally either decided, or were enabled, to breach the barriers to full participation in the local government of Colchester, their alternative hierarchies of authority and influence fell to the ground. Integration had operated on many different levels for decades, but only then, a century and a half after their arrival, was it complete.

NOTES

1   Colchester Record Office (hereafter CRO), Liber Ordinacionum, fo. 92, 24 Nov. 4 Eliz.
2   For sources for these totals see N. Goose, 'The "Dutch" in Colchester: the economic

influence of an immigrant community in the 16th and 17th centuries', *Immigrants and Minorities* 1 (1982), 263; for 1616, P. Morant, *The history and antiquities of the county of Essex*, 2 vols. (London, 1768), vol. 1, 78.

3   N. Goose, 'Economic and social aspects of provincial towns: a comparative study of Cambridge, Colchester and Reading, *c.* 1500–1700', unpublished D. Phil. thesis, University of Cambridge, 1984, 248–51.

4   The Exchequer lay subsidy of 1598 indicates the presence of at least one alien taxpayer in every parish but one: Public Record Office (hereafter PRO), E179/111/532.

5   PRO, E179/108/147; E179/108/162; E179/108/169.

6   W. G. Benham (ed.), *The Red Paper Book of Colchester* (Colchester, 1902), 85–92.

7   R. H. Britnell, *Growth and decline in Colchester, 1300–1525* (Cambridge, 1986), 174.

8   CRO, D/B 5, Court Rolls 4 HVIII, 11 HVIII, 3 & 4 EdwVI – 1 & 2 Eliz.

9   CRO, D/B 5, Court Roll 25 & 26 HVIII.

10 CRO, D/B 5, Court Rolls 29 & 30 HVIII; 4 & 5 Ph & M.

11 CRO, Liber Ordinacionum, fo. 92, 24 Nov. 4 Eliz.

12 T. Cromwell, *History and description of the ancient town and borough of Colchester*, vol. 1 (London, 1825), 80; J. C. Ward, 'The Reformation in Colchester, 1528–1558', *Essex Archaeology and History* 15 (1983), 84–5; L. Higgs, 'Wills and religious mentality in Tudor Colchester', *Essex Archaeology and History* 22 (1991), 87–100.

13 CRO, Liber Ordinacionum, fos. 83, 86, n.d. and 16 April 1562. For a valuable general appraisal see M. S. Byford, 'The price of Protestantism. Assessing the impact of religious change on Elizabethan Essex: the cases of Heydon and Colchester, 1558–1594', unpublished D. Phil. thesis, University of Oxford, 1988.

14 Occupational analysis from an examination of all Archdeaconry, Consistory and Prerogative Court wills: Goose, 'Economic and social aspects', 159–70; J. S. Cockburn (ed.), *Calendar of Assize records: Essex indictments, Elizabeth I* (London, 1978), 51.

15 CRO, Liber Ordinacionum, fo. 94, 24 Nov. 5 Eliz.; Goose, 'The "Dutch" in Colchester', 265 and refs. therein.

16 CRO, D/B 5, Court Rolls, 3 & 4 EdwVI – 1 & 2 Eliz I.

17 J. Pound, 'The social and trade structure of Norwich, 1525–75', reprinted in P. Clark (ed.), *The early modern town* (London, 1976), 138.

18 For a fuller discussion of the town's economy in this period see N. Goose and J. Cooper, *Tudor and Stuart Colchester* (Chelmsford, 1998), 78–81.

19 *CSPD 1547–80*, 525, 697; *Acts of the Privy Council 1575–77*, 161–2, *APC 1589–90*, 276–7, *APC 1590*, 127–8.

20 PRO, SPD 12/144/18.

21 *Acts of the Privy Council 1601–4*, 506; BL, Add. Ms. 11404.

22 PRO, SPD 14/26/4.

23 Cromwell, vol. 2, 287.

24 Goose and Cooper, Table I, 77 and 81–2.

25 *Ibid.*, Table III, 83.

26 *Ibid.*, 84–7.

27 PRO, SPD 12/103/34.

28 CRO, D/B 5 Gb1, Assembly Book, 17 Oct. 1580.

29 M. Backhouse, *The Flemish and Walloon communities at Sandwich during the reign of Elizabeth I (1561–1603)* (Brussels, 1995), 35–6.

30 PRO, SPD 16/208/58.

31 As noted in 1591: PRO, SPD 12/240/115.

32 Goose, 'Economic and social aspects', 366–9; Goose and Cooper, 93–6.

33 PRO, SPD 16/206/58.

34 A. Everitt, 'The marketing of agricultural produce', in J. Thirsk (ed.), *The Agrarian History of England and Wales* vol. 4: *1540–1640* (Cambridge, 1967).

35 CRO, D/B 5, Court Rolls 28 & 29 Eliz, 29 & 30 Eliz, 35 & 36 Eliz, 41 & 42 Eliz.

36 PRO, SPD 122/173/3.

37 PRO, SPD 14/105/114.

38 PRO SPD 14/17/66; and calculated from W. B. Stephens, 'The cloth exports of the provincial ports, 1600–40', *Economic History Review* 22 (1969), 245.

39 Goose and Cooper, 99 n.7.

40 CRO, D/B 5, Court Rolls 15 & 16 Jas. I.

41 CRO, Thursday Court Book 1630–1; Monday Court Book 1660; D/B 5 Gb6, Assembly Book 1693–1712, Index of Free Burgesses; HSQS 12, 137.

42 CRO, D/B 5 Gb2, Assembly Book 1600–20, 23 September 1617.

43 CRO, D/B 5 Gb6, Assembly Book 1693–1712, Index of Free Burgesses; Moens, 137.

44 CRO, D/B 5 Gb1–6, Assembly Books 1576–1712.

45 Moens, 95; CRO, D/B 5, Gb1, Assembly Book 1576–99.

46 CRO, D/A BW 16/275, Commissary Court of London, will of Wynken Greenrice, St Nicholas parish, Colchester, 1585.

47 CRO, D/B 5 Gb1–2, Assembly Books 1576–99 and 1600–20.

48 CRO, D/A CW 9/69, Archdeaconry of Essex, will of Hugh de Lobell, merchant, St Giles, Colchester, 1621.

49 CRO, CRO, D/B 5 Gb4, Assembly Book 1646–66, July 1659–Jan. 1660.

50 CRO, CRO, D/B 5 Gb4, Assembly Book 1646–66, Jan. 1660–Aug. 1662.

51 PRO, PCC wills, Francis Pollard, saymaker, St James, Colchester, proved September 1670.

52 CRO, D/B 5 Gb4–5, Assembly Books 1646–66, 1666–92.

53 PRO, PCC wills, John Tayspill the elder, saymaker, Colchester, proved 1657; George Tayspill, saymaker, proved April 1666.

54 CRO, D/B 5 Gb6, Assembly Book 1693–1712.

55 Personal communication, Dr Janet Cooper, Victoria County History, Essex.

56 CRO, D/B 5 Gb4, Assembly Book 1646–66, 4 July 1654.

57 J. Cooper (ed.), *The Victoria History of the county of Essex*, Vol. 9: *The borough of Colchester* (Oxford, 1994), 135–6.

58 See, for instance, CRO, D/B 5 Gb6, Assembly Book 1693–1712, 22/24 March 1696, where well over 2000 free burgesses are listed.

59 PRO, SPD 12/78/9.

60 Moens, 102–5.

61 PRO, SPD 12/190/2.

62 PRO, SPD 14/129/70.

63 Calculated from Moens, 1–10.

64 Goose, 'Economic and social aspects', 263–7.

65 PRO, E179/246/22; CRO, Morant MSS, D/Y 2/2, 41.

66 CRO, D/P 203/1/1.

67 L. F. Roker, 'The Flemish and Dutch community in Colchester in the 16th and 17th centuries', *HSP* 21 (1965), 24.

68 Goose, 'The "Dutch" in Colchester', 272.

69 PRO, PCC wills, John Rebow, merchant, St Mary at the Walls, Colchester, proved May 1699.

70 PRO, PCC wills, Andrew Fromanteel, St Martin's, Colchester, proved October 1687.

71 PRO, PCC wills, Thomas Reuse (Ruse), gentleman, St Nicholas, Colchester, drawn up Feb. 1688, proved June 1693.

10

'Mayntayninge the indigente and nedie': the institutionalization of social responsibility in the case of the resident alien communities in Elizabethan Norwich and Colchester

LAURA HUNT YUNGBLUT

The development of institutionalized charity in Elizabethan England has received increasing attention over the past two decades as part of a movement among social historians examining the origins of the welfare state in the formative traumas of the early modern period. This paper is a preliminary study for future work which will seek to increase understanding in this area by examining both the role of the resident alien communities in the development of poor relief policy in Elizabethan England and their place in the native landscape on the same issue.[1] The discussion centres on expectations of alien responsibilities from the perspectives of both the English and the aliens themselves, the latter's paradoxical inclusion in and exclusion from the implementation of poor relief, and the influence of the aliens on municipal poor relief solutions. A comparison of the poor relief systems of the Reformed congregations and emerging municipal schemes in Elizabethan Norwich and Colchester strongly suggests the possibility that the former had more influence on the latter than may have been previously credited.

The reign of Elizabeth I is famous for the development of a national poor law, which owed much of its inspiration to local experiments. Compulsory taxes for the poor were tried as temporary expedients in London, Norwich, Ipswich and York in the 1540s and 1550s, with Norwich establishing a permanent scheme of poor relief in 1570. As is well known, this earliest of the permanent local schemes included a detailed survey by parish residence of the city's poor, an attempt to delineate between classes of poor (the impotent poor, the labouring poor, and the able but wilfully unemployed), an increase in poor rates, expedients to find employment for the able poor, and detailed administrative procedures for implementation of the aforementioned measures.[2] In these details remarkable similarities to the poor relief practised by the stranger churches in England can be found, similarities which beg the question of how much inspiration native municipal authorities drew from the refugees.

Arrival of the aliens

Aliens fled to England in rapidly increasing numbers in the second half of the 16th century, largely (but not exclusively) to escape the disruptions caused by the civil-religious wars on the Continent. Despite the concerns over the size of the influx, Elizabeth I's government permitted the settlement of large numbers of aliens and actively worked to integrate them into several English cities and towns in the hope that the new skills they brought would stimulate the economy.[3] Many of the aliens did prosper by introducing new commodities, but many were poor. Only a small proportion arrived with substantial possessions, either due to the circumstances of their departure from their homelands or to their belief that their migration was temporary. Those who had an unusual or particularly valuable skill could earn a living and perhaps even become prosperous; others, however, either had no skills, or had skills in areas for which the demand was already adequately served by native artisans. The position of the unemployed was causing great anxiety in the period, so there was a not unnatural reluctance to receive aliens who might be a burden, or who by their competition might injure natives. Who would be responsible for the alien poor was obviously an important issue during a time when governments struggled to deal with dramatically (or at least what was *perceived* to be dramatically) increasing native poverty.

Overview of the poor relief conducted by the Reformed churches

Although some small variations in local practice can be identified, the broad outlines of poor relief conducted by the alien churches in the provinces mirrored those carried out in London. This similarity was reinforced by the similarities in practice between the Dutch and French churches themselves in London. Virtually from the moment in 1550 when the first stranger churches were established through the permission of Edward VI, maintenance of their poor was as important to the newly-arrived refugees as it was to the governors of their new home. Aliens settled and set up churches in south-eastern England from the 1560s; the circumstances of their settlements varied, and this influenced the interaction between these groups and the municipalities of their residences on the issue of poor relief, as well as on others. For example, despite fairly liberal provisions in the original authorization of their settlement in Norwich in 1566, the aliens were compelled to agree to a variety of restrictive provisions, including paying:

> to the church wardeyns of everye parryshe wherin ye do inhabite for the Dyschardge of all monnor of Dewetyes growinge to the preste or the clarke for the same parryshe ... after the rate that ye Do paye for yo[ur] houserente or fearme: That is to saye, of e+verye shyllinge a penye for the whole yere ... according as other Citizens Do vse.[4]

An overview of the aliens' internal poor relief and their participation (willingly or less than willingly) in municipal charity opens the door to a number of questions.

Discussing the origins of the poor relief system practised by the exile churches in London, Andrew Spicer points out that the Reformed churches on the Continent were 'excluded from existing local provision' for poor relief, and 'were therefore forced to develop their own distinct system'.[5] Need was reinforced by the belief of the Reformed that care for the poor of their own confessional community was a moral dictate, one which held that caring for the poor was 'basic to the task of the church', and 'went hand in hand with spiritual discipline' and the ensuring of 'doctrinal and moral conformity'. This emphasis on the moral rectitude of their members, which obviously only they could judge, was one of the factors why the aliens 'resisted civil control over . . . poor relief'.[6] It is just as well that they did develop their own system, for their English hosts were not willing to support indigent aliens. In fact, it was either assumed or explicitly stated in practically every place the refugees settled that they would maintain their own needy. The London congregations immediately established an internal poor relief scheme, and other settlements such as those in Norwich and Colchester did likewise. At least in the case of Colchester, this responsibility was part of the terms of settlement on which the city government insisted and to which the aliens agreed.[7] No explicit statement exists for Norwich, but we do know that they did 'sustaine all their owne poore people'.[8]

To the end of providing for their paupers, both the Dutch and French churches in London followed earlier Reformed precedent by creating a relatively elaborate system for the maintenance of the poor of their respective congregations.[9] This system, followed with some minor additions or variations by the stranger churches in the provinces, was based on a diaconate specifically responsible for 'the charge of the poor'.[10] The basic elements of the deacons' responsibilities were that they collected funds for the poor chest, visited the poor to assess their needs and evaluate their behaviour on a regular basis, distributed alms weekly to the presumably godly poor, and accounted monthly to the consistory.

Although direct monetary payments based on assessed need were made weekly, relief actually took a variety of forms. When regular payments were insufficient for an emergency, extraordinary disbursements were made. The aliens maintained their own poor houses for the infirm in London, as well as in Norwich and Colchester. Bread was distributed to the needy according to extant records for the congregations in London and Sandwich, and presumably in other congregations as well.[11] Various members of the congregations received funds for expenses associated with caring for, teaching to read, and training spiritually, the congregation's orphan children. The care of orphans is one area where there is some variation in practice. Individually appointed women of the congregation seem to have been the preferred caregivers in most of the stranger churches, but in Norwich, the 'Politic Men' of both churches acted in a supervisory capacity vis à vis the care of orphans.[12] Funds bought materials for 'setting the poor on work' for those who were physically capable but unable to find adequate employment.

The distribution of assistance was not indiscriminate. 'Admission to the Lord's Table' was a prerequisite, as was continuing evidence of upright moral behaviour as judged by the fairly strict standards of the consistory and reported by the deacons. The stranger churches went to lengths to require affidavits of membership in good standing from other Reformed churches and other assurances of eligibility for newcomers. *Passant*, poor members of the faith passing through on their way to another destination (increasingly common once English municipalities with communities of resident aliens passed a number of restrictions forbidding new strangers to settle), frequently received monetary assistance to get them to the next congregation on their travels. These issues were sometimes complicated, however, by the Dutch and French congregations' confusion over which community was responsible for which poor.[13]

Collections to pay for all of this activity were made primarily at regular services, with occasional extraordinary collections taken door-to-door, at special services and other church functions. Those who were able to contribute were expected to do so regularly, and if they fell behind in their duty to the congregation's poor, the deacons were under instruction 'humbly' to admonish each to contribute.[14] Funds for the poor in general were supplemented by a fairly regular supply of bequests, 'forfeits' and the occasional extraordinary gift that was not from a will. Bequests and other extra-ordinary gifts to the church were routinely divided between the poor and 'the service', except for those specified solely for the 'use of the poor'. Such gifts were especially important in times of great stress, such as in the wake of the St Bartholomew's Day Massacre or during episodes of plague. These gifts sometimes came from wealthy members of the foreign congregations, from other stranger congregations and occa-sionally from individual natives. Even the Queen herself donated £30 to the poor chests of the foreign churches in Norwich (£19 to the Dutch and £11 to the Walloons) after an outbreak of the plague killed nearly 2500 resident aliens in 1578.[15] Forfeits, or fines, were usually divided between the service and the poor chest as well, but some are recorded as going exclusively to the poor. Most of the forfeits were imposed by the consistory, although there were exceptions.[16] The *Book of Orders Concerning Wool*, which listed the regulations governing the manufacture and sale of textiles in Norwich, listed a variety of infractions which carried fines that were usually divided into thirds between 'the pore the science & the Baylye', although in some cases the strangers' poor chest received half or even all of a fine. For example, one item notes that 'all new Drapers ar bounde to pay so well Inglis Wallowns as Duch to paye on shilling stg [sterling] to the profit of the pore of the Duch church', a rare example of the English being bound to pay into the aliens' poor chest.[17]

The aliens' participation in municipal poor relief

Although being expected to maintain their own needy meant that the aliens did not benefit from municipal poor chests, they were expected to contribute to them, if of sufficient means to do so. In 1562 Colchester instituted the collection of alms at Sunday sermons for relief of the poor.[18] The strangers, arriving a few years later, were apparently not originally required to contribute to this municipal collection. In 1580, however, the council ordered that 'ev[er]ye howsholder beinge a stranger shall paye to the relieff of the poor in the p[ar]ishe where he Dwelleth according as the howse before hathe byn accustomed'. The aliens complained 'bitterly' about this new exaction, but to no apparent avail.[19] Evidence that it held, despite their complaint to the Privy Council, can be found in the *Colchester Contribution Book to the Poor, 1582–1592*, where individual 'Dewche' contributions ranged from 1d to 4d per collec-tion.[20] It is less clear in the case of Norwich whether the strangers' obligation to contribute to 'the Dyschardge of all monnor of Dewetyes' abovementioned included being assessed for the maintenance of the poor in the city. The aliens were commended in 1575 for being 'contributors to *all* (emphasis mine) payments as subcedies, taskes, watches, contrubusions, mynisters wagis, etc.', and this seems to hint that if assessment for poor relief became a regular charge on residents of Norwich in 1570, it would naturally be included in the 'contrubusions'.[21] Some doubt is cast on this conclusion, however, by the fact that a legal opinion rendered in a 1606 dispute held that these 'Dewetyes' included payments to the municipal relief system, the implication being that this was a new situation.[22] It is unclear from the sources whether this was truly a new situation being resisted, or that the aliens were protesting against a practice already in place.

The aliens' influence on Elizabethan municipal poor relief

Some important points are to be made when one examines the relationship between the internal poor relief systems of the stranger churches and the municipal poor relief schemes in the towns where they settled. Firstly, it is not a likely coincidence that the administrative features of both systems are so strikingly similar. Taking the famous Norwich scheme as the model, we know that these municipal schemes centred on a network of deacons who maintained lists of paupers' names, oversaw the collection of the poor tax, recorded the names of contributors, made regular weekly distributions, solicited extraordinary donations in times of need, established a poor house, and worked with 'select women' to oversee the 'care and correction' of the indigent.[23] Able-bodied men and women were provided with resources to be 'set on work', children were taught to read, and orphans were fed and clothed as well. These elements are nearly identical to those outlined above as used by the stranger churches, even to the point of providing relief only to those indigent who met acceptable moral standards. By the late 1560s and through the 1570s, one can see an increasing emphasis in the *Monday Court Book* in Colchester and in the *Mayor's Court Book* in Norwich that civic authorities were disciplining 'ungodly' behaviour. This emphasis on correction came approximately in the same period when their governors praise the resident aliens' moral example: 'The good example . . . bothe for liefe and religion generallie geeven bie the straungers duringe their abide in Colchester have ben comfortable to all those that be godlie minded'.[24]

A second point concerns the timing of the establishment of municipal plans. The strangers settled in Norwich in 1566, and presumably maintained their poor from the start in a system. The Norwich poor relief scheme began almost five years later. Muriel McClendon argues persuasively to connect the rise of Puritan influence on the aldermen of Norwich with their pursuit of poor relief and correction. She points out that their emphasis in the law's preamble on 'searching and correcting' the poor gives support to the argument that the 'godly' were influential, and that it coincided with Norwich's 'early reputation as a centre of Puritanism, with a growing demand for hot Protestant preachers', like John More, who arrived in 1573 and 'became the central figure among the city's Protestant clergy'.[25] But from where did that English Puritan element get its inspiration? More came to the city after the scheme was established, while the Reformed communities had brought together poor relief and behavioural control well before the founding of the Norwich scheme. The scholarship of Patrick

Collinson and others has pointed out that for many of those unhappy with the Elizabethan religious settlement, the Reformed congregations represented an ideal for which the English Church should strive.[26] It is not reasonable to assume that municipal authorities seeking to create a mechanism for dealing with their impoverished residents would have overlooked a model right before their eyes that was successful on *both* scores.

Lastly, and most briefly, all of the Reformed congregations were located in the south-east of England. This was, of course, natural for reasons of proximity to their north-western European homelands and to the capital, and for settlement in traditional textile centers to exercise their trades. The south-east was also 'the heartland of English dissent' in matters of religion.[27] It seems more than mere coincidence that the earliest compulsory poor taxes and welfare plans would all originate in areas that met all of these criteria.

While the aliens who fled to England and established Reformed congregations enjoyed a number of privileges, not least of which was the right to practise their own faith freely, they also suffered from a number of mostly economic restrictions. The ones I have been chiefly concerned with here were the requirements that they maintain their own indigent population and that they nevertheless contribute to all municipal charges, including the newly-established compulsory poor relief plans. I argue that the evidence strongly suggests the probability that the first requirement provided both inspiration and practical example to local civic authorities. Moreover, it is widely accepted that the Norwich scheme provided the inspiration for the Act of 1572, the basis for the development of the famous Elizabethan Poor Laws of 1598 and 1601. The Act of 1572 certainly incorporated many elements from the Norwich plan. The institutionalized charity of the Reformed churches can be seen as a sort of 'grandparent' to that pivotal development in the origins of the welfare state in England.

NOTES

1 Paul Slack notes briefly that in the Norwich census of the poor in 1570, 'foreign immigrants were excluded', but does not investigate the matter further: Slack, 'Poverty and social regulation in Elizabethan England', in Christopher Haigh (ed.), *The Reign of Elizabeth I* (Basingstoke, 1984), 231. Andrew Pettegree's *Foreign Protestant communities in 16th-century London* (Oxford, 1986) centres on the role of the foreign churches in London in immigrants' lives but recommends to others the analysis of the alien communities in the provinces. More recent work on poor relief, and the aliens' role in it, can be found in Ole Peter Grell's *Calvinist exiles in Tudor and Stuart England* (Aldershot, 1996) and in Andrew Spicer's 'Poor relief and the exile communities', in Beat Kumin (ed.), *Reformations old and new: essays on the socio-economic impact of religious change, c. 1470–1630* (Aldershot, 1996), which focuses on the French churches. This work owes much to Dr Spicer's work, but also attempts to ask and answer new questions on the issue.

2 *The Norwich Census of the Poor, 1570*, ed. J. F. Pound, Norfolk Record Society, vol. 40 (Norwich, 1971), 7–21 and *passim*.

3 Select details are taken from Laura Hunt Yungblut, *Strangers settled here amongst us: policy, perceptions and the presence of aliens in Elizabethan England* (London, 1996), unless otherwise noted.

4 Norfolk Record Office (hereafter NRO), 'Norwich Book of Orders for the Dutch and

Walloon Strangers', fo. 18v; HSQS 1, 19.

5   Spicer, 241.

6   Charles H. Parker, *The reformation of community: social welfare and Calvinist charity in Holland, 1572–1620* (Cambridge, 1998), 11, 108–109.

7   HSQS 12, vi–vii; Nigel Goose, 'Social structure', in Janet Cooper (ed.), *The Victoria History of the County of Essex*, vol. 9: *The Borough of Colchester* (Oxford, 1994), 97.

8   PRO, SP 12/20/49; R. H. Tawney and E. Power (eds.), *Tudor economic documents* (London, 1924), vol. 1, 315.

9   Given the degree of detail incorporated into the administration of the alien congregations' provision for poor relief, a somewhat surprisingly small number of sources are extant. In *The Huguenots in England: immigration and settlement c.1550–1700* (Cambridge, 1991), Bernard Cottret notes 'Unfortunately, we are not in a position to assess the extent of the financial contributions levied on [the] foreigners' (64). The detail reflected in those surviving documents indicate how exacting the record-keeping was at the time, but now the historian must extrapolate from what remains. The evidence can be found in official statements of policy, church records, and civic records documenting everyday life, but naturally care must be had not to confuse prescriptions of law and policy with the realities of life.

10 *Acta van het consistorie van de Nederlandse gemeente te Londen*, ed. A. J. Jelsma and O. Boersma (1993), 73.

11 *Ibid.*, 388; Spicer, 242, 248–9.

12 NRO, 'Register of the guardianship of orphans of the Norwich strangers, 1583–1600'.

13 *Acta van het consistorie*, 300, 693.

14 *Ibid.*, 73, 415.

15 NRO, 'Proceedings of the Mayor's Court', vol. 10, 299 (paginated, not foliated); F. Blomefield, *An essay towards a topographical history of the county of Norfolk* (11 vols., London, 1805–10), vol. 3; Spicer, 245–6.

16 *Acta van het consistorie*, 151, 159, 208, 279, 404–5, 643, 645–6; Spicer, 245.

17 NRO, 'Book of Orders Concerning Wool, 1577'.

18 Essex Record Office (hereafter ERO), 'Liber Ordinacionum', fo. 94v; Goose, 90.

19 ERO, 'Assembly Book' [D/B 5 Gb1], fo. 20v; Moens, *Register of baptisms*, vi–vii; L. F. Roker, 'The Flemish and Dutch community in Colchester in the 16th and 17th centuries', *HSP* 21:1 (1965), 18.

20 ERO, 'Colchester Contribution Book to the Poor, 1582–92', unfoliated.

21 PRO, SP 12/20/49; Tawney and Power, vol. 1, 315.

22 Spicer, 253.

23 Muriel McClendon, *The quiet Reformation: magistrtes and the emergence of Protestantism in Tudor Norwich* (Stanford, 1999), 231.

24 PRO, SP 12/144/19; Moens, *Register of baptisms*, vi.

25 McClendon, 231–51 and *passim*.

26 Patrick Collinson makes this point in 'The Elizabethan Puritans and the foreign Reformed churches in London', *HSP* 20:5 (1964), 528–55 and in *The Elizabethan Puritan movement* (London, 1967).

27 Grell, 56.

11

Melting into the landscape:
the story of the 17th-century Walloons
in the Fens

JEAN TSUSHIMA

This paper is in the nature of a 'work in progress' report from the Huguenot and Walloon Research Association's Fenland Workshop's project to transcribe, edit and publish the sources concerning the immigration of the Walloons and the Flemish to the Fens in the 17th century. This research has already helped us to unravel parts of this long and complicated history.[1]

'The Fens' is a vast area of eastern England, stretching from the Wash into Lincolnshire and then south into Cambridgeshire. They have always been subject to flooding on a large scale, so that life in this area has always been, and still is, a never-ending battle to keep the sea out and to contain the several large rivers within their banks. Embanking rivers and the sea coast and draining the flooded lands has been a constant concern in these areas for all time. Even the Romans made attempts to control the floods. Later the Fens, which were generally not conducive to settlement, proved attractive to hermits and later to religious orders who built abbeys in this desolate area – Crowland, Ramsey and Thorney being three of the best known.[2] The inhabitants of the Fens developed their own style of living, being dependent on the fisheries, the eel beds and water fowl. Rushes were grown and harvested and, along with dried eels and fish, were used for rents and tithes. In summer when the floods receded, a certain amount of grain could be grown and orchards were possible on the higher sandy ground. A delicate balance of trade with inland towns was established and the Fens provided a tolerable way of life for the independent and rugged people who chose to live in them. No great towns could develop, as the soil of the Fens would only support at best a small two-storied house, which could split in two if the ground shifted. There were few roads, and in fact, transport was very often by punt and shallow boats. While outsiders regarded the Fenland life with dismay and horror, to those who lived in them it was often seen as idyllic and free – free from landlords, magistrates and kings.[3]

All this was to change in the early 17th century. In Lincolnshire the never-ending work of controlling and maintaining the dykes was in the hands of Commissioners of Sewers who raised money locally and kept careful accounts. Occasionally the Crown financed large enterprises, such as when Henry VIII ordered the drainage of the silted-up Boston harbour, for which workmen were brought over from Calais in 1522. The Dutch, the greatest drainers of all, were often called to the Fens. But all this work was merely to maintain the rivers within their banks and to keep out the sea. In the early 17th century new projects materialized to drain great areas of the Fens in order to bring more land into cultivation – in short, land reclamation. Behind this idea was the desire to speculate and profit from the land thus reclaimed.[4]

These ideas had been in the air since the 1590s, and early surveying was carried out by Sir William Russell, younger son of the 2nd Earl of Bedford, who had lived in the Low Countries and had served as Governor of Flushing. James I was interested, but it was left to his perpetually impecunious son Charles I to get affairs moving, through his agreement in 1626 with the Dutchman Sir Cornelius Vermuyden, one of the most famous names in fen drainage.[5] Vermuyden is linked with two areas and periods of land reclamation in the Fens, the Isle of Axholme in north-western Lincolnshire during the reign of Charles I, and the vast area of the Bedford Level in Cambridge-shire during the Commonwealth.

In 1626 Charles I enlisted Vermuyden to drain the soggy wastes of the Isle of Axholme, including Hatfield Chase, where the first experiments of draining were carried out. Negotiations to begin work were protracted, partly because of the acute shortage of money and partly because the ownership of the land was disputed. The King was convinced that the Crown owned the lands in Hatfield Chase, while the people who lived there were equally convinced he did not. According to local belief the land had been granted in perpetuity to the people living in the area as common ground by Sir John de Mowbray in 1359. They could graze their cattle when the low ground was not flooded and they could fish, cut reeds, dig turf (their only fuel) and in general live their own way of life undisturbed by outside powers.[6] This legal clash over land was the basis for all the troubles that assailed the drainage work and the settle-ment, a confrontation that was not put down until the early 18th century. In the 90 years from the time the agreement was made with the Crown in 1626 the area was a constant scene of riots and destruction of drainage works. Houses and fences were torn down and the strangers' church at Sandtoft was destroyed at least once, if not twice, before its final destruction. Nothing remains of the church today.[7]

The little church at Sandtoft was one of the benefits Vermuyden was able to obtain in 1626. He was given permission to build churches or chapels for the foreign com-munity and workmen, provided they adopted the Book of Common Prayer service in their own language.[8] How much this was observed in practice is difficult to determine, for the church sent its minister to the Synod of Calvinist stranger churches in London in 1647 and repeatedly turned to the consistories of the French and Dutch churches for help and advice in running their affairs and in finding a suitable minister able to speak French and Dutch.[9] It was 10 years before a church could be built and in the meantime the settlers were advised to use the local churches – which they apparently did.[10] The church cost over £1000, though the unfortunate man who built it, Isaac Bedloe, was only ever paid a tiny part of this sum and his widow petitioned for years for payment of the outstanding debt. This sum also paid for a minister's house. The first minister was Pierre Berchet, a Frenchman from the Calais area, whose father and grandfather were well-known scholars at the Academy of Sedan. Berchet was con-sidered to be a bargain for the church as he could speak both French and Dutch, thus obviating the need to have two ministers and saving the tiny community £30 p.a.

What was the composition of the community he served? As soon as Vermuyden could start work he brought over a small army of men – surveyors, engineers and diggers from the Netherlands. They were Dutch and required a Dutch minister but nothing is known about whether they ever had one; they may have brought one over with them. The work was finished within two years and many of the Dutchmen probably went home as there is little trace of them in local registers. Several of the rich Dutch merchants who had invested their money in the drainage scheme – Corsellis, Vernatti, Van Valkenburgh, the Katz brothers – settled in the area but lived in some style, while the workers would probably only have had huts. The principal settlers were the Flemings and Walloons from the southern regions of the Low Countries, then largely under Spanish rule. It is they who were the first cultivators of the reclaimed lands.[11] There were riots from the very first days, and they continued when these settlers started to come into the area to lease the land and start cultivation. We do not know the conditions of their contracts with the 'prospectors', as the speculators who owned the land were called. However, as the drainage was not as successful as had been hoped, more work had to be done on a very large scale and the huge sum of £20,000 found to carry it out. The prospectors were hard pressed and were losing money fast, so they started to leave the area, some going to London and others returning to the United Provinces. Vermuyden was heavily involved in costly legal battles, both with the Crown – Thomas Wentworth, the President of the North, being firmly on the side of the local people in pursuit of the restoration of their ancient rights – and with many of the prospectors.

Riots continued and the settlers were regarded as 'King's men' although they were probably not so at all. In the 1640s the area was caught up in the Civil War, and the settlers were again in an unenviable situation. It is not surprising that the exodus from this wretched area started with some of the very first settlers, who went north into south Yorkshire. It is usually thought that some members of the community returned to their homelands and the remainder went to Thorney Abbey in Cambridgeshire. This is not strictly true, though the community did melt away by the end of the 17th century. Those who 'went home' were probably the Dutch workers, who would have been indentured workers for the most part.

But the Walloons and Flemish settlers had no home to go back to, as they had left their country for good. The constant rioting and destruction made life very difficult and there was a steady drift inland to other parts of Lincolnshire out of the Fens area. The eastern part of the county was strongly nonconformist and this would be a great attraction to these Calvinists. They can be found in the records of this area. In the 1650s the Sandtoft church was without a minister, and the community was in despair not only because of the lack of religious care and support, but because their children could not read French or Dutch. It is thus obvious that by that time the community was in decline, just as another foreign settlement was being established in the Fens of Cambridgeshire.

The idea of draining the vast area of the Fens known as the Bedford Level, just north of Cambridge, was eagerly discussed and debated during James I's reign, but was not followed up during the construction of the drainage works in Hatfield Chase. In spite of the dissatisfaction with Vermuyden's work in the Isle of Axholme, his legal cases (he was in prison at one stage), his financial mishaps and his debts – to say nothing of his abrasive character – he was the man chosen to oversee the great work. It was not easy to find backers as the costs were going to be unlike any other work of the age. In the end Francis, 4th Earl of Bedford came forward as the only man rich enough to take on the major share of the costs. Many Dutch investors came forward but they all withdrew as soon as it was clear there was going to be civil war. New backers had to be found and more money. At some point it was agreed that the settlers should be Walloons and Flemings from the Low Countries who were having an unsettled time under Spanish rule. In 1639 an agreement was drawn up with the Bishop of Ely for permission for the church and abbey of Thorney to be restored and put to the use of the foreign settlers for their own services, to be conducted in either French or Dutch, although they were required to use a translation of the liturgy of the Book of Common Prayer. The damage to the church of Thorney was extensive as many tons of dressed stone had been taken to Cambridge to build new chapels in Trinity and Corpus Christi Colleges. The Earl of Bedford paid for the rebuilding of the church and it was arranged for a French minister to be in residence with a stipend of £40 p.a., rising to £60. However there were many problems to be solved. The Earl and his investors had seen only too well the problems ahead if they did not have a clear title to the land, and years were spent in negotiating this. In the end an Act of Parliament was passed which made the conditions of ownership quite clear. But with the disruptions of the Civil War and the death of Charles I, it was later considered necessary, if not vital, to have a new act acceptable to the Commonwealth Parliament. This was duly drawn up and passed. At last in the early 1650s the work commenced, but there was still the problem of finding sufficient diggers for such a huge work. This was solved by employing – though it was forced labour – the Scottish prisoners of war taken after the Battle of Dunbar. They returned home after the peace treaty was signed – though it is said that some of them found life in the Fens preferable to life in Scotland and stayed in the Fens, which might account for some of the names found in the records. Recourse was had again to using prisoners of war. This time it was a body of Dutch prisoners taken after a naval battle in the First Anglo-Dutch War. They were difficult to control but did the work well; it may well have been work they were used to doing.[12] At no point were Walloons or Flemings (let alone 'Huguenots') used in the digging and dyking work of the Bedford Level.

Walloons did settle in the regions, however, to cultivate the reclaimed land, and they worshipped in the church at Thorney. The only register from the Thorney church that has survived is the baptismal register which starts in 1654, which has already been transcribed and published.[13] The last entry is for 1727, and there are several thousand names which occur through the 70 or so years of the church's history.[14] They are all common names from the Low Countries and what is now northern France; thus it is reckless to claim that they come from one particular place or another without impeccable supporting evidence. The community prospered, having had leases drawn up in detail with the Earl of Bedford's bailiffs. These leases will be the basis of the Fenland Workshop's next research project. Again, as in Hatfield Chase, very few settlers were rich enough to buy land of their own, although a handful did – among them the Bailleuls,[15] the de la Prymes[16] and the de la Forteries (though this family dated from a much earlier migration to Canterbury in the previous century).

At the Restoration the Corporation, by which name the investors in the Bedford

Level had become known, was once again faced with the problem of whether they had a clear title to the lands. Negotiations were started and yet another Act of Parliament was drawn up and passed. When this was achieved a great ceremony of thanksgiving took place in Ely Cathedral. A new licence to worship in Thorney Abbey using the French translation of the English liturgy was granted on 13 August 1662, Finally there was a feeling of security among the settlers. Over the years a vast area of land, possibly as much as half a million acres, came into cultivation – the largest land reclamation known in England, and probably only exceeded by the reclamation work in the Netherlands. The Walloons and Flemings brought their skills as husbandmen, which is one of the reasons why they were invited to come over, and their industry raised the food stock of the country. It was only at the end of the 18th century, when the drainage works were allowed to decay, that it became clear that the work of keeping the Bedford Level and all the other cleared fens in working order meant ceaseless vigilance and inspection.

The Walloon community in Thorney and the surrounding towns was a stable one, though its members started to marry into the English community fairly early, and thus appear in the records of the Church of England as well as in those of the French community. There was no rioting, the Bedfords were model landlords and the Walloons and Flemings model tenants. It does not seem that French refugees made their way to Thorney after the Revocation of the Edict of Nantes, and the idea that they did may be a confusion with the little settlement of French refugees that was established at Beaumont-cum-Moze and Thorpe-Le-Soken in Essex.

Did any Walloons come to Thorney from the disrupted settlements in the Isle of Axholme? One does have to be very cautious in determining this, as the surnames found in the two communities are very common in the Low Countries name-pool. But as the Fenland Workshop group has collected and transcribed all the wills we could find for these two areas, it is possible to see from the evidence provided that some families did move to Thorney. Several wills reveal continuing links of family or friendship between members of the Isle of Axholme and Thorney communities, as legacies and gifts were bequeathed by inhabitants of one community to members of the other. We have thus been able to prove that a dozen or so families did migrate from Sandtoft to Thorney. That the entire settlement did not abandon Sandtoft for Thorney can, however, be borne out by the fact that marriages and baptisms were carried out at Sandtoft right up to 1685. However, it is true that by the mid-18th century very few Walloon names are found in the parish registers of the churches in the Isle of Axholme – Wroot, Belton and Crowle, Epworth – though they are found further inland in Lincolnshire and to a certain extent in east Northamptonshire. Care has to be taken in looking at Lincolnshire records, as the settlement of Dutch, Flemish and even French people in the north of the county was extensive from the Middle Ages onward, and it is possible to confuse some of these earlier families with later Walloons and Flemings.

The Thorney settlements were certainly more stable as there was no rioting to cause distress and possible flight, but they too suffered long-term decline and fragmentation. As the reclaimed land was wholly agricultural there was little scope for trades and industry, especially as the unstable ground would not support large buildings. The towns were very small indeed and did not support much in the way of intellectual life, so that an able young man or one anxious for a more lively career was forced to leave the Fens. However, to this day Walloon names can be found in Thorney itself – and in some of the little towns nearby. Crowland had an early influx of Walloons and so did Parsons' Grove – where the parish church actually had a Huguenot pastor – and Whittlesey had many Walloons in the late 17th and early 18th centuries. A few place-names in the Thorney fenland remind one that the Walloons have been there, such as French Drove and Le Talle Farm. In contrast, in the Isle of Axholme there are surprisingly few Walloon names in the local registers in the 18th and 19th centuries, though some appear in civil records, suggesting that they had turned to nonconformist churches.

It is obvious that many of the Walloons in the Thorney area were also attracted to nonconformity, as is revealed by the 1723 Wisbech Oath Roll, edited by Laurel Phillipson, which lists all those claiming exemption from taking oaths. Naturally the roll includes many Quakers, although there were very few Friends' Meeting Houses in Cambridgeshire. In this list are about 50 names of unimpeachable Walloon origin. Were they Quakers? That is doubtful, but this document has revealed the large number of Walloons who had otherwise disappeared from the church registers of both English and French churches.[17] Our next project, then, is to make a thorough search of nonconformist records to further trace these strangers.

The number of Walloons and Flemings who immigrated has been one of the major questions about the Fens for two centuries. George Stovin, a Fenlander whose family had immigrated into Lincolnshire in the mid-16th century, took a great interest in the Sandtoft community. He knew the register of the church and extracted a list of marriages and baptisms. He stated that there were about 500 baptisms, but he published only about a third of this number.[18] For 200 years his list has been the only evidence for the names of the settlers.

The HWRA Fenland Workshop has set out to improve on this list. It has already been noted that the settlers were instructed to use the local Anglican churches until their own church was built. We have looked in these English records and, as expected, found them full of Walloon and some Flemish names. These have been culled from the local records by members of the HWRA team and will be published in due course. We then went to other civil records and found more names of the settlers. Thus with these and the Church of England records and Stovin's list we have probably retrieved the complete Sandtoft community, excluding, of course, the indentured Dutch workers. We are confident, though, that these will turn up in records in the Netherlands which we have yet to examine.

The next step was to see if there were wills, inventories and leases for the Isle of Axholme. We did not expect many, for it was a poor agricultural area. However, we were fortunate and have found a satisfactory number which confirm the data we have come across in the parish registers. We have also found inventories of great economic importance. The leases are yet to be found – if indeed they survive. As the Dutch speculators sold off their holdings and for the most part returned to the United Provinces, any surviving records will have to be looked for there. We have still to track down the English owners who bought the lands from the Dutch to see if any records survive in their estate papers.

The settlement at Thorney is a very different story. This was stable and relatively content Walloon settlement, the leases were in order and there was a more propitious agricultural enterprise. In this context it is much easier to track down the families and reconstitute the community. We have the leases, the wills and inventories and the local church registers, though we lack, as we do for the Isle of Axholme, contemporary evidence in the form of letters, diaries or newspapers. We still have to search non-conformist records for both communities, and also to do research in the Low Countries.

Our larger Fenland Wills project has set out to find all the wills for the settlers from about 1630 to 1750. We have taken 1750 as the date at which the two stranger settlements formally died out, marked by the closure of the French Church at Thorney Abbey in 1727. We have had to extend the search to wills in other parts of Lincolnshire, Northamptonshire, south Yorkshire, Cambridgeshire, west Essex and even London. I hope this account has made clear why one settlement was a success and the other a failure. However, whether the terms of their settlement were bad as in the Isle of Axholme, or satisfactory as in the Thorney area, the Walloon settlements, each according to its local conditions, eventually melted into the landscape and became indistinguishable from their Fenland neighbours. It is the aim of our research group to reconstruct the identities and lives of these 'strangers' from their earliest years in this country.

NOTES

1   I would like to thank the following members of the Huguenot and Walloon Research Association Fenland Workshop for their immense help with the collection of material and transcription: Alan Bullwinkle, Charles and Valerie Fovargue, Lynn Scadding and Michael J. Wood. Other members of the team who have helped us are Kate Fisher, Michael Barker, Robert Barker, Mrs M. Oldfield, Mrs K. R. Taylor, Sue Graves, Colin Tigedin and N. Delahoy. Grateful thanks are due as well to the archivists of the Cambridgeshire, Huntingdonshire, Lincolnshire, Northamptonshire and Bedfordshire Record Offices for their great help in obtaining wills, leases and transcripts of parish registers.

2   Many of these monks in fact originated from the Low Countries, the precursors to their compatriots who came over in the 17th century. For the medieval Fenland monasteries, see Sandra Raban, *The estates of Thorney and Crowland: a study in medieval monastic land tenure* (Cambridge, 1977). See also H. C. Darby, *The medieval Fenland* (Cambridge, 1940).

3   Joan Thirsk, *Fenland farming in the sixteenth century* (University of Leicester Dept. of English Local History Occasional Paper no. 3) (Leicester, 1953).

4   For a general history of this project see H. C. Darby, *The draining of the Fens* (Cambridge, 1940); Dorothy Summers, *The Great Level: a history of drainage and land reclamation in the Fens* (Newton Abbot, 1976).

5   J. Korthals-Altes, *Sir Cornelius Vermuyden: the lifework of a great Anglo-Dutchman in land-reclamation and drainage* (London, 1925): Lawrence E. Harris, *Vermuyden and the Fens: a study of Sir Cornelius Vermuyden and the Great Level* (London, 1953).

6   Joan Thirsk, 'The Isle of Axholme before Vermuyden', in Joan Thirsk, *The rural economy of England: collected essays* (London, 1984).

7   The extent of the lawlessness in the Fens area around Hatfield Chase is quite remarkable; a full account of the riots is given in Keith Lindley, *Fenland riots and the English Revolution* (London, 1982).

8   For the stranger community at Sandtoft and the Isle of Axholme, see H. G. B. le Moine, 'Huguenots in the Isle of Axholme' and W. J. C. Moens, 'The first 30 years of the foreign settlement in Axholme', *HSP* 2 (1887–8), 265–331.

9 HSQS 2, 103, 109.

10 Based on an examination of the microfiche copies of the registers of the local churches. Parishes examined include Belton, Wroot, Crowle, Hatfield Chase and Epworth.

11 Only very few of the Walloons and Flemings who came over to the Fens area actually had enough money to buy estates. The poorer settlers, the majority, were only lease-holders, and they were encouraged to come over and settle as their agricultural expertise was well-known and highly valued. For an English commentary on Low Countries husbandry, see Samuel Hartlib, *A Discourse of Husbandrie used in Brabant and Flanders* (London, 1652).

12 See the *CSPD* for the Interregnum years for these details.

13 HSQS 17. See also R. H. Warner, *The history of Thorney Abbey . . . from its foundation to its dissolution, together with some notes of the modern parish and Baptismal Register of the French Colony* (Wisbech, 1879).

14 The following surnames (from both Sandtoft and Thorney) appear in the pedigrees of the members of HWRA Fens Workshop: Le Fevre; Descou; du Bo; Blicque; le Pla; Massengarb; du Rieu; Brunnye; Tys; Tyssen; Smacq; Delahoy; Dewing; Fovargue; Tegredine; Hersain (Hairsine); Frushar; Mainee; Seinee; du Moulin (Dumberline/ Dimberline); Six (Sixt/ Cy); Maquille (Merkilley); Senschal (Snushal/ Snitchel); le Conte; Scribo; Amory; Beharrell (Barrel); Behague (Behagg); Ferry; Delanoy; Gouagy. The Walloon spelling varies even in the registers. There may be other names in their pedigrees which have not yet come to light, as there was considerable intermarriage.

15 The Baileys of Willow Farm.

16 *The Diary of Abraham de la Pryme, the Yorkshire antiquary*, ed. C. Jackson, Surtees Society no. 54 (Durham, 1870), concerns the life of the grandson of the original settler, but contains a 'Memoir of the family of De la Pryme' compiled by Charles de la Pryme.

17 Laurel Phillipson, *The Wisbech Quakers' Roll of 1723* (Cambridgeshire County Council).

18 George Stovin, 'A brief account of the drainage of the levels of Hatfield Chase (1751)', *Yorkshire Archaeological Journal* 37:147 (1950), 385–91.

Part III

Stranger craftsmen and artists

12

Insiders or outsiders? Overseas-born artists at the Jacobean court

KAREN HEARN

In 1644 the Czech engraver Wenceslaus Hollar, long domiciled in London, produced an engraving after a self-portrait by a deceased artist. The original painting is now lost, but the print (PLATE 3) bears a lengthy Latin inscription, which identifies the subject:

> MARCUS GARRARDUS PICTOR, *Illustrissimis & Serenissimis Principibus Beatae /*
> *memoriae Elizabethae & Annae etc magnae* Brittaniae Franciae & / Hiberniae Reginis
> *Servus, & Praestantissimo Artifici* Marco Garrardo / Brugensis Flandriae *filius, ubi natus*
> *erat. Obijt* Londini */January 19: Anno Domini 1635* [i.e. 1636]. *Aetatisq[ue] suae 74. /*
> *hic ipse Marcus depinxit A[nn]o 1627./ Wenceslaus Hollar Bohe[miae], fecit Londi[ni]*
> *1644. / acqua forti.*[1]

Hollar did not come to London until after Gheeraerts's death. Some of the accompanying information may have been inscribed by Gheeraerts himself on the lost original, but Hollar could also have gathered biographical details from surviving members of Gheeraerts's extensive family in London – for instance, his son Marcus Gheeraerts III, who was a freeman of the London Painter Stainers' Company.

It is a truism that the portrait painters who worked for the English court, and particularly for the monarchy, during the 16th and 17th centuries were generally born and, more significantly, trained overseas. This pattern had become established with the German artist Hans Holbein II, who during the 1530s created the image of Henry VIII with which everyone is familiar.[2] Following Holbein's death in 1543, the German-born and trained Gerlach Flicke arrived at court, where he was active from about 1545, the approximate date of his portrait of Thomas Cranmer (National Portrait Gallery, London) until his death in England in 1558.[3] Flicke clearly considered it worth emphasizing his alien status – he signed Cranmer's portrait 'Gerlacus flickus Germanus'. The former Habsburg court portraitist Gwillim Scrots appears to have acted as official portrait painter to Edward VI.[4] The Antwerp-born and -trained exile Hans Eworth seems to have fulfilled the same role for Mary I.[5]

This was not a situation that pleased the indigenous painters in the London Painter-Stainers' Company – who, as Susan Foister has observed, can regularly be heard 'sounding . . . a tediously shrill note of protest against foreign intrusion'.[6] In 1502 the

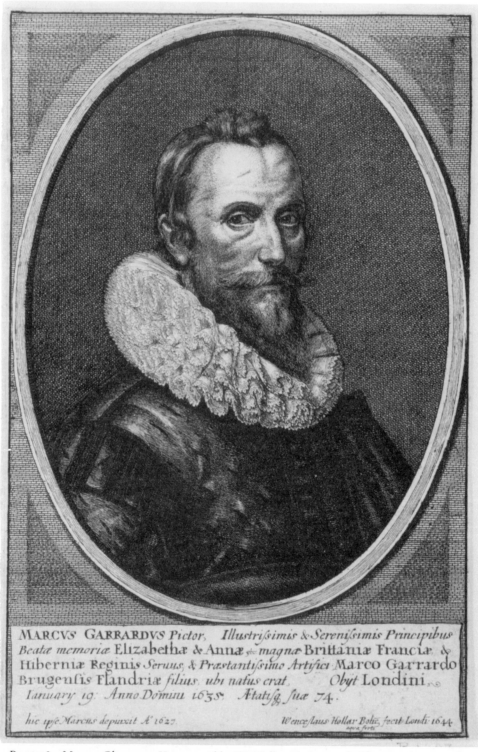

PLATE 3   Marcus Gheeraerts II, engraved by W. Hollar (© Copyright The British Museum)

companies of the Painters and the Stainers had amalgamated, and in 1532 the Company gained its own hall in the City of London. In 1581 – a major milestone – it was granted a royal charter. Unfortunately, almost none of its records prior to 1623 have survived. In broad terms, it was only able to exercise – or, rather, to attempt to exercise – its jurisdiction mainly within the City of London itself.[7] As in other trades, overseas-born craftspeople could establish themselves outside the City, or within those areas – such as Blackfriars – that were 'liberties', parishes that enjoyed special privileges.

It should be remembered that most of the painted work to be carried out at court was decorative – painting, or repainting, walls, windows, furniture, banners, bed-hangings, coaches, barges etc. Some of this would be carried out by members of the Painter-Stainers' Company – under the aegis of the Serjeant Painter. He was the official responsible for painted work required by the monarchy. The post seems to have carried a range of responsibilities, sometimes including the purveying of artists' materials, and the management and co-ordination of project teams. The Serjeant Painter would be a craft specialist, but until the appointment of George Gower, a gentleman of Yorkshire origin, midway through the reign of Elizabeth I in 1581, the post had not (as far as is known) been filled by a portrait-painter. But from then on the post seems to have gone wholly, or in part, to portrait painters. In spite of the large number of extant portraits of Elizabeth I – highly diverse in nature and quality – there is no definite evidence that she employed an official, named, portrait painter 'in large' (that is, as distinct from miniature-painting) apart from Gower.

In attempting to understand the oeuvres and careers of artists of this period, we run into various problems. It is clear that an immense number of paintings must have been lost – through the effects of time, natural wastage, and through deliberate destruction both during the Civil War and later. Those that survive very often do so in a damaged condition. Artists in early modern Britain seldom signed their works, so it can be hard to establish who painted what. We are faced with a tiny number of references in documents that cannot be tied up with surviving works, and extant paintings the names of whose makers we do not know.

Biographical information on artists and their family networks is equally rare. Many of the surviving archival records in this field were transcribed in the late 19th century by Sir Lionel Cust in a series of *Dictionary of National Biography* entries and subsequently in the *Proceedings of the Huguenot Society* in 1903 in an article, 'Foreign artists of the Reformed religion working in England'.[8] He published some of his expanded researches in the *Walpole Society* volume of 1914.[9] Rachel Poole's documentary researches on the De Critz and Gheeraerts families were also published by the *Walpole Society* in 1913 and 1914.[10] More recently Mary Edmond, in her 'Limners and picture-makers' paper in the *Walpole Society* volume for 1978–80, has added considerably to knowledge in this field.[11]

In discussing portraitists at the Jacobean court, 1603–25, I would, however, like to distinguish the differing phases of immigrant painting activity. Those initially employed were painters who had been born overseas, but who had apparently been trained largely in London within the incomer community, and who had come to prominence in the last years of Elizabeth I's reign. I shall highlight the two leading court portraitists – John de Critz I and Marcus Gheeraerts II. I shall contrast the trajectories of their careers in England from 1603 onwards, with those of the small group who arrive in London as fully trained adults from 1616 onwards. I want to emphasize how anomalous the careers of the former group were, in the context of court portrait-painting in that country.

John de Critz I was born in Antwerp in about 1551/2, and brought by his gold-smith father Troilus to Britain shortly afterwards, for on 10 March 1552, Troilus and his wife Sara gained denization. In 1571, it was noted that the family had come over 'for religeon' and were 'of the Douche churche'.[12] By November the same year, John had been apprenticed to the Ghent-born painter and poet Lucas de Heere 'of the Douche church', who is recorded as having come 'hither fyve yeres ago for religion'. De Heere had joined the community of Netherlandish Protestant exiles in London around 1566, signing the friendship albums of major merchant scholars in this com-munity – Emanuel van Meteren, Abraham Ortelius and Jan Radermacher. De Heere himself returned to the city of his birth after the Pacification of Ghent in 1576.[13]

From 1582 to 1588 De Critz was in the service of Sir Francis Walsingham, spymaster on behalf of Elizabeth I. A sole portrait type of Walsingham survives – and it does so in various versions, two of which are dated 1587 and 1589. The finest example is in the National Portrait Gallery, and it is presumed to have been painted by De Critz who, during this period, was regularly visiting Paris for Walsingham – perhaps on secret service business – whence it is recorded that he sent back paintings both by himself and by other, unidentified, painters.[14] The other image securely associated with De Critz is that of Robert Cecil, future 1st Earl of Salisbury – of which, again, numerous versions survive, the earliest one dated 1599. Cecil, Principal Secretary to Elizabeth, was a collector and a discerning patron of art.[15]

John de Critz was connected by marriage with the more accomplished, and more innovative, Marcus Gheeraerts II.[16] Marcus's grandfather Egbert had been enrolled as a painter in 1516 in Bruges, which, like Antwerp, was a major centre of artistic pro-duction. His father Marcus Gheeraerts I was an artist of some significance – a painter, but more especially an engraver and etcher. In 1561 the elder Gheeraerts was commis-sioned to finish a large altarpiece in the Church of Our Lady in Bruges by painting panels showing the Annunciation, the Nativity and the Resurrection. Unfortunately, the altarpiece was largely destroyed by iconoclasts in 1566. Other religious com-missions are also recorded. Gheeraerts was, however, very active on the Calvinist Council in Bruges, which suggests that he was able to separate his personal convictions from his professional activities.[17] Karel van Mander, writing in 1604, praised his abilities as a landscape painter.[18] This is interesting in view of the fact that one of his son's innovations was to introduce the landscape background to large-scale portraits in England. The elder Marcus's one certain surviving painting was pre-sumably made in England, or at least for the English market; it is a small signed image of Elizabeth I (private collection).[19] The fashion worn by the Queen in it dates it to between 1580 and 1585. The younger Gheeraerts was born in Bruges in 1561 or 1562, but in 1568 the family came to London, escaping the persecutions instigated by the Duke of Alva. The Return of Aliens for that year records the father as 'Markus Gerott of Bridgis, painter, Ducheman, came for relygyon'.[20] In 1571 he is noted as 'no denizon'. A handful of references indicate the family's presence in London. Presumably the younger Gheeraerts was trained, at least in part, by his father – in 1576 they are still recorded living in the same house. There is some suggestion that the widowed elder Marcus may have been a member of the Family of Love.[21] In 1571 he married Susanna, the sister of John de Critz. He is last mentioned in August 1586, standing godson to a nephew in London. He was among the earliest etchers – perhaps even the first – to operate in England.

In 1590 the younger Marcus married Magdalen de Critz, the sister of his step-mother, reinforcing his links with the De Critz dynasty. So, both Marcus and John grew up among the network of alien craftspeople in London who collaborated, took each other's offspring as 'servants' or apprentices, sourced materials from each other, intermarried, and generally negotiated routes through a not always welcoming in-digenous community.

It was during the 1590s that the younger Marcus's career took off, under the patronage of the courtier Sir Henry Lee. In the 1570s Lee had initiated for Elizabeth the annual public display of the Accession Day Tilts, over which he presided as the Queen's Champion.[22] He was an effective propagandist, and he appears to have picked out the younger Gheeraerts as capable of carrying out a series of elaborate emblem-atic portraits which he required, incorporating complex allegorical programmes; the most important of these is the immense 'Ditchley' portrait of Elizabeth I (PLATE 4).[23] In 1602 Lee and his mistress Anne Vavasour acted as godparents to one of Gheeraerts's sons, Henry. In spite of the caption to Hollar's print, surviving documents do not, however, seem to indicate that Gheeraerts had an official appointment to the Queen.

Some significant innovations are found in the work of the younger Gheeraerts: the use of canvas as a support, rather than wooden panel, and the inclusion of the land-scape background, emblematic in purpose. Both features are found in his large full-length of the 2nd Earl of Essex, c.1596 (Woburn Abbey) – the scene on the seashore behind the tall, elongated figure is thought to represent Essex's victory at Cadiz. The face pattern used for Essex relates closely to that found in the small images of the Earl painted by the miniaturist Isaac Oliver.[24] Oliver, too, was of an immigrant family – his father was a French Protestant goldsmith, who had brought his young family to London in 1568. The professional links suggested by this similarity were cemented in 1602, when Marcus the Younger's half-sister Sara married Oliver. Just to complete the craft dynastic picture, another half-sister, Susanna, wed the sculptor Maximilian Colt in London in 1604.[25]

In 1603 James VI of Scotland succeeded to the English throne, on the death of Elizabeth. Almost immediately John de Critz was appointed to the vacant post of Serjeant Painter to the King. He initially shared the role with the shadowy figure of Leonard Fryer, an English painter by whom no surviving works are known.[26] In Scotland, as in England, most of the court artists whose names are known seem to have been of Netherlandish origin. James had been portrayed as a boy by the Dutch artist Arnold Bronckorst.[27] By 1584 Adrian Vanson, originally from Breda, had become the King's official painter, a post which he retained until his death in 1602 (PLATE 5). In 1594 James specifically referred to him as 'our painter'.[28]

Anne of Denmark, James I's queen, also would have been accustomed to the notion that a court artist would be a Netherlander, for the leading court portraitists in Denmark were also part of the Netherlandish diaspora. A portrait of her brother, the future King Christian IV, from the early 1580s is attributed to the Flemish Hans Knieper.[29] The Dutchman Gerrit Corneliz. worked extensively for the Danish court from 1584 until 1601 – although no piece is definitely attributable to him. The principal painter to Christian IV following his accession, Pieter Isaacz., was of Dutch origin. He had been born at Elsinore, where his parents had come as religious refugees. Later, after training in the Netherlands with Cornelis Ketel, he returned in about 1608 to work in Denmark.

London records show that on 25 April 1604 'John de Critts born in Flanders and his heirs' were granted denization.[30] Having achieved his court post, De Critz had presumably decided that it was appropriate for him to take this formal step. Because John de Critz I held the post of Serjeant Painter, it is generally agreed that he must be the author of the first portrait-type of James I to be painted after his accession to the English throne. Certainly, in August 1606 De Critz was paid for a full-length of the King and for two others of his heir Prince Henry, to be sent to the Archduke of Austria.

Thus, a number of extant grand over-life-size images of James are assumed to have emanated from De Critz and his workshop. Versions of these, all slightly differing in costume and setting are now found at, *inter alia*, Dulwich Picture Gallery (PLATE 6), Loseley Park, the Pitti Palace in Florence (a half-length) and the Prado in Madrid.[31] They are in the mainstream international court tradition, which lays detailed emphasis on the sitter's jewellery, rich fabrics and accessories, and exaggerates his or her height in order to convey an image of authority. De Critz must have had a considerable studio, with a number of assistants to enable him to fulfil the regular orders for royal portraits, not only from the sovereign, but also from court members keen to display their loyalty; in October 1607, for instance, De Critz billed Robert Cecil for a picture of the King.[32] In 1611 and 1618 payments for images of James were also made to Marcus Gheeraerts II.[33] It is not now possible to distinguish these works, but it raises the possibility that the brothers-in-law may have worked in collaboration. Simultaneously, it should be remembered that De Critz was coordinating decorative painting, repainting and restoration activities at the various royal establishments.[34]

Anne of Denmark kept her own court. In 1605 she appointed Isaac Oliver, Gheeraerts's brother-in-law, her official limner (that is, miniature painter). Her husband, meanwhile, continued to use Elizabeth's favoured miniaturist, the English-born Nicholas Hilliard. During the early years of the reign, the images in large of Anne do not appear to have been particularly satisfactory. The De Critz studio seems to have been employed. A studio example, for instance, now in the stores of the Pitti Palace, may have been sent as a diplomatic gift to the Grand Duke Ferdinando de Medici.[35]

In about 1607, however, she seems to have appointed Marcus Gheeraerts II as her official artist. There were indigenous artists available – William Larkin and Robert Peake, to name but two – but she selected the foreign-born artist who had depicted Elizabeth at the end of her reign. A portrait of Anne of *c*.1611 in the Royal Collection (PLATE 7), of which there is a full-length studio version at Woburn Abbey, shows her apparently deliberately exploiting the visual parallels with Gheeraerts's earlier 'Ditchley' portrait of Elizabeth I of *c*.1592.[36] This must have been quite deliberate. At the beginning of their reign in London, James had insisted that Anne wear Elizabeth's gowns, not only because they were appropriately rich in quality and signifiers of royalty, but also because they must have provided, for English viewers, a sense of visual continuity. Anne was initially reluctant, but a decade later she was refusing to abandon the by-now rather old-fashioned wheel farthingale. So Gheeraerts's image is also a conscious throwback to a portrait of 20 years earlier.

For in 1611–12 the heir to the throne, Prince Henry, who had his own establishment, attempted to persuade the Delft-based portraitist, Michiel Jansz. van Miereveld, the favoured artist of the Dutch House of Orange-Nassau, to come and work at his own court in London. His was cutting-edge Dutch art – more sombre, more three-dimensional, the figure moulded by the use of shadow.[37] But the busy and successful Miereveld was reportedly unwilling to come to England for more than three months, and in the end negotiations broke down entirely.[38] England clearly did not appear a worthwhile career option to him.

Payments for royal portraits to De Critz and Gheeraerts continued. De Critz's eldest son, John II, followed in his professional footsteps, as did two other sons, Thomas (born 1607) and Emanuel (born 1608). Gheeraerts's second son, Marcus III, born 1602, also followed the career of a painter.[39]

The Miereveld initiative, however, was a foretaste of things to come. In 1617, the by-now old guard dropped rapidly out of fashion with the arrival of a group of Netherlandish artists seeking economic opportunity. These were men who arrived as adults, who had been trained on the Continent, and had established modest artistic careers there. Born in Antwerp in 1576, Paul van Somer had moved regularly in search of career opportunities – Amsterdam in 1604, Leiden in 1612–14, The Hague in 1615, Brussels in 1616. Reaching London in late 1616, he was immediately taken up by the most avant-garde court patrons, including the Queen, as demonstrated by his 1617 full-length of her in hunting attire in the Royal Collection.[40] Even James, notoriously unwilling to sit for his portrait, and content to use the same image of himself for over a decade, went to Van Somer for an image makeover.[41] Anne died in 1619, and Gheeraerts was mentioned among the artificers present at her funeral.[42] In c.1620 Van Somer portrayed James standing in front of a visually garbled version of the Banqueting House in Whitehall, in his scarlet and white robes of state.[43] For James this was a period of crisis, with the Spanish invasion of the Palatinate and the subsequent defeat and exile from Prague of his son-in-law Frederick and his daughter Elizabeth, subsequently to be known as the 'Winter King and Queen'. In early 1621 James was forced to call Parliament in order to have a chance of sending assistance to the Palatinate. When he was forced to dissolve it at the end of the year, this 'marked the eclipse of James as a potent and respected ruler'.[44]

Van Somer, who came to London with his wife, presumably meant to stay. However, he had the misfortune to die at the end of 1621. But his role was taken over by Daniel Mytens, who had reached London by August 1618. Born in Delft in about 1590, into an artist dynasty, Mytens is thought to have been a pupil of Miereveld. This connection may account for his taking the chance of seeking British patronage. It is not clear whether he came by invitation, but again he was immediately taken up by the top court patrons – the Earl and Countess of Arundel, the future Charles I and the Marquis of Buckingham. Mytens was the creator of the powerful, and last, image of James I of 1621 (PLATE 8). This paper closes with the end of James I's reign in 1625, but it should be remembered that on the horizon was the arrival of the Antwerp-born and trained Antony van Dyck in 1632 to take over all the major Caroline court portrait commissions, and to reinvent, once again, the public image of the monarchy.

Thus, by the time of Mytens's 1621 portrait, both De Critz and Gheeraaerts had lost their royal portrait patronage. De Critz was probably already wholly a manager, co-ordinating the painting of an extensive range of royal decorative commissions. Gheeraerts, however, continued painting portraits, his clients becoming increasingly less exalted. It may be worth noting that it was during this period of professional stress, in February 1618, that Gheeraerts finally applied for denization.[45] His known career continued until about 1630, three years after the making of his lost self-portrait. As was stressed earlier, artists at this period rarely signed their works. Only very occasionally did Gheeraerts do so, but, intriguingly, he sometimes appended a word that emphasized his foreign birth. His 1608 portrait of Louis Frederick, Duke of Württemberg, a royal commission, is inscribed 'gerardi Brugiense fece'.[46] Again, in 1624, he signed a modest head and shoulders of William Pope, Earl of Downe, 'Brugiensis'.[47] Does this suggest that he felt that the assurance that he came from Bruges conferred additional cachet on his artistic production?

One might consider it a continuing paradox of the English monarchy that it habitually used foreign-born artists to articulate its official visual image. In the careers of John de Critz I and Marcus Gheeraerts II, and their respective dynasties, we see the passage from stranger to citizen. Indeed, the third generation were to be wholly absorbed into the indigenous painter community. These personal trajectories were, however, the opposite of that customarily taken by English royal art patronage, which with the adoption successively of Van Somer, Mytens and Van Dyck (and indeed other, lesser, Netherlandish talents) reasserted its preference for overseas-trained portraitists – who were indeed veritable strangers.

NOTES

1 This may be translated as 'Marcus Gheeraerts the painter, in the service of the most Illustrious and Serene Princes, Elizabeth and Anne, of blessed memory, Queens of Great Britain, France and Ireland, was the son of the outstanding artist Marcus Gheeraerts of Bruges in Flanders, where he was born. He died in London on January 19th 1635 [Old Style] at the age of 74. Marcus himself produced this painting in 1627, which was engraved by Wenceslaus Hollar of Bohemia in 1644' (kindly translated by Dr Keith Cunliffe). See Rachel Poole, 'Marcus Gheeraerts, father and son, painters', *Walpole Society* 3 (1914), 6.

2 Hans Holbein II, *Henry VIII*, c.1536, oil on panel, Fundacion Coleccion Thyssen-Bornemisza, Madrid, reproduced in Karen Hearn (ed.), *Dynasties: painting in Tudor and Jacobean England, 1530–1630* (London, 1995), 43, fig. 23.

3 *Ibid.*, 48–9, catalogue no. 12.

4 Catharine MacLeod, 'Guillim Scrots in England' (unpublished MA report, Courtauld Institute of Art, 1990).

5 Roy Strong, *Hans Eworth: a Tudor artist and his circle* (Leicester, 1965); Hearn, *Dynasties*, 63, 66–7, catalogue no. 24.

6 Susan Foister, 'Foreigners at court: Holbein, Van Dyck and the Painter-Stainers' Company', in David Howarth (ed.), *Art and patronage in the Caroline courts* (Cambridge, 1993), 33.

7 Steve Rappaport, *Worlds within worlds: structures of life in sixteenth-century London* (Cambridge, 1989). I am grateful to Dr Claire Gapper for also discussing this issue with me.

8 Lionel Cust, 'Foreign artists of the Reformed religion in England, 1560–1660', *HSP* 7:2 (1903), 45–82.

9 Lionel Cust, 'Marcus Gheeraerts', *Walpole Society* 3 (1914), 9–45. The oeuvre that he there

proposes for the Gheeraerts is, however, unreliable. It contains works now recognized as being by other painters, such as Robert Peake.

10 Rachel Poole, 'An outline of the history of the De Critz family of painters', *Walpole Society* 2 (1913), 45–68; *eadem*, 'Marcus Gheeraerts, father and son, painters', *Walpole Society* 3 (1914), 1–8.

11 Mary Edmond, 'Limners and picturemakers: new light on the lives of miniaturists and large-scale portrait-painters working in London in the sixteenth and seventeenth centuries', *Walpole Society* 47 (1978–80), 60–242.

12 Poole, 'De Critz family of painters', 45.

13 Hearn, 154–5, catalogue no. 101.

14 *Ibid.*, 173–4, catalogue no. 118.

15 *Ibid.*, 174–5, catalogue no. 119.

16 Poole, 'Marcus Gheeraerts', 6.

17 Maximilaan J. Martens (ed.), *Bruges and the Renaissance: Memling to Pourbus* (Bruges, 1998), 231–3.

18 Karel van Mander, *The lives of the illustrious Netherlandish and German painters: from the first edition of the Schilder-boeck* (1603–4), ed. Hessel Miedema (Doornspijk, 1994), 290.

19 Hearn, 86–7, catalogue no. 41.

20 Poole, 'Marcus Gheeraerts', 3.

21 Edward Hodnett, *Marcus Gheeraerts the Elder, of Bruges, London and Antwerp* (Utrecht, 1971), 12.

22 Roy Strong, *The cult of Elizabeth* (London, 1977), 129–34.

23 Hearn, 89–90, catalogue no. 45.

24 *Ibid.*, 133, catalogue no. 80.

25 Poole, 'Marcus Gheeraerts', 3, 5.

26 Erna Auerbach, *Tudor artists* (London, 1954), 147–8.

27 Duncan Thomson, *The life and art of George Jamesone* (Oxford, 1974), 44–6.

28 *Ibid.*, 46–8; Hearn, 172–3, catalogue no. 117.

29 See *Christian IV and Europe, 19th art exhibition of the Council of Europe, Denmark 1988* (Copenhagen, 1988), 28, catalogue. no. 36, reproduced on 547, colour Pl. I.

30 Poole, 'De Critz family', 46.

31 Hearn, 184–5, catalogue no. 125.

32 Erna Auerbach and C. Kingsley Adams, *Paintings and sculpture at Hatfield House* (London, 1971), 72.

33 Edmond, 'Limners and picturemakers', 138, states that in the entry for 1611, Gheeraerts is described as 'His Ma[jes]ties Paynter'.

34 Poole, 'De Critz family', 49.

35 Marco Chiarini, *Visite Reali a Palazzo Pitti* (Florence, 1995), 51, catalogue no. 3, reproduced on 18; Lucy Wood, 'The portraits of Anne of Denmark' (unpublished MA report, Courtauld Institute of Art, 1971).

36 Hearn, 192, catalogue no. 130.

37 Hearn, 203–4, catalogue no. 137.

38 Timothy V. Wilks, 'The court culture of Prince Henry and his circle, 1603–1613' (unpublished D.Phil. thesis, Oxford University, 1987).

39 Edmond, 137–9.

40 Hearn, 206, catalogue no. 139; reproduced in Christopher Lloyd, *The paintings in the Royal Collection* (London, 1992), 26, fig. 3.

41 He was depicted in 1618 at full-length with the regalia on a table at his side: see Oliver Millar, *The Tudor, Stuart and early Georgian pictures in the Royal Collection* (London, 1960), text vol., 80–1, catalogue no.103; plates vol., plate 43.

42 Auerbach, *Tudor artists*, 165.

43 Lloyd, *Royal Collection*, 27, fig. 4.
44 David H. Willson, *King James VI and I* (London, 1963; reprinted 1971), 423.
45 Poole, 'Marcus Gheeraerts', 7. It seems probable that he also applied to become a member of the London Painter-Stainers' Company: Edmond, 137.
46 Roy Strong, *The English icon* (London, 1969), 272, no. 255.
47 *Ibid.*, 274, no.258.

13

A Dutch 'stranger … on the make': Sir Peter Lely and the critical fortunes of a foreign painter

JULIA MARCIARI ALEXANDER

When Paul Mellon, arguably the greatest recent American collector and philanthropist, passed away in February 1999, his obituaries featured a picture of him seated in front of Sir Antony van Dyck's full-length portrait of Mountjoy Blount, 1st Earl of Newport (1637–8; New Haven, Yale Center for British Art). Many who knew or worked for Paul Mellon felt this photograph was a particularly apt pictorial tribute at his death; it showed him before one of the nearly 40,000 works of art he gave as the core of the collection of the Yale Center for British Art, a centre whose sole purpose was to expose and educate American audiences about the visual and literary culture of Great Britain from the Tudors until today. Further, the photograph achieved precisely what such Grand Manner Baroque portraits aimed to do for their original patrons in whose homes they were displayed: it equated the glamorous and aristocratic Earl of Newport with its present-day owner, Paul Mellon, through the latter's proximity and – quite literally – ownership of the former. No matter how appropriate most found the photo and the associations made therein, the newspaper's choice to run this particular image with Mellon's obituary prompted a telling reaction from one of my colleagues, who loudly lamented its publication and exclaimed, 'Too bad he's not in front of an English painting!'

True, the Flemish artist Van Dyck was in no way a native of England nor even made a citizen. But can his paintings created in England for English patrons be dismissed so summarily as 'un-English', especially since his work is arguably the most important foundation for the mainstay of 'English' or British art: the Grand Manner portrait from Van Dyck to Sargent? I think not. This issue of definition, 'the history of art in Britain' versus 'the history of British Art' lies at the core of my paper.

Peter Van der Faes, known as Peter Lely, was born in Soest, Westphalia in 1618. He trained as a young artist in Haarlem in the workshop of Frans Pieter de Grebber. Little is known about his career prior to his coming to England, although various attempts to find works dating certainly to his 'Dutch' period have been undertaken.[1] Yet, Lely's artistic reputation did not depend on his 'Dutch' work; rather, it was only after his arrival in England sometime in the early 1640s that his name became an international artistic commodity.

Although many of his early paintings are of mythological, religious, or pastoral subjects – such as his *Sleeping Nymphs by a Fountain* (c.1645; London, Dulwich College Picture Gallery), Lely quickly saw the professional and commercial advantages of turning to portraiture. His insightful portraits of the English royal family, painted while Charles I was in captivity in 1647, demonstrate both the painter's artistic stature at the height of the Civil War and his virtuosity as a portraitist early in his career [PLATE 9]. Throughout the Commonwealth, Lely made his fortune and solidified his reputation by painting both prominent English nobles who had remained in the country during the Interregnum and many of the most important Commonwealth officials, among them the Protector himself. By the Restoration of Charles II in 1660, Lely was probably the most sought-after portraitist in England.

Shortly after Charles II's triumphant entry into London in May 1660 (and this despite the painter's associations with Cromwell and other notable Parliamentarians), Lely was awarded the post of Principal Painter-in-Ordinary to the King and sworn in on 20 June 1660; in October 1661, he received the first payment of his annual pension of £200, and the warrants indicated that this specific sum for the pension was the same as had been granted 'formerly to Sr. Vandyke'.[2] This enunciation of the Restoration painter's relationship to the earlier master must be seen as proof that Lely was appointed to the post primarily due to his skill as a portrait painter in oils and, more specifically, to his adherence to Van Dyckian modes of painting. This can be easily seen in a comparison between Lely's lovely portrait of the Capel sisters painted at the time of the Restoration in 1660 (c.1660; New York, Metropolitan Museum of Art) and Van Dyck's masterful, Thimbleby sisters, of 25 years earlier (c.1637; London, National Gallery of Art).

Whatever Lely's nationality by birth, his contemporary reputation, then, was not one of a usurper or a foreigner; and, indeed, as Katharine Gibson has shown in her monumental study of Charles II's iconography, the artist was in fact granted naturalization in May of 1662.[3] In fact, his contemporary chroniclers quickly asserted his status as a key member of the 'English' artistic community.

In his 1658 treatise, *Graphice: the use of the pen and pensil, or, The most excellent art of Painting*, William Sanderson attacked the issue of Lely's status as a 'forraigner' head on. He included Lely's name in his list of contemporary 'English' painters worthy of note, explaining:

> These now in *England* are not less worthy of fame than any forraigner; and although some of them be strangers born, . . . for their affection to our *Nation*, . . . we may mixe them together. Our Modern Masters [are] comparable with any now beyond seas. . . In the Life, Walker, Zowst [sic], Wright, Lillie [sic], Hayls, Shepheard, de Grange, [are] rare Artizans . . .[4]

Similarly, Bainbrigge Buckridge included Lely in his 'An Essay towards an English School of Painting', first published in 1706. Buckridge (along with his collaborator John Savage) was amongst the first – and, indeed, arguably the very first – to delineate and define an 'English' School of painting. In the work's dedicatory preface, Buckridge, like Sanderson, articulated a carefully thought-out defence for including in their 'English' School a number of 'foreign painters':

At present [the English school] is more than a match for the French; and the German and Flemish Schools, only excel it by the performances of those masters whom we claim as our own. Hans Holbein and Vandyck are as much ours as Sebastian of Venice belongs to the Roman school, Spagnoletto to the Lombard, or . . . de Champagne to the French . . . Nor have we a small title to Sir Peter Paul Rubens, for it was the protection and friendship of the duke of Buckingham that procured him the opportunities he had of distinguishing himself above others of his contemporaries. . . Why should we be so unjust to ourselves, as to think we stand in need of an excuse for pretending to the honor of a school of Painters? . . .[5]

These passages make plain that both Sanderson and Buckridge felt an imperative to undertake pointedly what amounts to the artistic naturalization of 'stranger born' or 'foreign' artists.

This rhetorical movement to define a more rigidly bound and inherently 'nationalist' artistic identity largely parallels political imperatives of Restoration and late Stuart England. Gone was the admission or understanding of the practical realities of artistic systems in which the great artists travelled throughout Europe gaining fame in court after court. In post-1688 Stuart England, colluding drives for national and colonial hegemony combined with the rise of oligarchy (as opposed to a perceived absolutist political state) to prompt a need to 'naturalize' – or in modern terms 'appropriate' – the 'stranger-born' artist. The conversion of 'strangers' into 'citizens' was necessary to the post-Glorious Revolution artist and critic; in fact, one of the aims of civic humanism was the creation of an aesthetic system for engendering indigenous artists of equal merit to those who were 'foreign born'.[6]

Lely's status as a 'stranger' became a liability especially to those of a later generation, who, among other things, felt he had failed to inspire a 'native' group of 'English' students. Entangled with his critical fortunes in the early 18th century, then, are two crucial issues: 1. the perceived need of critics to create a mechanism outside the traditional workshop system by which 'native' artists could be trained (in other words, England needed to create an English Academy); 2. an historically evident burgeoning disdain for the Restoration court to which Lely literally gave a face.

We are all familiar with the vehement advocacy, first of William Hogarth and, later, of Joshua Reynolds, to establish an 'English' Academy whose purpose would be to educate native-born artists who would establish a viable 'National' school of worthy painters. Certainly, the ebbing tide of Lely's critical fortunes in the 18th and 19th centuries was tightly bound up with his status as a non-native artist in a climate of intense and growing nationalism. Yet, for Lely's critics there seems to have been a second, equally forceful strike against him, one that joined with his status as a foreign painter to condemn him to the rung of second-tier artists: he was, in the mind's eye of later generations, the painter *par excellence* of the morally corrupt court of Charles II.

The reviling of the Restoration court clearly began as a tool of the Whig machine in the wake of the Glorious Revolution, despite the fact that the late Stuart queens as well as their Hanoverian successors were direct descendants and cousins of the allegedly depraved monarchs, Charles II and James II. In short, Lely's reputation as a masterful painter of virtuoso pictures quickly became replaced by his reputation as a painter of the wanton women of a lascivious court [PLATES 10 and 11].

Horace Walpole, for instance, admitted Lely's prowess with the brush, calling him 'the most capital painter of [Charles II's] reign . . .' but he also dismissed Lely's greatest commission, that of the Windsor Beauties as depicting 'the court of Paphos'.[7] Walpole's choice to equate the women of Lely's group with this legendary group of prostitutes (from amongst the many beautiful women of antique lore) indicated clearly both his own moral evaluation of Lely's sitters and his own clear disdain for that artist's unabashedly colourist style – the women of the court of Paphos having had the blood in their cheeks hardened to stone.

Indeed, from Walpole onwards, a gender-based contest arose between perceptions of Lely's female and male portraits; at the heart of this battle festered viewers' and critics' latent, misogynist nationalist tendencies to posit the female pictures as evidence of a transparent moral deprivation rampant at the Restoration Court. By contrast, Lely's male portraits were held up as potential, if somewhat flawed, representations of and representatives for a distinctly virtuous, and naturally 'English', moral dignity [see, for example, PLATES 12 and 13].

The critics' problem, however, lay in figuring out how best to reconcile their perception of Lely's ability to convey so convincingly the wantonness of the morally depraved English women with their desire to see his portraits of men as demonstrations of an upstanding 'English' male character (and I use 'English', as did the critics, as a synonym for morally superior character). The way out of this dilemma came in the writers' claims that, as a foreign painter, Lely did not convey the 'Englishness' of his sitters at all. In other words, writers could assert that the artist's status as a foreigner actually prevented him from capturing in full force of his sitters' moral – and typically 'English' – fortitude. Yet, within this complex system of demarcation, they were also able to claim that the male portraits were nonetheless successful since the sitters' inherent 'Englishness' was so powerful it actually imprinted itself on the picture.

This type of mapping of national, moral – or immoral – character on to Lely's portraits is illustrated best by passages from C. H. Collins Baker's *Lely and the Stuart portrait painters*, originally published in 1911. Collins Baker, despite his championship of Lely's abilities as a painter, remained firmly within the grip of nationalist sentiment in his discussions both of the female portraits and the male. In the case of the female portraits, he proclaimed that 'had Lely, with his great technical powers, been French, his development of the languorous syren [*sic*] type . . . would have been incomparably more piquant'.[8] In the case of the male, he lamented:

> Truly these hard seamen of the Dutch wars were a fine theme . . . No contemporary of Lely's, save the two great Dutch masters, could have painted these hardened seamen as truly as he. My one regret is that Lely's Dutchness prevented his painting their Englishness, for we hardly recognize our countrymen in them.[9]

Such an interpretation of portraits – and, by extension, of portraiture more generally – as windows into the soul of either a nation or a man tells us much more about the aspirations of the writers about portraits than about the paintings, the artists, or even the sitters themselves. Harry Berger has described this theory of portraiture as 'physiognomic art history' or, in other words, a history of the representation of the face as one that assumes the face is the visual index of the mind.[10] 'Physiognomic art history' assumes that both sitter and artist seek through a portrait to convey what the modern theorist might describe as 'the essence' of a sitter. This notion of the portrait as indicative of the essential is one that engenders an impetus for the artist to make and the viewer to seek visual confirmation in portraits of a national – read *moral* – character in portraits. In this equation the essence of both artist and sitter count equally: only a native 'Englishman' can truly capture what is 'good' or 'moral' – or 'English' – in his sitter. This formula clearly depends on the tight weaving together of political and moral character with evaluations of artistic taste and arguments about quality and style. In fact, the 'physiognomic' approach inherently pits the foreign-born portraitist against his native subject/sitter and, ultimately, dooms the 'stranger' to failure in his endeavour to paint a convincing portrait of the 'citizen'.

Few modern scholars are wont to embrace this theoretical approach, promoting portraiture as the effort of artist and subject to reveal an 'essential' self or 'true character' of the sitter. Instead, portrait specialists increasingly have come, rather, to view the historical practice of face-painting as one based on a transaction. According to the 'transactional' model of portraiture, a portrait seeks not to represent a 'true' internal self but instead, in reflecting the combined efforts of painter and sitter, imparts the sitter with a visual 'persona' – real or not real, it doesn't really matter.[11] In other words, a portrait is the result of an agreement between artist and subject to create a representation of the subject as he or she wished to be perceived by contemporaries and posterity. In this vision of portraiture as a transaction, the nationality of artist and/or sitter is necessarily irrelevant to the transmission of character since painterly construction of character is just that: simply an artistic construction. This is not to say that the transmission of 'national' character might not be the aim of the 'persona' depicted in any given portrait. But, in this model, Lely's birthright as a 'Dutch stranger' is irrelevant to his ability to create a distinct vision of the Restoration 'English' Beauty or Admiral.

That successive generations have spilled so much ink trying either to justify or to deny him a place within an 'English' art speaks more to the historical imperative to define a visually apparent 'national' or even 'native' character than it speaks to Lely's artistic acumen. Indeed, except for a few works painted in his early career and apart from a brief trip to the Continent in the 1650s, Lely did not produce a single work outside England during his mature career; with that in mind, can one claim him as a 'Dutch' artist any more convincingly than as an 'English' one? Clearly bound up with aims of nationalistic discourse, misogyny and moral/political disdain for the Restoration court combined to make Lely, the so-called 'Dutch stranger', both the perceived spokesman for and scapegoat of his artistic generation. Had Mr Mellon's picture shown him in front of Lely's glorious portrait of *Diana Kirke, Countess of Oxford*, [PLATE 10] in the Centre's collection, would it have been possible for my colleague to claim that Lely was not an 'English' artist?

In today's climate of multi-culturalism and the recognition and appreciation of difference within cultures and among cultures, just how should we consider this artist – as a 'Dutch stranger . . . on the make' as did Collins Baker or as a naturalized 'Englishman' whose art, regardless of his birth-citizenship, literally created the image of Restoration England? In fact, given his career history as a painter who lived and worked almost exclusively in London, should we consider his national 'essence' at all within our evaluations of career and his artistic prowess?

The larger issue, it seems to me, is determining how we can expect to gain understanding of the complexities of artistic and visual culture of early modern Europe if we continue to accept latent nationalism within art historical discourse. Indeed, we must ask ourselves if and why it is still viable to create institutions dedicated to – as is that in which I work – the promotion of the idea of 'The Englishness of English Art' (especially since it is now recognized that the socio-political structures of early modern Europe were as dependent on class as on national systems)? I am proposing here no answers to these questions. In raising them, however, I hope that we can begin the process of unravelling the tightly-woven canvas of art historical discourse, a discourse that sometimes insidiously and, more often, blatantly promotes a theory of portraiture that traps artists, sitters and viewers within a nationalist agenda. In so doing, perhaps we will be able to move away from a history of portraiture in Britain that perpetuates hitherto-accepted assumptions about a necessary elision between portraiture and national identity to one that celebrates the genius of strangers and citizens alike.

NOTES

This essay is published here as it was given at the conference on 6 April 2000, at a session chaired by Steven Parissien, Paul Mellon Centre for the Study of British Art. An expanded and revised version will appear in *Painted ladies: portraits of women at the court of Charles II, 1660–1685*, a catalogue accompanying the exhibition of the same title (London, National Portrait Gallery, 11 October 2001–6 January 2002 and New Haven, Yale Center for British Art, 25 January–17 March 2002).

1   See, for instance, Jacques Foucard, 'Peter Lely, Dutch history painter', *Hoogsteder-Naumann Mercury*, ed. Albert Blankert, no. 8 (The Hague, 1989).
2   Katharine Gibson, '"Best Belov'd of Kings": the iconography of King Charles II', unpublished Ph.D. thesis, Courtauld Institute, University of London, 1997, 116.
3   *Ibid.*
4   William Sanderson, *Graphice: the use of the pen and pensil, or The most excellent art of Painting: in Two Parts* (London, 1658), 20.
5   Bainbrigge Buckridge (and John Savage), *The Art of Painting with the Lives and Characters of above 300 of the most Eminent Painters* . . . (3rd edn., London, 1754), 5.
6   On the concept of 'civic humanism' and its role in aesthetic discourse, see especially, David H. Solkin, *Painting for money: the visual and the public sphere in eighteenth-century England* (New Haven, CT, 1993).
7   Horace Walpole, *Anecdotes of painting in England*, 4 vols. (reprint of the 1826 edition, New York, 1969), vol. 2, 91–3.
8   C. H. Collins Baker, *Lely and the Stuart portrait painters*, 2 vols. (London, 1911), vol. 1, 166.
9   *Ibid.*, vol. 1, 170–1.
10 For a more detailed elaboration of this definition, see Harry Berger, Jr. 'Fictions of the pose: facing the gaze', in *Representations* 46 (Spring 1994), 87–120.
11 For a broader discussion of the 'transactional' theory of portraiture, see Richard Wendorf, *Sir Joshua Reynolds: the painter in society* (Cambridge, MA, 1996), 4.

14

Foreign artists and craftsmen and the introduction of the Rococo style in England

Christine Riding

In general terms, the word 'Rococo' describes the elegant and fanciful decorative style introduced in France in the first half of the 18th century, which spread with varying degrees of influence across Europe and her colonies. In design, the Rococo was characterized by asymmetrical compositions and a distinctive decorative repertoire of *rocaille* and other natural motifs, and flowing S- and C-curves, and in fine art, by a bias towards the informal, the epicurean and the sensuous. In France, the Rococo developed from *c.*1710 and was the presiding aesthetic in art and interior design in the 1730s and '40s. But in England, its influence was tempered by the adoption from 1715 of the Palladian style, and later the fashion for the Gothic and Chinese styles. But the Rococo pervaded English design in the middle decades of the century, and informed British art production up to the 1760s, and arguably beyond.

Although there are numerous ways in which a style is appropriated, i.e. direct importation of goods and engraved designs, art patrons and artists travelling abroad to mention but two methods, this paper concentrates (albeit in brief) on foreign and immigrant artists and craftsmen, who, having settled in England, were instrumental in introducing and popularizing the Rococo style.[1]

This paper continues with a paradox. Historically speaking, France was the great national rival and in terms of armed conflict the traditional enemy. At the beginning, middle and end of the 18th century, England was at war with France. These wars had, however, resulted in substantial colonial and commercial gains for England and greatly enhanced Britain's reputation in Europe. But given this Anglo/French rivalry, and the nation's legendary xenophobia and in particular, francophobia, it may at first seem strange that a style so openly acknowledged as French – 'in the French manner' as it was termed – could achieve any success in England.

In the second half of the 17th century France had established its pre-eminence in all matters concerning taste and refinement, and its monarchy, surrounded by un-paralleled magnificence, was the envy of Europe. In contrast, despite its military successes, early 18th-century England was, as Derek Jarrett has observed, 'unsure of itself in many ways' with most Englishmen feeling 'a little awkward and self-conscious in the presence of the polished suavity of the French'.[2] The governing classes might rail against France and its absolutism, colonial ambitions, huge standing army, and its habitual support of the Jacobite cause, but for the social elite, a distinction could be made between the world of politics and empire and the world of fashion and taste.

Thus the reaction to France and all things French, was, in a word, ambivalent. Amongst the aristocracy, French culture was copied, often slavishly so. Gerald Newman remarks that 'there are signs that London was in some respects as much a cultural colony of Paris as Rome, Madrid, or St Petersburg'.[3] Wealthy tourists visited France and particularly Paris in their thousands, adopting the latest fashions and importing French luxury goods, designs and engravings, and occasionally artists and craftsmen. On the other hand, the onslaught of French culture provoked an exaggeratedly 'hale and hearty' mode of Englishness. Indeed it has been argued that it was during this period that the image of the free-born, fair-playing, plain-speaking, liberty-loving Englishman achieved currency across Europe, in part propagated by the observations of French travellers and exiles, such as the Huguenots Maximilien Misson (d.1721) and the Swiss-born César de Saussure (b.1705), and of course Voltaire (1694–1778).[4] These national attributes were often contrasted with popular perceptions of French society, the most resonant being 'papist superstition', 'governmental tyranny' and 'mass poverty'; all three were neatly visualized by William Hogarth in his unashamedly francophobic painting, O the Roast Beef of Old England ('The Calais Gate') (1749, Tate Gallery, London), engravings of which were reissued a number of times and achieved widespread popularity.[5]

Hogarth, of course, never tired of ridiculing the appropriation of French (and other foreign) customs and fripperies, which, in his opinion, led to affectation and foolishness; Viscount Squanderfield, the Frenchified fop in Marriage á-la-Mode, being a case in point (PLATE 14). In short, for many Englishmen, the French were either emasculated peacocks or scrawny, half-starved desperados.[6]

Between 1713 and 1744, England and France were in theory at peace, a period concurrent with the flowering of the Rococo style in France and its introduction into England. This situation encouraged numerous artists and craftsmen, including Frenchmen, to settle in London. Many proved instrumental in the appropriation of the new style. Inevitably, this paper focuses on London. London was the place to go for anyone, native or foreign, who had even an iota of ambition. By 1750 it held over one fifth of the total population and was at least ten times bigger than the largest of provincial towns. It was the financial centre of Europe, was the national centre of fashion and patronage, of luxury production and consumption. It provided the greatest access to cultural information from abroad, and was the hub of a growing press network, which created in turn a wealth of new work for engravers and illustrators. London had approximately sixty pleasure gardens, the most famous of which were Vauxhall and Ranelagh, 2000 coffee-houses, and a thriving theatre world. Of course, London was home to numerous immigrant communities. By 1720, for example, in the parish of St Anne's, Soho, three-fifths of the population was French, and the district was already known as the French quarter.

The Huguenots, of course, had an established reputation as innovative and highly-skilled craftsmen; as silk weavers, furniture makers, wood carvers, goldsmiths, watch- and clockmakers, and so on. At the turn of the century it was said that 'The English

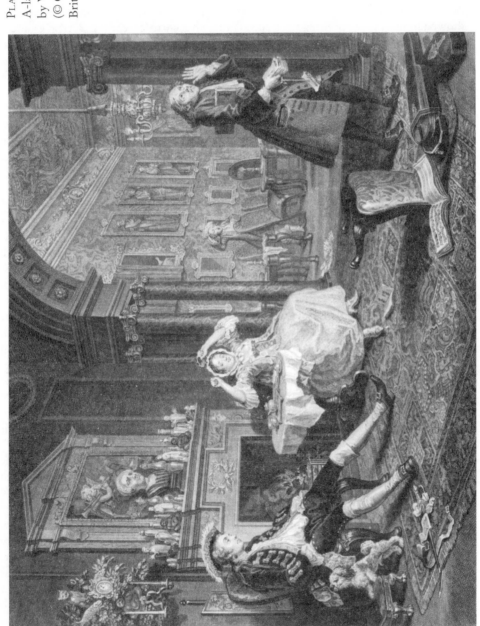

PLATE 14 Marriage-A-la-Mode Plate II by William Hogarth (© Copyright The British Museum)

have now so great an esteem for the workmanship of the French refugees that hardly any thing vends without a gallic name'.[7] As a close-knit community, ever mindful of their Gallic origins, and in communication with relatives living on the Continent, the Huguenots remained receptive to French fashions and abreast of the latest developments. Not surprisingly, Paul Crespin (1694–1770) and Paul de Lamerie (1688–1751), both second generation Huguenots and leading goldsmiths, were also pioneers in Rococo-style metalwork. De Lamerie registered his first mark in London in 1712 and showed signs of appropriating the budding French style in the early 1720s.[8] We should also not underestimate the Huguenots as patrons and cultivators of the new style. The Huguenot *emigré*, François Roubiliac (1702/5–62), who has been described as 'the greatest Rococo sculptor to devote his working life to this country',[9] received many of his earliest and most substantial commissions for portrait sculpture through this community.[10]

For British artists and craftsmen there seems to be a contradiction between patriotism and employing the Rococo style. However, their frustrations and complaints were levelled more pointedly at art connoisseurs and patrons, who seemed determined to buy imported goods and to ignore native talent, than against foreigners and their fashions *per se*. Generally speaking, native craftsmen can have had little argument against the Rococo itself. Its complicated, highly decorative vocabulary, once mastered, was labour intensive and increasingly in great demand. As a generous employer of craftsmen, the Rococo was thus extremely lucrative. This led to a few interesting contradictions. For example, the Anti-Gallican Society was founded in London in 1745 with the explicit aim of extending 'the commerce of England', discouraging 'the introduction of French modes' and opposing 'the importation of French commodities'.[11] Yet many of its members were craftsmen and patrons of the Rococo. As late as 1758 we find the designer and carver, Thomas Johnson (1714–after 1778), an Anti-Gallican, introducing his book of furniture designs with an elaborate dedication page (PLATE 15) replete with exuberant Rococo cartouches, surmounted by a triumphant Britannia (on the right), and a scowling personification of France relegated to the background (on the left).[12] Earlier, in 1752, a pamphlet entitled *Reflections on Various Subjects relating to Arts and Commerce: particularly the Consequences of admitting Foreign Artists*, recommended the immigration of French Protestant craftsmen for the benefit of the manufacture of English luxury goods, their Protestantism making them infinitely more acceptable than their Catholic counterparts. The pamphlet particularly praised the Chelsea porcelain factory, which from the 1740s was run by the Huguenot goldsmith, Nicholas Sprimont (1716–71), a native of Liège. Much of the factory's output during his directorship was in the Rococo style.[13]

The English artistic scene of the 1720s was, to use David Bindman's phrase, 'at a low point of provincialism'.[14] The English did not have a state-funded Academy like the French. There were very few places for formal training and there was no structure via which art was made accessible for the purposes of instruction or forums for artists to exhibit their own work. Although there was no shortage of interest in or money for buying art, patrons preferred the ready-made expertise of talented, well-trained foreigners. Even in the realm of portraiture, where one might expect English artists to have a fighting chance, they could find themselves trumped by a foreign artist. For example, the French court painter Jean-Baptiste Vanloo arrived in London in 1737, bringing with him a glossy, cosmopolitan style of portraiture that took London by

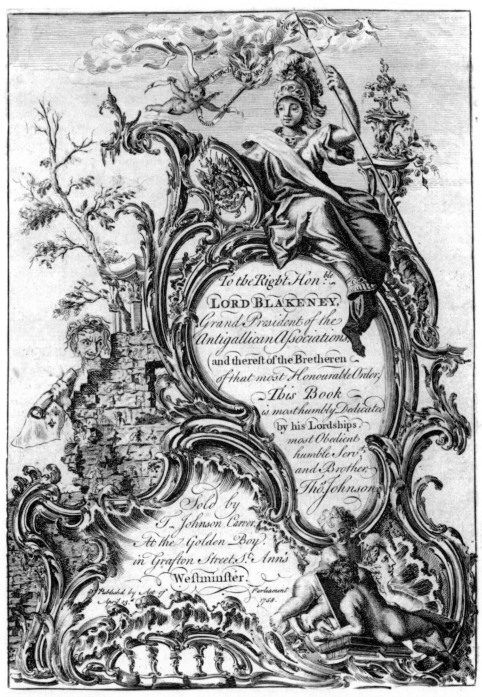

PLATE 15 Dedication page by Thomas Johnson (By courtesy of the Trustees of the Victoria
& Albert Museum)

storm. Native artists stood by helplessly as the great and the good scurried off to the Frenchman's studio.[15]

Undoubtedly a large proportion of foreign artists and craftsmen, whether French, Italian or Dutch, emigrated to England in order to exploit the prejudices of the art-buying public. However, in the early 18th century, we find native artists and craftsmen asserting their position and taking a very pragmatic approach to French style and the presence of foreign and immigrant artists. This manifested itself through serving apprenticeships in their workshops, absorbing and employing their innovations in style and technique, as well as utilizing their skill. As Jenny Uglow has pointed out, Hogarth himself, the 'obstinate patriot', when push came to shove, 'put nationalism second to quality'.[16] He did, after all, go to great trouble and expense to secure the services of three French engravers, Bernard Baron, Gerard Jean-Baptiste Scotin (see PLATE 14) and Simon François Ravenet, the most skilled and fashionable craftsmen he could find in London, to engrave the six canvases of *Marriage A-la-Mode* (1743–5, National Gallery, London), a series that has been described as 'one of his most Rococo conceptions'.[17] Hogarth's Modern Moral Subjects were in almost all cases engraved by Frenchmen, who 'imported a distinct French Rococo flavour to the more robust narrative style of the original picture'.[18]

The influence of French Rococo art in England is a complex subject and can only be hinted at here. One of the most significant developments in British painting between 1720 and 1740 was the new vogue for the 'conversation piece', which was introduced, and in no small part, popularized by foreign artists settling in London. Small in scale, and intimate in nature, these group portraits of families, friends and polite company were both civilized and fanciful, and constituted a break with the established portrait convention represented by the work of Sir Godfrey Kneller and his studio. While the origins of this genre are disputed, there is no doubt that the fashionable *fête galante* paintings of Antoine Watteau (1684–1721) and other French artists were of prime importance.[19] Thus the conversation piece, in combining portraiture with qualities of the *fête galante*, was the 'Anglicization' of a contemporary French genre. Watteau himself – a key figure in the development of the Rococo fine and decorative art in France – had come to London in 1719 to consult with Dr Richard Mead, the celebrated physician and art collector, who purchased two of his works. Watteau's paintings and those of his followers, Nicholas Lancret and Jean-Baptiste Pater, were greatly admired and sought after. His influence on English taste (as well as that of French art *per se*) was propagated by a group of French engravers and printers who had established themselves in London from 1712. These included the aforementioned Bernard Baron, as well as Claude Dubosc and Bernard Lépicié. Both Baron and Dubosc set up lucrative businesses importing and selling prints.[20]

The development of the conversation piece in England occurred in the 1720s and 1730s via the work of immigrant artists such as Pieter Tillemans (*c.*1684–1734), Joseph Van Aken (*c.*1699–1749) and Pieter Angillis (1685–1734), all of whom were Flemish, and the Huguenot, Philip Mercier (1689–1760), who was trained in Berlin and later Paris, before arriving in England in about 1716. Mercier, who is often credited with having produced the first conversation pieces in England (e.g. PLATE 16), was greatly influenced by Watteau's work – having engraved, pastiched and possibly forged numerous examples (for example, *A Conversation in a Park*, *c.*1720–5, in the possession of the Duke of Northumberland, and *A Music Party*, *c.*1737–40, in the Tate

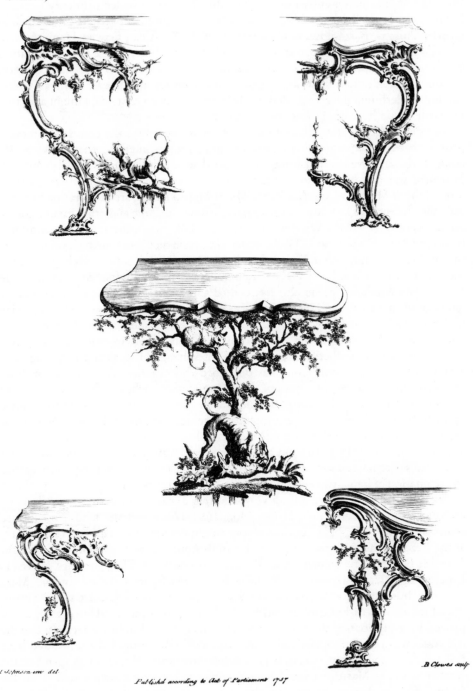

PLATE 17   Designs for pier tables by Thomas Johnson (© The Trustees of the Victoria & Albert Museum)

Gallery, London).[21] Between 1729–36, Mercier was Principal Painter to Frederick, Prince of Wales, and his subsequent career after 1739 was divided primarily between London and York. By the late 1720s and early 1730s a number of native artists such as Charles Phillips, Bartholomew Dandridge and the Scotsman Gawen Hamilton had speedily taken up the new portrait style; so did Hogarth. Indeed, his early conversation pieces, such as *Ashley Cowper with his wife and daughter* (1731, Tate Gallery, London), are executed with an elegance and intimacy that recall Watteau's *fêtes galantes* underlining the genre's debt to the French Rococo. Origins, I might add, that Hogarth would have been more than aware of.

Before we accuse Hogarth and others of gross hypocrisy, the conversation piece proved that contemporary French art and design was something that native artists could have a creative relationship with, rather than something to be blindly imitated. Nowhere was this better shown than within the artistic community that revolved around the St Martin's Lane Academy. The St Martin's Lane area was at this time not only the art centre of London, but also that of cabinet-making and other luxury goods. An offshoot of Kneller's Academy of Art (from 1711) and others, the Academy had been revived by Hogarth in 1735 and under his 'presidency' became the leading school of painting and graphic art in England until the 1760s.[22] By all accounts it began as little more than a life class, but by 1745 numerous artists and craftsmen were teaching classes. The Academy artists also frequented Old Slaughter's Coffee-house nearby (some of them earlier than 1735), which was described by the engraver and antiquarian George Vertue as 'a rendezvous of persons of all languages and Nations, Gentry, artists and others'.[23] Thus between the Academy and the informal environment of the coffee-house, a forum for aesthetic debate and the interchange of ideas and patronage was established. Indeed, David Coke has described this community as 'an amorphous group of artists, craftsmen, writers, actors and others whose ideas and work all contributed to an anarchic, destructive and unbalanced movement in all the arts, almost an early form of Dada; they were intent on the destruction of the old dogmas and taboos, of stylisation and intellectualism, and on bringing in a new freedom and tolerance'.[24] As many of the artists and craftsmen who frequented both venues were alive to the latest French fashions, the St Martin's Lane Academy has subsequently earned the reputation of being the 'seed-bed' of the Rococo in England.

Two French men played a leading role in this dynamic community: the designer and illustrator, Hubert-François Gravelot (1699–1773), and the before mentioned sculptor, François Roubiliac, both of whom taught drawing and sculpture respectively at the Academy. Gravelot was a pupil of Jean Restout and perhaps more importantly, François Boucher, the quintessential Parisian Rococo artist. Thus Gravelot arrived in London in 1732, well-versed in Rococo design and figure drawing. Indeed Mark Girouard has extravagantly opined, that 'If any single person can be said to have introduced the rococo to England, it was he'.[25] Clearly artists and craftsmen were in the process of appropriating the Rococo before Gravelot's arrival. But what Gravelot did introduce was a certain sophistication and delicacy, in the spirit of Watteau and others, to English art and design, particularly in book illustration. As a leading member and teacher at the St Martin's Lane Academy, and via his own drawing school off the Strand, he was able to disseminate the style to the next generation of artists and craftsmen (as well as designing directly for silver and goldsmiths and cabinet-makers). According to the miniaturist, André Rouquet, he was received 'as a kind of oracle'.[26]

Gravelot's most famous pupil was Thomas Gainsborough (1727–88), who was sent to London in 1740 at the age of 13 to train as an artist. Gainsborough is supposed to have studied at Gravelot's house under the Huguenot engraver Charles Grignion, as well as being taught by Gravelot and the painter Francis Hayman (c.1708–1776). In *A Conversation in a Park*, dated 1746–8 (Musée du Louvre), Gainsborough illustrates via the subject and the brilliant fluidity of the paint, how successfully he had appropriated the Rococo manner. Arguably it informed his artistic output for the rest of his career.[27]

The Academy's reputation in the field of decorative art was additionally enhanced by the presence of the chaser and enamellist, George Michael Moser (1706–83). Born in Switzerland, Moser had trained in Geneva and moved to London in about 1721, where initially he was employed by the cabinet-maker, John Trotter of Soho. His mastery of Rococo ornament can be seen in his designs for watchcases and *objets de vertu*. His reputation as the leading gold chaser in the capital and his activities as a designer and teacher, proved vital in the dissemination of the Rococo style. For example, the designer and furniture maker, John Linnell (1723–96), who produced some of the liveliest designs in the English Rococo period (PLATE 18), was taught at the St Martin's Lane Academy, most probably by Gravelot or Moser himself.[28]

It seems fitting to end this paper with a brief discussion of the Vauxhall Pleasure Gardens, which have been described as 'perhaps the most complete and convincing expression of the rococo in England'.[29] The Gardens had existed in the 17th century but had gained the reputation of being a 'rural brothel'. The entrepreneur Jonathan Tyers took over the run-down site in 1728 and reopened the refurbished gardens in the 1730s. By the mid-18th century, Vauxhall had become an immensely popular and highly fashionable summer venue, and patronized by its ground landlord, Frederick, Prince of Wales, for whom a special pavilion had been built. Given the nature of the enterprise, Tyers's enthusiasm for the avant-garde and the newsworthy, and his friendship with Hogarth and Hayman, it seems inevitable that a number of the St Martin's Lane circle would become involved with the decoration of the buildings or produced designs for the entertainments. These included a vast series of Rococo paintings for the supper-boxes, largely executed by Francis Hayman in and around 1740, and the rotunda built in the late 1740s with Rococo interiors by Moser.[30]

Gravelot further executed numerous Rococo-style vignettes and decorations for the music sheets of the popular Vauxhall songs, such as *The Invitation to Mira, requesting her company to Vaux Hall Garden*, dated 1738, which was engraved by George Bickham in the same year. But possibly the most revolutionary of the commissions, was also one of the earliest. This was Roubiliac's spectacular portrait sculpture of the celebrated composer, George Frederick Handel (PLATE 19), which was installed off the South Walk of the Gardens in 1738. It was the first of its kind and was an immediate success with the visitors. What makes this sculpture a supreme evocation of the Rococo style is less easily defined than with ornament. *En négligé* (informally attired) and seated crossed-legged, the latter-day Orpheus leans cheekily to the left, gently plucking at his lute, his whole body forming a gentle series of curves. What defines this work as Rococo is its informality and its humour; as Margaret Whinney has observed 'an example of that transitory mood, in change rather than in permanent ideal, which is a fundamental characteristic of the Rococo'.[31] Although Roubiliac had to wait some years before his career took off, this one sculpture established him as the most innovative and talented sculptor currently working in England, and greatly influenced the portrait painters of the St Martin's Lane circle.[32]

This paper has only scratched the surface of what is a vast and complicated subject. Even so, it is clear that those foreign artists and craftsmen mentioned here, and the many more living and working in London who have not been, were instrumental not only in introducing the Rococo style into England, but in a broader context were fundamental to the raising of standards in native design and craftsmanship and to the establishment of a national school of art.

NOTES

1 This subject, as well as the broader context of the Rococo in England, was covered by the ground-breaking exhibition at the Victoria and Albert Museum in 1984, *Rococo: art and design in Hogarth's England*, and its accompanying catalogue of the same name (London, 1984). The catalogue remains an important visual source for the work of a number of artists and craftsmen mentioned in the following paragraphs, and on which I have frequently drawn in preparation for this paper.

2 Derek Jarrett, *England in the Age of Hogarth* (New Haven, 1986), 166.

3 Gerald Newman, *The rise of English nationalism: a cultural history, 1740–1830* (London, 1997), 15.

4 *French travellers in England 1600–1900*, ed. R. E. Palmer (London, ?), x–xi; *A foreign view of England in the reigns of George I and George II: the letters of Monsieur César de Saussure to his family*, trans. and ed. M. van Muyden (London, 1902), 176–81.

5 For further discussion of the history and imagery of this work, see Elizabeth Einberg and Judy Egerton, *The Age of Hogarth: British painters born 1675–1709*, Tate Gallery collections vol. 2 (London, 1988), 131.

6 For further discussion of Anglo-French relations see Linda Colley, *Britons: forging the nation 1707–1837* (London, 1992).

7 As quoted in *The peopling of London: fifteen thousand years of settlement from overseas*, ed. Nick Merriman (London, 1993), 45.

8 Elaine Barr, 'Rococo silver: design', in *Rococo: art and design in Hogarth's England* [hereafter *Rococo*], 100.

9 Tessa Murdoch, 'The Huguenots and English Rococo' in Charles Hind (ed.), *The Rococo in England: a symposium*, proceedings of a symposium held at the Victoria and Albert Museum (London, 1986), 81.

10 David Bindman and Malcolm Baker, *Roubiliac and the eighteenth-century monument* (New Haven, 1995), 66–69. For a succinct account of Roubiliac's career see Margaret Whinney, *Sculpture in Britain 1530 to 1830* (2nd edn.,London, 1988), 198–226.

11 Quoted in Linda Colley, 'The English Rococo: historical background' in *Rococo*, 16.

12 Colley, *Britons*, 95. These designs were published with additions as *One Hundred and Fifty New Designs* in 1761.

13 For the role played by Sprimont at the Chelsea porcelain factory, and for French influence on style and Rococo models produced there, see Elizabeth Adams, *Chelsea porcelain* (London, 1987), 15–24, 25–38.

14 David Bindman, *Hogarth* (London, 1981), 18.

15 David Piper, *The English face* (London, 1992), 124.

16 Jenny Uglow, *Hogarth: a life and a world* (London, 1997), 320.

17 Elizabeth Einberg, *The French taste in English painting during the first half of the 18th*

century, catalogue of an exhibition at the Iveagh Bequest, Kenwood House (London, 1968), 16.

18   *Ibid.*, 33; see also Judy Egerton, *Hogarth's Marriage á-la-Mode* (London, 1997), 56–9 and David Bindman, *Hogarth and his times* (London, 1997), in particular 104–47.

19   David Solkin, *Painting for money: the visual arts and the public sphere in eighteenth-century England* (New Haven, 1992), 48–77.

20   Marianne Roland Michel, 'Watteau and England' in *The Rococo in England*, 48–9; Louise Lippincott, *Selling art in Georgian London: the rise of Arthur Pond* (New Haven, 1983), 13–14; for Watteau's influence on Rococo fine and decorative art see Katie Scott, *The Rococo interior: decoration and social spaces in early eighteenth-century Paris* (New Haven, 1995), 154–161 and Michael Levey, *Painting and sculpture in France 1700–1789* (New Haven, 1993), 29–43.

21   Uglow, 159; *Philip Mercier 1689–1760*, catalogue of an exhibition at the City Art Gallery, York and at the Iveagh Bequest, Kenwood House (London, 1969), 15–16.

22   For a concise history of the early London Academies see Rica Jones, 'The artist's training and techniques' in *Manners and morals: Hogarth and British Painting 1700–1760*, catalogue of an exhibition at the Tate Gallery (London, 1987), 19–22.

23   As quoted in Uglow, 260.

24   David Coke, 'Vauxhall Gardens' in *Rococo*, 80.

25   Mark Girouard, 'Coffee at Slaughter's? English Art and the Rococo' in Girouard, *Town and Country* (New Haven, 1992), 16.

26   As quoted in Uglow, 264.

27   Michael Rosenthal, *The art of Thomas Gainsborough* (New Haven, 1999), 122–136.

28   John Hardy, 'Rococo furniture and carving' in *Rococo*, 160.

29   'Coffee at Slaughter's', 20.

30   Brian Allen, 'Francis Hayman and the supper-box paintings for Vauxhall Gardens' in *The Rococo in England*, 113–33, and Brian Allen, *Francis Hayman* (New Haven, 1987), 62–70 and 107–9.

31   Whinney, 199.

32   Allen, *Francis Hayman*, 33–35.

15

The production and patronage of David Willaume, Huguenot merchant goldsmith

Eileen Goodway

David Willaume together with his son, also David Willaume, ran an eminent merchant goldsmith's business in the West End of London from the 1680s until the mid 18th century. Indubitably a man of stature in his native land and subsequently in his adopted one, David Willaume Senior received the Freedom of the Worshipful Company of Goldsmiths on the instructions of the Lord Mayor of the City of London within a few years of his arrival in England.[1] That near immediate acceptance conveyed status and thus patronage from Britain's aristocracy and gentry. Extant pieces of plate made by the Willaumes and engraved with the recipient's armorials show just how quickly they reached the heart of the society that had embraced them. This brief paper offers a glimpse of Willaume's personal and professional life and the close links between the two.

The archives at Metz in France confirm that David Willaume was born there in 1658. The son of a goldsmith, he was no doubt well established in his craft before his removal to England, probably in the late 1680s. The earliest original source that I have so far found that provides evidence about his residence and business in England appears in an issue of *The London Gazette* for the 9 March 1690.[2] He had placed an appeal which reads as follows:

> Lost, on the 4th instant, a ring with 7 diamond stones, the middle one is of a large bigness, having 3 little ones on each side, all inlaid in silver, The ring is of gold, fit for a little Finger, of the value of about 50 Lewis d'ors. Whoever brings it to Mr Willaume, a goldsmith at the sign of Windsor Castle near Charing Cross shall have a good reward.

This simple paragraph immediately tells us about his business. We know that he supplied silver but now we must consider him as a retailer, and a retailer of jewels at that. The use of French currency may also suggest that both he and his client are still living very much in the French manner and certainly he continued to write in French for much of his life. However it should be remembered that currency exchange was unneccessary, the coins in question being gold and therefore all that was required to convert one currency to another was a knowledge of the weight, easily determined with a pair of scales. Furthermore with the slight information given in the advertisement we are now immediately set wondering just exactly what his apprentices were being trained in. Was it solely the production of silver items as is generally thought or should we look more broadly and perhaps consider that apprentices were being trained in the art of salesmanship, the retailing of jewels, of gold and of silver and indeed banking? Moreover it would be of great advantage to Willaume's own expanding network to train men to be representatives of his firm. Certainly when Willaume appears in the various parish registers of the French Huguenot chapels he is listed not as a goldsmith but as a merchant goldsmith.

Over a period of 49 years the Willaume enterprise seems to have taken on apprentices two or three at a time. This would be consistent with having a couple of juniors working in a shop. Apprenticeship normally commenced at the age of 14 and lasted for seven years until the young men were made free of the livery company that had accepted them around the age of 21. They were then able to work as journeymen, frequently for their former master, or set up on their own account. Of the 25 apprentices that father and son took between them subsequently 12 registered their own silver hallmark and of these half again produced exceptional items of the highest quality. However that is not to say that the others did not play their part and it is to be wondered whether within the Willaume establishment various forms of apprenticeship were on offer. Certainly with the large influx of Frenchmen into England in the late 17th century anomalies arose, not all conformed to the usual pattern of apprenticeship. It was perhaps not a surprise then to find among Willaume's apprentices two who did not conform. One, Francis Vaillant, had a slightly unusual entry into apprenticeship but the other, John Petry, appears, as far as my present researches have revealed, to have been quite outside the practice of the day.

Francis Vaillant, was Willaume's first, and illegal, apprentice. Illegal because he was taken on three months before David Willaume himself had obtained the Freedom of the Goldsmiths' Company and therefore the date of freedom is registered only in the records of the City of London and not at Goldsmiths' Hall in Foster Lane.[3]

Francis Vaillant was the son of the bookseller of the same name. Originally from Paris, the family had moved to Saumur in the Loire valley where Francis was born around 1678. In 1685, just prior to the Revocation of the Edict of Nantes, Francis Vaillant Senior obtained permission to move his wife, children and all his goods to England. They were obviously of no mean status as the allowance of the removal of goods was not always given. Family tradition has it that they were smuggled to these shores in barrels but however they travelled, once here they settled in London in the Strand. They were retailers of second-hand books, French volumes and, as devout Protestants, religious tracts. Francis's elder brothers, Paul and Isaac, appear to have entered their father's business leaving their younger sibling to pursue a different career. There is no evidence as yet that the Willaumes and Vaillants were connected by marriage, unlike many of the other apprentices, but their respective premises in Charing Cross and Strand were very close so it would seem that this proximity was the reason that Francis entered the care of Willaume in June 1693.

As mentioned above, this apprenticeship did not quite conform and this is shown in the document or indenture stored at the City of London Record Office. It is not of the usual type, as it has no armorials on it – indentures carry the armorials of the particular livery company that represents the apprentice's intended trade or craft – and also the wording is rather different. It is, nonetheless, written in English and may be a translation of the French form. Francis Vaillant became free on 10 July 1700 and on the reverse of his indenture paper David Willaume has inscribed, in French, words to the effect that Vaillant has finished his time with all the fidelity required of an honest man with which he is very happy and satisfied. However Willaume does not appear to have accompanied Francis Vaillant to his freedom ceremony as the witness is another of David Willaume's apprentices, Lewis Mettayer.

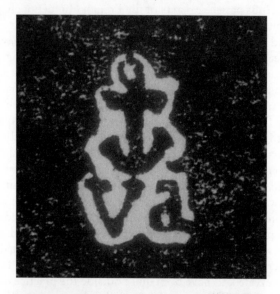

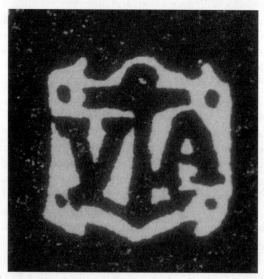

Two marks believed to be those of Francis Vaillant
Source: A. G. Grimwade, *London Goldsmiths, 1697–1837*, London 1990, nos. 3850–1

Willaume must have known that the apprenticeship was irregular and sure enough a few months later a query arises over the correctness of the apprenticeship and freedom. Court Minutes at Goldsmiths' Hall record that a letter had been received from the Chamberlain of the City of London noting that Vaillant had been apprenticed three months before his master took up his freedom but unless there was any other objection he could be made free of the company. Interestingly it is the apprentice rather than the master who is deemed to be at fault, officials of the Goldsmiths' Company deciding that Vaillant might have his freedom recognized on payment of a fine of three guineas. Vaillant paid forthwith.

Five years after his freedom was at an end, and presumably after working his time as a journeyman FrancisVaillant married Catherine Pearson at St Paul's, Covent Garden. They had five children but only two, William and Susan, appear to have survived for more than a few years.[4] He was living in New Exchange Court off the Strand in the early 1700s and according to his insurance policy with the Sun Insurance Company he moves with his goods to the Angel next door to Boyles Alley also in the Strand in 1710.[5] There he stays for two years before disappearing from London rate books and other records in 1712. In 1715 the two children William and Susan, are named as the beneficiaries of Vaillant's portion of his father's estate, implying perhaps that either he had predeceased his father or had gone away.[6]

As to Francis Vaillant's working career, it is briefly if unhappily recorded at Goldsmiths' Hall. At the time the use of the higher or Britannia standard silver was being enforced to prevent silver from being obtained by the clipping of the edges of sterling standard silver coins. But on Monday, 13 July 1709, at a meeting of the Court of Wardens of the Goldsmiths' Company Mr Vaillant appeared and submitted himself for judgement having made salt cellars that were worse than the required standard. He was excused on payment of a fine of 2s 6d.

So now we know that he worked as a silversmith or at least a retailer of silver but as with his irregular apprenticeship he did not formally register his mark at the Goldsmiths' Company. However, two hallmarks with the letters VA and an anchor have been noted on a few pieces of silver made in the first decade of the 18th century and I believe, admittedly on circumstantial evidence, that these are his.[7] Apart from the obvious use of the first two letters of his surname which was obligatory at the time he had every reason to include an anchor in his mark. First and foremost a branch of the Vaillant family of France included an anchor in their coat of arms. Secondly his bookselling family also had a nautical symbol, trading at the sign of the Ship, and, fortuitously the anchor is also the Christian symbol of Hope.

It may be that he also hoped to anchor himself in Britain having fled his native land but this seems to have eluded him. There is a mention of a Francis Vaillant, silversmith, residing in St Michael's parish, Barbados. As a first apprentice he does not seem to have added a great deal to the Willaume establishment although what is not known is whether he acted as an agent in the West Indies. At first glance it seems unlikely, though I have discovered a silver dish supplied by the Willaumes and on it are engraved the arms of a Governor of Barbados.

The other apprentice mentioned, John Petry, seems a rather more likely agent or, in modern parlance, sales representative. He was born in Heidelberg, Germany, a centre of Protestantism until sacked by the French in 1689, when it is to be presumed that Petry and his family fled.[8] His father appears to have moved to Hanover while

Petry himself may well have used the opportunity, if he had not done so previously, of joining a British regiment. He is noted that very same year as being the youngest lieutenant of the 2nd Troop of Life Guards.[9] He continued as an officer for a further ten years until he petitioned to become a naturalized Englishman and the following year, 1700, he entered the service of David Willaume. Assuming John Petry was the same age as his wife[10] he was probably in his late forties which seems extraordinary but even if that were not the case he was still a mature apprentice of at least 25 years of age. Maybe Willaume was trying to help a fellow Frenchman, as in the late 1690s Petry had moved to an army troop that was soon disbanded and he was placed on half pay. In any event he gained his freedom after seven years on 21 November 1707. That very same day he registered his mark at Goldsmiths' Hall giving the same address as his master, i.e. Pall Mall.

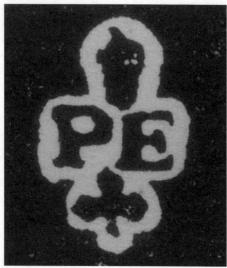

The mark of John Petry
Source: A. G. Grimwade, *London Goldsmiths, 1697–1837*, London 1990, no. 2170

Remarkably, during his apprenticeship his military advancement appears to have continued unabated. He was promoted Captain and Major and took part in and survived the battle of Blenheim in 1704 and, after further encounters, that of Malplaquet in 1709. While in Flanders, he received his promotion to Lieutenant Colonel of Horse in the Carabiniers from the Duke of Marlborough. You may be wondering why this diversion into John Petry's military career is relevant. Without written records it is difficult to ascertain why people patronized one goldsmith rather than another. Did Willaume recognize that as a reasonably high ranking officer in the British army, Petry was consorting with the leaders of British society? Or did he look favourably on English military men as they fought against the country that had rejected him? Was John Petry originally trained as a goldsmith before he entered the army or was this apprenticeship necessary to give him the knowledge to become the perfect envoy, a form of salesman, persuading his military colleagues to place orders through the Willaume establishment? The only other thought that comes to mind is that the army needed to be paid so was Willaume acting as its banker? Furthermore all officers had uniforms that included silver accoutrements of various sorts, including gorgets and buttons and lace. A list written in French in 1706 by a Huguenot commander of the contents of his campaign chest mentions six silver handled knives, six spoons and six forks, a pair of small candlesticks, a goblet and a salt cellar.[11] Given that the British army grew dramatically in size in the early years of the century was Willaume supplying bulk orders to the military?

Certainly quite a number of pieces of Willaume silver were supplied to military men, as can be seen by the armorials engraved upon them, and Petry may have been the link. For example a set of three sugar or spice casters supplied by Willaume in 1707, the same year that Petry obtained his freedom of the Goldsmiths' Company, are engraved with the arms of General Thomas Erle and his wife Elizabeth née Wyndham.[12] [PLATE 20] General Erle had served in Ireland, as had Petry, and General Erle's wife was a kinswoman of Brigadier General Hugh Wyndham, at one time Petry's commanding officer. Casters supplied by Willaume often have amusingly pierced tops. I do not know whether it was serendipity or suggested by the profession of the client but there are figures pierced on General Erle's casters and some are grasping what appear to be swords and shields.

Another connection that may have been forged by Petry was with one of his officers, his lieutenant in the same regiment, the Honourable Richard Ingram, son of Arthur, 3rd Viscount Irvine, the owner of Temple Newsam House in Leeds. There is no extant silver but bills that do survive that show that the Ingrams were certainly patrons of the Willaumes during the 1720s and they may well have received plate from them previously.

Regiments are mobile and prior to his apprenticeship Petry spent a considerable amount of time in Ireland. When he returned there is unknown but both he and his widow died in Dublin, he in 1723 and she in 1730. As has been previously mentioned, Petry consorted with other military men but it also seems more than probable that he would have known the leading Irish silversmith of the day, Thomas Bolton. According to records at the Dublin Assay Office Bolton far outstripped his competitors with the supply of plate and as with his London counterparts, sources other than his own workshops must have been necessary in order to fulfil large orders. Items bearing the marks of both David Willaume and Thomas Bolton bear remarkable similarities and it is to be wondered whether Petry was the intermediary. Interestingly one such item, a ewer now in the Boston Museum of Fine Arts, is engraved with the arms of Sir William Codrington, son of John Codrington who was both Colonel of the Life Guards, Petry's own regiment, and also a Governor of the Leeward Islands in the West Indies. Furthermore General Erle, the owner of the casters mentioned previously, also had sets of spoons made by both David Willaume and Thomas Bolton around 1710.

Although not a military man, another with Irish connections who patronized David Willaume was the Earl of Kildare. In 1720 Kildare ordered a toilet set for his wife who had just given birth to a son. [PLATE 21] This marvellous service, now in the Ulster Museum, comprises some 22 pieces made over a period of four years. Silver production is indeed a lengthy business. To put it in perspective a modern glass sculpture will be completed in a matter of hours whereas the casting, hammering and burnishing of the same object in silver may take up to a month. Each piece of the toilet service is hallmarked but some more correctly than others.[13] Those that have the full set of correct hallmarks range between 1719 and 1722. There are others however that have a Willaume maker's mark but the remaining hallmarks are earlier in date, for example 1698 and 1704, and so it would appear that those within the Willaume establishment were not melting down old plate from their store but were refashioning it and including the old hallmarks in the new object. I have found a number of other items supplied by the Willaumes that are also incorrectly hallmarked and they all appear to date from around 1720. Was there then trouble at the shop?

David Willaume Senior wrote his will on 13 June 1720[14] and it occurred to me that he may have done so because he had fallen ill at this time or that he was undertaking a significant journey and thus there was the possibility of his not returning. He might have temporarily relinquished control of the firm for practical reasons and this is further confirmed in that his new maker's mark, registered at Goldsmiths' Hall the same month, was signed David Willaume but it is his son's signature rather than his own.

Apart from the obvious reason of evading the payment of tax, illegal then as it is now, whoever was running the business may have had good reason not to send each piece for hallmarking which as yet we do not understand, but bearing in mind that Willaume was a banker, there is the strong possibility the business was feeling the effects of the South Sea Bubble. Whatever the reason, no doubt they were doing their best to keep the customer happy in trying circumstances! Willaume did not die until 1740 so presumably by 1722 either he or the business had recovered sufficiently to allow the last pieces of the Kildare service to be properly completed.

There are many influences on production and patronage, only very few of which have been touched on in this paper. Objects of silver are special amongst the arts in that they are frequently engraved with the symbols of ownership, revealing their provenance to the interested. In the absence of any ledgers describing the running of the Willaume establishment we cannot overestimate this rich resource. Having only just started to look at the many patrons of this man of distinction, I am absolutely certain that Willaume was at the forefront of the English commerce of his day.

NOTES

1   CLRO, CFI/73/146.
2   BL, Burney Collection, 102A, *London Gazette* no. 2643.
3   CLRO, CFI/164/101.
4   International Genealogical Index, under name 'Vaillant'.
5   GL, MS 11936, vol. 1, 19.
6   Family Record Centre (London), PROB 11/579/62.
7   A. G. Grimwade, *London goldsmiths, 1697–1837* (3rd edn., London, 1990), nos. 3850–1.
8   CLRO, CFI/239.
9   Charles Dalton, *English Army lists and commission registers*, vol. 3 (London, 1896), 19.
10 PRO Ireland, French Pensioners' Declarations.
11 General de Ainslie, *Historical Record of the First or the Royal Regiment of Dragoons* (London, 1887), 67–8.
12 Christie's (London), 18 March 1970, lot 152.
13 Sotheby's (London), Collection of the late Sir Harold Wernher, 24 May 1995, Lots 86–99.
14 Family Record Centre (London), PROB 11/715/38.

16

Worthy of the monarch: immigrant craftsmen and the production of state beds, 1660–1714

Tessa Murdoch

From the Restoration of Charles II in 1660 until well into the reign of Queen Anne, the most elaborate upholstery supplied for the royal palaces was – until recently – believed to be the work of visiting French upholsterers and resident French immigrants. The visiting upholsterers in the 1670s and 1680s included Jean Peyrard and Simon Delobel. Upholsterers who resided in London and are assumed to be of French origin included John Casbert (*d.*1677) and his son also named John, Jean Poitevin (active 1671–88), Francis Lapiere (1653–1714) who is recorded as in London from 1683, Etienne Penson (who was Poitevin's nephew and active in England 1704–13), and Philip Guibert (1692–1739). Specialist suppliers of accessories included the fringe-maker Peter Dufresnoy, recorded at Drayton House, Northamptonshire in 1700. Of these, Francis Lapiere was certainly a Catholic, so it cannot be assumed that these craftsmen had come to England as a result of persecution.[1]

Of these craftsmen, records in France (now in the Archives Nationales) are held for Jean Peyrard, Etienne Penson, and Simon Delobel who was active at Versailles in the service of Louis XIV in the 1670s and 1680s. Jean Poitevin died in France in about 1709, Francis Lapiere remarried in Paris in 1701. Many of the leading French upholsterers working in London maintained their links with France.

Not all the court upholsterers were of French origin. At the time of King Charles II's restoration, the native John Baker, junior, had enjoyed the position of court upholsterer for nearly forty years. His father had served in turn as upholsterer to Queen Elizabeth I and to King James I – indeed the term upholsterer is used for the first time in the royal accounts in 1603 to describe John Baker senior's occupation. John Baker senior also supplied upholstered furniture for the use of Charles I when Prince of Wales. Two successive generations of the same family indicate that there was a native tradition of court upholstery.

State beds are associated with court ritual, but it is rarely noted that they had an important role to play in the ritual associated with death as well as life. In September 1658 a wax effigy of the body of the Lord Protector Oliver Cromwell, clad in purple velvet, lay on a bed of state in what had formerly been the King's State Apartments at Whitehall Palace. On the death of Charles II, mourning was conducted in a similarly dramatic fashion to the death of the Lord Protector 27 years earlier. Charles II's Queen received all the mourning ambassadors lying in state in a black bed within a room hung with black cloth (the name of the upholsterer responsible has not been recorded in secondary sources). Ten years later, in 1695, Romeyn de Hooghe showed Queen Mary on her deathbed at Kensington Palace (PLATE 22). Whether this print is a record of the actual setting or imaginary, the Queen's bed is embellished with a royal crown and cypher on the head board above, royal arms on the sides of the tester and royal crowns and monograms on the corners, an accurate reflection of the decoration of state beds made for the monarch.

Jean Casbert

In 1661, John Casbert charged for 'Altering & fitting a Crimson damask bedde, bought by his Ma[jes]tie (Charles II) of a Frenchman'. It would be interesting to know the identity of this French supplier of the crimson damask bed. Was he a Frenchman resident in London or a French immigrant? For the Princess Royal, Casbert supplied a 'standing French bedstead of crimson velvet embroidered with strips of white satin and silver'. The four posts were cased in sleeves and plumes of feathers rose from the cups on top of them. In 1660–1 Casbert provided for royal use a 'crimson velvet French chair covered all over with gold and silver fringe and with a bagg filled with downe'.

In 1674 John Casbert spelt 'Caresbert' the elder and John 'Caresbert' the younger were appointed to the 'office and place of our Upholster of our Wardrobe of Bedds and of our Standing Wardrobe'. The duties included 'the making of all our standing bedds, Pallet Bedds, Canopies, Chaires, Stooles, Cushions, quilt Lynings of Counter-points, Cloathes of Estate, window Curteynes, fustian Blancketts, Cloth Blancketts, Gilt Sarge Cloathes, necessary Stooles, Straw cases, Downe Pillows, Cart, Carriages and alsoe all our Bedd Seates and Curteynes for all our Caroches, Litters and Charriotts, together with repayring & mending of all our Wardrobe Stuffe in all our severall wardrobes and to Serve and attend in all our Progresse, Journeys for repayring and mending of all our Wardrobe stuff from time to time.' The production of state beds was the most prestigious of the tasks demanded of the court upholsterer. A cloth of estate, supported the monarch on state occasions or in the Royal Presence Chamber consisted of a tester and valance – similar to those on the state bed and a back cloth – as shown in Romeyn de Hooghe's engraving of the coronation of William and Mary in 1689. In 1674 he also supplied a 'French chaire hollow in ye back and quilted of crimson damask'. Casbert also provided furniture for the French ambassador's lodgings at Somerset House.[2]

It has always been assumed that John Casbert was of French origin – his name could easily be French and as we have seen he is recorded as providing and altering 'French' beds, and 'French' chairs. But his will indicates that he was anglicized by 1677 (He lived in the parish of St Bartholomew Aldersgate) and the name John Casbert does not occur in the Huguenot church records for the 1660s and 1670s. Indeed there is no evidence to show that the Casberts were first generation French immigrants.

Jean Peyrard

Judging by the description, the Princess Royal's bed supplied by Casbert was similar to the bed surviving today at Knole, Kent which is known as the King's Bed (PLATE 23). It is believed that this was made for the wedding of James, Duke of York to Mary of Modena in 1673 as it bears the coronet of a royal duke on the headboard. Embroidered in gold and silver thread, with flowers which are raised in relief by being stuffed with horsehair over a leather foundation, the bed was lined with cherry coloured satin. It still retains some of the accompanying furniture, which consists of a pair of armchairs, four stools and a pair of squab-frames. The front stretchers and legs are carved with cupids holding a crown or bows and arrows, amongst billing doves. It is thought to be one of six beds supplied by the French upholsterer Jean Peyrard to Charles II between 1672 and 1675. It was acquired by the 6th Duke of Dorset in 1694 from Whitehall Palace after the death of Queen Mary.

In 1672 Jean Peyrard was paid £1,773 16s 6d for 'two Rich Beds bought in France and agreed for there by Our Lord Embassador Montague, one of them of Crimson Damaske Trimd with gold fringes of Goldsmiths worke with Chaires etc and hangings for the Above all suitable, the other of Yellow Damaske trimd with Silver ffringes of like Goldsmithes worke with chaires etc and Hangings. As also for two other Beds of Crimson Damaske trimd with Silke fringes with chaires etc.' Peyrard also charged for 'conveyance of the above named Goods from Paris to Whitehall with allowance to himself and Two Servants for that Journey to London and their returne to Paris'. The following year Peyrard brought over another crimson damask bed and a further purple state bed to London for royal use.

The state bed from Boughton House, Northamptonshire, given to the Victoria and Albert Museum in 1916, may be one of the beds commissioned from Peyrard by Ralph, Duke of Montagu in the early 1670s and delivered to London from Paris for the use of the royal family (PLATE 24). It has always been assumed that the Boughton state bed was commissioned by Montagu in readiness for a visit from William III in 1695. But if the bed dated from the 1670s, this would explain why it was in need of repair in 1705 when the leading London upholsterer Francis Lapiere (about whom see below) was paid £6 'for taking a crimson & gold damask bed all to pieces & new making it up again to go to Boughton'.

Jean Poitevin

Another extraordinary survival at Knole is the state bed with the arms of James II with hangings of blue-green Genoa velvet (PLATE 25) – this may relate to a royal warrant issued in August 1688 to the then Master of the Wardrobe, the Earl of Preston, to supply 'a bed of green and gold figured velvet (now faded to a rust colour) with scarlet and white silk fringe. The most likely supplier is the Huguenot Jean Poitevin who was the leading upholsterer during James II's reign. (His name is variously spelt Paudevin, Bodovine, Potvin, Popevine, Podvine, Potevine, Poictevine and Vaudvine in the official documents). The carving of the frames of the accompanying armchairs and six stools are attributed to the Royal Chairmaker Thomas Roberts. The bed bears the royal monogram, the royal crown and lion and unicorn feature on the tester of the bed. The chair frames are supported by four draped figures with trumpeting putti on the stretchers between. The earliest mention of Poitevin is in 1671. Like Casbert, Poitevin altered existing beds as well as supplying new beds. In 1678 he was paid for 'altering and Making a Crimson damask Bed into A New Fashion'. Poitevin had premises close to St James's Palace in Pall Mall. He supplied a bed of crimson mohair to Hamilton Palace, Scotland in 1688.

It was Poitevin who supervised the provisions of upholstery for the coronation of James II. But James II, like his elder brother, went to France for the highest quality of upholstery, commissioning from Simon Delobel in 1685 (Louis XIV's own up-holsterer) a crimson velvet bed with two elbow chairs and six stools en suite which cost a total of £1,515. This was delivered in August 1686, but needed adjustment and finishing. Poitevin was given the task of 'raising all the Curtains, making the new head-board, lineing the tester, vallance, Counterpoint and all ye Bases for ye sume of £250'. In the same year Poitevin also supplied a blue, white and gold bed embroidered with gold and silver for James II's Queen, Mary of Modena, for her use at Windsor. It is probable that the bed at Kensington Palace still associated today with Mary of Modena and the 'warming pan' incident – the birth of the Prince James Edward at St James's Palace in June 1688 – is in part that supplied by Poitevin in the mid 1680s. The hang-ings are of the original 1680s Genoa velvet, but the tester and headboard are thought to date from the 1720s. Jean Poitevin evidently returned to France as he died there in 1711.

François Lapiere

The fashion for elaborate state beds was of French origin and during the reigns of Charles II and James II the most luxurious examples were imported from Paris. Some French upholsterers recognized that there were exciting commissions to be gained at the English court, so they seized the opportunity to settle here. The Catholic Francis Lapiere is first recorded in England in 1683, when working for John, 5th Earl of Exeter at Burghley House, Stamford. By 1687 Lapiere was at Drayton House, Northamptonshire providing Henry, 2nd Earl of Peterborough with an elaborate bed.[3]

For the entertainment of foreign ambassadors in St James's Square in the mid-1690s Lapiere provided a wainscot bed hung with 'Mazarine' blue Genoa damask with six armchairs upholstered en suite. This cost £630 5s 9d. Perhaps it was no coincidence that a French upholsterer was given the commission to provide the French am-bassadorial suite. Lapiere certainly remained in touch with the latest French fashions as he remarried in Paris in 1701 when his father was described as Dominique Lapiere, a *marchand tapissier* of Paris and Francis Lapiere's own occupation was given as '*marc-hand tapissier*' of Londres. Ironically, by the late 1690s state beds made in London by French immigrant upholsterers were regarded as more sophisticated than those made in Paris. In a letter to William III from Paris in 1698. Lord Portland notes 'I am sure that the fashion of beds as they are made here will not please you, not approaching those that are made in England'.

The principal examples of state beds from the reigns of Charles II and James II were made for the royal palaces or to receive the King or Queen as at Powys Castle or Ham House. More research needs to be done to establish how many of the leading courtiers followed royal example and commissioned equally grand beds for their own use, and how exactly these state beds were actually used. 'Bedrooms' according to Mark Girouard 'became more public, though perhaps never quite as public as in France. They were decorated with the sumptuousness and furniture appropriate to important reception rooms. Their walls were lined with rows of richly upholstered chairs and stools; their occupant received visitors lying in bed framed by splendid curtains, under a tester decorated with plumes of ostrich feathers, and with his coat of arms carved or embroidered on the bed-head behind him'. Girouard goes on to explain that Princes of the Blood were allowed in, as were principal officers of state and privy counsellors, but for someone of lower rank, this was a notable compliment. John Evelyn notes complacently the occasions when he was received in this way by Charles II.[4]

Furthermore, although the names of leading upholsterers working in London are known through the Lord Chamberlain's accounts and the archives of the leading courtier houses, little work has been done on other upholsterers recorded in the Huguenot church records and further names which occur in contemporary accounts.

Although recent publications have concentrated on the leading court upholsterers who operated in the West End, notably in Pall Mall and Jermyn Street, the Upholders' Company was based in the City and thus native practitioners such as Nathaniel Carpenter, who supplied beds to the Earl of Melville and his son the Earl of Leven in 1690–1, were based there. Despite the restrictions of the guild system at least one Huguenot upholsterer attended the Threadneedle Street Church in London – Isaac de la Haye who worked from 1693 to 1705 in Frying Pan Alley, Stepney. Thomas Benoist, maker of fringes, received charity through the same church in 1681, Abraham David, maker of plumes, attended another City church that housed a Huguenot congregation, St Martin Orgars, in 1701.

Who, for example, was Francis Moran, upholsterer who was paid for his work at Boughton in October 1699? Was he one of Francis Lapiere's assistants? Lapiere was in Ralph Montagu's employ from at least 1698. Who was Mr Fountaine, upholsterer, also paid by Ralph Montagu's order in November 1700 (£45 3s)?

Upholsterers also acted as brokers furnishing rooms in their entirety. In 1682 John Poitevin supplied the Ambassador of the Savoy with a crimson damask bed, bedding and six caned chairs for six months at a charge of £36. In November 1688 Francis Lapiere furnished the Duke of Schomberg's apartments for 20 months with 'a crimson Genoa damask bed trimmed with crimson, green and white silk fringe and, six armchairs with matching cases, a Turkey carpet under the bed, and four pieces of Flaunders small figured Tapestry hangings'.

The court upholsterers did not just supply leading courtiers but lesser members of their households as well. Thus in 1702 Francis Lapiere was paid £20 6s in full for all the furniture of Mr Falaiseaux's Rooms (a member of Ralph, Duke of Montagu's household) at Montagu House, Bloomsbury. For the same house, individuals supplied tapestry for chair covers. In November 1703 Marie Pariselle was paid £20 for tapestry and the following month a further £10 for tapestry chairs, a further payment was made to her for the same in 1704 and again in 1705; to Ester Regneaux £8 was paid for two tapestry chairs in 1704. Was the Madame Justell paid in full for three silk and worsted needlework chairs in August 1705 related to the Mr Justell who supplied an easy chair for £10 in March 1699? All these references suggest there is a good deal of further research to be undertaken on the upholsterers and their suppliers during the reigns of William III and Queen Anne. Were these industrious women all members of the Huguenot community in London or were they French immigrants taking advantage of the taste for French workmanship and design in London.

It is probable that the women who supplied tapestry chair covers also supplied tapestry hangings for beds. Francis Lapiere charged Ralph Montagu 'making a bed of striped tapestry needlework' for his cousin Lady Sandwich consisting of 'curtains, valance, bases, cantoon, and tester headcloth, case post and counterpane' in 1705–6. This bed had moulded cornices and a fine carved tester with four cups. According to the bill, the cups and the cornices were made to designs drawn by 'Marrot'. This was almost certainly Isaac Marot, the younger brother of the architect Daniel Marot (1660–1752), although it was Daniel Marot who published designs for state beds in Holland in 1702. Lapiere's workshops made up the bed, but the tapestry needlework would have been supplied by a team of professional embroiderers. The tapestry needlework hangings of the Drayton state bed (PLATE 26) were made by Elizabeth Rickson and Rebekah Dufee, (in July 1700 they charged 22s a yard for the needlework) although the bed was made up by the French upholsterer Etienne Penson, Poitevin's nephew. Like Poitevin, Penson maintained his connections with France. His wife's father, Louis Dumoullier, was described as a *'marchand tapissier'* in Paris. Like the Lapiere bed supplied for Montagu, the needlework of the Drayton bed was made up in panes alternating with panes of green velvet. It is possible that tapestry or needlework bed hangings were considered more appropriate for a lady. Certainly Montagu's mad second wife had a tapestry bed because Lapiere charged in 1705 for 'taking downe my Lady Dutchess's tapistry Bed and Hangings for cleaning and safe storage'.

Such tapestry beds commissioned for the wives of leading noble courtiers mirror royal practice. Celia Fiennes, that intrepid Lady traveller, commented on Queen Mary's Chamber of State at Windsor Castle as 'all Indian Emboidery on white sattin being presented to her by the East India Company on it is great plumes of white feathers'.[5] In contrast Celia Fiennes noted that King William's Chamber of State at Windsor was 'equiped with a bed of green velvet strip'd down very thick with gold orrice lace of my hand's breadth, and round the bottom 3 such orrices and gold fring all round it and gold tassels, so was the cornish; at the head-piece was like curtaines fringed round with gold and tyed back with gold strings and tassels and soe hung down in the middle where was the Crown and Sypher embroyder'd; the hangings the same and another screen across the roome to secure the bed from the Common'. The adjacent Drawing Room of State was similarly hung with green velvet – the canopy was so rich and curled up and in some places 'soe full it looked very glorious and was newly made to give audience to the French Embassador to shew the grandeur and magnificence of the British Monarch – some of these foulerys are requisite sometymes to create admiration and regard to keep up the state of a kingdom and a nation.'[6]

It is likely that the King's bed at Windsor was supplied by Philip Guibert who petitioned in 1699 for payment of £1,695 worth of work in the King's bedroom and dining room there. Guibert, despite his French origin, was admitted into the freedom of the Upholders' Company in 1702 when his address was given as

St German's Street (Jermyn Street). He gave the Upholders' Company a triangular silver-gilt salt cellar. Although he was named a steward of the Company in 1705, by 1730 he was dependent on them for poor relief.

Celia Fiennes also visited Hampton Court where the King's bed in the Presence Chamber was of scarlet velvet with gold orrice. This was a second-hand bed acquired from Lord Jersey as King William was concerned that his state rooms should be furnished as cheaply as possible. Today the bed retains part of its original headboard and cornice but the curtains and counterpane were replaced after the fire at Hampton Court in 1993. The design is restrained and rectilinear and may indicate that the bed was bought in Paris during Lord Jersey's embassy there in 1688–9. At Hampton Court, Francis Lapiere was only given the task of supplying 'Five French bedsteads, for the Gentlemen and Groomes of our Bedchamber at Hampton Court and for our Staff Officers Rooms there'. French beds are thought to be those that have a wooden framework supporting hangings so as to form a plain rectangular box with curtains hung from the top rails.

The elaborate beds made or acquired to adorn the Royal Chambers of State produced a healthy crop of imitations ostensibly made in readiness to welcome the monarch. Evidence suggests that these were made after the death of Queen Mary in December 1694, when after a period of mourning, leading courtiers were justified in thinking that King William might be persuaded to grace their newly built country seats with a visit. Significantly the bed made to receive the monarch at the order of Thomas, Lord Coningsby for the King's Room at Hampton Court in Herefordshire was made up using the same crimson damask which was hung in the King's own dressing room at Hampton Court Palace.

In 1697, William, 1st Duke of Devonshire created an elaborate crimson silk damask four-poster bed at Chatsworth, of which the tester, headboard and backboard survive today at Hardwick; the headboard is adorned with his own cypher. The grand bed supplied by Lapiere to Belvoir in 1697 was created to celebrate the birth of an heir, marking the arrival of John, son of John Roos and his wife Katherine. In 1700 George, 1st Earl of Melville commissioned an elaborate bed for his newly built family palace Melville House, Fife, Scotland (PLATE 27). The bed, adorned with the conjoined cyphers of the Earl and his Countess, Catherine Leslie, marks the marriage of two titles the Earldom of Melville and the Earldom of Leven, which were to come together in their younger son, David, 3rd Earl of Leven.

Were all these so-called state beds really intended for the reception of the monarch? Why were the beds embellished with the cyphers and coronets of the patrons who had built or rebuilt the architectural settings in which they were housed? Were they not intended as a monument to their patrons and the climax of a series of state apartments, which albeit worthy of the monarch, were intended as a statement of the loyalty of the patron to that monarch, thus demonstrating the power and the influence of their owners.

The Royal Wardrobe continued to patronize English upholsterers and in 1714 an elaborate bed was ordered from Hamden Reeve, an upholsterer based in the Strand and active 1704–14. The bed was for Queen Anne's use at Windsor Castle. The silk velvet with a cream-coloured ground and a dull red and yellow-brown pattern was woven in Spitalfields. It was originally accompanied by a large armchair and eight square stools. The frame of the bed and seating furniture was made by Richard

Roberts, son of Thomas Roberts who succeeded his father as Royal Chairmaker. This bed can be seen today at Hampton Court Palace. Its accompanying armchair still survives. Thus in the year in which Francis Lapiere died, English upholsterers can be said to have taken over the task of providing appropriate state beds for use at the royal court.

Between 1660 and 1714 the fashion for elaborate state beds was dictated by France and thus French émigré and visiting upholsterers were much in demand. The designs for state beds provided by Daniel Marot and his brother Isaac spread the taste for elaborate upholstery which overtook the rectilinear French models. By the time Daniel Marot's designs for state beds had been published in Holland in the early 18th century, there was a team of English upholsterers able to provide the necessary skills for such confections. More research is needed to establish how such skills were passed from the immigrant upholsterers to the native practitioners of this craft. Certainly Francis Lapiere had at least one English apprentice or journeyman. Thomas Ebrington, aged 22 in 1711, witnessed his master's work for Ralph, Duke of Montagu to the Duke's executors.[7]

As a postscript I would like to draw attention to the remarkable bed hung with feathers which was made for Augustus the Strong's Dutch Palace and then transferred to the Japanese Palace in Dresden. Maureen Cassidy Geiger has demonstrated that the hangings were made in Putney by Nicholas le Normand-Quesnel, a native of Rouen, who maintained his ties with France.[8] His agents were London merchants of Huguenot origin named Bosquet and Clerembault. The link with the agents is confirmed in that in 1720 and 1728 a Marie Quesnel, wife of Nicholas le Normand stood as godmother to two Bosquet children baptized at the Threadneedle Street church. The bed hangings took 12 years to manufacture and appear to have been a unique achievement. The bed was advertised in the *Mercure de France* and thus attracted the interest of Augustus the Strong's agent in Paris. It appears to have been made as a speculative venture. The bed was accompanied by feather hangings en suite in the style of Daniel Marot's published designs. It is a supreme example of the way in which French models were developed in England. The more elaborate results commissioned for the monarch and his leading courtiers presented the ultimate status symbol. The English development of a French form was recognized abroad – in Paris – and re-exported to the Continent in a unique form.

NOTES

1   Much of this paper is based on the information, and the accompanying transcriptions of primary documents, in Geoffrey Beard, *Upholsterers and interior furnishing in England, 1530–1840* (New Haven, 1997). Also helpful and relevant is Peter Thornton, *Seventeenth-century interior decoration in England, France and Holland* (New Haven, 1978).

2   The principal archival collections which have been examined for this paper and from which extracts have been taken are: PRO, LC 5 (Bills to the Great Wardrobe) and LC 9 (Accounts of the Great Wardrobe); Boughton House, Household Accounts of Ralph, 1st Duke of Montagu.

3   For more on Lapiere, see Geoffrey Beard and Annabel Westman, 'A French upholsterer in England: Francis Lapierre, 1653–1714', *The Burlington Magazine* 135, no. 1085 (August 1993), 515–24.

4   Mark Girouard, *Life in the English country house: a social and architectural history* (New Haven, 1978), 130.
5   *The journeys of Celia Fiennes*, ed. Christopher Morris (London, 1949), 279.
6   *Ibid.*, 280.
7   Boughton House, Executors' Accounts of Ralph, 1st Duke of Montagu.
8   Maureen Cassidy-Geiger, 'The Federzimmer from the Japanisches Palais in Dresden', *Furniture History* (The Journal of the Furniture History Society) 35 (1999), 87–111.

17

Huguenot master weavers: exemplary Englishmen, 1700–c.1750

NATALIE ROTHSTEIN

My title reflects encounters for 45 years with virtuous Huguenots. The cut-off date of 1776 rests upon the fact that the negotiations for Eden's Free Trade Treaty in that year were the last occasion when the Weavers' Company played a role in a political decision and the Huguenot element was then still very important in the Company.[1] Moreover, the best information has come from the wills of hundreds of master weavers and others in the industry, for personal letters, diaries, and business records are sadly lacking. *Successful* Huguenots, anyway, did not die young. Their wills thus refer back to a far distant period. Published work on which this paper is based must start with the classic Survey of London volume on *Spitalfields and Mile End New Town* by Ison and Bezodis.[2] I have also raided my own published and unpublished work as well as the parish Vestry Minutes and the Sun Insurance policies compiled by the late Stuart Turner and his successors, led by Myrtle Mumford.[3]

Although divided into manageable portions, this study would not qualify as a serious work of social or economic history because it is primarily anecdotal – I can only use the evidence presented to me and I cannot claim it is exhaustive. I have not found any wicked Huguenots since the entertaining accounts published about late 17th-century smugglers.[4]

Family alliances and personal behaviour

Many years ago I was told that some Huguenots did not marry outside their own circle of friends before the 19th century but already in 1723 Colonel Peter Lekeux (who died, aged 73, in that year) left money to his two daughters and they had both married Englishmen, named Walker and Franks, respectively. Col. Lekeux was an important figure, both nationally and locally, as will be seen below. Matthew Hebert's will of 1739 mentions a son married to Judith Langham while the newspapers reported the marriage in 1746 of Mr Turner of Booth Street to Mrs Votier (Vautier) of Spital Square. All the other instances I have come across date from the third quarter of the 18th century. Families with grandchildren bearing English names include Dalbiac, Dupree,

Gobbé, Loy, Pilon, and Sufflee – in the latter case five English families are mentioned.

Apart from marriages, there are other personal connections. Peter Marescoe's will in 1710 was witnessed by Edward Peck, Christopher Baudouin, and John Hodgson. 'Rich old Mr Marescoe' was Col. Lekeux's father-in-law. Peck was a leading citizen of Spitalfields and a dyer, Christopher Baudouin was the leading designer of the time while Hodgson may be anonymous but is certainly English. Peter Campart the elder (plain silks) was a trustee under the will of the designer Anna Maria Garthwaite to whom she left a gold watch in 1763, while Abraham Jeudwine, who died in 1767, chose as his executors his 'good friends' Nathaniel Collyer of Amersham and George Popplewell of East Melford. Perhaps the nicest incident dates from 1776 when a thief, named John Davis, was caught robbing silk from James Louis Desormeaux. He was sentenced to death for the felony but Desormeaux wrote pleading for his life to the judge and the sentence was commuted to transportation. Davis's family wrote to thank Desormeaux – which is how we know.

Partnerships

Partnerships in the silk industry tended to be for only a few years but I have noted a minimum of ten with both English and Huguenot partners. One of the most interesting is that of Mary Chauvet, who also died in 1763. She referred in her will to her 'worthy partner', Isaac Gervaise, as well as to her other partner, James Rowlinson. *Both* received annuities. The partnership of Batchelor, Ham and Perigal lasted until the early 19th century with successive changes. They advertised from 1755 and in 1763 their production was listed as 'gold, silver, brocaded and flowered silks'; their address as White Lyon Street, Norton Folgate. John Perigal gave evidence to Parliament in 1765 'as a weaver of silks from the slightest to the roughest'; his partners were John Batchelor and John Ham.

The Weavers' Company

Although in the early 18th century Huguenot masters were exhorted to take English boys as apprentices, there is little evidence to suggest that such apprenticeships led to long-term associations. Generally, it is the sons or nephews who inherit, the other boys become free and graduate to journeyman status. Unfortunately for the Company, their perpetual battle – to control entry to the textile trades in London and eliminate 'non-freemen' – was never won. But there were some notable campaigns, the first in 1707 when the Company's new charter sought successfully to include all the weavers in Tower Hamlets – outside the City.[5] Many people subscribed to the petition protesting this move, 224 signing and a few making their mark. Many were Huguenots familiar in other contexts but there were, equally, many English weavers, so as both were resisting the Weavers' Company this was not a case of Huguenots against English.

Once recruited to the Company, all became loyal and even active members. The agitation against the import of Indian, East Indian and Chinese textiles and printed cottons was led by the Weavers' Company. They could be legally re-exported to the colonies or Europe but Daniel Alavoine and Company had to publish a denial in 1724 that they had built a warehouse to stock East Indian goods. James Leman, the weaver and designer, organized the pamphlet war in 1719–22 against printed cottons. The use and wear of printed cottons was prohibited in 1721 with a useful act in 1722 reducing the duty on imported raw silk when woven silks were exported.

In 1739–40, when the Weavers' Company was short of funds, 38 new Liverymen were nominated, instead of the usual six to twenty, and even more were chosen in subsequent years.[6] The majority were Huguenots but there were plenty of English masters. This ploy, possibly the suggestion of Alderman Sir William Baker, replenished the funds of the Company but also added to the personnel available for every kind of campaign. By 1754 they were able to defeat the last attempt at sumptuary legislation in England. Under the direction of the Upper Bailiff, Captain John Baker, eight of the committee they appointed were English, joined by four distinguished Huguenots.[7]

The real benefit to the Company of the 1739–41 recruitment came with the major campaign to prohibit French silks in 1765–6. A crisis in trade followed the end of the Seven Years War. Select Committees in Parliament were held in successive years to investigate and 21 of those who gave evidence were weavers, all members of the Company, several of them recruited in 1739–41. Witnesses included Lewis Ogier, Peter Ogier, Abraham Jeudwine, Stephen Paris, John Perigal, John Sabatier, Charles and Peter Triquet. By this point Huguenots were taking some of the highest offices in the Company, even those like Thomas Abraham Ogier, who had not even been born in England. They secured the total prohibition of French silks, a prohibition which lasted until 1826, and clearly identified themselves completely with their English colleagues.

Care for the industry and their staff

Those commanding the Company were weavers, as can be proved from insurance records, wills, directories, the Victoria and Albert designs and the records of the Vestry of Christ Church Spitalfields (which sometimes gave addresses and trades in the mid-century). A few demonstrated their concern for their business and specifically bequeathed 'the utensils belonging to my trade' or stipulated that legacies were to be delayed to prevent 'trade from stagnating'. Interest had to be paid but partners had time to adjust.[8]

Where the Huguenots do stand out is in their bequests to workmen and servants. Thus Louis Desormeaux, ribbon weaver, in 1748 left to his son Matthew 'all my tackling, looms and utensils in trade whatsoever, excepting the loombs which may be at the time of my decease lent to any of my Journeymen which loombs I give to such of my journeymen as shall have them in their possession' and there were others.[9] While some servants mentioned in wills are clearly domestic, it is notable how many were remembered with gratitude and money.[10] While the testators were of French origin the domestic servants were usually English.

Charities

The charities to which the master weavers subscribed are fairly predictable. At least 52 of the Directors of the French Hospital from 1718 to 1794 can be connected with the silk industry, including Peter Ogier (1761) and Lewis Ogier (1771).[11] Both Ogiers were very busy with the affairs of the Weavers' Company at the time. Naturally, there are both bequests to the Hospital in many wills and legacies to the French churches.

The French Church in Threadneedle Street was the most important, and bequests were made either for schools or, more frequently, for the poor. I have noted seven for schools run by the French Church, including one from Daniel Pilon (1762) for the support of one boy and one girl, but 17 for the poor. The church in the Artillery Ground attracted slightly smaller legacies and fewer of them.

Links with the past were sometimes continued; three Huguenot weavers bequeathed sums to the Walloon Church in Canterbury, while Daniel Booth left £5 5s in 1764 to each of 'the master weavers of Canterbury with whom he dealt before leaving'. Thus it was not only Huguenots who kept this connection with Canterbury alive and indeed London weavers owned property there and vice versa until late in the 18th century.[12] Peter Leman, father of the designer James Leman, was 'natif de Cantorberry' and his son employed several boys from Canterbury families – but there the connection ended. Several of the refugees from Bas Poitou left money to the Trustees of the Society of Saintonge for the poor.[13]

Several left money for the poor in the parishes to which they had retired, *but* most generous of all, Nicholas Garrat in 1725 left £1000 to the Wardens of the Weavers' Company for founding six almshouses in Norton Folgate, together with £600 to support them. The size of this bequest contrasts with those of the Huguenots but may reflect more upon his worldly success than upon any meanness on their part. Captain John Baker left £100 to the Trustees of the Charity School in Christ Church Middlesex and £400 in 3 per cent consol-dated annuities of the Bank of England to buy coals for the 'industrious poor', while two of the Ogiers served on the Weavers' Company Committee collecting relief in 1765.

Hospitals

I had hoped that the clearest comparisons in good citizenship could be made by looking at the records of the general hospitals which existed in the 18th century and which still exist today. In the event I was able to examine the records of St Bartholomew's Hospital, the Middlesex and the Foundling Hospital – now the Thomas Coram Foundation – and to compare these with those of the London Hospital, now the Royal London Hospital.[14]

Both St Bartholomew's and the Middlesex had aristocratic patrons, such as the Earl of Bute, and important merchants and financiers among their supporters. Thus in 1750 Jacob Bosanquet, described as a Hamburg merchant, paid £35 and became a Governor for Life of the Middlesex Hospital. Several of his family were silk importers but that is the closest I have been able to get to the silk industry. Chief contributors were people like Benjamin Mendes da Costa, who gave £50 and whose names heads most charitable lists in his lifetime. Several actors gave benefit performances for the Middlesex.[15]

The legacy registers of St Bartholomew's[16] lists Hannah Fromanteel in 1699, presumably a relative of Annesley Fromanteel, who mentioned St Bart's in his own will. Benefactors also included Sir Peter Delmé (1708), originally a factor who handled silks from Canterbury (and probably other goods). John Peck, the dyer, and a Governor, gave £200 for finishing new buildings, and Mozes Delahaize contributed £100 in 1749, but most contributors were what we would now call 'the Great and the Good'.

The annual subscription book of the Foundling Hospital includes legacies from 1739–1776.[17] Surprisingly – considering the attacks upon Thomas Coram in the *Gentleman's Magazine* (for encouraging loose living) – the Hospital was also supported quite generously by aristocratic patrons and by the King. The same people appear as in the records of the other two hospitals: Peter and John Delmé, David and Samuel Bosanquet and Benjamin Mendes da Costa. It was interesting, but irrelevant, to find William Hogarth and Sir Hans Sloane there as well. Daniel Booth (1747) was also a benefactor who may have been the earliest customer of the designer Anna Maria Garthwaite in 1732–3. A legacy of £500 was left by the merchant David Godin in 1763 to the 'hospital in Conduit Street for deserted and exposed young children dedicated by way of atonement if any oversights have occurred in any of my transactions'. While other Godins were important in the silk industry, regrettably I cannot find any connection for him. The Godins I am familiar with seem to have been admirable characters without any need for a guilty conscience.

The London Hospital

All these records are in a marked contrast with those of the London Hospital. Sermons at the Hospital, with a list of contributors, were printed from 1747 onwards. Governors for Life paid 30 guineas, plus annual contributions. Those listed include large numbers from the weaving industry, the overwhelming majority of them Huguenots. Peter Bigot, James Godin the elder, and John Luke Landon were all associated with its foundation. James Godin contributed £21 to the Building Fund in 1747, was Treasurer in 1757 and 1760, and a Steward and Governor for Life. The long lists of names are tedious,[18] but they do include several of the English master weavers who appear in other contexts: Daniel Booth (again! he left the Hospital £100 in 1764), George and Alexander Garrett, John Baker, the two Champions and Robert Turner. But by 1763 Robert, Lord Clive, had joined the list of Governors and in the next year Richard Barwell Esq., of the East India Company. It did not, however, lose its supporters from Spitalfields. It was also listed in the wills of Abraham Deheulle (1765, for £100), Annesley Fromanteel (1789, for £100), John Guillemard (1793, for £20), John Baker (1783, for £100) and James Maze (1795, for £100). I have probably missed others.

There are far fewer bequests to other hospitals. Members of the industry seems to have identified with the London Hospital which was, after all, on their doorstep.

Good Citizens

While a master weaver, (throwster or dyer), needed concentration to achieve success – and flair if working in the fashionable end of the trade – they also worked hard locally. Some of the jobs undertaken were not very exciting, such as paying for the leather coats for the watch in 1763[19] or auditing accounts.

Several were members of the Trained Bands – which is very useful for identifying them. Unfortunately, the relevant records have not survived. Colonel Peter Lekeux was the most distinguished. He was a JP for the Tower Liberty, a Commissioner for Sewers, Deputy Lieutenant for the Royal Hamlets, Lt. Col. of the First Regiment and Commissioner for the Land Tax for Middlesex. In addition, he was on occasion called to give evidence to the Commissioners for Trades and Plantations. At the same time he was a successful master weaver who employed the designer Christopher Baudouin. The Lekeux were important in the industry until the 1770s and his nephew, Captain Peter Lekeux, who died in 1743, was equally active, especially in the Weavers' Company. Only the third Peter Lekeux is absent, although he carried on the family tradition, working in the luxury end of the trade and concentrating on the most expensive silks for men.

In 1764, however, he was one of the Gentlemen on the Jury for the trial of the publisher of no. 45 of the *North Briton* (which led to the constitutional crisis over General Warrants).[20] Others in the Trained Bands included Captain James Dalbiac, who died in 1749 'an eminent black silk weaver very rich' and a man frequently at odds with the Weavers' Company. Five English master weavers can be distinguished, including Captain John Baker, who drilled his men in 1745 when expecting the Young Pretender to march south.

Huguenot master weavers supported their communities in various ways. Zachariah Agace (black silks and gauze) gave evidence to the Select Committee of the House of Commons on the Paving of Norton Folgate in 1759 together with Thomas Abraham Ogier.

In 1745, 134 'Loyal Manufacturers' offered men to fight the Young Pretender – the list was printed in the *London Gazette*, 5–8 October 1745.[21] Of these, 77 firms were certainly Huguenots, although the largest number of men was offered by some of the English firms. One of the English was the builder Samuel Worrall; every one else I have identified was involved in textiles. The Huguenots offered 1736 men, the English 1111. The best Huguenot offers were from Captain James Dalbiac, with 80 men, Peter Campart, with 74 men, and Daniel Gobbee, with 70 men. In both groups some of the offers were just for one or two men. Simon Julins, successful weaver of damasks, offered 22 men.

It could be said that the Huguenots had most to lose had the Young Pretender been successful, but it is clear that there was no division of opinion on this between the English and Huguenots.

Vestry Minutes[22]

While there were negative remarks both in the press and in the Weavers' Company minutes about *'the French'*, the Vestry Minutes of Christ Church and Norton Folgate suggest trust and integration from the third quarter of the 17th century. Already in 1674 one of the Overseers of the Poor in Spitalfields Hamlet was Joseph Dambrine, a factor for Canterbury weavers and himself from Canterbury. He was Constable in 1678, and fined for Churchwarden in 1684. Many names from the 1680s and '90s became familiar in the next 100 years – Lekeux, Duthoit, Dupree, Gobbee, Le Count, Alavoine – and they remain familiar because they attended town meetings and either served or fined for the various offices. Peter Marescoe, whose daughter married Peter Lekeux (Colonel), fined for Churchwarden in 1681. Christopher Baudouin, the designer, fined for Headborough in 1693, in 1702 was chosen as one of the Overseers of the Poor, and Sidesman for the year 1711. He was one of the 'Principal Inhabitants'[23] who signed the petition in 1714 which eventually resulted in the building of Hawksmoor's Christ Church. We can follow the eldest Peter Lekeux through the ranks of the Trained Bands, so diligent was he in attending the Vestry. As Major Peter Lekeux in 1703 he was excused all offices since he had been 'instrumental in procuring Charity Money' for the parish, on payment of a £10 fine, a fairly token amount.

A Committee was set up following a resolution in 1711 to petition for the hamlet to become a parish. It had eight English and five Huguenots, nearly all connected with textiles.[24] Thereafter, the number of names, whether English or French, of those who were also active in the Weavers' Company increases. Col. Lekeux (by this time) hardly missed a meeting. Such meetings included one in 1717 to deal with grievances: the regulation of the Watch, leases, a true survey of the town, and inspection of the accounts for the horse and cart. They resolved, indeed, to sell the horse and cart. Lekeux was a man called upon by the Commissioners for Trade and Plantations for advice – but along with a rich dyer, John Peck, the brewer (?) Joseph Truman, and others, he discussed the hamlet's horse and cart. The tradition of unpaid, tiresome, and time-consuming service to local government was well established by the early 18th century and continued to flourish.

There is a gap in the minutes until 1743 but no difference in representation. Huguenots served on the committees to repair the cracked north steps of Christ Church in September 1743 and to recast the cracked tenor bell four years later.[25] John Sabatier reported on workhouses he had investigated in other parishes on 15 November 1752, and a decision was made in 1754 to erect one in Spitalfields. John Sabatier, James Lardant senior, Isaac Roberdeau, Nicholas Jourdain, Abraham Dupree, William Jourdain, John Fremont and Peter Duthoit were eight of the 29 selected governors. Sabatier was Treasurer of the Watch and Lamps in the same year. He gave interesting biographical details about his career to Parliamentary Select Committees in 1750 and 1766 and continued a family tradition, for his father, of the same name, had fined for offices in 1718.[26]

The Vestry Minutes for Norton Folgate do not start until the 1720s but the Huguenots attending include some of the richest in the industry: Captain James Dalbiac, Obadiah Agace, John Luke Landon, James Godin, Peter Bigott, Thomas Abraham, Lewis and Peter Ogier (the successful family from Chassis l'Eglise in Bas

Poitou), and the designer John Vansommer, partner in the firm of Ogier, Vansommer and Triquet of Spital Square. Norton Folgate seems to have had fewer problems than existed in Christ Church next door, until the riots of 1763 and 1765, but the Huguenots were equally assiduous in their attendance. Five out of ten nominations for the Court of Conscience for Tower Hamlets were weavers – and all were Huguenots.[27]

Because there is a dearth of business evidence the success in worldly terms of the master weavers of Spitalfields has to be judged from their wills and their house insurance. We can, however, concentrate on two aspects, the desire for a country house and the actual sums of money bequeathed or the value of house property insured. Having the 'pad' in town and the 'des. res' in the country is emphatically not a 20th- or 21st-century ambition. As the second generation of masters (or fourth or fifth in such families as the Lekeux) made their way in the world it is evident that those who could moved out, generally to the east but occasionally further afield, sometimes retaining premises in town.[28]

Neither community re-invested in the textile industries. Their wills speak of government stocks, the Bank of England, and the East India Company. They wanted to be gentlemen – as the contingent from Bas Poitou had been in France – and, by and large, they succeeded, for bankruptcies were few.[29] Two cases are specially interesting, that of Andrew Ogier (bankrupt 1739), who is discussed by Mary Bayliss,[30] and Stephen Jeudwine, a loyal inhabitant of Spitalfields early in the century who also failed in 1739. He was left a pension by his successful son in the will drawn up in 1762, though by then Stephen was over 80.

House property seems to have been the chief investment for Captain Baker, the glorious exception, who invested £33,000 very profitably in Ben Truman's brewery (he had married Joseph Truman's daughter) and owned a string of pubs in and near Spitalfields, as well as extensive property in the City and in Buckinghamshire. I cannot find a comparable Huguenot property owner.

Looking at those in the industry who insured property valued at over £1000, I have found 220 English masters and 106 Huguenots, well above their proportion in the industry.[31] Among them are Peter Bigot, the Beuzevilles, Captain Peter Lekeux, Peter Ogier, John Sabatier, James Godin (whose house was 'finished in a grand manner') and Lewis Chauvet, the handkerchief weaver who had his windows broken by angry journeymen in 1765 and whose house sported 'enriched corniches . . . ornamental ceilings'. Peter Campart's will totalled £44,600 in bequests in 1772. Several master weavers of black silks as well as plain silks were among this prosperous group, for their products were always needed and did not suffer from changes in fashion.[32]

Conclusions

If we ignore the vitriolic sentiments expressed by the 18th-century equivalent of the modern tabloid newspapers, we see that some quite reasonable concerns were shown by the Commonalty of the Weavers' Company. A petition was presented to its Court on 29 June 1715 about the French employing non-freemen. A committee was formed, as usual, and Captain Lekeux (nephew of Colonel Peter) and a Mr Harlé were deputed to meet the Elders of the French Church. In January 1717 there was *again* a complaint about the employment of non-freemen but without specific reference to their being French. There were more complaints about the employment of *girls*!

By 1719 John Harris in his *History of Kent* spoke with slightly exaggerated admiration of the contribution made by Huguenots in Canterbury. In general, whatever their private thoughts, English and French worked together harmoniously. In *Postlethwayt's Universal Dictionary* (which contained much which was not a translation of Savary des Bruslon's) he acknowledged the contribution made by Huguenot immigrants in the late 17th century, but by his own day, in the 1750s, seems to have taken them for granted.[33]

Peter Bigot lamented in his will, proved in 1773, 'I do hereby declare that my motive for giving the said . . . estates to my grandnephews intailed . . . is that I have reflected on the Extravagance and Luxury of the present generation which inevitably occasions great fluctuation'[34] – this from a highly successful master weaver whose success *depended* upon the 'Extravagance' and 'Luxury' of his customers. The elder generation is always suspicious of the next generation, but few put these sentiments into their wills, unless there has been some family row, and certainly some can be deduced in the Huguenots' wills – interesting to speculate upon but irrelevant here. No difference in attitudes can be discerned between the masters of French origin and their English counterparts in this or in anything else.

NOTES

1   Natalie Rothstein, 'Huguenots in the English silk industry in the eighteenth century', in Irene Scouloudi (ed.), *Huguenots in England and their French background* (London, 1987), 126. In 1783–4 there were 1383 weavers in the Weavers' Company, of whom 173 were Huguenots; of the 28 members of the Court of Assistants and the officers, 7 were Huguenots; there were 40 Huguenots in a Livery of 210. Thus the total percentage of Huguenots in the Company was 12.5 per cent, yet they formed 25 per cent of the Court and 19 per cent of the Livery. Other industries wrote to the Weavers' Company to represent their interests in the negotiations surrounding the Treaty.

2   *The Survey of London* vol. 27: *Spitalfields and Mile End New Town*, ed. P. A. Bezodis and Walter Ison (London, 1957).

3   Natalie Rothstein, 'Canterbury and London: the silk industry in the late 17th century', *Textile History* 20:1 (Spring 1989), 33–48; Rothstein, 'The successful and unsuccessful Huguenot: another look at the London silk industry in the 18th and early 19th centuries', *HSP* 25:5 (1993), 439–50.; Rothstein, *Silk designs of the eighteenth century in the collection of the Victoria and Albert Museum* (London, 1990), esp. 300–44; Rothstein, 'Fashion, silk and the Worshipful Company of Weavers' in Simonetta Cavaciocchi (ed.), *La seta in Europa sec. XII–XX: atti della 'ventiquattresima Settimana di studi', 4–9 maggio 1992*, Istituto internazionale di storia economica 'F. Datini', Serie II, 24 (Florence, 1993), 465–85 (unfortunately many typographical errors were introduced in this paper by the proofreaders); Rothstein, 'The silk industry in London, 1702–1766' (unpublished MA thesis, University of London, 1961); *Indexes of the fire insurance policies of the Sun Fire Office and the Royal Exchange Assurance, 1775–1787*.

4   W. H. Manchée, 'Some Huguenot smugglers: the impeachment of London silk merchants in 1698', *HSP* 15:3 (1936), 406–27; Henry G. Roseveare, 'A Huguenot London merchant of the late seventeenth century and his circle', in Scouloudi, *Huguenots in Britain*, 72–88.

5   Rothstein, *Fashion, silk and Company of Weavers*, 469–70.

6　*Ibid.*, 470–2.

7　They were James Leman, Captain Peter Lekeux, James Godin and Daniel Gobbé.

8　For example, James Beuzeville (1763); his widow and brother Stephen were beneficiaries but 'my partners shall not be obliged to pay the same out of their trade until 2 years after my decease'. They were to pay interest to the legatees for these two years. James Brant (1740) left '£500 already given' and added the 'utensils belonging to my trade'. Abraham Jeudwine (1767) added third and fourth codicils to his will to try to prevent 'trade from stagnating', hence there was a delay in paying out his daughters' inheritances. But these were exceptions. Most turned their profits into house property or government stocks.

9　A customer of Anna Maria Garthwaite in 1745 left £100 to William Ward, Wood Street, Spitalfields, 'my late foreman'. Ann Byas (1767) left £100 to her son to 'distribute among my poor workpeople'. Annesley Fromanteel (1790), trusted by Abraham Jeudwine to run his business for the benefit of Jeudwine's sons (which he did), left 'to each of the journeymen that have worked more than 12 months £5 each'.

10　Peter Bigot (1773) gave 5 guineas and owed wages to each servant, as well as £10 10s for life to his housekeeper, Mary Bonner. Mary Chauvet (1763) left 10 guineas each to two servants; Gabriel Grellier (1740) £5 to all his servants. John Guillemard (1793) had lent £450 to the Commissioners entrusted with paving, lighting and watching the Old Artillery Ground at £4 10s p.a., the interest to be paid to his housekeeper, Mrs Jane Scott, widow of Walter Scott, for life. If the debt was repaid then the money should be re-invested to yield an annuity of £20 5s. Daniel Gwilt (1749?) left his servants £5 each but his 13 'good friends' who received mourning rings were all English – no mixing in this case. John Sabatier the elder (1745) left £10 to a servant; Robert Turner (1756) left an annuity to a servant for 'long and faithful service'. Edward Wollstonecraft (1756), handkerchief maker, left £10 each to his servants and also 1s each to the settled paupers of the parish of St Botolph. He was rich and the executors recieved £15 for their trouble.

11　The directors of the French Hospital are listed in alphabetical order in D. C. A. Agnew, *Protestant exiles from France in the reign of Louis XIV* (2nd edn., London, 1871) vol. 1, 76. In order of date those connected with the silk industry are: 1718–21 Benjamin Barroneau, René Baudouin, James Louis Berchère, James Baudouin(?), Philip Fruchard, John Perigal, Peter Reneu, Stephen Seignoret, Peter Triquet, Peter Seignoret, James Gaultier, Henry Guinand; 1741–2 James Massé, Peter Lemaitre, James Godin; 1748–51 John Jullian (?), James Fruchard, Nicholas Jourdain, James Landon, Isaac Roberdeau; 1753–6 Abraham Delamere, John Luke Landon, David Delavau, Daniel Pilon, Peter Auber, Simon Dalbiac, Henry Guinand, Peter Triquet, Daniel Vautier; 1758–61 Simon Dalbiac, Giles Godin, Zachary Agace, Peter Cazalet, John Sabatier, Peter Nouaille, Peter Alavoine, Peter Ogier; 1763–7 Obadiah(?) Agace, Stephen Barbut, Jacob Jamet, Jacob Agace, John Landon, Peter Auber; 1769–72 Philip Delahaize, Leonard Turquand, Peter Merzeau, Lewis Ogier, Capt. James Barbut; 1774–7 James Beuzeville, Stephen Beuzeville, Louis Chauvet, John Fremont, James Louis Turquand; 1779–86 James Auber, junior, James Maze, junior, John Perigal, John Peter Roberdeau.

12　Notably the Duthoit family, but also the Ferrys, James Boudry, the Jeudwines, Abraham Macaré, Samuel Six, Daniel Lepine, Arnold Facon, Dalbiac & Co. John Landon (1725–96) insured £1000 in goods in the house of James Gant in Canterbury. Altogether I have found about 30 such insurances.

13　John Chevalier (1752), Mary Chauvet (1763), Gabriel Grellier (1740).

14　I am very grateful to Marion Rea, Trust Archivist of St Bartholomew's Hospital, and to Mr M. F. Sturridge, archivist of the Middlesex Hospital who both replied very helpfully to my request and allowed me to visit their archives. When I first approached the London Hospital, as it was then, 40 years ago for my research I was also treated with both courtesy and efficiency.

15 Middlesex Hospital Archive, Ledger 1750–74, 111: 'produce of a play by Messrs Garrick and Lacy Dec. 21st 1757 £158 17s'.

16 St Bartholomew's Hospital Archive, HB 5/2 and HB 5/3.

17 London Metropolitan Archives, A/FH/B3/20/1.

18 The names are all very familiar and occur year after year, both Huguenot and English. The people concerned supported both the French Hospital and the London Hospital. Interestingly, some Huguenots only supported the London Hopsital: John Debonnaire and Daniel Gobbé in 1747, for example, or Peter Bigot, Peter Lekeux, Daniel Messman, Thomas Abraham Ogier, Peter Saubergue in 1752. From the next years, 1752–7, I have noted a number of widows or daughters, but also Charles Triquet (of Ogier Vansomer & Triquet), and in 1760, Daniel Cabanel junior, Abraham Deheulle junior, and Nicholas Hebert. From 1774 addresses are given, indicating that many had retired, such as Obadiah Agace, Esq., in Stratford Green. There are many English names familiar in the silk industry like Daniel Booth, Alderman Sir William Baker, the Turners, Col. George Garrett, John Batchelor, but not until 1774 does John Baker senior of Prince's Street, Spitalfields, appear. £31 10s was the set fee for becoming a Governor for Life of the London Hospital.

19 Christ Church Spitalfields, Vestry Minutes, vol. 88, 26 July 1763. John Sabatier paid for 18 leather coats for the Watch, as well as the cleaning of the Watch House.

20 Reported in the *St James's Chronicle* or the *British Evening Post* for Tues. 21 February–Thurs. 23 February 1764. I am ever grateful to Miss Wendy Hefford for spotting this.

21 I provide the complete list of names in my 1961 MA thesis, 'The silk industry in London, 1702–1766', 546–52.

22 I am very grateful to the archivists and librarians of Tower Hamlets Local History Library and Archives, Bancroft Rd, who have been as helpful and efficient in 2000 as their predecessors had been in 1960. The relevant Vestry Minute Books of Christ Church, Spitalfields, are vols. 83–8. The minutes for 1729–43 are missing. The Vestry Minutes for the Liberty of Norton Folgate begin in 1729.

23 Rothstein, *Silk designs*, 31–2.

24 The English were: Mr Doddington (the Church Warden), Alexander Garrett, Edward Peck (dyer), Charles Elliston, John Allen (possibly a master weaver), John Folwell (also possibly a weaver), Thomas Speare and George Arthur, who was to write the peitition. The French names are: Peter Lepipier, John Furniot, Samuel Hanrot, John Lekeux. I am not certain about Raphael Dubois for this is a name which could have originated before Huguenot immigration. He was in the Weavers' Company.

25 Christ Church Spitalfields Vestry Minutes for 14 April 1746, discussed in Rothstein, 'The silk industry', 212.

26 Rothstein, *Silk designs*, 337.

27 The five Huguenot weavers were James Godin, Peter Ogier, Thomas Abraham Ogier, Obadiah Agace, Daniel Messman.

28 Zachariah Agace, Edmonton, 1772; Samuel Alavoine, Tottenham, 1743; the Bigots, Upton West Ham; Stephen Cazalet, Clapton, Hackney, 1742; Mary Chauvet, Tottenham, 1763; Isaac Grou, Cowledge parish near Clare, Suffolk, 1734; Matthew Hebart, Walthamstow, 1739; the Jeudwines, Palmers Green as well as Basinghall Street; Sebastian Loy, Clapton as well as a house in Spital Square, 1772; Daniel Messman (black silk), Southgate, 1765; Lewis Ogier, Hackney, 1769, then emigrated to America c. 1775–6; John Ouvry, St John Hackney, 1774; Daniel Pilon, 1762, wished to be buried in Dagenham and had an estate in Barking; John Sabatier, 1770, insured a house in Sevenoaks but retained his own house (valued at £1000 in Church Street in 1773), but when he died in 1780 he was described as 'of Chichester, gent.'; Daniel Vautier, died in 1760 in Cheshunt, Herts. In 1747 this man or another of the same name was living in Bath when summoned by the Weavers' Company to serve as one of the Company's officers. Other places mentioned include Standford (*sic*)

Hill and Hoddenham. The lure of the country house is discussed in Rothstein, 'The silk industry', 203–5.

29 Rothstein, 'Successful and unsucessful Huguenot', 441–2.

30 Mary Bayliss, 'The unsuccessful Andrew and other Ogiers: a study of failure in the Huguenot community', *HSP* 26:2 (1995), 230–40.

31 Rothstein, 'Successful and unsuccessful Huguenot', 440. The worldly success of the master weavers and what they chose to do with their funds is discussed in Rothstein, 'The silk industry', 203–5.

32 There were periodic protests at the prevalence of official public mournings both in England and France. The *Black Branch* formed a distinct section of the silk industry, some of whose representatives signed the *List of Prices*, the earliest surviving trades union agreement in the industry, which gives piece rates for different kinds of silk.

33 Malachy Postlethwayt, *The universal dictionary of trade and commerce* (2nd edn., London, 1757), 736. In the article on engraving, he writes: 'After the Revolution [i.e. 1688] the French refugees settled the silk manufactures here in London, and particularly the flowered silks. The principal persons herein concerned were Mr Lauson, Mariscot and Monceaux, and the first designer and pattern drawer was Mr Baudouin'. Eulogies of the Huguenot community seem to begin in the middle of the 19th century.

34 Quoted in Rothstein, *Silk designs*, 303.

Part IV

Immigrants and intellectual life in England

18

Immigrants in the *DNB* and British cultural horizons, 1550–1750: the merchant, the traveller, the lexicographer and the apologist

Vivienne Larminie

As you may already be aware, the *Dictionary of National Biography*, as it appeared in the 1880s and 1890s, begins and ends with immigrants and, moreover, with immigrants active from 1550 to 1750. The first entry is Jacques Abbadie, born near Pau in south-west France, educated at Puylaurens, Saumur and Sedan, then pastor at Berlin, visitor to Holland, and finally preacher and apologist for Protestant Britain, living in London and in Ireland. The last entry is for the three Zuylesteins, members of an Anglo-Dutch family sprung from the House of Orange, who were soldiers, courtiers, politicians and English peers. That this should be so stands as a significant pointer to the part, or rather parts, played by immigrants in British life.[1] It also testifies to the width of cultural horizons both of those contemporaries who celebrated or patronized them (or, for that matter, vilified them), and of contributors to the original *DNB* who recognized, investigated and included them and their exploits in an official record of notable British lives.[2]

Armed with a general sense of immigrants' importance, I set about on a systematic search for them both in the *Old DNB* and among the subsequent entries which will appear in the consolidated and expanded *New DNB*, which is to be published by Oxford University Press in 2004.[3] The search was not without methodological problems, and was attended by the unsettling knowledge that it will certainly be an easier undertaking, and its findings will be more precise, once the *New DNB* is published. Then anyone with suitable equipment should be able to search electronically for, say, subjects born in Italy between 1600 and 1700. What follows is avowedly an interim analysis, based on combing through groups of subjects on the database who were recorded in January and February 2000 as definitely included in the new dictionary. Even leaving aside the certainty that more new subjects, some of them immigrants, have been included before the gates closed finally in 2001, for various reasons the results may underestimate immigrants. Proposals for new subjects, in particular, are often accompanied by incomplete initial data on birthplace, and inferences drawn from names alone of undelivered articles are insecure and potentially misleading.

The search was restricted to people deemed active between 1550 and 1750. In the *New DNB* terms this means those born between 1510 and 1710, or, if death date only is known, dying between 1570 and 1770. It thus immediately excludes a generation of early 16th-century humanists, reformers and printers, who may well swell the overall percentage of immigrants in the dictionary, but who, strictly speaking, lie outside the chronological scope of this volume. The decision was taken to exclude colonial blocks[4] and the sizeable number of subjects born abroad to British parents, including soldier's daughter Brilliana Harley, ambassador's son George Digby, and many children of royalist and Jacobite exiles.[5] Subjects born abroad to just one British parent were in general similarly disallowed, although subjects with a British grandparent were included. Included also were temporary visitors, who ended their lives abroad, but who nonetheless made a lasting impact on British life – people such as Simon de Passe (1595–1647), engraver, born in Cologne and died in Copenhagen; Henri Gascar (1635–1701), portrait painter, born in Paris and died in Rome; or Lorenz Natter (1705–63), engraver and medallist, born in Swabia and died in St Petersburg.

The results were, I think, striking. Around 412 immigrants active between 1550 and 1750 were recorded in the *Old DNB*. By far the greatest number of them are artists of one kind or another. If craftsmen, sculptors, architects, goldsmiths and jewellers are also included under this heading, then the majority is overwhelming. This seems understandable: it is symptomatic of the truly enormous contribution made to 'British' art at this period by non-native portrait painters, engravers, print-makers and the like. For the convenience of editing, articles in the dictionary are divided into blocks of like subjects: of 156 in one block of artists, 82 are foreigners, most of them in the *Old DNB*. Also well-represented are clergy, other religious leaders and controversialists, authors and soldiers, many of the last Huguenot refugees or Dutchmen in the train of William III. A testament to the inclusiveness, in certain respects, of the *Old DNB*, is the appearance, at the other end of the scale, of odd or obscure categories. There are people such as George I's brother Ernest Augustus, Duke of York and Albany and Bishop of Osnabrück, who was born in the bishopric in 1674 and died there in 1728, and of whom the contributor observes that, 'the fact of his existence was scarcely known to the British nation'.[6] He, like some others, for example John Drassier (1676–1763) of Geneva, medallist, may never have set foot in Britain. At least one other, Mary Carleton (1642?–73), the so-called 'German princess', may never have lived anywhere else: she claimed to come from Cologne, but her detractors suggested Canterbury.[7] Still others were 'reluctant' immigrants. Perhaps the most notable is Sir Théodore de Mayerne (1573–1655), born in Geneva, whose medical ministrations to Charles I and his court were so valued that he was repeatedly refused permission to leave and to take up residence on his newly-acquired estate at Aubonne in the Pays de Vaud.

Ascription of precise nationalities to *DNB* subjects is far from straightforward. Not only is there the problem of shifting international boundaries between 1550 and 1750, which affected, for example, natives of Calais, Alsace and Poland, but it is also evident that many immigrants in Britain came from families who had taken two generations to move northwards from their places of origin. Thus subjects might have been born to Portuguese families in France or to Italian families in Geneva.[8] Beyond observing that this adds to the truly cosmopolitan upbringing of many immigrants, and probably to their ability to adapt, survive and even assimilate, I have been unable so far to find a way of accommodating it in my figures: hence geographical findings are very broad-brush. Given the predominance of artists in the *Old DNB*, it is perhaps hardly surprising to find many Netherlanders – about 81 from the United Provinces, about 42 from the Spanish Netherlands, and a further five probably from the Low Countries – a total of about 128. However, running about equal are the French – a definite 117, and probably at least 126. They are prominent as artists but also as clergy, authors, scholars, physicians and soldiers. There are slightly more than half that number of Germans – 68 or 69 – many of them again artists, but proportionately more prominent among royalty, courtiers and musicians. Half as many again are Italian. Apart from 21 born in Switzerland – physicians, engineers, authors, merchants – there is a sprinkling from other European countries, headed by Poles, many of them, like the Portuguese, of Jewish origin. At this period there are few non-Europeans, exceptions being the Coptic scholar Abudacnus and, borrowing momentarily from the colonial blocks I have otherwise eschewed, Pocahontas, or Rebecca Rolfe, born in territory not yet British and buried in Gravesend in 1617.

Pocahontas is just one of many 'foreigners' from the *Old DNB* who will reappear in the *New DNB* at significantly greater length. This reflects greater knowledge of their backgrounds and greater appreciation of the extent of their impact on Britain and, in her case at least, on subsequent generations.[9] But the *New DNB* includes also a total of about 13,000 new subjects, an increase of about 35 per cent over the *Old DNB*, including supplements and *Missing Persons*. It has sought to promote the inclusion of categories of people whose contribution to British life was previously overlooked or underestimated. Some areas which have seen expansion, such as provincially significant figures and women, have drawn in relatively few first-generation immigrants. However, other areas, most notably merchants, musicians and diplomats, have seen a significant influx of those born abroad, and there has been a slight but palpable increase in the overall proportion of immigrants. Italian musicians (retrieved thanks to the renaissance in early music over the last quarter century), Venetian painters and Jewish merchants and community leaders are conspicuous here. The *Old DNB* included Handel; the *New DNB* adds the Spanish violinist Louis Grabu (*fl.*1665–94), the Neapolitan violinist Nicola Matteis (*fl.*1670–1710), the Paduan composer Angelo Notari (1566–1663), the German viol player Dietrich Stoeffken (*d.*1673) and the Bassano family, notable at the court of Elizabeth I. The *Old DNB* has Van Dyck, but the *New DNB* also has Rubens, a visitor whose impact was huge. It has Giacomo Castelvetro (1546–1616), gardener and extoller of vegetables and Signora Violante (*née* Larini, 1682–1741), rope dancer and theatre company manager. It encompasses group articles on Castilians in 1570s Edinburgh, on exotic foreigners, whose appearance in this country in the 18th century excited public comment, and on industrial spies, whose infiltration of the nation's infant engines of wealth drew fear and suspicion. At least 160 new foreign-born entrants, individual and collective, have joined the dictionary since the 1890s. In January and February 2000 they comprised about 4.25 per cent of the 13,436 articles on subjects active from 1550 to 1750. Abbadie and Zuylestein have not yet been toppled from their first and last places: in the unlikely event that they are displaced, it would probably have to be by other immigrants or their descendents.

As I hope has already been evident, immigrants may be in the *DNB* because they made a positive or a negative impression on contemporaries or subsequent generations. 'Foreignness' might be tangential to their public reputation or it might be central. For chef and cookery writer Vincent la Chapelle (*fl.*1733–6), French nationality was doubtless advantageous even then to his career and his celebrity. For his country-woman Mary Hobry (*d.*1688), who murdered her husband in 1687, the conjunction of her nationality, her religion (Roman Catholic), and her profession (midwife), ensured her instant notoriety: Londoners' habitual paranoia about husband killers was, if anything, exceeded by their conviction that James II was about to import French-style popish absolutism, and midwives, as in France, were an important part of this strategy. Diego Sarmiento de Acuña, otherwise known as Count Gondomar, was partly the victim of ready-made hostility to Spain. But he earns his place in the new dictionary thanks to widespread suspicion and hatred surrounding his embassy to James I's court and to a public vilification exemplified by his immediately recognizable personification as the arch-villain in Thomas Middleton's 1624 play, *A game at chess*.[10]

Largely, however, the *DNB* reflects both the positive contribution of immigrants to national life and the extent (sometimes underestimated) of British participation in wider European culture.[11] This is especially evident among scholars. The *Old DNB* had Isaac and Meric Casaubon, (1559–1614) and (1599–1671) respectively, Gerard and Isaac Vossius, (1577–1649) and (1618–89) respectively, the philologist Francis Junius (1591–1677), the Hebraist John Immanuel Tremellius (1510–80), and the librarians Henri Justel (1620–93) and John Verneuil (1582/1583–1647). The *New DNB* has added Hebraist and book collector Isaac Abendana (*d.*1699), historian of Essex Peter Mullman (1705?–90), writer on education, politics and theology Jean Gailhard (*fl.*1660–99), and the writer on the Church of England, ecumenist and associate of Archbishop William Wake, Pierre-François de Courayer (1682–1776). The *Old DNB* had Samuel Hartlib, but thanks to the recognition of the importance of his and of other intellectual circles, the *New DNB* also has educational reformer Comenius (Jan Amos Komensky) and philosopher Francis (Franciscus Mercurius) van Helmont (1614–98).

In order to explore some recurrent themes associated with immigrants in the *DNB* in general, and with their place in the enrichment of national culture in particular, I shall now present very briefly some cases studies of subjects on whom I have worked. As indicated earlier, merchants are a group who emerge more strongly in the new dictionary. Some combined commercial and scholarly interests – men like Jacob Vanderlint (*d.*1740), timber merchant and economic theorist, and Johannes de Laet (1581–1649), lexicographer and correspondent of many English scholars and antiquaries. Others , by their very financial success, affected markedly the character of the metropolitan society in which they largely moved – Philip Burlamachi (*d.*1644), the financier; Alvaro Jacob da Costa (1646–1716), the first naturalized Englishman of Jewish origin; Alvaro de Fonseca (1657?–1742), the diamond merchant; Sir Peter Rycaut (1578–1653); and Sir Horatio Palavicino (*c.*1540–1600), the diplomat. One man who illustrates as well as any the extent and the limits of integration and assimilation is Sir Peter Vanlore, another foreigner honoured with a title. Born in Utrecht about 1547, Vanlore had established himself in London as a jewel merchant by the late 1570s, and by the 1590s had an extremely lucrative business supplying the court.[12] In 1604 he purchased Tilehurst manor near Reading, and over the next two decades, despite some hostility from the Berkshire gentry, increased his estates locally to the point where, at his death in 1627, he owned one of the largest estates in the county. 'He possessed', concluded Chris Durston, 'a great potential influence over county affairs and a social parity with any of his fellow landowners'.[13] Yet he continued to straddle two communities, Dutch church and parish church, and even in old age did not feel secure in his adopted country. His daughters' husbands included, as well as the previously mentioned scholar-merchant de Laet, the second-generation immigrant and Master of the Rolls, Sir Charles Caesar (grandson of Dr Cesare Adelmare, *d*.1559) and the Master of Requests, Sir Edward Powell.[14] Connections with lawyers, though, were no proof against his prosecution in Star Chamber in 1619, along with other merchants of Dutch origin, for the illegal export of bullion. Brief imprisonment and a large fine followed, and John Chamberlain informed Dudley Carleton that Vanlore had recently 'said that when he had ended this busines he wold bid England farewell . . . he wold go to save his skin, for they that upon such witnes could take away his goods might, when they pleased, take his life'.[15]

Travellers are another group better represented in the *New DNB* who opened up cultural horizons, this time by offering the British, through their writing, a novel reflection of themselves and a window on the outside world. Voltaire is a new entrant, as are the Swiss Thomas Platter (*fl*.1590) and César-François de Saussure (1705–83). The latter came to London in the 1720s, significantly exploiting a network of ready-made contacts, and gave an account of English society complementary, in its analysis of civic, mercantile and low life, to Voltaire's more aristocratic contemporary work. It was in London that he was initiated into Freemasonry, and he subsequently took it with him back to Lausanne.[16] Another native of Lausanne, noticed in the *Old DNB*, emerges on reassessment as a significant example of a visitor who not only eventually stayed, but also built a notable reputation as an author and lexicographer. After travelling with the Earl of Carlisle and Andrew Marvell to Russia in 1663, a journey described graphically in *A relation of three embassies* (1669), Guy Miège or Miege (1644– died in or after 1718) settled in Panton Street, near Leicester Fields, London, teaching French and geography to the aristocracy.[17] His *The grounds of the French tongue* (1687) provided 'the basis of most of the French grammars published in English over the next 60 years',[18] while his *The English grammar* (1688) 'has the distinction of being the only grammar of English written in English by a non-native speaker'.[19] His various versions of a primer for learning English contained entertaining dialogues drawing on his observations of English life: coffee houses and clubs earn approval, but the weather is uncertain, the sun 'little seen' and the air 'gross and thick'.[20] His final publication was a collaboration with Abel Boyer in 1718.[21]

However, Miege is perhaps most striking as an example of the involvement of French-speaking Protestant immigrants in apologetics for the Glorious Revolution and the Hanoverian succession. His *The first part of the new state of England* (1691) endorsed the 'late Revolution', the downfall of popery, and the Church of England as a Reformed church. Consciously modelled on Thomas Smith's *De republica Anglorum*, 'improved and fitted to the present times', it celebrated the English as 'a free People, averse from Slavery', with a genius for invention and knowledge in experimental philosophy, divinity and literature, and with 'a most happy language'. He preached a monarchy under the law, abhorring James II, 'who strikes at the very Foundations of Government'. Parliament was for him 'one of the most August Assemblies in the World', and Charles I's breaking of its privileges in 1641 was noted as a cardinal error.[22] Edward Chamberlayne, whose father had previously published an analysis of England, was furious at the effrontery of a foreigner who not only plagiarized (as he saw it), but also adopted a Whig perspective. Undaunted, Miege published a robust reply in *Utrum horum? Oppression or moderation in answer to Dr Chamberlayn's High Church principles* (1705), a plea for 'the true and moderate Church of England' and for toleration of Protestant dissenters.[23]

Other immigrants were equally passionately involved in the defence of a Protestant church and state, and in spreading to the English the message of Louis XIV as cruel tyrant. Sometime in 1683 there arrived in London from Montpellier the suitably-named octogenarian pastor and patriarch Isaac Dubourdieu (1597?–1700?), with his son Jean Dubourdieu (c.1643–1720?) and numerous grandsons and nephews, mostly called Jean, Armand, or Jean-Armand. The resulting confusion in library catalogues has served to obscure their several contributions to political and religious apologetics. From the beginning the family served the conformist chapel at the Savoy, and gradually they were inducted to Church of England livings too.[24] They were eager to affirm their political loyalty, but not blindly. In his *A discourse of obedience unto kings and magistrates* (1684), Isaac expressed his profound thanks to 'a Monarch, who is the Sanctuary of the Oppressed and the refuge of the persecuted'.[25] He called on his fellow Huguenots to 'be examples of fidelity and subjection' to a king who had been established by the providence of God, and whom they could serve with purity of conscience.[26] His son Jean, incidentally one of a significant number of refugee clergy whose Gallicanism served to nourish the ecumenism of Archbishop Wake's circle, learned to be more wary of the Stuarts and more forthright in his condemnation of Louis XIV – 'the Adversary of God, the implacable Enemy of Goodness, and the Barbarous Persecutor of the Saints, who has everywhere declared war against Christ and his Church'.[27] In *The triumphs of Providence* (1707), an acclamation of Marlborough's victory at Ramillies, he coupled English 'false Protestants', who had opposed the war and government policy, with 'the idolaters of France' and 'the slaves of arbitrary power'. French refugees in England were exhorted to throw off the frequently-made insinuation that they were disloyal to the Queen, and to exult in the overthrow by God of a persecuting pharaoh, remembering that 'we are men, that we are Protestants . . . [and] this day England is our country'.[28]

Jean's sons and nephews came to England in their youth, attended English universities and, like Jean, found powerful friends and patrons among certain sections of the aristocracy and episcopate, but like him they combined Protestant zeal with insecurity. In *La faction de la Grande Bretagne caracterisée et confondue* (1716), originally preached in French to his congregation at the Savoy, but evidently with a wider audience in mind, Jean Armand Dubourdieu (1677–1727) expressed the horror of English political faction characteristic of many immigrant writers and the urgency with which many felt impelled to defend the Reformed foundations of the Church of England and constitutional monarchy. He anathematized false Anglican brothers who advocated passive obedience to the Stuarts, who countenanced Jacobite insurgency and who questioned the validity of the Huguenots' baptism, and even their very Christianity. That Archbishop William Laud should be singled out as 'le Patriarche de la Faction que nous combatons'[29] suggests that his was an agenda shared by his English patrons, but his reputation as a controversialist brought him enemies too. His *Mephiboseth, ou le caractère d'un bon sujet*, a sermon to mark the return of George I from Hanover in January 1724, was dedicated to an anonymous duke whose father had been a stalwart of the fight against popery, but who himself had limply refused to support king George. It was a paean to Protestant kingship limited by law and vested in the House of Hanover. In a furious reply, *A noble peer vindicated* (1724), D.F.R. attacked Dubourdieu's presumption. He was an 'Abhominable Sycophant', a 'wretched and ridiculous Flatterer' and 'an impertinent Frenchman'. His arguments are revealing and familiar:

> ought a Foreigner, a Frenchman, one who has the Mark and impression of the Shackle still remaining, who lives here, as it were, but on Courtesy; was it not the highest and most unpardonable insolence . . . to thrust himself uncall'd into a Controversy in which he had nothing in nature to do . . . [B]ecause thro' the extraordinary Charity and Indulgence of our Nation to him and his Countrymen, he enjoys the same Privileges and Advantages, and is in every Respect consider'd as a natural born Subject, he grows rude and insolent, and even abuses his Benefactors.[30]

Acceptance of immigrants by D.F.R. and some of his contemporaries, just as by some others since, was grudging. Often, criticism such as D.F.R.'s missed the mark. Dubourdieu spoke and wrote in his native language and officiated at his community's church, but he had arrived in England aged six and graduated from Oxford. Like other refugees, he gained a native patron (the Duke of Devonshire), an English wife and in 1701 a Church of England living (Sawtry Moyns, Huntingdonshire).[31] Like Vanlore and Miege, he lived in two communities, and his experience of the outside culture enriched his contribution to English culture. Both the *Old* and *New DNB* reveal and acknowledge the enormous contribution made by immigrants like them to British art, politics, religion, commerce and literary culture. With the help of the many contributors to the *New DNB* we hope to continue the tradition of public recognition of this fact.

NOTES

1   As Daniel Statt, *Foreigners and Englishmen: the controversy over immigration, 1660–1760* (Newark, 1995), 22, observes: 'The century after 1660 marks one of the great ages for immigration to England, and the challenge and promise presented by the foreign settlers helped to shape the fundamental changes that in these years transformed England into a commercial society'.

2   The latter may come as a surprise in the context of recent debates on national history and identity and on the nature of Britishness and Englishness, which have pointed to a failure among the population at large at the end of the 20th century to appreciate the diversity of the peoples who contributed to the past (and hence to the present) of our islands. For different statements of this, see: Linda Colley, review of N. Davies, *The Isles* in *Times Literary Supplement* (10 March 2000) and N. Davies, 'The decomposing of Britain: how Anglocentricity distorts our islands' changing history', *Times Literary Supplement* (6 October 2000), 15–16; J. Green, 'Before the *Windrush*', *History Today* 50/10 (2000), 29–35.

3   The author, who is a research editor for the 17th century area, wishes to acknowledge the considerable help and encouragement received from others on the project, especially Brian Harrison (editor), Elizabeth Baigent (research director), Rupert Mann (database manager), colleagues Anita McConnell, Annette Peach and Tim Wales, and former colleague Robert Armstrong.

4 The colonies, established at different times through the period and fluctuating in extent and form, present formidable problems when, for the purposes of a paper such as this, one comes to assign nationality or immigrant status to individuals who found themselves either within their borders or travelling to the British Isles, especially when the full information is not yet available. The *New DNB* itself is a comprehensive project, and it considers as a potential candidate for inclusion anyone who *either* made a notable contribution to the life of Britain and its dependent territories (embracing between 1550 and 1750 England, Scotland, Wales and Ireland, and at various times Calais, Tangier, parts of North America, the Caribbean and India) *or* was born in any of these places and then made a name elsewhere in the world. Thus, for example, there are places for the Scottish soldiers who replenished the Swedish nobility and for the Irishman William Lamport (*c.*1611–59), swordsman and spy in Spanish service, who having been burnt at the stake in Mexico in an *auto da fé*, was resurrected in novel and film as 'Zorro'.

5 For example: Brilliana Harley (1600?–43), born at Brill in the Netherlands, daughter of Sir Horace Vere, commander of the English forces there; George Digby (1612–77), later second Earl of Bristol, born in Madrid, where his father John Digby was on embassy; Charles Killigrew (1655–1725), later theatre manager, born in Maestricht of an English royalist father and a Dutch mother; Cornelius Evans (*fl.*1648), imposter of Charles, Prince of Wales, born in Marseilles of a Welsh father.

6 A. V., 'Ernest Augustus (1674–1728)', *Old DNB* (1888).

7 On Carleton see, E. Graham, H. Hinds, E. Hobby and H. Wilcox (eds.), *Her own life: autobiographical writings by seventeenth century Englishwomen* (London, 1989).

8 E.g. Theodore Diodati (1573–1631), physician.

9 The *New DNB* is keen to include comment on subjects' 'afterlives' in literature and films. See also William Lamport above (n. 4).

10 See J. Briggs, *This stage-play world: English literature and is background 1580–1625* (Oxford, 1983), 155–6.

11 The *DNB* gives the lie, for example, to the supposition that the English Reformation resulted in cultural isolationism.

12 W. H. Rylands (ed.), *Visitations of Berkshire*, Harleian Society 56 (1907), vol. 1; HSQS 10; *CSPD 1591–1594*, 568.

13 C. G. Durston, 'Berkshire and its county gentry 1625–1649' (unpublished Ph.D. thesis, University of Reading, 1977), 209.

14 PRO, PROB 11/152, sig. 88.

15 J. Chamberlain, *The letters of John Chamberlain to Sir Dudley Carleton*, ed. N. E. McClure (Philadelphia, 1939), 279–80. For background see: W. J. C. Moens (ed.), *The marriage, baptism and burial registers . . . of the Dutch Church, Austin Friars* (1884), xxxii–xxxiii; R. Ashton, *The Crown and the money market 1603–1640* (Oxford, 1960) and *The City and the court 1603–1643* (Cambridge, 1979).

16 Société Vaudoise de Généalogie (ed.), *Recueil des généalogies vaudoises* (Lausanne, 1950), vol. 3, 161–3; César de Saussure, *Lettres et voyages de Monsr César de Saussure en Allemagne, en Hollande et en Angleterre 1725–1729*, ed. B. van Muyden (Lausanne, 1903); W. de Charnière de Sévery, 'César de Chaussure et la société des francs-maçons de Londres en 1739', *Revue historique vaudoise* (1917), 353–66.

17 Archives cantonales vaudoises, Lausanne, Eb 71/3, 34 and Bdd 106, 97. Miege's life emerges through his publications, most notably *Utrum horum?* (1705), 26 ff. and *A relation of three embassies* (1669).

18 G. Miege, *The grounds of the French tongue, 1687: a facsimile*, English Linguistics 1500–1800 no. 157 (Menston, 1969), preface.

19 G. Miege, *The English grammar: a facsimile*, English Linguistics 1500–1800 no. 152 (Menston, 1969), preface.

20 G. Miege, *Nouvelle méthode pour apprendre l'Anglois, avec une nomenclature Françoise et Angloise* (1685), 88–9.

21 A. Boyer and G. Miege, *A new double grammar French-English and English-French* (Amsterdam, 1718).

22 G. Miege, *The first part of the new state of England* (1691), bk. 2, 2, 6, 61, 65, 96; bk. 3, 1.

23 G. Miege, *Utrum horum?* (1705), 24.

24 W. J. DuBourdieu, *Baby on her back: a history of the Huguenot family DuBourdieu* (Lake Forest, IL, 1967); D. Agnew, *Protestant exiles from France chiefly in the reign of Louis XIV* (3rd edn., Edinburgh, 1886), vol. 2, 345–6; HSQS 58, 123; HSQS 26, 28, 32, 36, 40; HSQS 27, 65; Venn and Venn, *Alumni Cantabrigienses*; Foster, *Alumni Oxonienses*; PRO, PROB 11/575, sig. 173 (will of Jean or John Dubourdieu).

25 I. Dubourdieu, *A discourse of obedience unto kings and magistrates* (1684), 1.

26 *Ibid.*, 15.

27 J. Dubourdieu, *A sermon preached on the 7th day of September* (1704), 22.

28 J. Dubourdieu, *The triumphs of providence* (1707), 21.

29 'The patriarch of the faction which we are fighting': J.-A. Dubourdieu, *La faction de la Grand Bretagne characterisée et confondue* (1716), 22.

30 D.F.R., *A noble peer vindicated* (1724), 6, 8–9.

31 Venn and Venn, *Alumni Cantabrigienses*.

19

Maps, spiders, and tulips: the Cole–Ortelius–L'Obel family and the practice of science in early modern London

Deborah E. Harkness

Scholars have long known that highly skilled individuals joined the flood of religious and economic refugees who came to England during the reign of Elizabeth I, bringing with them new trades and European techniques that stamped the goods and services produced in London and other English cities with the impression of Continental style.[1] 'Strangers' knowledgeable about the natural sciences also joined the throng seeking a more secure life for their families, including physicians, surgeons, scientific instrument makers, apothecaries, and others interested in the myriad properties of the natural world.[2] As immigrants, they were often denied a place within appropriate institutional frameworks such as the Barber-Surgeons' Company and the Royal College of Physicians. In addition, strangers found it difficult to gain membership in guilds such as the Grocers (whose membership lists included both apothecaries and instrument makers) and the Blacksmiths (the guild with which many English clockmakers were affiliated).[3] Though a few strangers became limited members of the guilds and companies as foreign brothers, the vast majority of stranger science practitioners were forced to operate outside the guild system. Some found refuge from the City of London's officials – who made efforts to curb the activities of guild non-members – under the aegis of royal letters patent, others in the old ecclesiastical liberties such as the Blackfriars and the Tower of London, but most engaged in a life-long struggle to practise their trades and occupations with the threat of arrest or prosecution hanging over them.

Despite these handicaps, stranger science practitioners played a major role in the development of natural science prior to the Scientific Revolution. Their success rested heavily on the extensive family networks that gave them intellectual, institutional, legal, and financial support. These networks, which stretched across London, over the Channel, and into many European cities, could become a circuitous route by which stranger science practitioners in London gained wider acclaim and supportive friends and clients in their new home city. Strangers in London could ask friends and family in Antwerp to recommend them to a patron or potential client in England, for example. Contact amongst distant members of a practitioner's support network could be maintained through active epistolary connections over significant distances despite wars, religious conflicts and bad roads. More than just letters and packages travelled in the mailbags of the foreign postmasters: careers and reputations also journeyed in search of willing ears and appreciative eyes.[4]

In addition, as with many trades and occupations, natural science knowledge and experience were often transmitted across generations, creating notable natural science dynasties over time. While this was true for both English and stranger science practitioners, these dynasties could be especially crucial to the success of the immigrant population. One prominent Tudor-Stuart example was the De Laune family: physician William de Laune's (*fl.*1582–1610/1) son Gideon (*fl.*1585–1659) was an apothecary to James I, and his daughter Sara married the famous stranger surgeon credited with the invention of the forceps, Peter Chamberleyn (*fl.*1565–1631).[5] The Noway family of Brabant, known in court circles for their skill in watch and clock making, had at least two family members active in London during the Elizabethan period.[6] But the most internationally and locally renowned stranger natural science family revolved around James Cole (1563–1628), a silk merchant who lived in Lime Street in early modern London.

James Cole

James Cole, christened Jacob Coels or Cools, was born in Antwerp in 1563 to James Cole the Elder (*d.*1591) and his second wife Elizabeth (*d.*1594).[7] James the Elder made his fortune in the silk trade and established an outpost of his Antwerp business in London, possibly as early as 1541.[8] In 1568 James Cole the Elder and his family were living near the Thames in the parish of St Botolph's Billingsgate, between the Tower of London and London Bridge, in the heart of the mercantile district. At that time Cole the Elder claimed that he had been in England since 1551, and had resided in the Billingsgate Ward since 1557.[9] As their son James was born in Antwerp in 1563, it is clear that the family did not settle permanently in London until after that date. By 1568 Cole the Elder had been made denizen, which gave him additional privileges and marked a rise in his socio-economic status.

The Cole family remained in St Botolph Billingsgate for a number of years before relocating by 1576 to a more prestigious central location, Lime Street: an expanse 'of fair houses for merchants and others' in the parish of St Dionis Backchurch.[10] In Lime Street the Cole family joined their cousin, the historian and Dutch postmaster Emmanuel van Meteren (1535–1612), and the well-known Dutch apothecary Peter Tipoots (*d.*1582). Other strangers who lived on this twisting street included friends of the family such as the artists Marcus Gheerhaerts the Elder (1516–1604) and his son Marcus Gheerhaerts the Younger, and the wealthy merchant Abraham van Delden.[11] By 1583 James Garret (*fl.*1583–1610), another Dutch apothecary with an interest in natural history, also lived in Lime Street.[12]

In addition to their immediate neighborhood, the Cole family had a strong network of family and friendship ties among the merchants, artists, and intellectuals of London.

Other members of their family living in London included Daniel Rogers (1538–91), who was a diplomat and clerk of the Privy Council for Elizabeth I, and the merchant factor Johannes Radermacher (1538–1617) who remained in the city from 1567 until 1580, when he relocated to Middelburg.[13] The Coles were also on good terms with the Hoefnagel family of merchants and artists, including the famous botanical artist George (or Joris) Hoefnagel (1545–1600), who lived for a time in London in the 1570s before travelling to join the court of the Emperor Rudolf II in Vienna.[14]

James Cole and Abraham Ortelius

While London networks of friends and family were important throughout the life of James Cole the Younger, it was his mother's family in Antwerp that provided him with access to highly-esteemed European scientific circles. Elizabeth Ortels Cole was sister to the famous Dutch cartographer and author of the highly regarded *Theatrum orbis terrarum*, Abraham Ortelius (1527–98), who exercised a profound influence on his nephew. Prior to her marriage she worked in her brother's cartography shop mounting the maps on linen and hand colouring them (along with her sister Anne) according to the wishes of each buyer.[15] After her marriage she and the Cole family remained in close contact with her brother in Antwerp, receiving and sending numerous letters and gifts assisted by friends and extended family members. Even a parcel of smoked tongue made it safely across the Channel with the help of Marcus Gheerhaerts.[16] In 1577 Ortelius visited the Cole family in London before travelling throughout England and Ireland accompanied by their cousin, Emmanuel van Meteren, in search of ancient maps and other antiquities.[17] Ortelius and Van Meteren were especially close, as the cartographer had been orphaned at a young age and raised in the Van Meteren household.[18] The two had remained in regular contact since Van Meteren had emigrated to England; the first extant letter between them is dated 1556 when Ortelius wrote assuring him that the maps of Europe he desired to be sold in London would be sent from his workshop immediately.[19] Following this visit to England Ortelius and George Hoefnagel set forth from London to tour the Holy Roman Empire in pursuit of similar items.

James Cole the Younger showed signs from an early age that he possessed the intellectual curiosity and abilities of his uncle, and the two fostered their intellectual and familial closeness through occasional visits and regular correspondence. This correspondence reveals that James Cole was not just the son of a silk merchant, but also a well-read Latinist with an avid interest in plants, fossils, old coins, and other curiosities. In addition, the Ortelius–Cole correspondence enables us to see how family connections enabled this extended Huguenot family to occupy a prestigious place within the European Republic of Letters, and how the position Cole occupied in European intellectual circles made him a desirable contact for English natural science practitioners.

Abraham Ortelius's first surviving letter to his nephew is dated 25 May 1575. Though Cole was only 12 at the time, his uncle wrote to him in simple Latin sentences, and sent him a parcel of books for his use by way of the famous publishers and booksellers, the Birckmans, who had a shop in London. Included in the parcel were Greek works, since Ortelius knew young James was labouring to master that language.

Ortelius's desire to remain an active force in his nephew's intellectual life was made clear when he wrote: 'If you want anything in the way of literature, write to me: regard everything I have as your own. Farewell, and diligently cultivate the Muses (to whom I commend you) in your youth, as so you will receive fruit from them in your old age'.[20] Ortelius's next surviving letter to Cole was dated 9 January 1586. Cole's intellectual interests had developed substantially in the intervening decade, and he now shared Ortelius's love of natural history, antiquities and numismatics.

Though the two were separated by age, geography, religion and politics, this 1586 letter demonstrates Ortelius's and Cole's belief that family and intellectual ties made them part of a community of interests and associations. Ortelius reported that his nephew's letter, along with a letter from the Polish merchant Martin Frolich (who also lived in London, and would soon marry James's stepsister, Suzanna) had been opened and read by the Margrave, because they came from a hostile country. It was good that they contained nothing offensive, Ortelius continued, but such things must be endured in these troubled times. Cole must have told his uncle earlier (in a letter not extant) that the latest edition of his monumental geographical work, the *Theatrum orbis terrarum*, was selling in London, which pleased Ortelius.[21]

We can determine more about the contents of Cole's non-extant letter from other matters that Ortelius mentions – nearly all of which relate to their shared intellectual interests. Cole must have asked Ortelius to lend his assistance to his English friend and near neighbour in the parish of St Andrew Undershaft, Thomas Penny (*fl.*1569–88/9), since he and his work are discussed in the 1586 letter. Penny was a physician and natural historian who was particularly interested in the insect kingdom.[22] At the time of the letter from Ortelius to Cole, Penny was gathering his notes on insects, and asked his friend if Ortelius might have any specimens to add to the project. Ortelius, sadly, had no insects to send Penny, save 'some common flies, and a spider, called tarantula by the Italians, sent to me from Naples.' Unfortunately, Ortelius continued, 'Matthiolus has figured it from life in his Dioscorides.' Nonetheless, Ortelius praised Penny's project, which he thought would make a unique contribution to learned society.[23] In addition, Ortelius asked to see James's sketch of a rhinoceros horn, because he thought he had seen a man hawking the object in the Antwerp market. Finally, Ortelius praised his nephew's st udy of ancient coins, which he promised was 'not so barren as it appears', asked James to see if the French publication of Charlemagne's book *De imaginibus* was available in England, and requested that his good wishes be extended to their relative Daniel Rogers.[24]

A great deal of business, intellectual exchange, and accounts of present activities appears in this letter, and in every letter that Ortelius and Cole wrote to one another. A total of 21 letters between Ortelius and Cole survive from 1575 to Ortelius's death in 1598 (see table 19.1). Only three of Cole's letters to his uncle have survived, but, since many of the letters feature queries and responses similar to the 1586 letter, they provide great insights into Cole's knowledge of natural history. Like the letter discussed above, most of the correspondence focuses on books and their publication (19 letters), botany (10 letters), geography and maps (10 letters), various branches of natural history (four letters), and numismatics (seven letters). Throughout the letters Cole emerges as a serious and apt student of natural history, one of the most popular branches of natural science in the early modern period.[25]

Table 19.1 Subjects included in the correspondence between Abraham Ortelius and James Cole, 1575–97

All numeric references correspond to those assigned by Hessels in vol. 1 of the *Ecclesiae Londino-Batavae Archivum.* Numbers from the Sotheby's sale catalogue (*Catalogue of highly important correspondence*) are in brackets. Letters without Sotheby's numbers were written by Cole to Ortelius and sold in a single lot containing all of Cole's letters to a variety of correspondents, lot 94. Cole's letters were not individually described.

Letter No.	Date	Subject(s)
57 [13]	25 May 1575	books, education
144 [16]	9 January 1585/6	books, natural history [entomology], numismatics
149 [18]	19 January 1586/7	books, botany, geography, numismatics
164 [20]	15 May 1589	books, botany, natural history [paleontology]
184[23]	25 August 1590	books, geography
192	25 January 1590/1	books, botany, numismatics
196 [24]	2 May 1591	books, geography
199 [24a]	6 June 1591	books, botany, geography
212 [25]	8 April 1592	books, botany
214 [26]	6 May 1592	books, botany
228 [28]	27 January 1592/3	books, botany
229 [29]	March 1593	books, natural history
261 [30]	4 January 1594/5	books, maps
265 [31]	2 February 1594/5	books, botany
278 [32]	18 October 1595	books, botany
286 [33]	23 March 1596	books, maps, numismatics
294	October 1596	books, botany, maps
303 [34]	3 April 1597	books, maps, numismatics, travel
309	18 October 1597	antiquities, astrology, geometry, maps, museums, natural history [petrology], numismatics, travel
314 [35]	24 January 1597/8	travel
322 [36]	3 June 1598	books, numismatics

Not until 1588, after Cole had lived for a time with his uncle in Antwerp, did he begin to underscore his connections to his uncle by styling himself in his correspondence as 'Jacobus Colius Ortelianus'. He was 25, and seemingly eager to make a name for himself in Ortelius's powerful intellectual circles. During his stay with Ortelius, Cole studied diligently, as his uncle reported to his father: 'your son, my nephew, is with us, he does not waste his time but studies every day, which pleases me and, I believe, will also please you'.[26] While under his uncle's care Cole began to formulate his own ties to the European Republic of Letters, but always followed in the footsteps of Ortelius. It is not surprising, therefore, that a lifelong friendship with Francis Raphelengius (1568–1643), one of the heirs to the Plantin printing house, stemmed from this time in Antwerp and was facilitated by his uncle's friendship with Christopher Plantin, with whom he shared Familist religious beliefs.[27] The two young men had common interests in botany and numismatics; once Cole asked Raphelengius to send him a rare pure white tulip if he could find one.[28]

After Cole's return to England, Ortelius was in a position to draw Cole more deeply into his intellectual web since he was acquainted first hand with his nephew's abilities and interests. It is clear from these letters that Cole and Ortelius had spent some time gardening in Antwerp; Ortelius reported in some detail to his nephew about the state of the garden where they had planted specimens sent by the pre-eminent botanist of the period, Joachim Camerarius.[29] Ortelius asked Cole pointed questions about Richard Hakluyt's *De orbe novo Petri Martyris Anglerii, decades octo* published in Paris in 1587, requiring to know if there was anything new and original in the work or whether it was a simple reprint. Ortelius also replied at some length to queries Cole sent him concerning the nature of fossils, sparring with his nephew about his original theories and making it clear that this was an ongoing conversation between the two which pleased him greatly.[30]

Subsequent letters discuss Cole's plans to publish his own works on botany, Ortelius's need for certain books and maps that he could not procure in Antwerp, news of friends and likeminded people with whom Cole had yet to make an acquaintance. In 1597, following the death of his first wife, Cole decided to tour Europe and wrote to his uncle of his plans. Ortelius, delighted by news of Cole's forthcoming tour, urged him to write a narrative of his travels. 'If in your journey you should come across any books, maps, or coins related to my studies', Ortelius wrote in early April 1597, 'especially such as contain the names of places, you may buy them for me'.[31] Ortelius went on to provide a dazzling list of his friends that Cole could ask to meet including the botanist Joachim Camerarius in Germany, the naturalists Marcus Velser and physician Adolphus Occo (1524–1606) in Augsburg, and one of the two leaders of the Neapolitan Academy Giovan Vincenzo della Porta.[32]

Cole never wrote a travel nattarive recounting his experiences, but the Republic of Letters tracked his progress carefully, and informed Ortelius of his nephew's successes and his snubs. In early June 1597, for instance, Cole was with Camerarius in Nuremberg. The two had conversed pleasantly, and Camerarius wrote letters on Cole's behalf to speed his travels into Italy.[33] On his way to Italy Cole stopped in Augsburg. There Cole saw Marcus Velser, one of his uncle's closest intellectual companions, who showed him a map of Britain, Aquitaine, Africa, Rome, Constantinople and Antioch. 'I have gladly seen that most civilized young man Cole [who bears] your name,' Velser wrote to Ortelius, 'I offered my labour in his travels if he may be able to use it, but it is of no use to him.'[34] Such disrespect on Cole's part reflected badly on Ortelius, and the uncle grew increasingly fretful about his nephew and his progress.

It was in Italy that Cole made the most of his uncle's contacts and their offers of help. By early autumn 1597 Cole was in Venice, whence he travelled to Verona, Mantua, Ferrara and Bologna. In that esteemed university town Cole called on the house of the astronomer and University of Bologna professor Giovanni Antoni Magini (1555–1617) to seek out a map his uncle desired.[35] Cole arrived to find that Magini was in Rome, and so moved on to Florence, where he met with notable artists, Siena, and finally arrived in Rome in October. Cole was met in Rome by Johannes L'Heureux and Fulvio Ursino, two of his uncle's friends and fellow enthusiasts of natural history. L'Heureux made a particular effort to help Cole navigate the tricky political territory between Rome and Naples, and wrote to Ortelius that he had seen to it that his nephew 'will be recommended by letters from Wenzel Coberger our artist through the Belgian merchants . . . so that . . . he might survey the city [of Naples] and one Stelliola'. L'Heureux held 'little hope' that the meeting with the encyclopaedist and polymath Nicol Anton Stelliola could be arranged, but felt that if anyone could manage it Coberger could, 'as he alone through friends liberated him from Rome's prison.'[36]

Having safely arrived in Naples Cole had the opportunity to share in the collaborative spirit of science that was a hallmark of the Neapolitan intellectual scene in the late 16th century. Home of the Lincean Academy, Naples was a centre of natural history of all kinds. Well-known naturalists like Niccolo Stelliola and Ferrante Imperato, as well as polymaths like the della Portas, drew in visitors from all over Europe.[37] Cole was dazzled by Giovanni Baptista della Porta's mathematical studies on the quadrature of the circle, and Giovanni Vincenzo della Porta's work on the judicial astrology of Ptolemy, but their museum of rare coins and some recently discovered marble statues found near their villa made an equally strong impression. Cole was able to meet Stelliola, who complained bitterly about the confiscation of his scholarly notes and maps by the Neapolitan authorities.[38]

Six months after Cole's return from Europe in December 1597 or January 1598, Ortelius had died and left to his nephew the coins, medals, maps, antiquities, correspondence and library that remained as a testimony to the great geographer's intellectual life. It would be another eight years before Cole was to link his already distinguished name to another equally distinguished naturalist, Matthew L'Obel.

'Jacobus Colius Ortelianus' and Matthew L'Obel

In December 1606 James Cole married Louisa L'Obel, the daughter of one of the two most important botanists of the 16th century, Matthew L'Obel (1538–1616).[39] Known for his pioneering work on botanical taxonomy and his collaboration with Pierre Pena on the *Stirpium adversaria nova* (1571), L'Obel first resided in England between 1569 and 1571. Then, in 1585, he returned to London to take up permanent residence near Cole at the southern end of Lime Street. As with most of the important intellectual companions in Cole's life, it was probably his relationship with Ortelius that facilitated his friendship with L'Obel. In 1577, Joachim Camerarius wrote to Ortelius from Nuremberg to ask whether or not L'Obel was now living with Ortelius.[40] It may be that L'Obel was told about the Coles and the Van Meterens by Ortelius before he fled the Low Countries in 1585, though no letter containing such information survives.

Once in England L'Obel made his living as a physician as well as a botanical consultant to men such as Edward St Loo, Lord Zouche. Lime Street provided a warm and welcoming atmosphere, as it boasted many physicians, apothecaries and botanists from the Low Countries. Once L'Obel resided on the street there is little question that young Cole would have sought out his illustrious neighbour, who shared his interests in rare botanical specimens. It was over 20 years later that Cole finally made a formal alliance with the L'Obel family, and the dynastic significance of the Cole–L'Obel marriage was seen immediately by the European Republic of Letters, and couched in particularly intellectual terms. Cole was congratulated by friends at home and abroad for choosing a wife who was not only 'beautiful and loving,' but also the daughter of a 'more diligent searcher after plants than Dioscorides'.[41] When Johannes Radermacher sent his congratulations on the match from Middelburg he went so far as to surmise that the marriage must make Cole the Younger especially 'happy as you have obtained a father-in-law with whom you can continually converse on a part of your studies'.[42]

The L'Obel family appears to have warmly embraced their new member. After their marriage, Cole and Louisa L'Obel travelled to Antwerp in autumn 1607. While in Antwerp they fell ill, and their families at home feared they would not return safely to England. Among the letters Cole received in Antwerp were two from his L'Obel brothers-in-law, Paul and Matthew the Younger.[43] Paul shared many interests with Cole, as he was an apothecary interested in botanical medicines as was his father Paul L'Obel's note to Cole contains, besides wishes for the couple's improved health, news of changes in the royal household's apothecary staff. In this instance, both the king's and the queen's new apothecary were either related or soon became related to the L'Obel family: Louis le Myre married Mary L'Obel, and Johann Wulf Rumler married Anne L'Obel.[44] These matches lent even greater prestige and influence to the Oretlius-Cole–L'Obel dynasty.

James Cole's ties to the L'Obel family made it possible for him to befriend one of the most notable figures of the Scientific Revolution, Nicholas Fabri de Peiresc (1580–1637).[45] Peiresc visited England in late 1608 or early 1609 and visited both Matthew L'Obel and James Cole. During his visit he might have shared reminiscences with Cole about their different experiences in Naples, which Peiresc had visited in 1601.[46] The French experimental philosopher wrote to Cole on 2 February 1608/9 from Aix-la-Chapelle where he led a group of likeminded experimenters including Pierre Gassendi. He feared that his earlier letter, to which he had no reply, had been lost. Since Peiresc was about to send some shrubs to his father-in-law Matthew L'Obel, he had once again taken up his pen. In addition he sent some of the same shrubs to Cole, plus some specimens of styrax, 'tagacanthe', and 'tartouraire' (possibly tartar root, or American ginseng discovered earlier in the 16th century) which grew well in France but were not common in England. To please Cole further, Peiresc included some newly-arrived double narcissus from Algiers with the promise that he would send more if desired. Peiresc assured Cole that he would be pleased if anything he sent to London would be good enough to plant in his 'beautiful little garden'. Pereisc had returned to France with a list of Roman medals that Cole wanted to add to his now extensive collection, and he was able to tell his friend that one of his relatives would travel to London in the spring and bring them to Cole.[47]

Because L'Obel and Cole lived in such close proximity and did not need to rely on epistolary communications, only two letters survive from L'Obel to Cole regarding observations he made and specimens he collected in northern England and Wales in 1609. Forced by the plague to remain in Chester treating friends among the local gentry, L'Obel is grateful for the help that Cole gave to his wife, Elizabeth L'Obel, when travelling northward. It is clear from this letter that L'Obel saw in Cole someone who could act *in loco parentis* to his son Paul, who had just returned from a tour of Europe that included stops in Montpellier (where his father had received his degrees), Nuremberg (where he saw one of his father's greatest friends, botanist Charles de L'Ecluse), and Antwerp. 'Tell him it is not wise to spend all his wealth in travelling', L'Obel commanded Cole, continuing, '[and] tell him to take care of the notes and books that I gave to his late brother Matthew'. After signing off, L'Obel took time to scrawl two more lines: 'I don't have enough time to write more. I discover many beautiful simples in the mountains.'[48]

After nearly a year had passed L'Obel was still in Chester, and still studying the local flora to further his botanical insights. His letter to Cole of 7 June 1610 requested an update on the political affairs in Europe, reported his botanical adventures, boasted of his fine accommodations and the attentions of his patrons, and asked that the rest of their luggage be sent on. L'Obel gave no sign, in short, that he was in any haste to leave the North of England. Knowing that Cole would share his excitement at the new plants he had found, he shared these finds in some detail including their location and their rareness. On this occasion, L'Obel was thrilled to have found two new varieties of well-known plants: a yellow-flowered pulsatilla and a blue-flowered butter wort. His feelings towards his son Paul had not changed, however. He asked Cole to 'Give my great affection to my children [Louis] Le Myre, his wife [Mary L'Obel], [Johannes] Wolf [Rumler] and his wife . . . [and] your wife; don't forget Paul.'[49]

But the illustrious Cole–Ortelius–L'Obel dynasty, once so prominent in European intellectual circles, was not able to continue making such remarkable dynastic marriages, nor was it able to foster in future generations strong similarities in intellectual outlook and interest. Matthew L'Obel, who is still remembered as one of the first botanists to attempt a workable taxonomy of plants, died in Cole's house in 1616. Paul L'Obel never managed to reclaim his status at court or in the city of London, and died a few years later in 1621. James Cole, like his uncle before him, died childless in 1628 and passed his natural history cabinet and books to a nephew, Abraham Bush, of whom we know little.

But it is more valuable to focus on how significant this Huguenot science dynasty was, than how it faded into obscurity. Between 1589 and 1629, Lime Street was the centre of natural science knowledge in England. Moreover, it was *known* to be the heart of such enterprises by such luminaries as Clusius, Occo, the della Portas, and Peiresc whose names are more familiar to us today. For an astonishing four decades James Cole's house in Lime Street received letters and packages, plants and fossils, sketches and maps from all over the world. In return Cole sent news of English naturalists and his fellow Huguenots in London throughout the European Republic of Letters. Though not well-remembered today, like his father-in-law and uncle, James Cole played an instrumental role in furthering of natural science in early modern England.

NOTES

1   For the foreign population in early modern England see: HSQS 10, 4 vols.; Irene Scouloudi (ed.), *Huguenots in Britain and their French background, 1550–1800: contributions to the historical conference of the Huguenot Society of London, 24–25 September 1985* (Basingstoke, 1987); HSQS 57; Andrew Pettegree, *Foreign Protestant communities in sixteenth-century London* (Oxford, 1986).

2   For more information on my use of the term 'natural science' rather than 'natural philosophy' and the broader impact of stranger immigration on natural science in the Elizabethan period, consult Deborah E. Harkness, 'Strange ideas and English knowledge: natural science exchange in Elizabethan London', in Pamela Smith and Paula Findlen (eds.), *Merchants and marvels: commerce and the representation of nature* (London, forthcoming 2001).

3   For the relations between strangers and guilds in London, see: Ian Archer, *The pursuit of*

stability: social relations in Elizabethan London (Cambridge, 1991), esp. 131–8; Joseph P. Ward, *Metropolitan communities: trade guilds, identity and change in early modern London* (Stanford, 1997), esp. 2, 145. For the guilds and science in early modern London, see: Michael A. Crawforth, 'Instrument makers in the London guilds', *Annals of Science* 44 (1987), 319–77; J. Aubrey Rees, *The Worshipful Company of Grocers* (London, 1923); Arthur Adams, *The history of the Worshipful Company of Blacksmiths* (London, 1937); G. N. Clark, *A history of the Royal College of Physicians of London* (Oxford, 1966); William Munk, *The roll of the Royal College of Physicians of London* (London, 1878); Sidney Young, *The annals of the Barber-Surgeons of London* (London, 1890).

4   For the importance of epistolary relationships in early modern intellectual culture, see Giuseppe Olmi, '"Molto amici in varii luoghi": studio della natura e rapporti epistolari nel secolo XVI', *Nuncius* 6 (1991), 3–31.

5   Information on the De Laune family can be found in the heralds' visitation of 1633 which outlines the descent of the family: Joseph Jackson Howard (ed.), *The visitation of London anno Domini 1633, 1634 and 1635*, Harleian Society 15 (London, 1880), 225. The family resided in the parish of St Anne Blackfriars, along with many other Huguenot families including the Chamberleyns, and the registers for that parish include many entries for the De Laune family: GL, MS 4508/1, 4509/1, and 4510/1.

6   For information on the Noway family in London, especially Andrew, Michael and Francis Noway see: HSQS 10, vol. 2, 12, 34, 179, 212, 253, 254, 276, 318, 355, 410; W. J. C Moens (ed.), *The marriage, baptismal and burial registers, 1571 to 1874 . . . of the Dutch Reformed Church, Austin Friars* (Lymington, 1884), 53, 124; Brian Loomes, *The early clockmakers of Great Britain* (London, 1981), 415; Guildhall Museum of the Clockmakers Company, no. 5; GL, MS 4508/1 (the parish register of St Anne Blackfriars).

7   The most detailed description of the Cole family can be found in J. H. Hessels (ed.), *Ecclesiae Londino-Batavae Archivum* vol. 1: *Abrahamii Ortelii, geographi Antverpiensis et virorum eruditorum ad eundem et ad Jacobum Colium Ortellianum epistulae* (Cambridge, 1887), lvi–lix. Further details concerning James Cole the Elder's children and property can be found in his will, PRO, PCC wills, 27 Sainberbe (27 April 1591).

8   A James Cole of St Martin-le-Grand parish was assessed as having goods worth 20 shillings in the 1541 lay subsidy: HSQS 10, vol. 1, 52. Other early entries for James Cole include references from 1544–9 to a James Cole living in the parish of St Anne Blackfriars, assessed for the lay subsidy at increasingly large sums over this five year period: vol. 1, 83, 129, 173. The first definite reference to Cole the Elder comes in 1568, when James Cole and Elizabeth his wife of the parish of St Botolph Billingsgate stated that they had been in England since 1551, and in the Billingsgate Ward since 1557: HSQS 10, vol. 1, 444.

9   *Returns*, vol. 1, 173. Living with the Cole family at that time were John Dobloys, servant and denizen, and Esseken his maid. Later in 1568, servants Garrett Johnson and Ellen Benardes were living with the family: HSQS 10, vol. 3, 355.

10   John Stow, *A Survey of London* (1598, reprinted London, 1994), 169. James Cole the Elder remained in Lime Street until his death in 1591. See HSQS 10, vol. 2, 168, 214, 233, 271, 336, 341.

11   Marcus Gheerhaerts signed Emmanuel van Meteren's *album amicorum*, though the illustration is now missing: BL, MS Douce 68. Abraham van Delden served as overseer to James Cole the Elder's will, PRO, Prerogative Court of Canterbury wills, 27 Sainberbe (27 April 1591).

12   For James Garrett, see Charles E. Raven, *English naturalists from Neckham to Ray* (Cambridge, 1947); R. S. Roberts in F. N. L. Poynter, *The evolution of pharmacy in Britain* (London, 1965), 165–86; Charles Webster and Margaret Pelling, 'Medical practitioners' in Charles Webster (ed.), *Health, medicine and mortality in the sixteenth century* (Cambridge, 1979), 178

13 For Johannes Radermacher, see K. J. S. Bostoen, *Bonis in bonum: Johan Radermacher de Oude (1538–1617), humanist en koopman* (Hilversum, 1998). His *album amicorum* has been published as *Het album J. Rotarii: tekstuitgave van het werk van Johan Radermacher de Oude (1538–1617) in het Album J. Rotarii, handschrift 2465 van de Centrale Bibliotheek van de Rijksuniversiteit te Gent* (Hilversum, 1999).

14 For more on the Hoefnagel family in England (Willem, Giles, Jacques, and his son George) see *Returns* vol. 1, 284, 332, 339, 384; vol. 2, 84, 155, 202, 213; vol. 3, 395. George (Joris) Hoefnagel signed Emmanuel van Meteren's *album amicorum* in Antwerp on 6 December 1575: BL, MS Douce 68, fo. 5r. George Hoefnagel dedicated his *Traité de la Patience*, ed. Robert van Roosbroeck (Antwerp, 1935) to Johannes Radermacher, one of the Cole family's cousins. See also: Marjorie Lee Hendrix and Thea Vignau-Wilberg, *Nature illuminated: flora and fauna from the court of the Emperor Rudolf II* (Los Angeles, 1997); Marjorie Lee Hendrix, 'Joris Hoefnagel and the Four Elements' (unpublished Ph.D. thesis, Princeton University, 1984).

15 The James Cole/Abraham Ortelius correspondence was published as the first volume of J. H. Hessels (ed.), *Ecclesiae Londino-Batavae* (4 vols., Cambridge, 1887–97) and reprinted as J. H. Hessels (ed.), *Abrahami Ortelii, geographi Antverpiensis et virorum eruditorum ad eundem et ad Jacobum Colium Ortelianum, epistulae* (Osnabrück, 1969). Because the letters were sold by Sotheby's auction house in 1955, it has been impossible to trace their present whereabouts. All references to the letters, therefore, are either to them as transcribed by Hessels in *Ecclesiae Londino-Batavae Archivum*, vol. 1 [hereafter *Ortelius correspondence*] or according to the translated excerpts which appear in the Sotheby's *Catalogue of the highly important correspondence of Abraham Ortelius (1528–98)* (London, 1955) [hereafter *Catalogue*]. This letter is *Ortelius correspondence*, no. 334 (7 January 1603/4), 787–91.

16 The six smoked tongues, a gift to Ortelius from Emmanuel van Meteren, reached him after passing through the hands of both Marcus Gheerhaerts and Gerard Troyls. *Ortelius correspondence*, no. 108 (17 July 1581), 260–1.

17 *Ortelius correspondence*, xxvi.

18 Giorgio Mangani, *Il 'mondo' di Abramo Ortelio: Misticismo, geografia e collezionismo nel Rinascimento dei Paesi Bassi* (Ferrara, 1998), 19–20.

19 Ortelius in Frankfurt to Emmanuel van Meteren on Somers Key, London: *Ortelius correspondence*, no. 6 (8 April 1556), 13–14.

20 *Catalogue*, 9.

21 *Ortelius correspondence*, no. 144 (9 January 1585/6), 331–3.

22 Penny's work on insects was not published during his lifetime, but was included in Thomas Moffett's posthumous publication, *Insectorum sive minimorum animalium theatrum olim ab Edoardo Wottono, Conrado Gesnero, Thomaque Pennio inchoatum* (London, 1634).

23 *Ortelius correspondence*, no. 144 (9 January 1585/6), 331–3.

24 *Ibid.; Catalogue*, 9.

25 Many historians have written on natural history's place in the Scientific Revolution, including William B. Ashworth, 'Natural history and the emblematic world view', in David Lindberg and Robert Westman (eds.), *Reappraisals of the Scientific Revolution* (Cambridge, 1990); Harold J. Cook, 'Physicians and natural history', in Nicholas Jardine, James A. Secord, Emma Spary (eds.), *Cultures of natural history* (Cambridge, 1996), 115–49; Lorraine Daston and Katharine Park, *Wonders and the order of nature, 1150–1750* (New York, 1998); Paula E. Findlen, *Possessing nature: museums, collecting and scientific culture in early modern Europe* (Berkeley, CA, 1994).

26 Quoted from *Catalogue*, no. 19, 10; see also *Ortelius correspondence*, no. 161 (30 September 1588), 375–6.

27 For the correspondence between Cole and Raphelengius see *Ortelius correspondence* no.

165 (8 July 1589), no. 193 (1 February 1591), no. 336 (16 December 1606), no. 346 ([1608]), no. 361 (16 October 1613). Giorgio Mangani's *Il 'mondo' di Abramo Ortelio* focuses a great deal on Ortelius's connections to Plantin and to Familism. For Familism, see Christopher Marsh, *The Family of Love in English society, 1550–1630* (Cambridge, 1994) and Jean Dietz Moss, *'Godded with God': Hendrik Niclaes and his Family of Love* (Philadelphia, 1981).

28 *Ortelius corrrespondence*, no. 165 (8 July 1589), 395–7.

29 For Camerarius, see Frank Baron, *Joachim Camerarius (1500–1574): Beiträge zur Geschichte des Humanismus im Zeitalter der Reformation* (Munich, 1978).

30 *Ortelius correspondence*, no. 164 (15 May 1589), 393–5; *Catalogue*, no. 20, 10.

31 Quoted from *Catalogue*, no. 34, 13; see also *Ortelius correspondence*, no. 303 (3 April 1597), 714–15.

32 *Ortelius correspondence*, no. 303 (3 April 1597), 714–15.

33 *Ibid.*, no. 304 (6 June 1597), 716–17.

34 *Ibid.*, no. 306 (2 July 1597) 719–21. The original Latin reads: 'Humanissimum iuvenem Colium cum tuo tum suo ipsius nomine libens vidi, operam meam si aliqua illi in re usui esse possit, detuli, sed in nulla usus est'.

35 *Ibid.*, no. 309 (18 October 1597), 726–9.

36 *Ibid.*, no. 310 (25 October 1597), 730–2. 'Dum Roma Neapolim transvolat, effeci ut literis commendaretur a Wenzel Coberger pictore nostrate . . . mercatoribus belgis, eorum ut opera commodius et viseret urben, et una Stigliolam conveniert uti fecit, sed parum spei audio esse . . . . Multum apud eum potest Coberger ut qui juverit, et e carcere romano fere exemerit solus per amicos'. For Stelliola, see Saverio Ricci, *Nicola Antonio Stigliola, enciclopedista e linceo* (Roma, 1996).

37 For the Lincean Academy, see Giuseppe Olmi, 'La colonia lincea di Napoli', in F. Lomonaco and M. Torrini (eds.), *Galileo e Napoli* (Naples, 1987), 23–57; Findlen, 226–9.

38 *Ortelius correspondence*, no. 309 (18 October 1597), 726–9.

39 For details on L'Obel and his work see Edward Lee Greene, *Landmarks of botanical history* (2 vols., Stanford, 1983), vol. 2, 876–937; A. Louis, *Mathieu de L'Obel 1538–161: épisode de l'histoire de la botanique* (Ghent-Louvain, 1980).

40 *Ortelius correspondence*, no. 70 (3 June 1577), 166–7.

41 For a song written by Peter Petit in honour of the marriage of James Cole and Louisa L'Obel, see *ibid.*, no. 337 (16 December 1606), 796–800.

42 *Ibid.*, no. 338 (1 March 1607), 801–3.

43 Matthew L'Obel the Younger's letter is *ibid.*, no. 344 (9 October 1607), 814–15. In the letter, he offered to provide practical assistance to the couple in their voyage home, as he had just finished a tour of France. For Paul's letter see below, n. 44.

44 *Ibid.*, no. 343 (8 October 1607), 812–13; no. 355 (8 October 1610), 836–7.

45 For Peiresc, see Peter N. Miller, *Peiresc's Europe: learning and virtue in the seventeenth century* (New Haven, 2000).

46 Findlen, 227–8.

47 *Ortelius correspondence*, no. 348 (3 February 1608/9), 823–4.

48 *Ibid.*, no. 352 (10 September 1609), 831–2. The original French reads: 'J'entens que mon filz Paul est arrivé, je vous prie le saluer de ma part, et luy dire quil soit sage, il ne devoit pas estre si prodige en voyagant: je n'ay pas despendu le quart en voyageant [sic] et ay plus veu at et apprinz que luy. Il faut qu'il recompense ses superfluitez en bon service. Dictes luy quil face bonne garde de quelques escritz et lives qu'ay preste a son feu frere Matthis, affin qu'ilz ne se perdent;' 'Je n'ay pas eu le temps descriere d'avantage. Je descouure des beaus simples aus montaignes'.

49 *Ibid.*, no. 353 (7 June 1610), 832–3. This displeasure of the father towards the son was not mitigated when Paul found himself, in 1612, disgraced and accused of poisoning Sir Thomas Overbury with one of his medicinal preparations. Cole was instrumental in reconciling the

two following the trial, as can be seen in a letter between Alexander Reed and James Cole, *ibid.*, no. 356 (31 January 1611/2), 838–9. For the Overbury case, see Anne Somerset, *Unnatural murder: poison at the court of James I* (London, 1998).

20

The Huguenots and Medicine

HUGH TREVOR-ROPER

There is no specific Huguenot medicine, but by the accidents of history and the polarization of ideas in the age of the Reformation the Huguenots became the carriers and disseminators of certain new ideas in those areas of medicine in which improvements could be made at a time when the true nature of disease was still undiscoverable. Those ideas were in chemical remedies, surgical methods, palliative drugs and therapy, and they had been propounded, aggressively, by the great German-Swiss physician Paracelsus.

Seen in retrospect, Paracelsianism consists of these medical ideas, but seen in its historical context it was an ideology, that is, a total philosophy which claimed to answer all the major questions of religion, cosmology, science and politics, and thus challenged all entrenched orthodoxies. It is the nature of ideologies that after generating great power and great opposition, they dissolve, leaving their particular claims to be adopted, adapted or rejected by the particular sciences to which they belong.

Since Paracelsus was a medical man, the concrete residue of his philosophy was in medical practice, but in his own time it was a religion – a heretical religion – which challenged not only the official teaching of medicine but all the reigning orthodoxies. As such it was a third force, a rival to Lutheranism in divided Germany.

The works of Paracelsus, locked in the German language, at first circulated only in Germany. There they were disdained by the medical establishment but embraced by surgeons and apothecaries, the depressed class of the medical world, the physicians of the poor, and were soon recognized as offering an alternative medicine which found patrons among the secular rulers and free cities of that fragmented political system. Afterwards they were translated into Latin and published, mainly in Basel, an enlightened and tolerant city where Paracelsus himself had briefly taught. They thus reached other countries, where the same pattern was repeated. The disciples of Paracelsus were condemned by the established institutions as quacks and charlatans (which many of them often were) but patronized by the Valois court and by independent grandees – especially Huguenot grandees – and the towns and colleges under their protection. The grandest of these grandees was the Huguenot leader, Henry of Navarre, and the grandest of such colleges was the University of Montpellier, the hated rival of Paris – which, like Basel, remained liberal and tolerant even while the Wars of Religion hardened attitudes on both sides.

It was during the wars of religion, and through religion, that Paracelsian ideas invaded France. Debarred by their religion from the great national universities, ambitious Huguenot students went to study in Protestant Germany or Switzerland. Here they discovered Paracelsianism and on their return to France sought the protection of Huguenot grandees. The ablest, or luckiest, of them gravitated to the court of Henry of Navarre at Nérac. As King of Navarre, Henry always had Huguenot physicians. He was also the great patron of the University of Montpellier, where he founded a professorship in anatomy and biology and another in surgery and pharmacy. In 1593, having defeated the forces of the Catholic League, he became King of France.

Germany, the French Wars of Religion, the University of Montpellier, Henry of Navarre – these formed the context which shaped the early life of Theodore de Mayerne, the Huguenot who brought a new kind of medicine to England. Of course he did not do it alone. Other immigrants had prepared the way at a lower level; some Paracelsian texts had been translated into English, and there was one native physician who had made his mark. This was a Scot, Thomas Mouffet who had obtained his doctorate at Basel with a provocatively Paracelsian thesis. He had become physician to *avant garde* members of the English *élite* – the Earl of Pembroke, Sir Philip Sidney, Sir Francis Drake – and a member of Parliament.[1] But he died in 1604, before Mayerne visited England. It was Mayerne who continued and completed his work

Theodore de Mayerne, originally Turquet, came of a migrant family.[2] His grandfather, Etienne Turquet, had migrated from Turin to Lyon, where he had founded a silk-manufactory. His father, Louis Turquet, had become a Protestant and had been disowned by his Catholic kindred: when the Massacre of St Bartholomew came to Lyon, his two houses there were burned by the mob and he fled with his wife to Geneva. There his son Theodore was born in 1573. His godfather was the Pope of the Huguenots, Calvin's successor, Théodore de Bèze. He was educated at the Calvinist University of Heidelberg and then studied medicine at the University of Montpellier. In his doctoral thesis, like Mouffet at Basel, he boldly defended chemical, i.e. Paracelsian, remedies. Neither at Montpellier nor at Basel was chemical medicine officially taught. Whence then did Turquet derive his interest in it?

I have no doubt that his prime source was his father's personal friend, his own lifelong patron and colleague, Joseph du Chesne. Du Chesne was a Huguenot from Gascony who had gone to Germany and discovered Paracelsianism there. He had practised as an army surgeon and been patronized by German princes. He was a total Paracelsian, in religion and philosophy as well as in medical practice, a prolific writer, controversialist and poet. After many adventures, amorous as well as medical and chemical, he settled in Lyon and became a friend of Louis Turquet, whom he afterwards followed to Geneva. There he stood godfather to Theodore Turquet's younger brother Philippe.[3] Like Louis Turquet, he became a follower of Henry of Navarre and acted as the king's secret diplomatic agent among the German princes, raising money and troops for the wars of religion. Active in the politics of Geneva, the confidant of German princes – particularly of Moritz the Learned, Landgrave of Hesse, who founded a chemical laboratory at Kassel – he was also the most famous Paracelsian writer of his time. Several of his works were translated into English.[4] Ennobled as sieur de La Violette, he provided, in the multiplicity of his interests, a rôle model for his friend and disciple Theodore Turquet.

In 1593 Henry of Navarre, having victories in the war, agreed to become a Catholic in order to secure the crown of France. But he kept his Huguenot doctors: they were, he thought, less likely to poison him. He liked Huguenot cooks too, for the same reason. His *premier médecin*, who accompanied him from Nérac to Paris, was Jean Ribit, sieur de la Rivière, who had come from Savoy to Geneva and had then become physician to the Huguenot grandee the duc de Bouillon.[5] Having accompanied the Duke on an embassy to Germany for Henry of Navarre, he had made a careful study of Paracelsianism and adopted much of its teaching. Henry now also summoned to Paris Joseph du Chesne as *médecin ordinaire*, and soon afterwards we find Theodore Turquet in Paris too, summoned, no doubt, by du Chesne. In 1599 the King took notice of Turquet and appointed him to accompany his own young cousin, Henri, duc de Rohan, afterwards famous as the warrior-hero of the last Huguenot revolt, on a grand tour to Italy. On the journey Turquet had discussions with German and Italian doctors and made notes on mineral deposits and mines, on baths and hospitals, laboratories and pharmacies. In a long stay in Florence, where the Grand Duke of Tuscany was a patron of Paracelsianism, he also gave lectures and demonstrations at the hospital. He travelled with Rohan as far as Naples but seems then to have returned independently to Paris, while they went on to Austria, the Netherlands, England and Scotland. He became a lifelong friend and admirer of Rohan as a pattern of Huguenot virtue. On his return to Paris the king made him – against competition – one of his *médecins ordinaires* and thus a colleague of du Chesne.

To the Faculty of Medicine at the University of Paris, the powerful corporation which controlled the profession, this was perhaps the last straw. It was certainly the beginning of a new campaign. All through the civil wars of France, the three central institutions of religion, law and teaching – the Church, the Parlement and the University – had stood together as the guardians of stability against heresy and revolt on one side and the weak and vacillating Valois kings on the other, and when they finally made their bargain with Henry of Navarre, they did not intend to be content with a mere personal conversion in the plural society envisaged by the Edict of Nantes. Not merely the king but the whole authority and patronage of the crown was to be committed to the cause of unity, order and orthodoxy. Now they saw the king, still surrounded by Huguenot grandees and counsellors, his former companions in arms, appointing yet another royal doctor, who like La Rivière and du Chesne, was a heretic in religion and medicine and not a doctor of the University of Paris. Worse still, he was a doctor of Montpellier, that 'stinking bog of ignorance and prejudice' as the most learned doctor of Paris, Guy Patin, would call it. So began a campaign which would continue throughout the reign, and indeed beyond, until its final victory in the Revocation of the Edict of Nantes. It was fought, with varying success, on several fronts. It would entail the humiliation of Jacques-Auguste de Thou, author of the Edict, the remorseless pressure to convert the Huguenot intellectuals, and a running war against the Huguenot royal doctors.

The first shots in this war were fired in 1603 when the Faculty published a ferocious denunciation of du Chesne and Turquet, ordering them to leave Paris and forbidding apothecaries to compound their poisonous drugs or patients to consult them. Prudently the name of La Rivière was omitted but implicitly he was condemned too, for the three men worked as a partnership, and a highly successful partnership too: the *beau monde* of Paris, Catholic as well as Protestant, resorted to them. The victims defended themselves, Turquet himself writing an *Apologia*, and received support from the Huguenot doctors of Orléans, which no doubt increased the fury of the metropolitan monopolists. The affair turned into a controversy over the use of chemical medicines and Turquet scored a triumph by bringing in the great German chemist Andreas Libavius who crushed the Paris doctors with a massive tome. In the end, after five years of battles, they were obliged to surrender and consoled themselves by persecuting a weaker enemy, Pierre Le Paulmier, whom, as a crypto-chemist, they expelled from their society.[6]

This controversy did not harm du Chesne and Turquet in the least. Their practice and reputation continued to grow and in the autumn of 1605 Turquet had a great stroke of luck. An English nobleman, Lord Norreys of Rycote, who had gained importance by marrying into the Cecil family, returning from a special embassy to Spain, was struck down by an epidemic in Paris. The Paris doctors called in could not save him, so the king sent Turquet. Norreys then recovered, and next spring asked the king for permission to take Turquet to England to attend the Queen, Anne of Denmark. Norreys probably took him to his country seat, Wytham Abbey, near Oxford, for he was taken to visit the University. He arrived simply as a tourist but the Vice-chancellor had presumably been tipped off and he was captured and made a doctor of the University as 'the Queen's doctor'. He stayed in England for a month and made some useful contacts. Back in Paris he received a tentative invitation which could only have originated with King James I. He declined it, for the present, but did not forget it. It might come in useful later.

In 1609 Turquet's career in Paris reached a critical stage. In that year du Chesne died. La Rivière had already died in 1605. So Turquet was now isolated at court, and the partnership broken up. But in the same year the king's new *premier médecin* also died and the king was determined to have Turquet as his successor. However, the Catholic *convertisseurs,* led by Cardinal du Perron (himself a convert) and the king's Jesuit confessor Père Coton, were now in full cry and insisted that, to qualify for the post, Turquet must be converted. Under their pressure, Turquet wobbled. But his old father, whom (as he would afterwards claim) he had never disobeyed, pressed him never to yield, and prevailed. The king then decided to stand firm too. But the Jesuits knew a trick or two and approached the Queen, Marie de Medici, the patroness of the *dévots.* That turned the scale. A sound Catholic doctor was appointed. Next year the king was assassinated by a Catholic fanatic; under the Regency of the Queen the *dévots* took power; Turquet's career at court was blocked, and he decided to cash the blank cheque dangled before him from England.

He managed the affair very skilfully. He obtained excellent terms from King James. At the same time he continued to keep his position at the French court. Although his old father had just published a blistering attack on the Regency and the feminine rule he persuaded the Queen Regent to continue his appointment as *médecin ordinaire* on the assumption that he was merely on temporary loan to the English court: he would appoint a deputy for the routine business and make periodic visits for important occasions. He was a perfect courtier and particularly successful with the ladies. He was also fond of money. His emigration served him in another way too. In 1609 he had been registered as 'noble'. This enabled him to discard the ignoble surname Turquet and style himself 'sieur de Mayerne'. In France the old name stuck, but in England he began anew as Theodore de Mayerne and would never acknowledge any other name.

So under this new name Mayerne began a new career in a new country, and began it at the very top. He was the king's 'chief physician'. It was not, at first, plain sailing. The courtiers were critical, the other court doctors jealous, and the medical establishment, the Royal College of Physicians, was almost as suspicious of Paracelsians as the doctors of Paris. He had some bad luck too: the deaths first of the Lord Treasurer, the Earl of Salisbury, aged 49, then – worse still – of the Prince of Wales, the nation's favourite, at 18, were held against him – especially the latter, although the king explicitly cleared him. In 1611, soon after his arrival, there was an unfortunate episode when a pamphlet against a notorious medical quack was published. It was puffed by all the grandees of the Royal College soon after his arrival and dedicated to the king. The king accepted it gracefully, but when he read the dedication he was furious, for in it he was urged to follow the good example of the Paris Faculty, which had decreed the expulsion from the city of the similar quacks, du Chesne, Le Paulmier 'and others'. 'Others', of course, meant Mayerne. The king, we are told, demanded that the doctors be punished and apologize to Mayerne; but Mayerne wisely made light of the affair.[7] He had his reward. Within four years, thanks to his tact and professional success, and to the favour of the king, he was himself a member of the College, accepted and respected by all his colleagues.

By then his new career was made. King James, himself an intellectual, open-minded toward novel ideas, was delighted with him, and he with the King, '*mon bon maistre duquel l'oeuil a tousjours esté très favorable envers moy*'. For the rest of his long life he remained firmly based in London. The French rulers, in agreeing so readily to his emigration, had thought that he would be a useful spy for them. They soon realized their error. Successive French ambassadors watched him suspiciously. Was he not the king's agent among the malcontent Huguenot grandees? They were all his patients and he continued to see them. When he visited France in 1618 – a critical year in France and in all Europe – he was immediately, and without explanation, ordered out of the country. That caused a great row and the breach of diplomatic relations. In 1626, in the aftermath of the 'bedchamber crisis', when Charles I dismissed all his queen's French attendants, Richelieu sought the dismissal of Mayerne and his replacement by a medical spy of his own. Henrietta Maria, who doted on Mayerne, absolutely refused. Next year, when England and France were at war, the French government arbitrarily terminated Mayerne's appointment as *médecin ordinaire*. That caused another row: Mayerne bombarded Richelieu and the French ministers with furious letters until he ultimately received compensation. In 1638 feelers were put out to Mayerne to discover whether he could be lured back to France. The offer, in very guarded terms, came to him through his Huguenot apothecary and banker in Paris, Pierre Naudin. It probably originated with the King of France or Cardinal Richelieu, for who else could outbid the King of England? But Mayerne evaded it. Their British Majesties were so kind to him, he said, that he could not leave them.

In fact Charles I was far less kind to him than his father had been. It was politics that separated them. Charles I had no sympathy with the Huguenots or the causes for which they were fighting in Europe, and Mayerne, whose ideas were formed in the French civil wars, was a political Huguenot. Though his profession made him a courtier, his ideas, like those of his father, were semi-republican, at least Whiggish. In his private letters he would complain of the servility of court life and he dreamed of retiring to the castle in Switzerland which he had bought under the indulgent James I and which Charles I, from the very beginning of his reign, had forbidden him to revisit. When the English Civil War broke out, Mayerne refused the king's order to his physicians to join him at York. He stayed firmly with his rich patients. The Parliament appointed him to care for the health of the younger royal children, who had stayed in London. The royalists accused him of desertion, but in fact he remained true to the Whiggish principles of his father and of his friends the Huguenot grandees, *princes qui règnent sur eux-mesmes* as Agrippa d'Aubigné called them. He combined courtly manners with an independent spirit and hoped consistently for 'settlement'. He remained true to his own economic interest too. Twice during the civil wars the Parliament threatened to tax him. Twice he replied by packing his bags and threatening to emigrate once again – this time to Holland. Each time the Parliament surrendered: the country, they agreed, could not afford the drainage of such a brain.

It is tempting to speak of Mayerne's extra-curricular activities. Under James I, who took his position as the crowned head of European Protestantism seriously, they were semi-political. He was the king's confidential agent in foreign affairs. He had contacts in France and Germany, Switzerland and the Netherlands. Almost all British ambassadors were his patients, as were several foreign ambassadors in England. His two wives were both Dutch – one the sister, the other the daughter of important Dutch ambassadors. He was the official agent in London of the city of Geneva and the canton of Berne, head of the Swiss Confederation. Even when Charles I had broken with International Protestantism, this network remained. When a special envoy of the court made an unwise proposal to raise a coalition against Richelieu, Mayerne's patient Sir Isaac Wake, ambassador in Savoy, wrote to the secretary of state, Lord Conway, urging him to consult Mayerne; and Conway, another patient, assured him that this would always be done in such cases.[8] Through his ambassadorial contacts Mayerne was able to plant his *protégés* in the courts or camps of the Tsar of Russia and the King of Sweden. Under Charles I he became a connoisseur of art and collected material on the chemistry of painting and the techniques of artists;[9] and he championed the Huguenot churches in England against the pressure of the all-powerful Archbishop Laud.

But these are marginal interests: his central activity was always as a physician. What was his particular contribution in medicine? Like his mentor du Chesne he was a total Paracelsian: that is, his practice was inspired by the ideology of Paracelsus. His personal papers show that he accepted the cosmological and eschatological theories and the Hermetic philosophy which gave that ideology its explosive power. He came to chemistry through alchemy. In Paris he was, with du Chesne, a member of an alchemical coterie which sought to achieve 'the great work' of transmutation. This group was dominated by a Huguenot physician from Orléans, Guillaume Le Normand, sieur de Trougny, whom, as their leader, they designated 'Hermes'. After his emigration, Mayerne remained in touch with Trougny. In the critical year 1621, under the protection of the duc de Bouillon in the Huguenot citadel of Sedan, he discussed with Trougny the imminent coming of 'Elias Artista', 'Elijah the Alchemist' who was 'to make all things new'; and he sought to secure for Trougny, if necessary, asylum in England.[10] Back from his Grand Tour with Rohan, Mayerne tried to secure the patronage of the Duke of Württemberg for du Chesne's book on the true Hermetic medicine; and thirty years later, when planning a medical career for his second son James, he ruled that after learning surgery in Paris (which he generally conceded was the best school for it) he should master the true Hermetic foundations of medicine

But if Mayerne's Paracelsian metaphysics would soon be obsolete, dispersed in the ideological explosion of the 17th century, his medical method looks forward. Like the best of the Paracelsians he concentrated on those areas of science in which real progress could be made. He was always the ally of apothecaries and surgeons. He was a practical chemist and anatomist. When he first visited England, his precursor there, Thomas Mouffet, had just died. His efforts had failed to secure changes in the London Pharmacopœia. Mayerne resumed them. He discovered Mouffet's apothecary and acquired his papers – among them the manuscript of Mouffet's great compilation on insects, which he would publish and dedicate to the College. Once established there, he would give a lead in reform. In alliance with the Huguenot apothecary Gideon de Laune he would sponsor the emancipation of the Society of Apothecaries from their subjection to the Grocers. He would preside over the production of the new Pharmacopœia which included a section on chemical remedies. In the wake of the plague of 1630 he would submit a plan for a central London hospital like those he had known in France and Italy.[11] In many ways he was in tune with Francis Bacon, who despised Paracelsus for his bombastic language but was, as he said, 'partial to poticaries'; for he believed in the observation of nature, personal experiment and human reason. In 1605, in his *Advancement of Learning*, Bacon had regretted 'the discontinuance of the ancient and serious diligence of Hippocrates which used to set down a narrative of the special cases of his patients and how they proceeded and how they were judged by recovery or death.' That discontinuance was ended by Mayerne. His regular records, which survive and are a valuable source for historians, were admired at the time by his patient Sir Henry Slingsby, who also noted that his consulting room was dominated by a picture of 'Hippocrates, that great physician'.[12] In 1635 Mayerne sat for his portrait by John Hoskins. In that portrait (one of seven primary portraits, which include a medallion by Nicolas Drist and a miniature by Jean Petitot, both Huguenot *protégés*), he is represented holding a bust of Hippocrates which rests on a book labelled 'Hermes' – the models, respectively, of his practice and philosophy.

The subtitle of this conference is 'from strangers to citizens'. I have to admit that Mayerne, in his own person, does not represent the full transition. When he migrated to England in 1611 he was naturalized and wrote to the British ambassador in Paris that he would now become '*à tout escient anglais*'. But although he lived in England for the next 44 years, he never completed this transformation. He did not really like England. He despised the frivolity of the courtiers amongst whom he moved with apparent ease, and the idle life, as he saw it, of the gentry. His closest friends were foreigners – French, Swiss and Dutch – and among them especially, artisans and craftsmen. Only necessity would force him to use the English language: he would write to the royal family and the courtiers in French, to clergy, lawyers and scholars in Latin. He would never buy property in England. His ambition was to retire to his castle in Switzerland and there write a great work on medicine, and then 'after my death, but not before' to establish his family as a baronial dynasty there. In fact he did neither. All his children died young, without issue, and in the protracted quarrels of his remoter kinsmen his huge fortune melted away. His disorderly notes would be published only 45 years later, when they had become irrelevant. But what of this? The useful function of immigrants is to mediate between two cultures, not to be absorbed into one. That can be left to later generations.

NOTES

1 On Mouffet see 'The Paracelsian movement' in my *Renaissance essays* (London, 1985).

2 The main sources for the career of Mayerne are his medical papers among the Sloane manu-scripts, and in Additional MS. 20921, in the British Library. I do not think it necessary in this paper to give precise references to individual manuscripts.

3 Recorded in the register of the cathedral of St Pierre, Geneva.

4 A list of his works (*s.v.* Quercetanus) can be found in J. Ferguson, *Bibliotheca Chemica*, 2 vols. (Glasgow, 1906).

5 On La Rivière see ' The Sieur de La Rivière' in my *Renaissance essays*.

6 The controversy is documented in the manuscripts of the Paris Faculty in the Ecoles des Médecins, rue des Ecoles, Paris. Le Paulmier was a friend of Mayerne, who afterwards obtained his papers.

7 Matthew Gwinne, *In assertorem chymicae Fra. Antonium adversaria* (London, 1611). The episode is described with some relish by the French ambassador.

8 *Negotiations of Sir Thomas Roe in his Embassy to the Porte, 1621-28*. Ed. Samuel Richardson (London, 1740), 694, 719.

9 For Mayerne's artistic interests see my essay 'Mayerne and his manuscript', in David Howarth (ed.), *Art and patronage in the Caroline courts* (Cambridge, n.d.).

10 See the King's instructions to the Earl of Doncaster in BL, Egerton MS. 2594, fo. 198. An allegedly successful transmutation carried out by Trougny (Trugnianus) is described in *Theatrum Chemicum* (Strasbourg, `1659).

11 PRO, SP16/187/60. The proposal was made officially by the royal doctors collectively, but the document is in French and in Mayerne's hand throughout.

12 On this portrait compare n. 9 above.

21

'That great and knowing virtuoso':[1] the French background and English refuge of Henri Justel

GEOFFREY TREASURE

The Rue Neuve des Petits Champs in Paris: any Thursday morning in the mid-1640s at 8 a.m. A group of scholars waits for the gates of the Palais Mazarin to open. They will go up the stairs to the vaulted reading room of one of Europe's most famous libraries. It is the first French library to open its doors to the public. Here, under the eye of Mazarin's librarian Gabriel Naudé,[2] may be seen, among others, Grotius, Gassendi, Pierre Dupuy, and, often enough, Christophe Justel, savant, canonist and *sécretaire du roi*. He has already secured (1636) the transfer of his prestigious office to his son, Henri, born in 1620.[3] It will give him valuable privileges, exemption from the *taille* and some access to government circles. He will be an insider. Growing up in this milieu, he may feel at ease, a freeman in the city of European scholarship, breathing an air of tolerance, livened by the spirit of enquiry, growing bolder in subjects tackled and questions asked. The political climate is unsettled, the king a boy and his first minister widely mistrusted, but an end to European war seems imminent and with it, surely, an end to the notion that religious conformity can be imposed by force.

January 1649: Henri Justel attends the wedding of Henri de la Trémouille, to Emilie of Hesse. Here is Protestantism as an international interest; a dynastic match and the climax of a stay in Holland, made possible by peace (Münster, January 1648) and recognition of the United Provinces as an independent state. The Fronde has broken out (August 1648) and Paris is under siege, France in turmoil. For Justel, Christiaan Huygens, the precocious young Dutch mathematician and physicist whom he has met during his stay in Holland, and their convivial circle, there is another dimension to this 'time of shakings': that of the world of ideas. With well connected fathers and ample means they can look forward to exciting intellectual journeys. Disciples of Descartes, like Huygens, may feel that deductive reasoning offers the ideal method for testing accepted beliefs. Those of Mersenne and Gassendi[4] – like Justel – tending more to the empirical, working from evidence, still have grounds for optimism; if Huguenots, reason to feel secure.[5] Does not the cultured, far from dogmatic outlook of the Italian-born first minister, though frowned upon by *dévots*, hold out hope for continued toleration? Will the art and music-loving boy whom he is training to be king not look favourably on his talented Huguenot subjects? Does not the cluster of Huguenot financiers, like Barthélémy Hervart (soon to be praised in a royal decree),[6] suggest that they are indispensable? Huguenots are prominent too in the creative arts which Mazarin rates so highly, which Colbert will see as enhancing *la gloire*. Justel should feel at ease in high Parisian circles when Valentin Conrart is still Secretary to the Academy (till 1674), Louis Testelin, Secretary of the new Academy of Painting (1648). What should be feared from *dévots* when Sebastien Bourdon is invited to paint the revered Monsieur Vincent?

Henri Justel had a head start. His father stood well with the Huguenots around Henry IV and later became secretary to the duc de Bouillon, head of the family whose fortress city of Sedan owed allegiance to the Emperor. While Bouillon was occupied in the plots that allowed Catholics to paint Huguenots as *mauvais français*, his secretary was busy collecting the books which would come to form the library of the Huguenot academy of Sedan. A peaceful man, like most Huguenots after the Grace of Alais, he was content to live a decorous, bookish life. Canon Law was his deepest study, an area where Catholics and Huguenots could seek common ground, leading Richelieu's *patron*, Cardinal du Perron, to hope he might become Catholic. Even if he had been so tempted the convictions of his wife, Olympe de Lorme, would have deterred him. In this faith, home-nurtured through the Bible, women had a significant role. Without their support more men might have hesitated before taking wife and children to exile.

Henri Justel's life will be seen to reflect his parents' values. There were other models, like Pierre Dupuy (1582–1651), the first to catalogue the royal archives, who (with his brother) travelled around France collecting 20,000 books and manuscripts before presenting them to the king. His speciality – the legal rights of the crown *versus* Pope and Emperor – would commend him to the king. Unlike Valentin Conrart he was no Huguenot, rather, indeed, a sceptic, like a growing number of French intellectuals. It is Conrart who is the key figure to understanding Justel and his milieu. Like Justel he was a *sécretaire du roi* – and rich enough to buy the office himself. From 1629 a literary group met regularly at his house. Richelieu (tending to distrust what he could not control) saw Conrart as the ideal man for his projected *Académie*, committed to conformity in the use of language: literature in the service of absolute monarchy. Conrart was acceptable both to Charenton (where he was an elder), and to the *Palais cardinal*. His friend Guez de Balzac was a stylish advocate for the passive obedience to royal authority which some Huguenots saw as their main hope (though others saw it as fatally compromising to Calvin's ruling idea, the absolute sovereignty of God. There lay the deep rift within Huguenotism till 1685 – and calamity.) Meanwhile Conrart's example of faith and conduct, tolerant, and tactful, showed Justel's generation how they might live and prosper.

Another scene: Count Lorenzo Magalotti (as he records in 1669) is taken by Justel to hear a funeral sermon at Charenton. He is struck by the beauty of Marot's psalms, recently translated by Conrart into classical French. Afterwards Justel invites him to sup with him and the consistory 'to enjoy some Huguenot wine' – maybe, says Magalotti, 'to turn his coat?'[7] The suggestion is hardly serious. Justel is no proselytizer.

In the '60s and '70s we see Justel centrally placed in Paris, at 'the intellectual centre of Europe',[8] an influential and respected figure. His name appears on Colbert's lists of subsidies, along with such notable French recipients as Racine and Boileau, and several foreigners, Huygens among them. One name that figures is that of Paul Pellisson. His very different career shows what possibilities were open to men in Justel's position: from Huguenot upbringing, service to Fouquet and consequent spell in the Bastille, then conversion; from Dutch War service as royal historiographer (with much inventive flattery) to the management of the notorious *caisse de conversions*. Justel's steadier path surely had its temptations. The appeal of the Establishment, court and Catholic, was great. Nor was he critical of the regime – at least until the renewal of anti-Huguenot legislation after 1678. He enthused about Versailles, its magnificence and the cornucopia flowing to favoured artists.

Justel was now a regular correspondent for the Royal Society in London, usually through its Secretary, Oldenburg.[9] That sympathetic interest between the two countries could endure in the realm of ideas, despite persecution and war, is attributable to Colbert's patronage. It also testifies to the overriding intellectual concerns of those whom he enlisted for their propaganda value: in the case of Justel, showing too the minister's broader vision, 'à cause de commerce qu'il entretien avec la plupart des savants hommes de l'Europe'.[10] Justel might be forgiven for seeing himself as secure, under the wing of Versailles. He was also a frequent guest of Condé at Chantilly where he would experience *libertin* talk that would push to the margins the time-worn concerns of theologians about the nature of sacraments or the place of purgatory.[11]

At Versailles or Chantilly, or among the 7000 books of his library, Justel may seem to have been inclined to cautious conformity. Yet we may wonder whether that is how his intimate friends and foreign visitors saw him. Did he already have the feeling of living on borrowed time? Men so attuned to the scientific and cultural discourse of the time would surely see mixed blessings in the new political climate. Enlightened patronage was just one aspect of the official programme for a more prosperous – and stronger state; it was an early casualty of wartime budgets. With its rationalist, information-based ethos went a distinct chauvinism. The cult of glory could be seen as beneficent. There was, however, another side of absolutism, appealing increasingly to Catholics, offering common ground for Gallicans to stand with Ultramontanes; for rival Jansenists and Jesuits at least a chance to move, by different routes to the same end. Conformity was an essential part of the absolutist message and unity much spoken about and envisaged by its most persuasive advocates in Catholic terms, whether as heartfelt aspiration or as a rule to be defied by heretics at their peril. As if trying to stay within the culture some Huguenot ministers were sounding increasingly erastian.[12] Calvinist purists buckled on their armour. Meanwhile divisions within European Protestantism were exposed by approaches to reunion between Catholics and Lutherans. Bishop Bossuet was prepared to discuss the possibility with Leibnitz and Paul Ferry, pastor of Metz.[13]

So we come to anxious days. It is early in 1681. Since 1677 Justel has been a married man: Charlotte de Lorme is a cousin, many years younger than he. There are two children. He has decided to sell his books, He has received a letter written at the behest, he assumes, of his friend, ambassador Henry Savile (2 December 1680) from Charles II, inviting him to come and sort out the royal collection of manuscripts which are in disorder. Justel is already confiding to friends that he sees no future for Huguenots in France, that the king has already decided to act against them. 'Our extirpation is decreed', he tells Hickes.(*c.*November 1680).[14] That may be news to Louis's ministers.

Justel, who has been made to surrender his office, may hear gossip but now has no privileged access. Neither Colbert, concerned for the economy, nor Louvois, for the discipline of the army, wants such an outcome. Louis will act empirically to the end, guided by events in Europe and by changing assessments of the Huguenot position in the provinces. *Le roi dévot* is also *le roi politique.* But the trend is ominous. The conversion of the great Turenne (1667), who earlier refused the Constable's sword rather than abjure, has served early warning. The marquis de Ruvigny is left to champion the Huguenot cause at court: his stout advocacy is respected by the king but he is an increasingly isolated figure. Till 1678 Louis has been distracted by the Dutch War but now the Huguenots are high on his agenda. There is a clamour in southern provinces about the tax burden, increased, it is believed, by concessions to *nouveaux convertis.* Bishops denounce 'the synagogues of Satan'.[15] Some *intendants* seek to impress the king or to win support in local power struggles. In this year, 1681, Marillac tries billeting dragoons on Poitevin Huguenots. A flow of edicts (10 from 1661 to 1679, 85 from 1679 to 1685) is driving Huguenots from public office, bringing penury and unease. Mme Justel, fearful for her children, supports her husband's decision – some say is pressing him to leave. They will not starve in London; they have well-connected English friends. But such a sacrifice! His books, representing a lifetime's work and interest – and his father's; congenial Paris, the fellowship of colleagues, not all Huguenots; an honoured position among them.

Next we see Justel in his chamber at St James's Palace – or is it his house in Piccadilly? (Soon he will be giving it up for Soho and Huguenot neighbours). He is reading a letter from Saint-Evremond, Anglophile and long-term exile, fine flower of gentlemanly scepticism, engaging epicurean. Saint-Evremond holds that a man of breeding should concern himself only with ethics and polite letters. He stands aloof from the intellectual cross-currents of the age. Anticipating a later sensibility he hopes that faith will shift from 'the curiosity of our spirits to the tenderness of our hearts.'[16] It will be too much to hope to translate the ideal of the *honnête homme* to English soil but he looks benignly on the transmission of ideas: 'The salt of the earth are the French who do the thinking, and the English who put it into words.' He loves these 'talking libraries' but finds the latest cross-channel traffic puzzling – perhaps embarrassing. He sits loose to dogmatic faith and professes not to understand why Justel is hankering after his native France. He is reminded of 'those poor Israelites weeping for Jerusalem beside the waters of the Euphrates.' His advice is brisk: 'Either live happily in England, and with a clear conscience, or make some accommodation with the slight religious difficulties in your country in order to enjoy all the conveniences of life.' Then, for good measure: 'The rage of opinions and the stiffness of parties are surely nothing to a man as wise as you.' Plainly a misjudgement there. Is Justel, *dépaysé*, offended, amused – or a little sad?

Such scenes mark the areas, social, political, religious, within which Justel's career may be followed, which offer clues to contemporary attitudes and indicate questions we may ask. What sort of man was this privileged, and early, *émigré*? What was his place in Louis XIV's France, and in the England of Locke, Boyle, Evelyn and Wren?

He would know the passage when Gassendi quotes Cicero, with approval: 'What pleasures don't a thinking mind enjoy, employed night and day in contemplation and study. What extraordinary delight to observe the motions of circumferences of the world.'[17] He was missionary in zeal to promote discoveries. With boundless curiosity he wanted 'to know all, understand all, register all.' He was fascinated by the voyages, like those of his fellow Huguenot Jean Chardin, which were to contribute to European man's 'crisis of conscience',[18] introducing a disturbing relativism to history – and a theology already under rationalist scrutiny by such as Simon (one correspondent) and Leibnitz (another). In particular he wanted to know what John Covel had found in the Ottoman empire. His letters to Henry Compton (future bishop of London who will be so useful) show him sharing his enthusiasms: for botany, old texts and enlightened faith; also his aversions, pedantry and narrow dogmatism. John Locke was a specially appreciative visitor, sharing his taste for the curious and practical, for statistics and mechanisms. His Journal[19] records the diversity of table-talk at Justel's house: eider-downs (the down from Norway);[20] the memoirs of Sully (deemed unreliable);[21] the 'pipiness [sic] from whence all the king's gardens are supplied';[22] the best French Bible – 'that in folio of Elsevier but notes not very good';[23] 'a leafe of Palimpsestus or in French peau d'asne . . . what is written on it with inke may be blotted out again';[24] the Duke of Hanover's coach 'which at night he turns into a tent and which will serve also for a boat'.[25] Like so many in this time-conscious age (and as befitted the friend of Huygens) Justel was interested in the construction of clocks. He enthused about Papin's experiments with steam but seems, typically, to have been interested most in his pressure cooker device 'to cook without fire' and its possibilities as a way of dispersing fog.[26]

There was a light-hearted side which must have been part of his appeal to visitors as different as Pufendorf and Pepys. He liked to introduce friends to the romances of Mme de Scudéry. But he was a pedestrian writer, lacking the light touch which enabled Fontenelle, for example, to captivate the beau monde with his Entretiens sur la Pluralité des Mondes (1686), designed to bring the new astronomy 'within the bounds of the feminine intelligence.'[27] Yet he would approve the objective and sympathize with Fontenelle's law: 'Make sure of the facts before you bother about their cause.' A dutiful translation of his father's book on Canon Law was not enough to win Justel renown.[28]

His métier was that of the middle man, or enabler. A recommendation from or to him was a kind of passport. Francis Vernon, for example, attached to the embassy in 1670, went to see him the day after his arrival, carrying books and letters from England, and often returned. He kept a hospitable table, brought people together, provided introductions and instructions. He helped Boyle with his experimental air pump at the Académie des Sciences. He sent Oxford (through Dr Hickes, in 1674) the 7th century Greek manuscript of the Canones Ecclesiae Universalis, which earned him a Doctorate of Civil Law. He provided Locke with a list of the 22 fine houses in Paris that could be visited (it survives in his handwriting). Writing in 1669 Magalotti called Justel 'the most helpful and amiable man in Paris'.[29] From this 'prince among men' the aspiring savant could receive advice and help. 'He is involved in a hundred different occupations and wholly fitted for each.' His English was limited and would need improving when he came to England; English friends in the main seem to have coped with French. He sought them out but the attraction was mutual. Justel's device was otio dives. The leisure was busy and fruitful. The wealth was banked in the hearts of his friends.

Research and invention might be, for a Huygens or a Boyle, a compelling vocation; Justels's was connecting and collecting. In his wide acquaintance and weekly evenings the two pursuits were complementary, those of scientist and intermediary, pursued in a spirit of mutual appreciation. In an important letter to Oldenburg Justel wrote: 'the dealings that one has with capable people serve, and contribute advantageously to the sciences and arts, each man striving to find something new'.[30] The connecting role was furthered through a vast correspondence. Justel the collector was evident in his work of many years for a projected book on commodities and the practical inventions peculiar to different countries that made life easier or more productive. We cannot tell how far the work progressed since it has not survived. He expressed misgivings about the enormity of his task. Leibnitz was among those who encouraged him to persevere. Was he only half-serious in this ambitious project? Was to travel enjoyably as important as to arrive? The daily search for things useful and curious, what he could not wait to impart to his friends – was it from relish in the chase for its own sake (*la chasse à courre* crops up in table talk) as much as any ambition to secure a place alongside Bayle as a father of the encyclopaedia? Did he lose heart before the mountains of his own notes? Perhaps he knew his limitations as a writer: There was enough in his life to satisfy his desire to be useful and valued.

Justel's actions during the 12 months before his arrival in England suggest a long-term plan, now activated by recent royal edicts. He could also see an opportunity. Anglo-French relations were friendly after the Oxford parliament of April 1681 and Louis XIV's renewed subsidy to Charles. The succession crisis had left the Catholic Duke of York as heir; as king he would hardly look with favour on Huguenot refugees. Meanwhile, however, despite a reaction to the excesses of the Popish Plot, anti-Catholic feeling ran high and darkened the image of the Bourbon king, already seen to be grasping in foreign policy. The year which saw Justel come to England saw also the annexation of Strasbourg and the first use of dragoons as an instrument of persuasion against the Huguenots. So there was shrewd calculation but also dismay, as of a man feeling the ground slipping beneath his feet; a man too who had always lived comfortably, an adventurer only in his books. He had been thought a prudent bachelor. About to marry, he confided to a friend that he should not have to worry about his young wife: he would be more likely to need her help. Now he was concerned for her, and for their children. His son was two, his daughter ailing: she died in March 1681. His letters appeal for sympathy and material support. 'As I have sold my books I only buy those which are good and useful. We are in so pitiable a state that we have no heart to read, nor to think about *curiosité* . . . If you can give me some good advice as to how I can deposit safely some small sum, that would please me'.[31] It was now, as in that letter to Locke (June 1681), that he could appeal to those whom he had befriended. Henry Compton, now Bishop of London, was one. Justel begs him 'to deliver me and my family from a country where Protestants can no longer live' and declares that he would be eternally indebted 'if under the pretext of some employment Monsieur Savile should receive an order to ask that I be allowed to leave the realm and to sell my goods'.[32] He did secure such an order and he was given leave to travel. On 15 September 1681 he told Findekeller that he was 'gone to make a little voyage'. He might be surprised because 'you know that I am not by temperament a man to run and that a sedentary life and an honest leisure are much to my taste'.[33] From London he wrote: 'I have left Paris to avoid execution of the declaration against children and the sick . . . The king has given me leave. I had resolved to leave because of the great number of declarations made against those of my religion which prevents them from dying in peace and being able to live and to earn a living.'

Now he was so able – and in a position of honour and respect. It cannot have mattered that he was not formally naturalized till 1687. He set up house in Piccadilly. He was cordially received by the king and charged, but as assistant only to Keeper Thynne, to work in the library at St James. He called on Hickes (an exciting journey surely, past the scaffolding and stone of the city's rebuilding to his house on Tower Hill) to remind him of his prediction. On 7 December 1681 he was elected by unanimous vote to the Royal Society which, before 1720, would extend that honour to no fewer than 15 other Huguenots. His proposer, grateful no doubt for earlier favours, now engaged on the greatest of architectural commissions, was Christopher Wren.

The 12 London years were busy, useful ones. We have occasional glimpses of his enthusiasm for life and its novelties. A valued friend was John Evelyn. He accompanied him during the great frost of 1684, to the frozen Thames. It bore stalls, braziers, coaches – and a printing press where people could buy souvenir cards for 6d a name: so one survives:

> Mons. Et Madame Justel. Printed on the river Thames being frozen. In the 36th year of King Charles II, February 5th 1683. [34]

Justel – how typical of this good European, meticulous about detail – his date being 15 February, added *V.S. (vieux style)*. On 3 December Evelyn notes that he took Justell and Slingsby, Master of the Mint, to see Mr Sheldon's collections of medals: important people, collections and commemoration – surely irresistible.[35]

In March 1691 Evelyn records: 'went to visit Mr Justell and the library at St James in which that learned man had put the MSS (which were in good number) into excellent order, they having lain neglected for many years, divers medals having been stolen or embezzelled.'[36] He was by then Assistant Keeper. He assumed the keeper's title only in August 1689 – for a salary of £200. He would die in office – of the stone, in agony we may guess. He was buried at Eton. His wife was granted a pension. His son, Henry, went to Oxford, became chaplain to the Duke of Montagu (son of an earlier ambassador in France be it noted); thence to a living, Clewer in Berkshire, as is recorded at the time of his marriage in the French chapel of St James's Palace in 1721, to Charlotte Françoise de la Croix. A memorial at Clewer records his death in 1729. They had two surviving daughters. His sister, Olimpia Urania died unmarried. So the name (in England at least) died. But the reputation is pleasant to record: a decent man remembered by friends with affection; a man of prodigious learning, of generous instincts, not possessive over his material. Is that enough? Was he more than the 'very ingenious man but far from learned' of Hearne's rather patronizing account[37] or even Wood's more generous 'most noted and learned'?[38]

He was first in a line of distinguished Huguenot librarians.[39] It is not his chief claim to notice. A man who works mainly through other people, and serves scholarship in bringing them together is hard to assess. He has to be traced through his surviving letters. But set him in his place and time, 'entre le grand savant et le grand seigneur' in the ferment of ideas that characterizes the years between Descartes and Newton; see him putting Boyle, the great experimenter, in touch with the work of Gassendi; see him ensuring that Bayle, the encyclopaedist, who pressed him to contribute to his *Nouvelles philosophiques,* become *au courant* with English science; see the infectious love of truth and accuracy and the search for what was unusual – but possibly useful

– that accorded so well with the ideas of Locke; see the flow of information that fed alert minds in the Royal Society; see his correspondence with the great Leibnitz, advocate of reunion of churches. Hear too contemporary voices: of Fontenelle describing Justel's 'circle of rebels who conspired against ignorance and the dominant prejudices',[40] and of Bayle: 'Justel was so enquiring, so learned, so well-informed in all concerning the republic of letters'.[41] We may then judge that Henri Justel (blazing a trail for Voltaire) was a most important intermediary of English ideas to Frenchmen, and that he well earned a place in the company of those who created the Early European Enlightenment.

NOTES

1   *The Diary of John Evelyn*, ed. E. S. de Beer (Oxford, 1955), vol. 4, 365–6.
2   For Naudé and his milieu of *érudits* and bibliophiles see J. A. Clarke, *Gabriel Naudé, 1600–1653* (Archon, CT, 1970).
3   By the end of the century, despite Colbert's abolition of 215 such offices there were 340. By the convenient device of the *paulette*, like other offices they could be secured for an heir by payment of an annual premium.
4   Marin Mersenne (1588–1648) anticipated Justel in his role as a central store of information and channel of communication, Pierre Gassendi (1592–1655), writer of scientific biographies, in his encyclopaedic knowledge. The latter's ideas, opposed to the rationalism of Descartes, were grounded in the doctrines of Epicurus and Lucretius and faithful to the philosophy of experience. Mid-century French intellectuals still generally thought in Gassendi's way, interested in facts and in the research which could discover more, suspicious of systems and willing to let men arrive at their own conclusions. It would only later become evident that this tendency – that of Justel's circle – could be viewed as subversive.
5   R. Mettam, 'Louis XIV and the persecution of the Huguenots', in Irene Scouloudi (ed.), *Huguenots in Britain, and their French background* (Basingstoke, 1987) points out that Louis's *Mémoires,* listing the 'disorders' at the start of his personal reign, makes no mention of the Huguenots.
6   For 'saving the crown for the king'.
7   Quoted from *Delle lettere familiare del Conte Lorenzo Magalotti* (Florence, 1769) by C.-E. Engel in 'Henri Justel', *XVII Siècle* 61 (1963), 18–30.
8   Henry Butterfield, *Origins of modern science* (London, 1949), 75.
9   Henry Oldenburg was an original member of the Royal Society. As Joint Secretary he edited its *Philosophical Transaction*, 1664–77, and, alongside Justel, maintained an extensive correspondence with Leibnitz, Spinoza and Bayle.
10   Along with many others: the lists and amounts for the years 1665–72 (pensions abruptly curtailed with war) are cited in P. Clément (ed.), *Lettres et Mémoires de Colbert* (Paris, 1861–82), vol. 3.
11   Chantilly was the nearest approach to an alternative court: the soldier had proved his loyalty; the philosopher-grandee remained slightly suspect to government.
12   For example Pierre du Bosc of Caen declared that before 'Louis of miraculous birth' scrutiny of the rights of God and Caesar must be irrelevant 'for they belong alike to him'.
13   As Justel would know well as correspondent of Leibnitz, also of William Wake, future Archbishop of Canterbury, eirenist, friend of leading French churchman and keen protagonist of reunion of churches.
14   M. Ancillon, *Lettres choisis de M. Simon* (Amsterdam, 1730) vol. 1, 37. Here see also Justel's relationship with the Oratorian Richard Simon, author of the daring *Histoire critique de*

Vieux Testament (1678) and Justel's project for a non-sectarian translation of the Bible (which gave offence to Bossuet).

15   For these and similar intemperate words, coming mainly from the Church Assembly, see J. Orcibal, *Louis XIV et les protestants* (Paris, 1951), 20–2.

16   For Saint-Evremond, this episode and the following quotations see E. R. Briggs: 'Some Huguenot friends of Saint-Evremond.' *HSP* 23 (1982), 7–18.

17   See above, note 4.

18   From the title, P. Hazard, *La crise de conscience Européenne* (Paris, 1935).

19   J. Lough, *Locke's travels in France, 1675–9* (Cambridge 1953).

20   *Ibid.*, 181.

21   *Ibid.*, 197.

22   *Ibid.*, 273.

23   *Ibid.*, 255.

24   *Ibid.*, 176.

25   *Ibid.*, 175–6.

26   Denis Papin (1647–1712), French-born English physicist who assisted Huygens with his air-pump experiments, went to London in 1675 to work with Robert Boyle. His career typifies the scientific network of which Justel was a key member. See Robert Boyle, *The works of Robert Boyle*, ed. Michael Hunter and Edward B. Davis (London, 1999–2000), vol. 9, xix–xxii, 121–263.

27   For the importance of Bernard de Fontenelle in the kind of scientific and literary debates that engaged Justel and his circle – like the quarrel of the Ancients and Moderns – see A. Tilley, *The decline of the age of Louis XIV* (Cambridge, 1929), particularly 397–428.

28   Henri Justel, *Bibliotheca Juris Canonici veteris, in duos tomas distributa* (Paris, 1661).

29   Engel, 'Henri Justel', for quotation from Magalotti, *Delle lettere familiare del Conte Lorenzo Magalotti* (Florence, 1769), 23

30   *Ibid.*, 24.

31   *Ibid.*, 26.

32   *Ibid.*, 27.

33   *Ibid.*, 27.

34   *Diary and correspondence of John Evelyn*, ed. William Bray (London, 1906), vol. 2, 426n.

35   *The Diary of John Evelyn*, ed. E. S. de Beer (Oxford, 1955), vol. 4, 396.

36   *Ibid.*, vol. 5, 44.

37   Thomas Hearne, antiquarian, writing in September 1710: *Remarks and Collections of Thomas Hearne*, ed. C. E. Doble (11 vols., Oxford, 1885–1921), vol. 2, 545.

38   Anthony Wood, *The Fasti or Annals of Oxford University*, ed. Philip Bliss (4 vols., London, 1813–20), vol. 2, 350.

39   I am indebted to Mr Stephen Massil, Huguenot Society Librarian, for showing me a draft of his paper on Huguenot Librarians, setting Justel in the context of a distinguished tradition. See *HSP* 27 (2000), 370, 372–6, 381.

40   A. Adam, *Grandeur and illusion: French literature and society 1600–1715*, trans. H. Tint (London, 1972), 135.

41   Pierre Bayle, *Nouvelles de la république des lettres*, entry for March 1684.

22

Huguenot self-fashioning: Sir John Chardin and the rhetoric of travel and travel writing

S. Amanda Eurich

In 1686 the Huguenot jeweller-cum-scholar, Sir John Chardin published the first edition of his memoirs, *Travels in Persia*, simultaneously in English and French with the London printing office of Moses Pitt.[1] Three editions of Chardin's *Travels* followed in rapid succession, culminating with the publication in 1711 of the definitive three-volume edition, which firmly established the jeweller's reputation as one of the most shrewd interlocutors of Persian culture in 18th-century Europe.[2] His meticulous chronicles of his two journeys to Persia and clear, even-handed descriptions of Persian culture and society earned him the praise of Gibbon, Montesquieu, and Voltaire, all of whom consulted *Travels in Persia* to authenticate their own analyses of Persian literature and culture.

Jean Chardin's career and literary production reveal the complexity of the 17th-century European-Asian exchange which introduced early modern Europeans to cultures which could not be easily configured in the language of the civilizing mission inherent in colonial discourse. In Safavid Persia, the young Huguenot merchant encountered a society which he characterized as more hospitable, more civilized, and more tolerant than his native France.[3] As Chardin explained in the preface to his *Travels*, his journeys to the East offered him the opportunity to transcend the boundaries of class and confession which restricted his opportunities for advancement in France. 'In the Indies', wrote Chardin, 'where trade is an Imployment so considerable, that even Soveraign Princes publickly follow it, I could, without altering my Religion, or abandoning the Condition of a Merchant not fail to gratifie a moderate Ambition'.[4] As this essay will argue, travel and travel writing allowed the Huguenot merchant, adventurer, and refugee to refashion a new identity as a gentleman-scholar which facilitated his assimilation into the highest circles of English society.

Chardin's early life and journeys to Persia

Born in Paris on 16 November 1643 and baptized at Charenton eight days later, Jean Chardin was the eldest son of the prosperous Protestant merchant-jeweller, Daniel Chardin, and his wife Jeanne Guiselin, who, like her husband, issued from among the ranks of the Huguenot commercial elite.[5] At the tender age of 21, Chardin began his international apprenticeship, journeying in 1665 with one his father's associates, the Lyonnais merchant Antoine Raisin, to Persia, where the two managed during the course of their 10-week sojourn at the Safavid court in Ispahan to sell jewels and ornaments worth 15,000 livres to Shah Abbas II as well as secure lucrative commissions from the Shah for more jewelry and finery. After a scouting trip to India, Chardin and Raisin returned again to Persia in 1666 and witnessed the coronation of Abbas II's eldest son and successor, Suleiman III, before returning to Paris in 1670, almost six years after they had set out on their commercial pilgrimage to the Orient.

As Chardin explained in his *Travels*, the increasingly repressive policies of the Bourbon state toward Protestants, as well as the success of this first Persian venture, encouraged him to mount a much more ambitious expedition with Raisin to the Safavid empire a mere 15 months after his return to France.[6] With the precious jewels and ornaments sewn into his clothing and saddles, the 26-year-old Huguenot merchant began the nine-year voyage that would cement his reputation as one of the foremost Orientalists of 17th- and 18th-century Europe. Negotiating the perils of international commerce – the duplicity of the Grand Vizier in Constantinople, the danger of the Black Sea and the Muscovy pirates who patrolled it, and the inevitable corruption of Persian officials in the hinterlands – Chardin and Raisin reached Ispahan in June 1673 with their cargo largely intact, only to spend weeks haggling with the new sultan, Suleiman III, who refused to honour the favourable terms of sale offered by his father several years earlier.

For the next five years on a self-described quest to penetrate the mysteries of the East 'in as great a Degree or perhaps even greater than those that have visited the Country before me',[7] Chardin travelled extensively, often in the company of his boon companion, Herbert de Jaeger of the Dutch East India Company. Combing the streets and back alleys of Ispahan with de Jaeger, Chardin claimed that he became more familiar with the Persian capital than with Paris and as comfortable in the Persian language as he was in his maternal tongue. He even employed two mullahs to provide him with full descriptions of the mosques of Ispahan, which he was forbidden to enter as a non-Muslim.[8] From 1677 to 1679, Chardin expanded his base of operations to India, where he signed an *acte de separation* with his partner Raisin on 15 December 1679 and boarded an East India Company ship bound for London.[9]

The various accounts of Chardin's first encounters with polite society after his second voyage to Persia reveal the aura of exoticism which surrounded Europeans who had plumbed the mysteries of Persia and the Asian subcontinent. Jean Chardin returned to Paris in the summer of 1680 a minor celebrity, sought after by both court and salon society alike. Agents of the press described the Huguenot adventurer less as a purveyor of jewels than as a purveyor of those exotic novelties which excited the imaginations of 17th-century European elites and filled their *wünderkammern*.[10] In June 1680, for example, the *Mercure Galant* heralded Chardin's Paris homecoming by delineating in delirious detail the cargo of curiosities which he had acquired on his travels, from an ancient Bible written in Malabar on palm paper to several tortoises weighing more than 250 pounds each from the Ascension Islands.[11] When Chardin travelled to London a month later to recover the bulk of his belongings still aboard the English East India Company ship, he immediately attracted the attention of the Royal Society, whose members dispatched John Evelyn, Joshua Hoskins, and Christopher Wren to visit the 'French stranger, one Monsieur Jardine . . . to salute him, & let him know how glad they should be to receive him'.[12] According to John Evelyn who recorded the details of this first meeting in his *Diaries*, Chardin impressed his guests as a reliable chronicler, who was, in Evelyn's words 'not inclin'd to talke Wonders'. However, it is clear from the rest of Evelyn's entry that Chardin assiduously cultivated his image as a gentleman-adventurer, greeting his visitors in full Persian dress and regaling them with fabulous tales of his encounters with the barbarous *Igniculi* who still worshipped the sun and fire as Gods, the pale-skinned odalisques from Georgia and Mingrelia who serviced the sexual needs of Eastern pashas, and the race of Amazon women who only a century earlier had 'given themselves to war'.[13] As Leslie Pierce has asserted, 17th-century travellers in Asia struggled to embrace the strict empiricism demanded by intellectual Cartesianism, while continuing to shape their travel narratives according to the moral imperatives of an earlier humanist tradition which perpetuated enduring Western images of Eastern sensuality, cruelty, and sexual decadence.[14] Thus from his very first meeting with the Englishmen who would become his patrons, Chardin was caught between the desire to offer a critical eyewitness account of his travels and the temptation to satisfy the expectations of European elites, steeped in classical tradition and the wonderbooks of the Middle Ages.[15]

Chardin's meeting in London with members of the Royal Society could not have been more timely given the growing legal restraints imposed on Huguenot communities in France. While in Paris, Chardin had met the English envoy, Henry Savile, who was surreptitiously using his Court appointment to serve as a kind of broker for wealthy Protestants in France anxious to relocate their families, talents and capital to England. In correspondence with his brother, the Marquess of Halifax, Savile argued that it was precisely 'such men as Sr. John Chardin [who] should be encouraged' to ply their trade in England. With letters of recommendation from Savile, Jean Chardin emigrated in the spring of 1681 to England, where his expertise and experiences catapulted him to the very centre of English *haute société*. Knighted by Charles II in April 1681, elected to the Royal Society in November 1682, and appointed as the East India Company's representative to the Dutch in May 1683, Chardin settled into the life an English gentleman-entrepreneur and set about trying to capitalize on his travels in the fluid circles of Court society, science and commerce in which he circulated. He tirelessly attended salons, wrote letters, dined with friends and dignitaries, and began compiling his memoirs with the assistance of John Evelyn.[16] He also became an important fixture in the Huguenot émigré community, an energetic patron of his fellow exiles, and a close associate of the former French ambassador in London, the marquis de Ruvigny, who had also served as Deputy-General of the Protestant churches in France.[17]

Nevertheless, solid political preferments still eluded the Huguenot émigré. Failure to pay his subscription to the Royal Society led to Chardin's expulsion four years after his election to that venerable institution, while constant quarrelling with Sir Josiah

Child, the wily and ambitious governor of the English East India Company, eventually frustrated any career designs he harboured in conjunction with that august body.[18] With the publication of his memoirs in 1689, Chardin claimed the public renown and influence that he had so clearly desired to wield in his adopted country and cast himself as a key player in the nascent commercial trading empires of the East.[19]

Chardin and the linguistic imperative

For Chardin, the originality and reliability of his memoirs lay in his relentless and exacting quest to penetrate the subtleties and mysteries of the Persian language. In later, expanded, editions of his *Travels*, for example, he refused to write about his two-year tour because, as he explained, 'I understood only Vulgar Languages, without the knowledge of the Brahams'.[20] Throughout his writing, Chardin repeated his conviction that linguistic precision was pivotal to the success of any European power endeavouring to establish stable and profitable commercial ties with Persia. In so doing, he repeatedly positioned himself as a crucial broker in the developing European trading monopolies in the East. Two examples illustrate his rhetorical strategy.

Chardin described the circumstances surrounding the arrival of the first envoys of the French East India Company, who appeared at the Court of Shah Abbas II in November 1666 bearing only a letter of recommendation from Louis XIV. The unusual composition of the embassy – composed as it was by a rather motley assembly of merchant adventurers – and Louis XIV's failure to send requisite gifts to the Shah and his servants offended the entire Safavid Court. Only Chardin's timely intervention, if we are to believe his chronicle, redeemed the mission from total failure. Playing the role he clearly relished as broker between his native and adopted culture, Chardin explained to his host the curious European custom of deputing travellers and merchants to be royal ambassadors without much thought to foreign protocol. Appeased, Abbas II granted the Company exemption from tolls and customs for three years, in accordance with the trading privileges extended to the Dutch and English.

Chardin also detailed the considerable advantages that he enjoyed at the Safavid Court during his second tenure in Persia because of his careful attention to the customs of courtly language and deportment. In his first audience with the Nazir, for example, Chardin recorded that he used no interpreter and endured the interminable circumlocutions of Persian court protocol with the consummate skill of a diplomat. Seated in the immobile posture required by Persian custom (and reproduced in print), he distinguished himself from other European travellers who 'have naturally a motion or Gesticulation about them' which engendered the Persian practice of referring to anyone who stirred in the presence of a courtier or official as 'a Fool or a Frenchman'.[21] On the strength of this interview, Chardin was pressed into service as an erstwhile translator by the Nazir and propelled to the very centre of the vigorous diplomatic exchange between the Safavid Court and the various European governments anxious to establish trading monopolies.

The system of employing translators ad hoc upon which Abbas II depended to carry out his dealings with European powers rendered the Persian system of gathering information vulnerable, and Chardin was not slow to underscore the potential commercial and diplomatic advantages available to any power that could dominate the translation trade. During the course of his second sojourn in Ispahan, Chardin noted that he was summoned frequently to translate petitions and letters of recommendation, where his mastery of several languages allowed him to counter the influence of Portuguese and Dutch agents who had insinuated themselves into the Shah's service. He took particular pleasure in relating how he translated diplomatic dispatches from Charles II, which neither the Shah's personal translator nor the Arab interpreter employed by the Dutch East India Company could decode. Shrewdly manipulating the anti-Dutch sympathies of his Anglo/French audience, Chardin described how very anxious the Arab translator was 'to have those Letters in his Hand, that he might give a Copy thereof to his Masters who are very curious to know the Affairs of other People, but more especially those with any relations to theirs and any-wise concerned with commerce'.[22]

Religion and the rhetoric of tolerance

Chardin's experiences in Persia separated him from his fellow Huguenot émigrés, many of whom had suffered in France at the hands of the very religious orders who offered him refuge and protection during his eastern travels. His analysis of the complex religious geographies of the Middle East and Asia re-examined the veracity of standard European conventions concerning Islamic culture, many of which had been deeply incised into the European consciousness since the Crusades. In his relative tolerance toward Islamic thought, Chardin was not alone. The reasoned discourse of philosophical scepticism, the growth of European travel and trade in the East, and the collapse of the Turkish military threat in the Mediterranean all contributed to a resurgence of interest in Arabic literature and language among 17th- and 18th-century European elites.[23] According to Ahmad Gunny, European Protestant writers, in particular, penned glowing descriptions of the relative tolerance of Islam and Islamic rulers toward religious dissidents as part of a larger polemical strategy which implicitly vilified the putative intolerance of Roman Catholicism.[24]

In his discussions of religion, Chardin called into question the fundamental confessional divide upon which 17th-century European politics and diplomacy rested. In the opening chapter of his *Travels*, the Huguenot merchant reminded his readers of the peculiar circumstances of Christian communities in the East which rendered the religious distinctions and confessional controversies of the Western world meaningless. Living in the shadow of powerful political Muslim majorities, he argued, 'Christians learn to be at Peace in the East, and keep a good Correspondence one with another', since the dominance of Islam reduced the 'thousand Sects' of eastern Christianity to one simple dichotomy, 'Christian and the Mohumetan'. Yet even this simplified taxonomy, Chardin revealed, was confounded within the first few days of his departure from European shores when the fleet of six trading vessels and two men-of-war with which he and his Catholic trading partner were travelling encountered one of the Christian corsairs whose 'impious and barbarous Crimes' threatened Mediterranean trade and their co-religionists along the Adriatic.[25] Thus, from the beginning of Chardin's voyage to the East, the fluid boundaries of identity along the eastern trading routes redefined, relativized, and even inverted conventional European categories of meaning. Christians were impious and barbarous; Muslims were pious and civilized; and Catholic missionaries from the very religious orders in the vanguard of Huguenot persecution in France became Chardin's most indispensable allies.

The dangerous conditions of travel through the Black Sea, over the Caucasus, and through the Persian hinterland repeatedly rendered Western travellers completely dependent upon Theatine and Capuchin missionaries who had established a series of mission outposts along eastern maritime and overland trading routes by the 17th century.[26] Time and time again Chardin recorded how their ministrations saved his cargo and his life. In Colchis, where the princess's overt sexual overtures made Chardin suspect that he was the target of the nefarious white slave trade or of a robbery attempt, the Huguenot jeweller went so far as to assume the guise of a Capuchin monk to save himself. When the armoured henchmen of the princess appeared at the mission the following day, Chardin scuttled out the mission window with 6000 livres of jewelry while a Capuchin lay-brother valiantly held off the armed thugs.[27]

In Mingrelia, where the eruption of hostilities with the Turks undermined plans for overland travel, the Theatine Father Zampi, a lay-brother and a servant helped Chardin find passage on a felucca and provided him with company and safe conduct.[28] In Georgia, Theatines provided the Huguenot jeweller with letters of recommendation that allowed him to take refuge in the castle of a Georgian Muslim turned Christian. In the Caucasus, Chardin appealed to Capuchin missionaries from the Congregation de Propaganda Fide to help him retrieve both his partner and the goods left in Mingrelia. They in turn urged him to recover his friend by donning the cowl of a Theatine friar.[29] Even in Ispahan, Chardin was forced to appeal to Capuchins, who functioned as crucial intermediaries in his first efforts to gain access to Court officials.

The irenic – even generous – tone that Chardin employed toward the Theatine and Capuchin missionaries who proved to be invaluable colleagues stopped short of the Eastern Orthodox patriarchs or *catholicos*, whose ignorance, immorality and barbarism figured prominently in his analysis of eastern Christianity in its many variations.[30] The graphic catalogue of abuses which Chardin ascribed to the *catholicos* drew from both anti-Catholic and anti-Protestant polemical traditions with which he would have been familiar. Drunkenness, desecrations of the Host, disregard for sacraments, and even the sale of children to the Muslim slave trade figured among the sins of the eastern priests whose fundamental indifference and ignorance stood in stark contrast to the evangelical fervour and refinement of the Catholic missionaries of Chardin's acquaintance.[31]

Conclusion

Throughout his writings, Sir John Chardin positioned himself as one of the most important arbiters of European expansion into Persia, a traffic which he legitimated by appealing to the intrinsic paradoxes of the Persian culture which he came to admire. Although he ultimately failed in his bid to play a key role in English overseas expansion, through his writings Chardin refashioned a new identity as a gentleman, scholar, and diplomat in his *pays d'adoption*. Furthermore, he constructed an image of Persia into which his fellow Englishmen could easily insinuate themselves as crucial brokers, supplying the requisite energy, acumen, and capital to reinvigorate and revitalize the Persian economy and wrest Safavid Persia from its fatal decadence.

NOTES

1 Jean Chardin, *The Travels of Sir Jean Chardin into Persia and the East Indies* (London, 1686); *idem, Journal du voyage du Chevalier Chardin en Perse, & aux Indes Orientales (par la mer Noire et par la Colchide)* (London, 1686).

2 The English version was reissued as *idem, The Travels of Sir John Chardin into Persia, and the East Indies... to which is added The Coronation of this Present King of Persia, Solyman the Third* (London, 1689); *idem, The Travels of Sir John Chardin into Persia and the East Indies* ... (London, 1691). The first edition of *Le Couronnement de Soleiman Troisième* had appeared in France in 1671 and included a fulsome dedication to Louis XIV, lavish praises of the two 'sun-blest' monarchies of France and Persia, and generous prognostications concerning trade between the two countries, which Chardin hoped to facilitate. Jean Chardin, *Voyages... en Perse et autres lieux de l'Orient* (3 vols., Amsterdam, 1711). A four-volume edition of Chardin's *Voyages*, along with his *Couronnement de Suleiman*, was further published in Amsterdam in 1735. Passages critical of the Catholic Church which were omitted in the 1711 publication were included in this posthumous edition as well as the 1811 ten-volume edition which has become the standard reference text for most specialists. For a lengthy discussion of the publishing history, see Jean Chardin, *Voyages... en Perse et autres lieu de l'Orient*, ed. L. Langles, vol. 1 (Paris, 1811), preface. Much of my discussion is also based on an early 20th-century abridged edition of Chardin's *Travels* published by Sir Percy Sykes: Sir John Chardin, *Travels in Persia*, ed. Sir Percy Sykes (London, 1927).

3 According to Mary Louise Pratt, 19th-century European travellers to Latin American frequently praised South American elites for their hospitality, aristocratic civility and appreciation of Europeans, while indicting society generally for its backwardness, indolence and pre-capitalist economies. Mary Pratt, *Imperial eyes: studies in travel writing and transculturation* (London, 1992), 150–5.

4 Chardin, *Travels* (1689), 2

5 For a careful chronology of Jean Chardin's career and ancestry, see Laleh Labib-Rahman, 'Sir Jean Chardin, the great traveller (1643–1712/3)', *HSP* 23:5 (1981), 309–18. Chardin's paternal grandfather, François, settled in Sainte-Marie-aux-Mines, then part of the Holy Roman Empire, around 1588, and fathered ten children. The eldest, Daniel, settled in Paris in the early 17th century and married Jeanne Guiselin, whose father was a Protestant merchant from Rouen. For the most recent biography, see R. W. Ferrier, *A journey to Persia: Jean Chardin's portrait of a seventeenth-century empire* (London, 1996), 11–20.

6 Jean Chardin, *Journal du voyage* (1686), iv.

7 Chardin, *Travels* (1689), 2.

8 David Morgan, *Medieval Persia, 1040–1797* (London, 1988), 140.

9 Labib-Rahman, 310–11, 316. Chardin's sojourn in India and subsequent contacts with members of the East India Company in England encouraged him to establish a branch of the family business in India. In 1686, he formed a partnership with his brother Daniel. See Edgar Samuel, 'Gems from the Orient: the activities of Sir John Chardin (1646–1713) as a diamond importer and East India merchant', *HSP* 27:3 (2000), 351–68.

10 On the evolution of the *Wünderkammern* in Renaissance Europe, see Oliver Impey and Arthur McGregor (eds.), *The origins of museums: the cabinet of curiosities in sixteenth- and seventeenth-century Europe* (Oxford, 1985). Leonard Helfgott has argued, however, that Islamic goods rarely figure in the inventories of early modern *Wünderkammern* because the late medieval revival of East-West trade had already familiarized and desensitized Europeans to their rarity and worth. Leonard Helfgott, *Ties that bind: a social history of the Iranian carpet* (Washington, DC, 1993), 110–13.

11 *Mercure Galant*, June 1680, 266, as quoted in Labib-Rahman, 310.

12 John Evelyn, *The Diary of John Evelyn*, ed. E. S. de Beer, vol. 4 (Oxford, 1955), 212–14.

13 *Ibid.*

14 Leslie Pierce, *The imperial harem: women and sovereignty in the Ottoman Empire* (Oxford, 1993), 114–15. See also Rana Kabbani, *Europe's myth of the Orient* (Bloomington, 1986), 14–29, and Alain Grosrichard, *The Sultan's Court: European fantasies of the East*, trans. Liz Heron (London, 1998), 123–47. Both argue that the seraglio was an obligatory *topos* in Western travel writing which perpetuated the archetype of the cruel and vengeful Eastern male. For a trenchant discussion of the evolution of history and travel writing, see Erika Harth, *Ideology and culture in seventeenth-century France* (Ithaca, NY, 1983).

15 For a recent critical discussion of the pervasive influence of the medieval tradition of wonder books in early modern European travel writing, see Mary B. Campbell, *The witness and the other world: exotic European travel writing, 400–1600* (Ithaca, NY, 1988), 47–161. Campbell argues that the demystification and domestication of the Middle East by crusaders and chroniclers pushed the boundaries of European exotic imagination further east. From the 13th century onward, Europeans transposed the fabled landscapes and peoples of their imaginations upon Persia, India, and China.

16 Evelyn, *Diary*, vol. 4, 372. Evelyn, it appears, was instrumental in helping a number of French travellers translate their memoirs for an English audience, including François de Chassepol's *Histoire des grands vizirs Mahomet Caprogli-pacha et Achmet Caprogli-pacha* (1677).

17 Chardin's connections at Court encouraged Huguenot communities across England to seek his help and intervention on their behalf. See, for example, a 1683 letter from one Chauvin, a French merchant in Norwich, imploring Chardin to use his credit at Court to defuse religio-economic tensions which had prompted repeated attacks on Huguenot refugees, whom locals accused of being 'papists': *CSPD Charles II, July–September 1683* (London, 1934), 363. See also Chardin's generous legacy of £500 to 'poor Huguenot refugees' and £1000 to the Society for the Propagation of the Gospel (PRO 11/530, sig. 231). See Ferrier, 12.

18 In 1688, acting as agent for the Armenians who were the crucial brokers between Persian and European merchants, Chardin negotiated an agreement with Sir Josiah Child which promised to give the East India Company a virtual monopoly over the growing Persian maritime trade with Europe. Within five years, however, the directors of the Company recognized that their expectations had not been realized and attempted to draft a new agreement without Chardin's help. As Robert Ferrier has argued, Chardin's diminishing credit with the English government and the East India Company may owe as much to the increasing deterioration of the Safavid economy and the inability of the English to establish stable ties with the Armenian merchant community in Ispahan as it does to his own thorny relations with Child (Ferrier, 12–16). Chardin, however, continued to serve as an agent for the Armenian 'nation', as his 1691 petition on their behalf to import swords into England attests. *CSPD William and Mary, 1690–1* (London, 1969), 380.

19 The 1686 edition stopped short of his journey to Ispahan.

20 Chardin, *Travels* (1689), 112.

21 Chardin, *Travels*, ed. Sykes (1927), 12–13.

22 *Ibid.*, 98–103.

23 Paul Hazard, *La crise de la conscience européene, 1680–1715* (Paris, 1934); Pierre Rétat, *Le Dictionnaire de Bayle et la lutte philosophique au XVIIIe siècle* (Paris, 1971).

24 Ahmad Gunny, 'Protestant reactions to Islam in late seventeenth-century French thought', *French Studies* 40:2 (April 1986), 129–40.

25 Chardin, *Travels* (1689), 3. While they emerge unscathed, the experience furnishes Chardin with the opportunity to recount the tale of a French captain who asked an Adriatic corsair if he feared for the salvation of his soul given 'the Robberies, the Murders, the Sacriledges,

which you dayly commit'. To which the belligerent pirate purported responded, 'Not at all. I am a Lutheran, I do believe not a tittle of any such thing'. This, I would argue, is not some interconfessional jest at the Lutherans' expense.

26 Under the leadership of Père Raphael du Mans (1644–96), whose mastery of the Persian language and customs made him an invaluable contact for French travellers and diplomats, the Capuchins flourished in Persia during the late 17th century. In 1660 du Mans composed his *Estat de la Perse* for Colbert, who with characteristic thoroughness was interested in collecting data on Persia before forming the French East India Company in 1664. See Peter Jackson and Laurence Lockhart (eds.), *The Cambridge History of Iran* vol. 6: *The Timurid and Safavid periods* (Cambridge, 1986), 397–8; Roger Savory, *Iran under the Safavids* (Cambridge, 1980), 120–1.

27 Chardin, *Travels* (1689), 127–8.

28 *Ibid.*, 150.

29 *Ibid.*, 170.

30 *Ibid.*, 93. As Chardin argues, it is the product of 23 years of experience.

31 *Ibid.*, 93–104, 192–3.

23

Jean-Théophile Desaguliers: d'une intégration réussie à l'Europe des savoirs

Pierre Boutin

───────

The role of Jean-Théophile Desaguliers (1683–1744) in popularizing the scientific thought of Isaac Newton and in furthering the development of the Freemason movement in Britain is well known. This paper discusses his successful integration into English society and the important influence he exerted in the emergence of the British and European 'Enlightenment' of the 18th century. It reveals some of the networks he established with the Continent in order to communicate there the scientific and Masonic ideas he espoused. Yet in addition to proselytizing Newtonian science in the princely courts and learned societies of Europe, he also advocated the ideal of religious toleration, which he considered a necessary condition for the development of technical and social progress throughout Europe and Britain.

Desaguliers was born in La Rochelle, but came to England with his Huguenot father at a very young age. After moving to London from his studies in Oxford in 1713 he made his name and fortune through a series of highly popular public lectures, in which he demonstrated and explained the principles of Newtonian physics. In 1714 he was elected a Fellow of the Royal Society, and its President, Sir Isaac Newton, appointed him Curator of Experiments. As an active member of the Society, Desaguliers was influential in furthering contacts with scientists on the Continent and exchanging scientfic ideas with them. The Society saw an increase in foreign admissions during the period of Desaguliers's influence, and he was instrumental in having important works, such as Newton's *Optics* and Mariotte's work on hydraulics, translated into French and English respectively.

He was also significantly involved in establishing Freemasonry in England, becoming the first Grand-Master of the London lodge in 1719, and helping to draw up the first constitution of the fraternity, the Constitutions of Anderson, in 1723. He also played a role in spreading Freemasonry throughout continental Europe. In 1735, for example, he was in France and, representing the authority of the then London Grand-Master Thomas Thynne, helped to constitute a new Masonic lodge in Château d'Aubigny.

He furthermore advocated religious toleration, both as an ideal in itself and as a means of ensuring technical and scientific progress. To this end he argued strongly for the substitution of the outdated Julian calendar, still followed in Protestant Britain, by the Gregorian calendar, observed on the Continent since the late 16th century. The differences in calendar systems, he believed, impeded scientific and technical communication, and thus social progress. In addition, he thought that asking Protestant Britons to adopt a calendar system originally developed by the Papacy would help further religious toleration in Europe, as it would force both Catholics and Protestants to accept their doctrinal disputes as legitimate and unalterable differences and to set them aside in order to help facilitate communication between Britain and Europe for a larger good.

Because of his integration into English society, Desaguliers was able to contribute to the propagation in Europe of Newtonian science, of Freemasonry, and of the ideal of religious toleration. In this way, he occupies a unique and important place in the history of ideas during the Enlightenment.

La contribution de Jean-Théophile Desaguliers (1683–1744) à l'*Enlightenment* n'a guère retenu l'attention des chercheurs. Cet essai nous offre l'occasion d'évoquer, certes à grands traits, l'exemple qu'il peut représenter d'une intégration réussie à la société anglaise, mais aussi l'apport qu'il en déploya à l'émergence de l'Europe des savoirs.

L'on connaît de Desaguliers sa pratique de l'expérimentation en matière d'optique, aux côtés de Newton, les cours qu'il dispensa en matière de physique, et son comportement d'entrepreneur des sciences.[1] L'on sait aussi qu'il fut l'inspirateur du premier texte constitutionnel de la confraternité maçonnique de Londres. Sans prétendre traiter ici de son volontarisme scientifique et politique,[2] nous essaierons de montrer quelques-uns des liens qu'il établit en matière de communication des savoirs avec le reste du continent. En effet, s'il propagea la science newtonienne dans les cours princières et les cercles savants de l'Europe, il y exposa aussi les idées de tolérance religieuse et de paix. Celles-ci, déclarées à l'égard de l'Eglise catholique romaine, lui paraissaient représenter un préalable au développement du progrès technique dans les nations de l'Europe. Ainsi, saisissant le prétexte de la nécessaire substitution du calendrier grégorien au julien, il évoqua, dans *Leap-Year: Cambria's Complaint*, 'l'augure à la paix de l'Europe' que représenterait cette décision.

Rappelons quelques éléments des débuts de la carrière du jeune Jean-Théophile, témoins de son intégration réussie dans la société britannique des savoirs. Né à La Rochelle, il quitte la France avec son père huguenot à un très jeune âge. Il fait ses études universitaires à Oxford, et commence sa carrière d'expérimentateur en y devenant assistant de John Keill. Il lui succède en 1709 dans la fonction de 'lecturer' et démonstrateur. Puis, il entre dans les ordres de l'Eglise anglicane, y est ordonné diacre en 1710; il sera ordonné ministre en 1717. En 1710 il est chapelain de James Brydges. Après avoir obtenu une rente de William Cowper, Lord Chancellor, il se rapproche de la famille royale. Installé à Londres depuis 1713, il peut acquérir très rapidement une solide expérience en matière d'expérimentation, dont la réputation atteint les cercles de la *Royal Society*.[3] Le décès en avril 1713 de Francis Hauksbee, alors démonstrateur (*curator*) des expérimentations, ouvre une place que Newton, président depuis 1704, ne peut laisser inoccupée. John Keill l'informe de la compétence de son ancien étudiant. La candidature de Desaguliers, comme sociétaire, est présentée en juillet 1713 par Hans Sloane. Parrainé par Newton, il est élu sociétaire en 1714. Auparavant, il avait présenté de nombreuses expérimentations à la société savante; en particulier, celles portant sur la physique du rayon lumineux et des couleurs. L'élection de Desaguliers coincide avec la ré-émergence qu'il a permise de l'*experimentum crucis* du rayon lumineux et des couleurs. Dès juillet 1714 il reprend devant les membres de la *Royal Society* les expérimentations sur le prisme, démonstrations dont il maîtrisait parfaitement l'exercice pour les avoir faites de nombreuses fois en public à la fin de 1713. Newton a probablement pu, dès ce moment, apprécier combien la popularité scientifique de Desaguliers pourrait servir à la propagation de ses acquis. En particulier, il intégrera à sa quatrième édition de l'*Opticks* des résultats issus directement des expériences de son collaborateur. Pédagogue efficace, Desaguliers fournit à Newton la plupart des résultats d'expériences en optique dont il a besoin. Dans des cours dispensés à des publics vivement intéressés, il illustre l'existence des forces attractives, explique la gravitation comme un principe universel inhérent à la matière, et la cohésion des particules comme une 'attraction de nature électrique'.[4] Soulignons que Desaguliers compléta en 1718 son cursus universitaire du titre de docteur en droit.[5] De cette formation, l'on retrouve plus que des traces dans les *Constitutions d'Anderson* promulguées en 1723, texte fondateur de l'institution maçonnique londonienne.[6]

Le rayonnement en Europe de l'activité maçonnique de Desaguliers est fort bien connu, comme l'est sa carrière au sein de la confraternité londonienne dont il fut élu Grand-Maître en 1719. Ainsi, s'il inspira l'élaboration des premières Constitutions d'Anderson, il en permit le rayonnement en Europe, de même que celui de la confraternité.[7] Attardons-nous sur quelques-unes de ses visites. A La Haye en 1731 il participe à des tenues. En France en 1735, représentant l'autorité du Grand-Maître Thomas Thynne, il constitue une loge au Château d'Aubigny. Le journal *The Whitehall* des 18–20 septembre de la même année relate que Desaguliers a présidé récemment les travaux de la loge en l'Hotel de Bussy, rue de Bussy à Paris. En d'autres occasions, il effectua de nombreuses visites dans des loges françaises.

En matière de philosophie naturelle, Desaguliers a largement contribué à la propagation en Europe des acquis nouveaux issus des travaux réalisés au sein de la Royal Society, des siens propres, et de ceux de la science newtonienne. Ainsi, de passage en France,[8] en février 1715, il demande à Pierre Coste de traduire l'*Opticks* en français. L'ouvrage est publié à Amsterdam en 1720. De nombreux rapports des *Philosophical Transactions* donnent à lire qu'il poursuivit le programme entrepris dès les débuts de la société par Oldenburg.[9] A cet égard, il contribua à maintenir les normes d'une politique éditoriale que celui-ci avait conçue et fondée sur le développement et la densité des réseaux nationaux et internationaux de philosophes de la nature. Desaguliers a contribué, comme Oldenburg, à faire des correspondants des *Philosophical Transactions* d'authentiques auteurs, substituant ainsi à la fonction du prince mécène, celle d'une corporation de savants interdépendants qui devenaient la première instance de légitimation. Georges Lamoine a relevé les noms et nationalités de 571 admissions d'étrangers pour la période de 1662 à 1800, soit 21 pour cent du total des membres répertoriés. Bien que l'auteur ne puisse assurer l'exhaustivité de ses itérations, l'on doit constater que pendant les années au cours desquelles Desaguliers fut particulièrement actif au sein de la société savante et fit rayonner en Europe autant l'institution maçonnique que la science newtonienne, les admissions furent particulièrement nombreuses: par exemple, 12 en 1715, 13 en 1730, 11 pour chacune des années 1724, 1736, 1738, et 13 en 1740. Le recrutement le plus important eut lieu, relève Lamoine, à partir de 1721.[10] Certes, l'on ne peut porter de façon certaine toutes ces admissions ni leur nombre croissant au crédit de Desaguliers.

En revanche, l'on ne peut nier l'intérêt qu'il portait aux travaux des scientifiques étrangers; par exemple, en 1719 il rend compte à la *Royal Society* de l'invention par Vilette d'un aimant artificiel.[11] Parfois, il discute les résultats et annote la traduction qu'il en fait. Très tôt intéressé par les questions portant sur le vide et les mouvements des fluides, il publie en 1718 une traduction de l'ouvrage d'Edme Mariotte, membre de l'Académie Royale de Paris, portant sur les mouvements de l'eau et autres fluides.[12] Plus tard, il prêtera ses compétences en matière d'hydraulique à la conception de réseaux de distribution d'eau. Ainsi, la contribution de Desaguliers peut-être observée aussi comme représentant un vecteur de communication des savoirs entre les nations continentales et l'Angleterre.

Du point de vue religieux, il n'apparaît pas que le ministre Desaguliers ait exercé une activité pastorale soutenue, ni n'ait laissé d'écrits théologiques majeurs. Peut-être, faut-il, comme nous l'avons relevé ailleurs,[13] noter que son volontarisme scientifique prend quelque appui sur les théories physico-théologiques, alors très en vogue, de l'allemand Nieuwentyt (1654–1718).

En 1738 Desaguliers publie *The Newtonian System of the World the Best Model of Government: an allegorical poem*.[14] A sa suite, dans un court texte, il présente un authentique réquisitoire, certes sous la forme d'une allégorie, contre le maintien de ce qu'il appelle le style julien (c'est-à-dire, le calendrier julien), alors en vigueur en Angleterre. Il l'intitule *Leap-Year: or, Cambria's Complaint against the intercalary Day*.[15] Arguments financiers et économiques à l'appui, il suggère de substituer le style grégorien au style julien (vers 65–92):

> Si nous avions dû subir un tel abîme du temps,
> Bénis, comme nous le sommes, de l'opulence et du commerce,
> Quel aurait été chez nous l'embarras
> Des propriétaires terriens et des rentiers !
> La date des documents de facturation, papiers financiers et locations aurait glissé ,
> Fournissant d'étranges débats aux tribunaux;
> Les locataires auraient protesté à l'approche de l'échéance,
> Et tous nos titres auraient perdu deux *pour cent*.
>
> Comme je voudrais me comporter avec prudence, et avec souplesse
> Envers les consciences scrupuleuses et sensibles;
> Comme je voudrais accomplir un pas de réconciliation avec *Rome*,[16]
> Sans rapporter chez nous un lambeau de papisme;
> Introduire une formule commune de calcul,
> Tout en maintenant la tolérance en usage.
>
> Hâtez-vous donc, mes patriotes, de regagner vos Sièges,
> Et lorsque vous y serez rassemblés au complet,
> *Décidez*, sans un seul non contradictoire,
> D'exercer ma vengeance sur ce jour de traîtrise;
> Avec rigueur contraignez le scélérat à disparaître,
> Proscrit et banni de l'année *britannique*.

Néanmoins que justice lui soit appliquée, alliée à la grâce,
Et que, pénitence appropriée accomplie, il reprenne sa place.
Qu'aucune [année] Bissextile ne soit ici revue,
Avant que George n'ait égalé le règne de la Grande Elizabeth.[17]

Cela rendra imperceptibles les différences
Entre les deux calendriers opposés.
Et puissent nos fermes intentions faire cesser leur querelle,
Et représenter une sûre augure à la paix de l'*Europe*.[18]

Desaguliers recommande une normalisation calendaire, comme l'on dirait de nos jours, dans l'Europe chrétienne. Après avoir réfuté les arguties des protagonistes du style julien (vers 65–68), il expose des arguments juridiques (vers 70) et économiques (vers 72). Certes, liée aux intérêts intérieurs de l'Etat, leur pertinence l'est tout autant à l'égard des relations entretenues avec les autres nations. Pour Desaguliers, entrepreneur en sciences mécaniques et hydrauliques, à une exportation accrue du savoir-faire technique britannique doit correspondre la réduction des obstacles qui en limitent le profit technique et finalement financier; pour lui, le style julien est un obstacle. Puis, il explique qu'une réduction des différences entre les styles de calendrier n'impliquerait pas une résurgence des querelles doctrinales en présence. Si, pour lui, les doctrines en matière de religion ne doivent pas être modifiées, la pérennité de la tolérance devra cependant être assurée (vers 78). Mais, de quelle tolérance s'agit-il, sachant qu'elle doit favoriser le développement et la propagation en Europe du progrès technique? Le pasteur Desaguliers ne souhaite-t-il pas que soit témoignée à l'Eglise catholique romaine la reconnaissance de l'altérité de ses spécificités dogmatiques, comme l'on dirait de nos jours? Sollicitant le terme 'reconciling', c'est-à-dire rapprochement, voire estime et/ou reconnaissance ('reck'ning'), il donne, certes, à comprendre aux anti-papistes que la tolérance calendaire n'implique pas l'introduction en Angleterre du papisme. Maie cette précaution n'altère nullement l'idée qu'il se fait de la reconnaissance d'une altérité catholique romaine. Certes, il ne peut évoquer ici l'idée d'une paix religieuse en Europe. Cependant, présentant, quelques vers plus loin, la réconciliation des calendriers comme une 'sûre augure à la paix de l'*Europe*', il ne peut ignorer qu'un préalable majeur en est la réduction des conflits toujours effervescents entre les tenants des doctrines religieuses.

On le constate, si en matière de physique, la contribution de Desaguliers à la *Royal Society* et aux sociétés savantes continentales est indiscutable, son engagement en politique pourrait sembler mineur. Pourtant, la lecture de l'ensemble de ses travaux invite à nuancer cette position. Comme nous avons tenté de le montrer par ailleurs, l'influence qu'il a exercée au sein de la franc-maçonnerie anglaise et européenne, nous paraît devoir être considérée aussi comme un engagement de caractère politique. De telle sorte que sa contribution à l'Europe des savoirs apparaît comme un prolongement étroitement lié à la réussite de son intégration dans la société civile anglaise.

Le regard que nous venons de jeter sur quelques aspects du rayonnement des travaux de Desaguliers reste trop elliptique. Il permet cependant de dresser un constat provisoire et une invitation. De son intégration à la société anglaise, il a pu contribuer, en Europe, à la diffusion de la science newtonienne, à la propagation de l'idée de tolérance religieuse et à sa concrétisation politique. A cet égard, il occupe dans l'histoire des idées de l'Europe des Lumières une place unique. L'invitation est que, en ce qu'elles permettraient de reconstituer quelques pans restés dans l'ombre de l'environnement newtonien, ses contributions à la société anglaise et à l'Europe des savoirs méritaient que l'on prête attention au caractère volontariste de l'ensemble de ses travaux.

NOTES

1   Dans le chapitre 'Desaguliers and the usefulness of philosophers' de *The rise of public science: rhetoric, technology, and natural philosophy in Newtonian Britain, 1660–1750* (Cambridge, 1992), Larry Stewart présente l'étude, à ce jour la plus complète, de la carrière scientifique de Desaguliers. Nous lui sommes redevables des éléments biographiques rapportés ici. Consulter aussi A. Rupert Hall, 'Desaguliers' dans *Dictionary of scientific biography*, vol. 4 (New York, 1971), 44–6. Pour Margaret E. Rowbottom, 'Il fut un ferment actif des prémices de la révolution industrielle': 'John Theophilus Desaguliers (1683–1744)', *HSP* 21 (1968), 196–218.

2   Nous avons étudié le volontarisme politique de Desaguliers dans notre ouvrage, Pierre Boutin, *Jean-Théophile Desaguliers: un huguenot, philosophe et juriste en politique* (Paris, 1999). Retenons ici que le volontarisme de ce moment tient principalement dans l'idée que les buts et les fins sont les produits du désir humain lors de l'expression de la pensée rationnelle. Cette vision fut sans aucun doute encouragée par la dominance de la cosmologie mécaniste. Etroitement lié au subjectivisme, ce volontarisme fut fortement promu par la cosmologie newtonienne. Il représente une attitude qui confère à la raison une place particulière dans les affaires humaines. A l'époque médiévale, la capacité de l'homme à aimer Dieu et à connaître son nom était exprimée comme la source principale de la dignité humaine. A partir du 17ème siècle, l'idée se fait jour que la découverte des phénomènes de la nature et la possibilité pour l'homme de conduire les affaires du monde peuvent être une autre source de sa dignité. Voir à ce sujet Philip T. Grier, 'Modern ethical theory and Newtonian science: comments on Errol Harris' dans Philip Bricker and R. I. G. Hugues (eds.), *Philosophical perspectives on Newtonian science* (Cambridge, MA, 1990), 232–4.

3   Pour l'étude des débuts de l'institution et du contexte scientifique qu'elle connut jusqu'à la fin du 17ème siècle, consulter les ouvrages de Michael Hunter, en particulier *The Royal Society and its fellows, 1660–1700: the morphology of an early scientific institution* (Chalfont St Giles, 1985), *Science and society in Restoration England* (2nd edn., Aldershot, 1992), *Establishing the new science: the experience of the early Royal Society* (Woodbridge, 1989).

4   J. T. Desaguliers, *Physico-Mechanical Lectures* (London, 1717), 72–3.

5   Titre daté du 16 mars 1718: Bodl., Rawlinson MSS, J, fo. 3.

6   *The Constitutions of the Free-Masons, Containing the History, Charges, Regulations, etc. of that Fraternity . . . 1723* (London, 1878).

7   Boutin, *Jean-Théophile Desaguliers*, en particulier le chapitre 'L'acte juridique de Desaguliers', 126–84.

8   Rupert Hall a explicité les tenants scientifiques de ces visites en France dans 'Newton in France: a new view', *History of Science* 13 (1975), 243.

9   Mario Biagioli, 'Le prince et les savants: la civilité scientifique au 17ème siècle', *Annales* 50:6 (Nov.–Déc. 1995), 1417–53.

10   Dans 'L'Europe de l'esprit ou la *Royal Society* de Londres', *Dix-huitième siècle* 25 (1993), 167–98, Georges Lamoine montre que la société savante londonienne fut le lieu de 'la rencontre des esprits les plus éclairés de l'époque . . . leurs réflexions souvent transcrites dans les *Philosophical Transactions*, contribuèrent à une diffusion rapide des idées et des découvertes par le biais des réseaux de correspondants d'un pays à l'autre'.

11 Royal Society, Journal Book (C), vol. 11 (1714–20), 393–4, pour 5 nov. 1719.

12 *The Motion of Water and other fluids. Being a Treatise of Hydrostaticks, written originally in French by the late Monsieur Mariotte, Member of the Royal Academy of Paris* (London, 1718).

13 Boutin, 75.

14 *The Newtonian System of the World the Best Model of Government: an allegorical poem* (Westminster, 1728) (BL shelfmark 643.K.3.(5)). Nous remercions Antony McKenna, Professeur à l'Université de Saint-Etienne, et Directeur de l'UPRES 5037 du CNRS, de l'attention qu'il a bien voulu porter à la traduction que j'ai faite en français de ce texte.

15 *Ibid.*, 35–46.

16 *Ibid.*, 44. Note de Desaguliers: 'Les styles Romain et Anglais peuvent certainement être réconciliés, sans qu'aucune doctrine religieuse papale ne pénètre en Angleterre'.

17 *Ibid.*, 45. Note de Desaguliers: 'Si sa présente MAJESTÉ règne aussi longtemps que la Reine Elizabeth, c'est à dire 44 ans . . . notre situation avancera de 11 jours, et ajustera notre style à celui du Grégorien: et si sa MAJESTÉ règne plus longtemps, ce que nos voeux illimités peuvent nous faire espérer, il vivra pour voir (si notre politique le permet) un même Style en usage sur toute la partie Chrétienne de l'EUROPE'.

18 *Ibid.*, 43–6.

24

Emanuel Mendes da Costa: constructing a career in science

GEOFFREY CANTOR

Although the Jews who settled in England in the late 17th and early 18th centuries were predominantly poor, they included a small number of wealthy families who sought legitimation within the elite strata of English society and culture. Members of several of these families joined the Royal Society of London, the leading scientific society of the day. Science provides a particularly interesting site for studying the assimilation of the stranger since science in general and the Royal Society in particular espoused a non-denominational ideology, operated no religious bar and was open to foreign members. The Jews who joined the Royal Society were principally upwardly-mobile medical men such as Issac Samuda (FRS 1723), Meyer Schomberg (FRS 1726) and Jacob de Castro Sarmento (FRS 1730) or wealthy merchants like Alvaro Suasso (FRS 1735) and Joseph Salvador (FRS 1759). These men enjoyed the status conferred by the letters FRS, while membership also enabled them to forge social and economic alliances with other Fellows. As Todd Endelman has noted, such 'face-to-face . . . encounters – rather than the reflective or polemical writings of a handful of self-conscious observers – . . . constitute the entry of the Jews into English society'.[1] Although none of the above-named was particularly active within the Society, the 18th-century Jew who created for himself a career in science was Emanuel Mendes da Costa, one-time Assistant Secretary to the Royal Society. Da Costa is best-known for having been dismissed from his post and imprisoned owing to financial irregularities, yet my focus today is on the way he constructed his scientific career. Da Costa's papers in the British Library provide much insight into his determined pursuit of patronage during his rapid and at times uncertain upward trajectory. The question posed in this paper is: How did this social outsider create for himself a career in science?

Da Costa was born in 1717 into a Sephardi family that had recently moved from France to London – although he liked to give his family a longer and more respectable pedigree. His father appears to have been a wealthy merchant and Emanuel claims to have been educated by a private tutor. As he later informed one correspondent, 'the persuit [*sic*] of Natural History first gained Access to my thoughts about the year 1736 when I became patronized by' such eminent individuals as Sir Hans Sloane (President of the Royal Society 1727–41), Martin Folkes (President of the Royal Society 1741–52), the Duke of Richmond, Dr Richard Mead, the Duchess of Portland and the Bishop of Exeter (Charles Lyttelton). How he first encountered these patrons is one of the many outstanding questions surrounding da Costa's early life.

Late in 1745 his name first appears among the visitors to the Royal Society, usually the guest of the Quaker Peter Collinson but sometimes invited by more elevated members, even the President himself. In mid-1749 he was proposed and elected to the Royal Society, his proposers including Collinson, Folkes (PRS) and six other members. It is significant that his proposers shared his interest in both antiquities and natural history, and were members of the Society of Antiquaries and the Royal Society. Da Costa regularly attended meetings of the Antiquaries and was elected to that august body four years later.

By the mid-1740s we find him building up networks of patronage across Europe and commencing his business trading in shells, fossils and minerals. What is so remarkable is his tenacity and enthusiasm. A high proportion of the two and a half thousand items that comprise the extant da Costa correspondence are drafts of letters addressed to the great and the good, the powerful and the rich – and sometimes the not-so-rich – urging them to enter into philosophical correspondence with him and to exchange or purchase specimens. Catalogues, fossils and shells flew back and forth, not only across the length and breadth of Britain but the whole of Europe. His correspondence is remarkable because it shows how an entrepreneur lacking social position could enter science by creating a network that linked dukes and duchesses, country clergymen, Fellows of the Royal Society, lowly quarry workers and the likes of Linnaeus and Sir Hans Sloane. It was an astounding feat. Soon he was widely acknowledged as one of the most knowledgeable experts on shells, fossils and minerals and his advice was frequently sought. On a number of occasions he was entertained by wealthy and noble landowners who sought his advice on local fossils, on the composition of mineral deposits (including their commercial value) and on the specimens to include in their cabinets. Thus, for example, when the Duke of Richmond was constructing 'a wild receptacle for fossils', he invited da Costa to his estate at Goodwood.[2]

With his extended web of correspondents and patrons da Costa proved a very useful acquaintance. He frequently advised those who were about to travel – informing them whom they should meet, where they should stay, what collections to see, which natural phenomena to observe and which specimens to collect. He often provided letters of introduction that enabled the traveller to gain access to other naturalists. For example, the Warrington physician Thomas Percival expressed his gratitude to da Costa whose letters resulted in his receiving a warm reception from leading naturalists in Leiden, Amsterdam and Paris.[3] Most importantly, da Costa assisted his friends and patrons in gaining election to the Royal Society through collecting signatures to support their candidatures. Thus he first broached the question of a Fellowship for his Cornish friend Revd. William Borlase in September 1749 and shepherded the certificate through to Borlase's election in the following May.[4] Da Costa also acted as London agent for many of his correspondents who frequently received information from him about the proceedings of the Antiquarian and Royal societies, and purchased books and other items on their behalf. For example, when one of his correspondents wanted a statue carved in London da Costa supervised this work. As a Jew he was especially useful to his antiquarian friends, being frequently consulted on such matters as a strange (apparently Hebrew) inscription on a stone found in Canterbury, an early deed from Dorset written in Hebrew and the history of the Jews of China – a topic which he helped open up.[5]

Scientific correspondence often shaded into business and he tried to combine the roles of philosopher with that of trader. He collected an impressive cabinet but was continually offering his correspondents items either from his own collection or ones that he could obtain from other sources. He frequently distributed hand-written catalogues of fossils and shells, often with several dozen entries accompanied by detailed descriptions and prices. Since he was dealing in merchandise that was geographically specific he could entice a customer living in Cornwall with fossils from Derbyshire and a Swedish correspondent with mineral specimens from Cornwall. When an established collector died valuable items would often be released on to the market through auction sales, which da Costa attended in order to obtain specimens either for himself or for one of his patrons. His entrepreneurial activities also extended to trading in manuscripts and rare antiquarian items where he again combined the roles of trader and also member of the republic of letters. He was, for example, involved in collecting and handling the manuscripts of the 17th-century geologist Edward Lhuyd, which William Huddesford subsequently published.[6]

In 1750 da Costa married his cousin, Leah, and also entered into a business relation-ship with her brother Abraham Prado. Prado was engaged in supplying His Majesty's army with provisions, and in the late 1740s accompanied a military campaign against the French in the Netherlands.[7] Da Costa spent almost a year with his brother-in-law at 's Hertogenbosch, but also took the opportunity to travel on the continent in order to increase his natural history cabinet and contact other naturalists and potential customers. For reasons that are far from clear, this business venture resulted in his serving a two-year prison sentence. As he explained to Borlase, 'these misfortunes . . . proceed from family dissensions as the only Cause of my present Confinement on account of some unfortunate family affair' – presumably of a financial nature. Writing from prison to Turberville Needham he commented: 'I have made my confinement a Monastic Life, for my Cabinet & Library being with me I have intirely dedicated all my time to study and have by that means near compleated my work'.[8] The work to which he referred was his *Natural history of fossils*, volume 1, part 1 of which eventu-ally appeared in 1757, with a subscription list of 98, of whom 38 were Fellows of the Royal Society.[9] He experienced some difficulty generating subscriptions and claims to have made a financial loss of nearly £200 on this volume.[10] As with so many of da Costa's projects, it was not concluded satisfactorily – in this case the much-trumpeted part 2 never appeared.

It appears that by the time da Costa reached his thirties his family's financial position had declined significantly and proved insufficient to support his passion for scientific and antiquarian pursuits. He thus became increasingly dependent on his own earnings. Although on many occasions he sold cabinets of specimens for between 20 and 30 guineas, his commercial success is difficult to assess. Against such income must be set not only the cost of specimens but also the outlay involved in establishing and maintaining patronage. In order to attract potential customers and patrons he frequently plied them with gifts, such as a few unusual fossils for their cabinets. However, unless such presents resulted in a remunerative sale he would make an overall loss. It also needs to be remembered that specimens that ended up in his own cabinet represented savings, not income. Thus one patron and friend congratulated da

Costa as 'one who can collect & hoard up with so much Philosophical avarice, . . . [but was] at the same time . . . so generous & communicative'.[11] Yet his effectiveness as a trader is also open to question since he seems often overwhelmed by the demands made on him. There are also several instances of his quarrelling with purchasers because he failed to fulfil their orders and/or his promises – or so they claimed.

Another source of income was the courses he delivered on fossils and shells – usually charging 2 or 3 guineas for a series of 27 lectures. In many letters preserved in the da Costa collection he tried to drum up subscribers for his books or his lecture courses. He even appears to have offered one series of lectures to boys in the Sephardi community.[12] Again, presumably in order to improve his financial situation, he was admitted to the Society of Scriveners and undertook notarial work.[13]

Being frequently in debt some of his closest friends came to his aid, one of whom paid off the considerable debt he had incurred in publishing his *Natural history of fossils*. His co-religionist the merchant Joseph Salvador and the Quaker doctor John Fothergill were among those who made substantial loans; for example, between 1753 and 1762 Fothergill loaned him £168 against which specimens, mainly fossils, to the value of £69.16.0 had been supplied.[14] '[O]ft necessitous' was how Fothergill described da Costa to a correspondent.[15]

Although some contemporaries clearly disliked da Costa,[16] many others portrayed him as cultured, well-informed and a fellow member of the republic of letters. Despite trading in natural history specimens he was no mere tradesman but a true philosopher respected for his extensive knowledge and his willingness to assist others in their pursuit of natural history. Thus Josiah Wedgwood reported that Thomas Percival 'is very high in his incomiums of da C[osta]– as a very sensible Man, of the most extensive knowledge, & equally extensive correspondence, with the Literati all over Europe, amongst whom the Dr [Percival] says he is very much esteem'd'.[17] As his correspondence shows da Costa was also held in great esteem and affection by many of his long-term friends and patrons.

In the 1750s and early '60s da Costa appears to have been caught in the following predicament. By dint of hard work he had earned his credentials as a naturalist and antiquarian who could rub shoulders with men and women of wealth and power. They respected him for his expertise and acknowledged him as a fellow philosopher. However, unlike many of the naturalists in the Royal Society and antiquarians in the Society of Antiquaries, da Costa had to scrape a living from science. As one of his friends commented, he 'has hitherto laboured in the vineyard of literature and curiosity to his own undoing'.[18] A paid position in science would rescue him from this uncertain financial situation. When the post of Curator of Natural History at the newly-founded British Museum became available in 1760 da Costa expressed keen interest and gained the patronage of 'the Dukes of Argyle & Portland & the Hon[our]able Charles Stanhope Esqr [,] Mr Watson the great Botanist and [a] great part of our Royal Society'.[19] However, he was not appointed because 'my religion was an obstacle' (or so he claimed).[20] Subsequently he frequently criticized the British Museum for failing to provide adequate access for the public.[21]

Then, providentially, early in 1763, the death was announced of Francis Hauksbee, junior, who had served as Clerk – otherwise known as Assistant Secretary – to the Royal Society for the previous 40 years. Council rapidly moved to find a replacement and da Costa canvassed his friends for votes. Despite the recent death of his 'most tender and affectionate Father, whose obsequies by my religion I must strictly attend to',[22] over a four-day period da Costa approached at least two dozen friends and patrons in the Royal Society to solicit their support in his bid for one of the very few paid science-related posts in mid-18th-century Britain. Through these letters we see how da Costa was able to mobilize votes in his favour.[23] One of da Costa's initial concerns was whether his religion would bar him from the post; an issue he broached with his closest advisers but was pleased to discover that it offered no impediment. The aged William Stukeley wrote to a colleague:

> My Friend Da Costa must get a paper for his friends to sign recommending him to be clerk and house-keeper to the Royal Society, in place of Francis Hawksbee, deceased, to be exhibited next Thursday to the Council. The choice is in the Society, Thursday se'nnight. I know he has very many friends. All my corner of the room unanimous: Sir William Brown, [Peter] Collinson, [James] Parsons, [Henry] Baker, [Samuel] Clark, [John] Van Rixtel, &c. &c.[24]

At its meeting of 27 January 1763 Council considered da Costa and five other applicants:

> His Application and Letter to the President, written by himself, are in a good, plain, steady and intelligible hand. Besides English (his Mother Tongue) he can speak Spanish, Portuguese, Italian, French, German & Latin; understands a little Greek, and Hebrew & Chaldee very well. Mr Da Costa's various Communications to the Society and Publications to the World, have fully evinced his Skill in natural History. He is conversant in Libraries, and has put several of considerable Consequence into Order. He says he has no Skill in Mathematics, or Mechanics; is a married Man, but without a Family: And can give any Security, by Persons of undoubted Credit.[25]

In the ensuing election da Costa attracted 52 votes in his favour and only 18 against.[26] His lobbying of friends and patrons was so successful that he far outstripped the other candidates. Two sureties each of £500 were appointed, one being the Sephardi merchant Joseph Salvador. In early February 1763 da Costa and his wife moved into the Royal Society. He was obviously delighted that at last he could combine his work with his scientific interests. 'He writes as one thoroughly happy', commented one of his friends soon after his appointment.[27] Living and working at the Royal Society he was now at the very centre of British science. His letters overflow with his enthusiasm for the post and the honour he clearly felt in gaining this formal position in the scientific world. Presumably he also thought that his financial worries were over.

This turned out not to be the case, and he 'borrowed' money from the Society's coffers presumably to help finance his many scientific ventures. Although I am unable to pursue this biographical narrative any further in this paper, there are several points I would like to offer by way of a conclusion.

(1) The first concerns the effectiveness of da Costa's search for patronage. His patrons appear to have been drawn from many different social, political and religious groups; Indeed, da Costa seems to have taken every opportunity to draw into his net everyone who might prove useful to his scientific career – fellow Jews, antiquarians, the gentry and nobility, Whigs, Tories, even Anglican clerics and bishops. He proved an effective connector, as well as a respected collector.

(2) However, what I find most interesting is that while he was patronized by

Anglicans, some of his most constant friends and supporters – even after his 'fall' – were drawn not only from the Jewish community but also from Christian dissenters. The Quaker John Fothergill was foremost among these as was Peter Collinson, a Quaker who traded in plants and seeds. Likewise, later in life probably his leading supporter was the botanist Richard Poulteney, also a dissenter. Among his closest friends and clients were several Huguenot merchants including Thomas and Samuel Fludyer and especially Isaac Romilly, with whom he engaged in a charming correspondence which displays a particularly close friendship between the two men. This suggests that dissenters and Huguenots were particularly sympathetic to the trials and tribulations of a fellow 'outsider' trying to forge a career in science.

(3) We should also reflect on his dependence on patronage. As I have stressed patronage networks were difficult, time-consuming and often expensive to construct and maintain. Although it is not clear how he attracted his first patrons much of his extant correspondence is devoted to the business of patronage. Yet, he was dogged by financial insecurity since patronage could suddenly end for any of a number of reasons – the patron's death, loss of wealth, loss of interest in science or by an insult (real or imagined). Moreover, the patronage he managed to attract proved insufficient to maintain his life in science. He, like a number of his correspondents, suffered from the 'Philosophical dropsy'[28] – that ill-understood disease which we might call an extreme enthusiasm for collecting natural history specimens.

(4) My final point relates to the conflicting demands of da Costa's various roles – as philosopher, tradesman and, from 1763, servant of the Royal Society. In respect to the first two we witness not only a clash of interests but also of social status. Jews have traditionally been traders, although rarely of scientific specimens. However, in adopting the role of philosopher and joining the ranks of the republic of learning da Costa undertook a new role. While Moses Mendelssohn in Germany is usually cited as the paradigm example of an enlightened Jew, da Costa was one of the very few English Jews who, as David Ruderman has pointed out, self-consciously participated in the *Haskalah* (Enlightenment).[29]

NOTES

Note: The Da Costa correspondence in the British Library, Add Ms 28534–44, is cited below as Corr., vol. 1 . . . vol.11.

1 T. M. Endelman, *The Jews of Georgian England, 1714–1830: tradition and change in a liberal society* (Ann Arbor, MI, 1999), 249.

2 M. Folkes to da Costa, 9 August 1747: J. Nichols, *Illustrations of the literary history of the 18th century* (London, 1822), vol. 4, 635–6.

3 T. Percival to da Costa, 19 September 1765: Corr., vol. 7, fo. 193.

4 Da Costa to W. Borlase, 21 September 1749 and 20 February 1750: Corr., vol. 2, fos. 33, 47.

5 See, especially, da Costa to unknown, n.d. BL, Add Ms 29868, fo. 4.

6 W. Huddesford, *Edvardi Luidii apud Oxonienses cimeliarchae Ashmoleani Lithophylacii Britannici ichnographia . . .* (London, 1760).

7 On Prado see C. Roth, 'The Jews in the defence of Britain', *Transactions of the Jewish Historical Society of England* (hereafter *TJHSE*) 15 (1939–45), 1–28; A. Hyamson, *The*

Sephardim of England (London, 1951), 103; E. Ironside, *History and antiquities of Twickenham* (London, 1797), 107; Horace Walpole to Lady Ossory, 14 September 1774: *The Yale edition of Horace Walpole's correspondence*, ed. W. S. Lewis (London, 1937–), vol. 32, 205–8; H. F. Finsberg, 'Jewish residents of eighteenth-century Twickenham', *TJHSE* 26 (1952), 129–35.

8   Da Costa to Turberville Needham, 31 March 1755: Corr., vol. 7, fo. 84.

9   E. M. da Costa, *A natural history of fossils* (London, 1757), vol. 1, pt. 1.

10   Da Costa to J. A. Schlosser, 29 March 1762: Corr., vol. 9, fos. 137–8.

11   W. Borlase to da Costa, 7 October 1760: Corr., vol. 2, fo. 115.

12   Da Costa to I. M. Belisario, 10 July 1766: Corr., vol. 1, fo. 206.

13   E. R. Samuel, 'Anglo-Jewish notaries and scriveners', *TJHSE* 17 (1953), 113–60.

14   Statement of account of da Costa's loans from Fothergill, 1753–62: Corr., vol. 4, fo. 143.

15   J. Fothergill to J. Morgan, 7 December 1765: B. C. Corner and C. C. Booth, *Chain of friendship: selected letters of Dr John Fothergill* (Cambridge, MA, 1971), 250. Writing to Charles Lyttelton on 28 December 1767, William Borlase claimed that da Costa 'has been necessitous ever since I [first] knew him': P. A. S. Pool, *William Borlase* (Truro, 1986), 139.

16   For example, Josiah Wedgwood called him 'the most disagreeable mortal, who bore the name of a Philosopher, that I had ever known'. J. Wedgwood to unknown, n.d.: Wedgwood Papers, University of Keele, Ms 18552–25, fos. 1–2.

17   *Ibid.*

18   W. Borlase to C. Lyttelton, April 1763: Pool, *William Borlase*, 238.

19   *Ibid.*

20   Da Costa to T. Needham, 18 March 1760: Corr., vol. 7, fo. 93.

21   Da Costa to W. Borlase, 14 July and 23 August 1759: Corr., vol. 2, fos. 99, 103.

22   Da Costa to Earl of Macclesfield, 19 January 1763: Corr., vol. 6, fo. 202.

23   Among those approached were Henry Baker, Thomas Birch, William Brown, Samuel Chandler, Samuel Clarke, Peter Collinson, Andrew Ducarel, George Edwards, Georg D. Ehret, James Empson(?), Samuel Felton, Martin Hubner, Charles G. Hudson, William Hudson, Gowin Knight, Earl of Macclesfield, Matthew Maty, Philip Miller, Charles Morton, James Parsons, John van Rixtel, Joseph Salvador, Noah Sherwood, William Stukeley and William Watson.

24   W. Stukeley to unknown, 21 January 1763: Nichols, *Illustrations of the literary history*, 506.

25   Royal Society, Minute Books, vol. 4, fo. 348.

26   *Ibid.*, fos. 581–9.

27   W. Borlase to C. Lyttelton, April 1763: Pool, *William Borlase*, 238.

28   J. S. Budgen to da Costa, 7 July 1761: Corr., vol. 2, fo. 285; W. Borlase to da Costa, 12 August 1765: Corr., vol. 2, fo. 161.

29   See D. B. Ruderman, 'Was there an English parallel to the German *Haskalah*?', in M. Brenner, R. Liedtke and D. Rechter, eds., *Two nations: British and German Jews in comparative perspective* (Tübingen, 1999), 15–44.

Part V

The 'Other' in Protestant England:
Jews, Muslims, Africans and Orthodox
Christians in Britain

25

London's Portuguese Jewish community, 1540–1753

EDGAR SAMUEL

After the expulsion of the Jews from Spain in 1492 many of them settled in Portugal where, in 1497, King Manoel I ordered their baptism by force and their renaming as 'New Christians.' Since any Jews willing to become Christians had stayed in Spain, it is not surprising that those who had left their property and native land for religion's sake were very strongly attached to their faith and continued to practise it in the privacy of their homes. The Portuguese Inquisition was set up in 1535 and an active persecution started in 1540. This caused many New Christians to leave the country. Where they could they often returned to Judaism. A small group of some 70 people took refuge in London and attended a secret synagogue in the house of one Luis Lopes,[1] but they had to be wary, because Henry IV's statute *De haeretico comburendo*[2] made it a capital crime in England for any baptized Christian to practise Judaism. In February 1542 the Privy Council ordered the arrest of a number of merchant strangers 'suspected to be Jews' and the sequestration of their property. Because this disrupted the marketing of the King of Portugal's pepper, the Queen of Portugal wrote to her sister, Queen Maria of Hungary, Regent of the Netherlands, protesting at some of the arrests and the Spanish ambassador procured the release of several men and their property. Others left the country.[3]

In 1540 Elizabeth Rodrigues, widow of Jorge Anes,[4] arrived in London from Lisbon with her family, household goods and a cargo of merchandise.[5] She took a house south of Lombard Street and was endenizened in the next year. Her letter of denization states that she was then aged 60, was 'born in the dominions of the Emperor' – a strange circumlocution for Spain – and had been resident in England for 20 years,[6] which we know was not true. Her son Gonsalvo changed his name to Dunstan, almost certainly by being confirmed by the Bishop of London, and in 1548 married another Portuguese New Christian, Constance, daughter of Simon Ruiz at the parish church of St Nicholas Acon.[7] They had 14 children and outwardly conformed to the established Church, while practising Judaism in the privacy of their home.[8] In 1557 Dunstan Anes obtained the freedom of the City of London and of the Grocers' Company on the recommendation of Queen Mary Tudor and of King Philip, who was then in London. For this he had to pay £40, half of which was returned to him.[9] Under

Elizabeth I the little colony in London increased to about one hundred.[10] In 1568 Dunstan Anes registered his arms at Herald's College, describing himself as 'Purvyor and Marchant for the Queen's Ma[jes]tis Grosery for the Howseholde'.[11] In about 1582 his son Jacob and two of his daughters migrated to Turkey. The English traveller Thomas Coryate reported that he visited:

> The house of a certain English Jew called Amis born in Crutched Friars in London, who hath two sisters more of his own Jewish religion . . . likewise born in the same place . . . This aforesaid Amis for the love he bore to our English nation, in which he lived till he was thirty years of age, being at the time of my residence in Constantinople sixty, received me with very courteous entertainment.[12]

Dunstan's son William stayed in London and carried on the business as a spice merchant until his death in 1630, 90 years after his grandmother had arrived here.

As well as the merchants, the Elizabethan community included medical men. Hector Nunes was physician to Lord Burleigh.[13] He traded to Spain and Portugal[14] and provided Burleigh with intelligence on the preparation of the Spanish Armada.[15] Dr Rodrigo Lopes married Dunstan Anes's daughter Sarah and became physician to St Bartholomew's Hospital, to the Earl of Leicester and finally to the Queen's household. Both were graduates of Coimbra University and Fellows of the College of Physicians. In 1594 the Earl of Essex falsely[16] accused Lopes of plotting to poison the Queen. He was convicted of high treason, together with two other Portuguese, and was hanged, drawn and quartered at Tyburn.

James I ended England's war with Spain in 1604. This led Jewish merchants in Amsterdam to send agents to London to trade with Portugal in English ships. The General Pardon of past heresies in Portugal, in 1605, caused further immigration. We know of a Passover service attended by seven people in a house in Aldgate Ward, in that year.[17] In 1609 James I expelled most of the Portuguese Jews.[18] However, Francisco Pinto de Britto, who had married Dr Lopes's daughter Anne,[19] remained in England until his death in 1618.[20]

The founder of the modern Jewish community, Antonio Fernandes Carvajal, settled in London in 1635. He was born in Fundão in Portugal, and had lived in the Canary Islands and in Rouen. He was a wine importer, and used to attend Mass at the Spanish embassy. In 1641 the Long Parliament repealed the Act Concerning the Burning of Heretics. In 1654 Cromwell declared war on Spain. Carvajal and his sons then took English nationality and converted to Judaism.[21]

The Dutch had allowed the Jewish refugees from Spain and Portugal to settle in Amsterdam with freedom of worship. In the 1650s they brought a very valuable trade with Spain and South America with them. This caused some Englishmen and especially the Baptist clergy to advocate their admission to England.[22] The Commonwealth's ambassadors had visited Amsterdam's Portuguese Synagogue in 1651 and met its junior rabbi, Menasseh ben Israel. In 1654 Oliver Cromwell invited him to come to England to petition publicly for the admission of Jews to the country and convened a conference at Whitehall Palace to consider the proposal, where to everyone's surprise, the judges ruled that there was now no law against Jews living in England.[23] Cromwell allowed the Portuguese Jews, headed by Carvajal, to meet privately for prayer, to lease a cemetery and to settle in the English colonies, but immigration was limited to recommended individuals.

When Charles II was restored to the throne in 1660, the City of London petitioned to have the Jews expelled, complaining that they were exporting cloth at lower rates than English merchants.[24] The government thought this no crime and ignored the petition. In 1664 the Secretary of State wrote to the leaders of the Jewish community that:

> They may promise themselves the effects of the same favour as they formerly had, so long as they demean themselves quietly and peaceably with due obedience to his Majesty's laws and without scandal to his Government.[25]

This meant no proselytizing and no religious disputes or publications in English. The Synagogue's earliest regulations state that:

> This Congregation . . . shall serve for the Jews of the Portuguese and Spanish Nation, who are at present in this city and later may come to it; and the Jewish persons, who may come here from other nations, will be allowed to he admitted to prayers, if it seems fit to the *Mahamad* that shall be in office.[26]

The first immigrants were mostly Portuguese refugees from Spain, like Carvajal. Several came from France and some directly from Portugal. There were also some professing Jews from the Netherlands. After Charles II's marriage treaty with Portugal gave England trading rights in the Portuguese empire, immigration increased because of both trading opportunities and persecution.

In 1674 a Grand Jury at the Quarter Sessions at Guildhall found a bill against the Jews for riotous assembly in their synagogue. The community petitioned the King, and the Attorney-General stopped the proceedings.[27] This incident made it clear to the community that the Lord Mayor of London needed to be placated. From 1679 to 1779 the Portuguese synagogue made a gift of plate to each Lord Mayor upon his investiture. This was usually a silver tray, filled with Portuguese pastries and decorated with 'The Arms of the Tribe of Judah, given them by the Lord.' It was never considered necessary to submit this Divine grant of arms for approval by the College of Heralds. In later years a silver loving cup filled with chocolate was given instead. Until 1738 the elders of the French Church and the Dutch Church also presented the new Lord Mayor with two matching silver flagons, one from each church.[28]

In 1689 the rural landowners who ran Parliament had the bright idea of levying a tax of £100,000 a year on the Jews of London. It was not ever enforced, but it caused the Jews to explain their circumstances in a petition to the House of Commons. They claimed that their community consisted of between 60 and 80 families, most of the merchants among them being endenizened.

> About a fourth part of these have Moderate Estates of their own. Another fourth part have very indifferent Estates: And the other half consists, partly of an industrious sort of People, that assist the better sort in the management of their Commerce, and partly of indigent poor people, who are maintained by the rest, and no ways chargeable to the Parishes.[29]

The community at that date depended upon about 20 successful merchants for its prosperity, the maintenance of the poor and the upkeep of the synagogue. In 1695 London's Jewish communities consisted of 560 Portuguese Jews and 200 German

Jews.[30] By then the German Jews, whose leaders came from Hamburg, had started their own synagogue.[31]

The expansion of the community in the 18th century was far more rapid. The persecution of the Portuguese New Christians in both Portugal and Spain increased in the 1720s. Portugal was then England's largest trading partner and many ships sailed between Lisbon and London. The community's leaders let it be known on the Royal Exchange that they would pay the passage money to any English captain who brought refugees from Portugal.[32] By 1753 there were some 2000 Sephardi (the medieval Hebrew word for 'Spanish') Jews in London (there was no other Sephardi community in England) and 4000 Ashkenazi (the medieval Hebrew word for 'German') Jews.[33] These numbers are far smaller, of course, than the 50,000 French Protestants, who had been welcomed to England in the late 17th century.[34]

The prosperity and leadership of the community were supplied by a small clique of successful foreign traders and specialist brokers. The merchants' trade was concentrated in areas where they had advantages of language, kinship or personal experience. The Francia family continued Carvajal's business as a wine importer.[35] Jewish merchants exported English wheat and cloth to Portugal and imported sugar, dyestuffs, and bullion.[36] The diamond trade was a Jewish speciality. Coral beads made in Leghorn were exported to India and diamonds were imported. London replaced Lisbon as the main European staple for unpolished diamonds.[37] Trade with the Caribbean colonies was important. Even in 1688 there were two synagogues in Barbados, one in Nevis and one in Jamaica.[38] In the early 18th century there were established colonies of Sephardi merchants on the North American continent – in New York, Newport, Rhode Island, and Philadelphia – who traded with their relatives in London. Trade with European Sephardi communities at Hamburg, Bordeaux, Bayonne, Leghorn and Amsterdam was also continuous.

In 1697 the Court of Aldermen ruled that in future only sworn brokers should deal on the Royal Exchange. They determined that there should be one hundred English brokers, six from the Dutch Church, six from the French Church and 12 Jews.[39] At the time it was a reasonable provision, but it was not altered when circumstances changed. Because of Dutch investments in the English funds, the volume of business conducted by the 'Jew brokers' increased dramatically in the course of the 18th century and the restriction on their numbers caused hardship. When a broker died the Lord Mayor had the nomination of his successor. If a son wanted to carry on the business, he would have to pay him as much as £2000 for the broker's medal in order to prevent it being sold to a competitor.[40] In 1753 there were two Ashkenazi and ten Sephardi brokers.[41] Most, but not all, were stockbrokers, some were diamond and pearl brokers,[42] and some were marine insurance brokers. Abraham Mocatta was bullion broker to the Bank of England and to the East India Company.[43] The Lindo family were sworn brokers for 200 years without am interruption.[44] The most successful Jewish broker was Samson Gideon, the government's adviser on the floatation of new loans.[45]

Linked with the brokers were the public notaries, a small profession, who translated and certified documents. Jews could not become solicitors or barristers, because the practitioners excluded them,[46] but the Archbishop of Canterbury appointed notaries and he saw no reason to impose a religious test on these secular officials and even gave notarial faculties to two rabbis, Isaac Nieto and Isaac Mendes Belisario. Notaries made a substantial cultural contribution to their community. Until he was sacked for embezzlement, Emmanuel Mendes da Costa, notary public, conchologist and fossilologist was Secretary of the Royal Society.[47]

Medicine was a respected Jewish speciality in Spain and Portugal. Jews and Dissenters were excluded from the universities and so could not qualify in medicine in England without renouncing their religion. Dr Jacob de Castro Sarmento was able to improve upon his M.B. from Coimbra University, however, by obtaining an M.D. by correspondence with Marischal College, Aberdeen,[48] one of those Scottish universities which, in Dr Samuel Johnson's words, 'grew wealthy by degrees'. He was physician to the Portuguese ambassador. He published books informing the Portuguese medical profession about the introduction of *variolation* against smallpox. He was elected to the Royal Society and contributed to its *Philosophical Transactions*. He also proposed the founding of the Portuguese Jewish community's 1748 infirmary. This had ten beds and a dispensary and a part-time medical staff of three physicians, a surgeon, and an apothecary.[49]

The London Sephardi community was too small to train its own rabbis and cantors, so they were imported along the trade routes from Leghorn and Amsterdam and exported to the colonies. The job of the *Haham* was to preach and teach and to rule on matters of Jewish Law, but the government of the community was in the hands of the merchants and brokers who staffed the *Mahamad* and the elders. Their most distinguished *Haham* was David Nieto, a native of Leghorn and a doctor of medicine, who was versed in philosophy and intensely interested in mathematics and astronomy. Unusually for a rabbi, his Hebrew and Spanish book, *Matteh Dan y segunda parte del Cuzari* (1714), discusses the possibility of life on other planets.

The immigrants brought with them a wide range of occupations. There were engravers, confectioners,[50] embroiderers, tailors,[51] a silk thrower,[52] a fencing master, diamond cutters,[53] several translators and language teachers, and hawkers. But because even English-born Jews were excluded from the freedom of the City of London, they were precluded from opening shops there or engaging as principals in any craft regulated by the livery companies. Added to this were the restrictions imposed by Judaism against working on Sabbaths and festivals. The best job opportunities for most were in the service of the merchants and brokers, as warehousemen, bookkeepers, and clerks. The silversmith Abraham Lopes de Oliveira (1657–1730) stands alone as the one 18th-century London Jewish artisan of distinction. He was born and trained in Amsterdam, where a Jew could serve an apprenticeship providing he practised his craft elsewhere. Oliveira came to London in 1685 to join his uncle, who was an established merchant, and probably worked as a journeyman.[54] The nine ceremonial pieces in tbe Jewish Museum which he made are of high quality.

The community had a tradition of helping the poor, but never on a generous scale. Often the poor were assisted to migrate to Georgia or the Caribbean colonies, or if they were not refugees, sent back to their place of origin. During the late 1720s, with heavy immigration of destitute refugees from the Iberian Peninsula, finding work for the immigrants was very difficult. Sometimes a man would be helped to become self-sufficient by being lent money to start out in business as a pedlar or as a buyer of second-hand clothes.[55] More typical was the trade in imported fruit, including hawking oranges.

The period 1700–50 was one of cultural achievement rooted in economic prosperity. It saw the publication of Daniel Lopes Laguna's *Espejo Fiel de la Vida*

(1720), with introductory sonnets by members of the community in Spanish, Portuguese and English, and of sermons, erudite dictionaries and prayer books. The charity and educational system was developed, including dowries for poor brides, charity schools and apprenticeships. The girls of the Villareal School were taught sewing, flower-designing and embroidery, to count in English and to read and write in English, Hebrew and Portuguese or Spanish.[56]

Between 1540 and and the mid-18th century there was a substantial improvement in Jewish civil rights in England. It was no longer a capital crime for a New Christian to revert to Judaism or illegal for professing Jews to live in England. They had at first been admitted as merchant strangers, but then open Jewish communities in England and the colonies enjoyed full religious freedom. Yet Jews were excluded from retail trade in the City of London and from all public offices above parish level. In the 1750s, at the request of Joseph Salvador, the Government brought in an Act allowing Jews to be naturalized. The Opposition campaigned fiercely against it, defeated the government candidate at the Oxfordshire by-election in 1753 and the Act had to be repealed.[57] In 1753, though, the Sephardi community was still largely a Portuguese-speaking village in Aldgate Ward of fairly recent immigrants. Sermons and all synagogue meetings and records were in Portuguese. Jews could practise medicine and could qualify as notaries but not as barristers or solicitors. They could be endenized but not naturalized, except in America. There was far more social acceptance in Britain than in most European countries, including admittance to Masonic Lodges,[58] to the Royal Society and to the Society of Antiquaries, but full citizenship was not attained for another hundred years.

NOTES

1   I am grateful to Prof. Aron di Leone Leoni for this information based on his researches in the Archives du Royaume in Brussels, which have corrected some of the misreadings of this episode found in Lucien Wolf, 'The Jews in Tudor England' in *idem, Essays in Jewish history* (1934), 71, 90.
2   'Concerning the burning of heretics', 2 Henry IV c. 15.
3   I am grateful to Prof. Aron di Leone Leoni for this information.
4   'Anes' is a common Portuguese surname meaning 'son of John'. It is pronounced 'Annish' or 'Annis'.
5   Archives du Royaume, Brussels, Etat et Audience, Liasse 11772 (abstract of Francisco Anes letter of 24 October 1540 from Lisbon to Dominique Mendes in Antwerp). A resumé is in University College London, Lucien Wolf MSS, CC12/27.
6   HSQS 8.
7   GL, MS 17621 (Marriage Register of St Nicholas Acon).
8   The deposition of Pedro de Santa Cruz, Madrid 4 July 1548: 'sabe por ser publico y notorio en londres que todos son judios de nazion y como tales en sus casas es fama que biben en sus rritos judaycos y en publico van a las yglesias luteranas y oyen los sermones y toman el pan y el vino en la forma y manera que los demas Herejes lo hazen' Lucien Wolf, 'Jews in Elizabethan England', *TJHSE* 11 (1924–7), 46, citing Archivo General de Simancas, Secretaria de Estado, Legajo 839, fo. 183.
9   CLRO, Repertories for 1557, 515v; GL, MS 1159r (Admissions to the Freedom of the Worshipful Company of Grocers).
10 Wolf, 'Jews in Elizabethan England', 33–5.

11   J. J. Howard and G. J. Armytage (eds.), *The Visitation of London in the Year 1568 taken by Robert Cooke, Clarenceaux King of Arms*, Harleian Society 1 (London, 1869); H. Stanford London (ed.), *Visitation of London, 1568*, Harleian Society 109, 110 (London, 1963).

12   Samuel Purchas, *Hakluytus Posthumus or Purchas his Pilgrimes* (Glasgow, 1905).

13   Conyers Read, *Lord Burleigh and Queen Elizabeth* (London, 1959), 261.

14   Charles Meyers, 'Debt in Elizabethan England: the adventures of Dr Hector Nunez, physician and merchant', *TJHSE* 24 (1970–3), 125–140.

15   Detailed in a letter of 27 February 1588 of Francisco de Valverde and Pedro de Santa Cruz from London to Don Bernardino de Mendoza in Paris: *CSP Spanish* and Wolf, 'Jews in Elizabethan England', 36.

16   This was the opinion of Bishop Godfrey Goodman, *Court of James I* (1839) and of Count Gondomar, *Documentos ineditos para la historia de España* (Madrid, 1936).

17   Edgar Samuel, 'Passover in Shakespeare's London' *TJHSE* 26 (1974–8), 117–18.

18   Edgar Samuel, 'Portuguese Jews in Jacobean London', *TJHSE* 28 (1981–2), 171–226.

19   James I's letter to the Lord Mayor requesting the freedom of the City for Francisco Pinto de Britto states that his wife and children were born in England. We know from her Chancery suit that her name was Anne Lopes. Anne, daughter of Dr Rodrigo Lopes was born in London 1579. The probability is that Anne's uncle, William Anes, had arranged the marriage of his niece with Pinto de Britto of Amsterdam, who received the *poortersrecht* citizenship there in 1602 . *Ibid.*

20   30 December 1618, 'Francis Pintoe a portingall died and was carried ov[e]r seas to be buried', Bruce Bannerman (ed.), *Records of St Olave Hart Street*, Harleian Society 47 (London, 1916).

21   Lucien Wolf 'The first English Jew: notes on Antonio Fernandes Carvajal', *TJHSE* 2 (1894–5), 14–45.

22   Edgar Samuel, 'The readmission of the Jews to England in 1656 in the context of English Economic policy' *TJHSE* 31 (1988–90), 153–69.

23   Lucien Wolf, *Menasseh ben Israel's mission to Oliver Cromwell* (1901) and David Katz, *Philo-Semitism and the readmission of the Jews to England 1603–1655* (Oxford, 1982).

24   Text published by Lucien Wolf in *TJHSE* 4 (1899–1901),186–8 citing GL, Remembrancer 9, 44, fos 1–8.

25   Reply to the petition of Emmanuel Martines Dormido, Elias de Lima and Moses Baruh in the Spanish and Portuguese Synagogue's archives, reproduced in Lionel D. Barnett, *Bevis Marks Records being contributions to the history of the Spanish and Portuguese Congregation of London* (Oxford, 1940), pt. 1, 9.

26   Lionel D. Barnett, *El Libro de los Acuerdos* (Oxford, 1930), 3.

27   Lionel D. Barnett, *Bevis Marks Records*, pt. 1.

28   Wilfred S. Samuel, 'The London Jews' yearly gift to the Lord Mayor', *Miscellanies of the Jewish Historical Society of England* 3 (1937), 99.

29   *The Case of the Jews stated*, published in *TJHSE* 9 (1918–20), 44, citing *CSPD 1689*, 318.

30   Maurice Woolf, 'Notes on the Census Lists 1695', *Miscellanies of the Jewish Historical Society of England* 5 (1948), 175–7.

31   Cecil Roth, *The Great Synagogue, London, 1690–1940* (London, 1950).

32   A. S. Diamond, 'Problems of the London Sephardi Community 1720–1733', *TJHSE* 21 (1962–7), 40: 'There was an understanding that masters of British merchant ships embarking refugees from Portugal would be paid fare and freight on arrival in England and in 5488 [1728/9] £254 4s was laid out on that account'.

33   Todd Endelman, *The Jews of Georgian England 1713–1830: tradition and change in a liberal society* (Philadelphia, 1979), 171 discusses the difficulty in estimating the population with any accuracy.

34 Robin Gwynn, *Huguenot Heritage: the history and contribution of the Huguenots in Britain* (London, 1985), 35.

35 Maurice Woolf, 'Foreign trade of the London Jews in the seventeenth century', *TJHSE* 25 (1973–5).

36 Edgar Samuel, 'The Jews in English foreign trade: a consideration of the *Philo Patriae* pamphlets of 1753' in John M. Shaftesley (ed.), *Remember the days* (London, 1966), 123–44.

37 Gedalia Yogev, *Diamonds and coral: Anglo-Dutch Jews in eighteenth century trade* (Leicester, 1978).

38 *Ya en seis ciudades anglas se publica*
    Luz de seis juntas de Israel sagradas
    Tres en Nieves. London Iamaica;
    Quarta y quinta en dos partes de Barbadas
    Sexta en Madras Pâtan se vérifica
    Daniel Levy de Barrios, *Historia Real de la Gran Bretaña* (Amsterdam, 1688), 55–6.

39 Dudley Abrahams, 'Jew brokers of the City of London', *Miscellanies of the Jewish Historical Society of England* 3 (1937), 85.

40 James Picciotto, *Sketches of Anglo-Jewish History* (1956), 171.

41 Abrahams, 'Jew brokers'.

42 Solomon Dormido was a pearl broker: Amsterdam Gemeente Archiefdienst, PA334/677/608–9 (Letter of David Gabay in July 1660). Isaac de Paiba and Abraham de Paiba were diamond brokers: R. D. Barnett (ed.), *Bevis Marks Records Part IV: The circumcision register of Isaac and Abraham de Paiba (1717–1775)* (1991), 13.

43 Gedalia Yogev, *Diamonds and coral*, 52.

44 Their brokers' medals are in the Museum of London.

45 Lucy S. Sutherland, 'Samson Gideon: eighteenth-century Jewish financier', *TJHSE* 17 (1951–2).

46 H. S. Q. Henriques, *Jews and the English Law* (Oxford, 1908), 205.

47 Edgar Samuel, 'Anglo-Jewish notaries and scriveners', *TJHSE* 17 (1951–2).

48 P. J. Anderson , *Records of Marischal College and University* (Aberdeen, 1898).

49 Richard Barnett, 'Dr Jacob de Castro Sarmento and Sephardim in medical practice in 18th century London', *TJHSE* 29 (1982–6), 84–114.

50 Leonor de Morais was employed by the congregation to make *bôlos de amor, rosquilhas, quejados and masapoins* (marzipans) for part of the gift to the Lord Mayor. Oral communication from Miss Miriam Rodrigues-Pereira, Hon. Archivist, Spanish and Portuguese Jews' Congregation.

51 Abraham Duque, tailor, is mentioned in the Minute Book of the Mahamad in 1739: A. M. Hyamson, *The Sephardim of England* (1951) 88.

52 Aubrey Newman (ed.), *Migration and Settlement* (London, 1971), 52, no. 65.

53 CLRO, 1692 Poll Tax Return, Assessment Box 56:19 lists Joseph Robles, Benjamin Franco and 'Mr Alivars' as 'diamond cutters'. Several others are to be found in the 18th century apprenticeship records.

54 Miriam Rodrigues-Pereira, 'Abraham Lopes de Oliveira, silversmith', *The Jewish Museum Annual Report* (1992).

55 Betty Naggar, 'Old-clothes men: 18th and 19th centuries', *TJHSE* 31 (1988–90), 171–91.

56 Hyamson, *Sephardim*, 85n.

57 Thomas W. Perry, *Public opinion, propaganda and politics in eighteenth century England: a study of the Jew bill of 1753* (Cambridge, MA, 1962).

58 J. M. Shaftesley, 'Jews in English Regular Freemasonry 1717–1860', *TJHSE* 26 (1974–8), 50–209.

26

Embarrassing relations: myths and realities of the Ashkenazi influx, 1650–1750 and beyond

Michael Berkowitz

This paper seeks to provide an overview of the history of early modern Ashkenazi Jewry in England. The main question I shall address is: why should we even bother, for this period in which Anglo-Jewry seems so clearly to be dominated by Sephardim, to talk about the Askenazim? In short, the answer is two-fold: we should include them because they were indeed significant, and because their significance often has been misunderstood. In explicating these points, [1] primarily am indebted to the scholarship of Todd Endelman and David Katz,[1] who themselves stand on the shoulders of historians such as Moses Shulvass, Gedalyah Yogev, Harold Pollins, Cecil Roth, Vivian Lipman and Albert Hyamson.[2] In addition to applying their insights, I wish to illuminate how the non-Jewish community, which did not necessarily differentiate Sephardim from Ashkenazim, tended to view the Jews in its midst. Here I enjoin the scholarship of Bernard Glassman, Frank Felsenstein and the burgeoning Shylock 'industry', on the evolution of the Jewish stereotype in England, which predates both the debate over the 'Jew Bill' and the readmission.[3] I aspire to synthesize my contemporaries' socio-economic and cultural-historical approaches, in the hopes of problematizing the very categorization of pre-modern Anglo-Jewish history as 'Sephardi' versus 'Ashkenazi'.

In the lands of the West, it is common for students of Jewish history to refer to brittle tensions between relatively established communities of Jews and the next group to reach the same destination. The popular historian Steven Birmingham separates American Jewry as 'our crowd', a shorthand for those who came mostly in the early and mid-19th century from Central Europe, and the 'the rest of us', the mass migration from Eastern Europe beginning in 1881. Interestingly, Birmingham's first foray into Jewish history was *The Grandees: America's Sephardic elite* (1971).[4] Two books about the German-Jewish reception of their brethren from Eastern Europe have the word 'stranger' in their titles, in order to emphasize the extent to which the waves of immigrants coming from the East were unable to merge easily with the existing German Jewish community.[5] To be sure, Judaic tradition implores Jews to empathize with strangers in their midst, which some Jews have read as a prescription of how to treat the newest immigrants.[6] Yet more often it has been the case that Jews evince deep ambivalence about the next group of Jewish settlers to come to, and invariably unsettle, the situation they have cultivated for themselves. Moreover, in America, and to a certain extent Central Europe, Sephardim have been imagined as a founding cultural and economic elite, which Ismar Schorsch has called 'the myth of Sephardic supremacy'.[7]

Hence it is not surprising that the 'arrival' of Ashkenazi Jewry to England typically has been cast in dark, if not ominous shades. In H. P. Stokes's *A short history of the Jews in England*, for instance, the author emphasizes the abject poverty of Ashkenazim in contrast to Sephardim, and that 'their relationship to the older and wealthier section led sometimes to difficulties'.[8] Stokes goes on to describe the 1720s to 1750s as a time when 'the Jews in London were increasing in numbers, especially in the German section; indeed, after a while we shall find that, although the Sephardim still retained much of its Spanish prestige, the Ashkenazim came to dispute ascendancy'.[9] Here we have the kernel of the myth: that the affluent and intellectual Sephardim were eventually overwhelmed by the sheer numbers of incoming Askenazim. A main thread of my argument is that while this is not an untruth, it is far from the whole truth, and in some respects misleading.

Although Ashkenazi Jews were often treated as 'second-class citizens' by the Sephardi majority, this attitude is not totally indicative of the reality. David Katz writes that '[a]lthough the blanket prohibitions of 1678–9 were softened in 1682, it was clear that the Sephardim of London did not see themselves as serving the interests of the Jewish people as a whole, but only those who conformed to their rite and maintained a certain standard of wealth, power and influence'.[10] Nevertheless, taking a step back we can see that Sephardim were beholden to certain myths about the Ashkenazim and themselves that were in some respects anachronistic.

To fill out some of Stokes's broad assertions, let us turn to Vivian Lipman's classic and still useful *Social history of the Jews in England 1850–1950*. By 1690, Lipman writes, the Jewish population in England had risen to about '350 to 400 individuals', including a number of Ashkenazim who had begun immigrating from mid-century due to the violence of the Chmielnicki revolt (1648–9) and the disturbed state of Central Europe in general. By 1707 the Ashkenazim community was so large that there were two separate synagogues to minister to its members. Lipman continues that:

> The Ashkenazim were, in the mass, far poorer than the Sephardim and less distinguished in their lineage; there were in the early years very few rich Ashkenazi families. But the Ashkenazim immigrated steadily and, though in 1677 there were only two Ashkenazi names among the 50 Jewish names in the first London directory, they out-paced the Sephardim in numbers from the beginning of the eighteenth century onwards.

Lipman estimates that in 1734 the Anglo-Jewish population stood at 6000, 'and of these half at least must have been Ashkenazim'. By 1753 the population had risen to about 8000, and Lipman looks to a number of pogroms and expulsions that took place in Central Europe in the 18th century to explain the increased Ashkenazi immigration to England,:

causing not only a rise in the total number of the Jewish population but also stimulating its dispersion into the provincial centres. It resulted also in the swelling of the Ashkenazi poor by large numbers, who found a regular livelihood, or any livelihood at all, difficult to earn, and this caused some to turn to a life of crime.[11]

We are now in a position both to appreciate and to challenge Lipman's survey. It begins with the almost organically rooted character of post-Readmission Sephardim, and ends with the precarious mass of Ashkenazim, whose marginal status is exemplified by the unmistakable stigma of criminals in their midst. First, let us ask: how insubstantial, or not, were the Ashkenazim in London at the end of the 17th century?[12] There were, as is well known, sufficient numbers to found a synagogue by 1690. But this does not necessarily indicate a miniscule or impotent community.[13] As Cecil Roth and then David Katz inform us, non-Sephardi Jews – especially if they were up-and-comers – tended to join the Sephardi synagogue. There even were some, especially those from Hamburg, who were membersof both the older, Sephardic synagogue and the new, Ashkenazi, one.[14]

So the founding of a specifically Ashkenazi congregation did not simply mean that there was a *minyan*, a prayer quorum of ten men, but that there was pressure to recognize and assert a separate identity. When the frame of reference is such a small community, the establishment of even a single *shul* (temple), able to secure its own premises, is far from negligible. But the affairs of the community suggest that early Ashkenazim were not just a community of *Luftmenschen*.[15] One of the first important, schismatic quarrels before 1700 featured 'Abraham [Nathan] of Hamburg, a man both rich and learned . . . and Marcus Moses . . . the son-in-law of Glückel of Hameln, the German-Jewish female Pepys'. Albert Hymanson continues, '[I]n addition to the political reasons for an absence of sympathy between these two men, there were personal ones. Both were East India merchants and trade rivals'.[16] Clearly, against the stereotype of impoverished Ashkenazim, these were 'men of substance and wealth, influential merchants, bringing considerable capital into the country'.[17] At that time, '[t]he most important overseas trade of the Jewish community . . . was in Indian diamonds'; the leading traders counted Sephardim and Ashkenazim.[18]

Although I do not intend to indulge the 'great man' theory of history, we must acknowledge that this was a period in which individuals mattered a great deal to the life of the small community and its image to the world at large. Surely Benjamin Levy, from Hamburg, was one of Anglo-Jewry's heavyweights. A broker on the Royal Exchange, he had his hand in 'almost every significant area of English commercial enterprise. He was the second name on the register of the newly organized East India Company in 1698, and was a very considerable shareholder. From 1688 he was a member of the Royal African Company. Indeed, [he] was a prominent figure not only among Jews, but in the Gentile business community as well . . . The very financial prominence of Bejamin Levy . . . was a communal problem in the making'.[19] Only furthering his prominence in the community, Levy's family had, according to Cecil Roth, connections to 'some of the best-known Rabbis of the age'.[20]

Down the social ladder the surname 'Pollack' became very common, indicating the growing Polish-Lithuanian origins of the community.[21] In addition, there were numerous unregistered families, especially from Poland, 'who did not immediately settle in new homes permanently . . . but lived successively in various countries in the

West'.[22] Indeed, it is often forgotten there were many notable areas of Jewish settlement containing appreciable numbers of Sephardim and Ashkenazim, such as Amsterdam, Budapest, Vienna, Trieste, Istanbul, Bucharest and Sofia.

In Lipman's précis, although the existence of Ashkenazim is taken into account, it is underscored in contrast to the Sephardim, particularly by their supposed vast disparity in wealth. But there also were poor, even destitute Sephardim in the first generations.[23] A major share of Sephardi synagogue income went into local poor relief among their own; others formed a pre-industrial, static lumpenproletariat.

> The most concentrated influx of poor Sephardim came in the period 1720-35 as a consequence of renewed activity on the part of the Inquisition in Spain and Portugal. During these years, approximately fifteen hundred new Christians arrived directly from the peninsula – an enormous addition to the local Sephardi community, which numbered only a little more than one one thousand persons in 1720.[24]

Todd Endelman shows that rather than being exclusively elite, Sephardim followed the supposedly quintessential Ashkenazi pursuits, such as street traders, beggars, itinerant peddlers and crooks – who were ubiquitious in the Sephardi world of the 17th and 18th centuries.[25] Of the less than 3000 Sephardim who came to Britain in the 18th century, the clear majority were impoverished. Although most of the Ashkenazi immigrants were very poor, by the 1740s, there had been a significant number of Ashkenazim who had arrived in England with 'Shutzbriefe from German governments and thus entered the ranks of the local Jewish "aristocracy".'[26]

I shall conclude by recalling some major characteristics of the Ashkenazi community proper. By the third decade of the 18th century, Endelman argues, the Ashkenazim already outnumbered the Sephardim. In 1750, there were around 7000 Jews in the country, with Ashkenazim estimated at two-thirds to three-quarters of the total. Vivian Lipman estimates that before 1750, around 6000 Ashkenazim had come to Britain. Therefore, these robust numbers allowed for the maintenance of the community, as opposed to the earlier, lower numbers of Sephardim – which might not have assured the continuity of Jewry in England. As Moses Shulvass writes, there was a huge population of destitute Jews in the German states, some 10,000, who provided a share of the immigrants moving westward. Even if they were not desperate, most of the Jews in the early Georgian period arrived with neither capital nor specific skills. As Endelman details, they engaged primarily in buying and selling old clothes and other secondhand goods.[27] In some respects Endelman is the Jewish social historian par excellence, in painting a vivid picture of Jewish social structure and life in his discussions of 'peddlers and hawkers' and 'pickpockets and pugilists'. His emphasis is on the life of Jewry beneath the level of the bourgeoisie. Indeed, it was these Jews, and these vocations, precarious as they were, that helped determine the character of Anglo-Jewry – much more than the inherited patterns from the Sephardi world.[28]

Endelman writes that 'as troublesome as the Sephardi poor were to the synagogue authorities, their arrival in England never became a matter of concern to the non-Jewish public. The popular image of the Sephardi Jew was an opulent stockbroker and that of the Ashkenazi Jew a ragged old-clothes man'.[29] What seems to have actually happened, however, was that poor Sephardim tended to merge, in Jewish and non-Jewish popular consciousness, with the growing masses of Ashkenazim, and the wealthy Ashkenazim were lumped together with the Sephardi upper echelon. Endelman infers that the popular view of the Sephardim was largely positive, or at least innocuous, contrasted with that of the Ashkenazim, whose influx was seen as pernicious. Most likely, though, Frank Felsenstein is more accurate to add that 'The awareness among anti-Semitic writers of the period of the distinction between Sephardim and Ashkenazim is at best superficial, but it is a distinction that is deployed to show that Jews, irrespective of their background, whether rich or poor, are everywhere the same in their love of gain and grasping nature'.[30] Moreover, although one may dwell on the important distinctions between portrayals of Sephardim verus Ashkenazim, the fact remains that both were seen as 'distinctly un-English'.[31] Likewise, whether Jews were perceived as having a constructive or destructive influence in the economy through speculative trading, such as in the little-studied South Sea Bubble affair, the very facts of their visibility and leading roles were readily and publicly denounced.[32]

There was indeed a separation between Sephardim and Ashkenazim, but it was not based on as rigid criteria of wealth and *yichus* – that is, pride in one's esteemed forebears – as is often claimed. To no small extent, the Jews at the extreme ends of the social spectrum were judged by conventions and stereotypes that they found ready-made: not only was the Shylock myth in place before the return of the Jews, but the vagabond thief type, who spoke a bizarre 'cant', also emerged on the English cultural scene before real live Jews entered on to the stage.[33] But most importantly, it probably is mistaken to see the notables of the Sephardim as Anglo-Jewry's founders, as they generally went over the brink into what Todd Endelman has called 'radical assimilationism'.[34] With impetus from a number of directions, the fates of the two communities would forever be intertwined, while the biological basis of Anglo-Jewry, the font of its continuity, would ultimately derive from the Askenazim. But the myth of Sephardim, as elite and avant-garde for the most part holds firm, in England and beyond. As Yosef Hayim Yerushalmi has written, academic history, such as that of Endelman and Katz, seems to have had little influence on popular consciousness.[35] Neither component of the community, however, should be thought to have had a monopoly on either the sages or scoundrels of their time. What Ismar Schorsch has termed 'the romance of Spain'36 served and continues to serve Anglo-Jewry as a means to distance itself from its East European origins, from which it is prone to recoil.

NOTES

1   Todd M. Endelman, *The Jews of Georgian England, 1714-1830: tradition and change in a liberal society* (Philadelphia, 1979) and David S. Katz, *The Jews in the history of England, 1485–1850* (Oxford, 1994).

2   Moses Shulvass, *From East to West: the westward migration of Jews from Eastern Europe during the seventeenth and eighteenth centuries* (Detroit, 1971); Gedalyah Yogev, *Diamonds and coral: Anglo-Dutch Jews and eighteenth-century trade* (Leicester, 1978); Harold Pollins, *Economic history of the Jews in England* (East Rutheford, NJ, 1982); Cecil Roth, *The Great Synagogue, London, 1690–1940* (London, 1950); Vivian Lipman, *Social history of the Jews in England 1850–1950* (London, 1954); Albert M. Hyamson, *A history of the Jews in England* (London, 1908; repr. 1928).

3   Bernard Glassman, *Anti-Semitic stereotypes without Jews: images of Jews in England,*

1290–1700 (Detroit, 1975); Frank Felsenstein, *Anti-Semitic stereotypes: a paradigm of otherness in English popular culture, 1660–1830* (Baltimore, 1995); James Shapiro, *Shakespeare and the Jews* (New York, 1996); John Gross, *Shylock: a legend and its legacy* (New York, 1994); Martin D. Yaffe, *Shylock and the Jewish Question* (Baltimore, 1997).

4 Stephen Birmingham, *'Our Crowd': the great Jewish families of New York* (New York, 1967); Stephen Birmingham, *'The Rest of Us': the rise of America's East European Jews* (Boston, 1984); Stephen Birmingham, *The Grandees: America's Sephardic elite* (New York, 1971).

5 Steven Aschheim, *Brothers and strangers: the East European Jew in German and German Jewish consciousness, 1800–1923* (Madison. WI, 1982); Jack Wertheimer, *Unwelcome strangers: East European Jews in Imperial Germany* (New York, 1987).

6 Max J. Kohler, 'The Unamerican character of race legislation', originally in *Annals of the American Academy of Political and Social Science* 84:2 (1909), 275–93; reprinted in Max J. Kohler, *Immigration and aliens in the United States: studies of American immigration laws and the legal status of aliens in the United States* (New York, 1936), 131–8.

7 Ismar Schorsch, 'The myth of Sephardic supremacy' in *Leo Baeck Institute Year Book* 34 (1989), 47–66.

8 H. P. Stokes, *A short history of the Jews in England* (London, 1921), 77.

9 *Ibid.*, 80.

10 *Ibid.*, 180–2.

11 Lipman, 5–6.

12 Katz, 180.

13 Shulvass, 73; Hymanson, 190ff.

14 Hymanson, 191.

15 Katz, 204ff.

16 Hymanson, 192. The 'Memoirs' of Glückel von Hameln provide details the affairs of Jewish families in Hamburg, many members of which settled in London.

17 *Ibid.*, 190.

18 Katz, 176–7, citing Gedalyah Yogev and Harold Pollins.

19 *Ibid.*, 180–1.

20 Roth, 4.

21 Shulvass, 42–3.

22 *Ibid.*, 63.

23 Endelman, 167–71.

24 *Ibid.*, 168.

25 *Ibid.*, chap. 5.

26 Shulvass, 74; Anton Rexhausen, *Die rechtliche und wirtschaftliche Lage der Juden in Hochstift Hildesheim* (Hildesheim, 1914), 130, 151–7; *Festschrift zum 200 jährigen Bestehen des israelistischen Vereins für Krankenpflege und Beerdigung Chevra Kaddischa zu Königsberg* i.Pr. (Königsberg, 1904), 6.

27 Endelman, ch. 5.

28 *Ibid.*, 166–226.

29 *Ibid.*, 171.

30 Felsenstein, 52.

31 *Ibid.*, 53.

32 Stokes, 77; see Edward Chancellor, *Devil take the hindmost: a history of financial speculation* (Basingstoke, 1999).

33 Thomas Harman, *The Groundworke of Conny-catching; the manner of their Pedlers-French, and the meanes to understand the same, with the cunning flights of the Counterfeit Crank* (London, 1579); Juan Hidalgo, *Romances de germania . . . con el volcabulario por la orden del a.b.c.* (1609); Captain Charles Johnson (i.e. Captain Alexander Smith), *A general*

history of the lives and adventures of the most famous highwaymen, murderers, street-robbers, etc. from the famous Sir John Falstaff to the Reign of K. Henry IV (London, 1736), 9, 373, 384; see Michael Berkowitz, 'Unmasking counterhistory: an introductory exploration of criminality and the Jewish Question', in Richard Wetzell and Peter Becker (eds.), *The criminal and his scientists in the nineteenth century* (forthcoming).

34   Todd Endelman, *Radical assimilationism in English Jewish History 1656–1945* (Bloomington, IN, 1990).

35   Yosef Hayim Yerushalmi, *Zakhor: Jewish history and Jewish memory* (Seattle, 1996).

36   Schorsch, 47.

27

Slaves or free people? The status of Africans in England, 1550–1750

PETER D. FRASER

The status of Africans in England in the two centuries before 1750 seems to be straight-forward. The normal assumption is that Africans in England were slaves. In this paper the argument is that such an assumption should not be made so easily; that the historiography has contributed to this assumption but that it arises from a particular perspective on the relations between Europe and Africa which over-emphasizes the slave trade and misreads in the case of England the timing of slavery in the Atlantic colonies; that a more refined chronology is possible and that only a closer examination of the surviving records of African people in England can bring us closer to an understanding of the status of Africans in Britain. What follows re-examines the secondary literature though it does look fleetingly at some original sources.

The slave status of Africans in Britain has been a consistent theme of the literature. In the first work on Africans in Britain, Edward Scobie's pioneering effort, we read: 'There were slaves in the British colonies of the Caribbean and in British North America; but more important, at least as far as this work is concerned, these Britons were slaves in Britain . . . These Britons were black . . . And it is with them that much of *Black Britannia* deals.'[1] Walvin's work, which appeared a year later, starts with the voyage of John Lok in 1555 and his importation of five slaves into England. It situates the arrival of Africans in England in the context of the developing slave trade of the Iberian powers and English interest in it.[2] Shyllon, in *Black slaves in Britain,* questions Walvin's assumption that the African men brought back to England by Lok's voyage were slaves (he thinks they were translators) but continues, 'But those Africans who followed them were slaves and formed the first permanent black settlers in Britain'.[3] In his second work, *Black people in Britain, 1555–1833,* Shyllon provides a more nuanced analysis. Here he points to the uncertainty of status until the early 17th century and the real development of English involvement in the slave trade coinciding with the success of Caribbean plantations.[4] Fryer briefly introduces a longer association with Britain, points to the sporadic nature of the trade and then moves on to the Atlantic context.[5] His second chapter is introduced by a section subtitled 'Sugar and Slavery' which amplifies this context.[6] Ramdin explicitly links the slave trade with the presence of Africans in Britain. His first chapter, entitled 'Profits, Slavery and the Black Poor', starts with two sections 'Slavery' and 'Profits' and then deals with black servants in England.[7] The most recent work, Gerzina's *Black England: life before emancipation*, follows Fryer closely in sketching in the early history and settling on transatlantic slavery as the defining issue for the status of Africans in Britain.[8] What we have is fairly universal agreement that the status of Africans in Britain in these centuries was from the beginning determined by the existence of slavery in the Americas and of the slave trade to the Americas. Since slavery existed there the Africans in Britain could only be slaves in Britain, since the only reason that they were in Britain was slavery and the slave trade.

Indeed given the importance of the 18th century, for both the development of the plantations and the beginnings of anti-slavery, most attention is devoted to that century. Gerzina's book, in fact, concentrates on it but even the more general histories and Shyllon's two books on the period to emancipation in 1834 pay more attention to this century, especially the second half. Hence the earlier period and any attempt to analyse the development of the status of Africans in Britain are neglected.

This interpretation of Africans in Britain is reinforced by discussions of what is really a separate issue. The image of Africa and Africans in travellers' writings and imaginative literature from the earliest contacts had stressed African distinctiveness.[9] What is often not noticed is how these descriptions commonly precede fairly mundane accounts of ordinary trading relations with Africans. The 1554/5 voyage of John Lok is famous because of the 'certain black slaves' brought back by him. The account of the voyage contains many disparaging comments on Africans but dwells on the great quantity of gold and ivory obtainable there[10] and comments on the Africans he had to deal with, 'They are a very wary people in their bargaining, and they will not lose one sparke of gold of any value. They use weights and measures, and are very circumspect in occupying the same. They that shall have to doe with them must use them gently: for they will not traffique or bring in any wares if they are evill used.'[11] The mixture of negative images and fairly complimentary descriptions of the Africans they actually encountered is a feature of these writings. Near the end of the century Richard Rainolds and Thomas Dassel would be interested in what commodities different regions or towns had, and were less impressed by the Portuguese and the Spaniards than by the Africans they encountered. At the end of the account they mention Spanish and Portuguese involved in the trade 'resident by permission of the Negros'.[12] These early accounts do not present Africans as extraordinary beings.

The need to examine closely the nature of European relationships with Africans in order to understand the status of Africans in Britain can be seen if we examine two important elements of the argument. First the context of English New World slavery and then the context of the slave trade with Africa. The first point to make is that slavery had ceased to exist in England at the time of the 16th-century voyages of discovery, plunder and slave trading. The re-creation of this status in the Americas becomes very important as it is the transatlantic existence of slavery that makes Africans slaves in England. An examination of the history of slavery in the American colonies produces some well-known but, in the context of slavery of Africans in Britain, neglected features. In Virginia for instance the slave status was not defined in a way that marked it off from that of contract labourers definitively until the end of the 17th century. Though Africans were treated differently from European contract labourers in that they served for life rather than a fixed term of years, it was not decided until the 1690s that their status was different in that it was inherited by their children. In the Caribbean islands, not settled until the 1620s by England, slavery took some time to establish itself. The initial source of labour was indentured servants from the British Isles; when in 1626 some Africans were taken to St Kitts they worked along-side indentured servants and their status was not defined differently. The 1640s and 1650s when sugar was introduced marked the real change in the source and status of labour in the English Caribbean. The Barbadians had in 1636 considered the status of Amerindians and Africans and decided that both were bound for life. They had thus anticipated the effects of the sugar revolution. In 1638 only a tenth of the 2000 servants in Barbados were Africans; by 1660 Africans outnumbered Europeans there and were classed as slaves. The Dutch had introduced both sugar and the slave work force from Brazil. The Barbadians had established that difference much more quickly than the Virginians, taking a few decades rather than nearly a century, and influenced attitudes in the Carolinas, which were settled from Barbados.[13] The conquest of New York by the British had produced a similar hardening of boundaries compared to the previous Dutch status.[14] So one element of the chronology is this: before the mid-17th century the pressure from the colonials to define the status of Africans in Britain (or at least those brought to Britain from the colonies) would not always have consisted of an attempt to claim ownership, rather than to assert the contractual relationship between master and servant. The American colonies did not all have the same legal status for Africans before the end of the 17th century.

The context of the slave trade with Africa provides a second important element in constructing a chronology. The early northern European traders with Africa were interested chiefly in gold and ivory, not slaves since for them slaves could only be smuggled into Iberian colonies.[15] Up to 1580 the best estimates suggest only 1000 Africans transported in British vessels to the Americas; from 1580 to 1640 only 4000 in British vessels to British colonies. From 1640 to 1700 371,000 were trans-ported, 271,000 of them to British colonies. In the first six decades of the 18th century the figures reached 1,286,000, of whom 971,000 went to British colonies.[16] As Colin Palmer writes, 'the English were relative late-comers to the trade in human beings'; very few people following John Hawkins's pioneering efforts of the mid-16th century.[17] The database of slave voyages confirms this: it shows 13 voyages from British ports in the 16th century, none in the quarter century to 1625, three between 1626 and 1650, [18] in the next quarter century and 468 in the last. The quantity of gold exported continued to increase in the course of the 17th century and Eltis[19] writes that 'Overall, commodity exports were much more valuable than their slave counterparts in the last third of the 17th century.'[20] From the beginning of the 18th century the export of slaves quickly established a primacy that was unmatched until the 19th century. The implications of this are that New World slavery was not the only, or even the most important, economic setting for European/African relations for three-quarters of these first two centuries. To the mercantile and shipping inter-ests Africa did not immediately mean slavery in this period as it would in the 18th century.

If we turn to the slave trade itself an important feature tends to be neglected. The *demand* for slaves was driven by the European colonies in the Americas and the transatlantic trade was in the hands of Europeans. Europeans, however, did not *control* the African side of the trade. Africans controlled trade down to the coast. Klein notes that the early experiences of traders stealing Africans for the slave trade were isolated and soon ceased.[21] The Europeans most in contact with Africans in Africa had to deal with them as superiors or equals, until, that is, they purchased them as slaves and transported them across the Atlantic. We have already noted John Lok's Africans described as slaves: as Shyllon correctly points out they were interpreters for the traders rather than commodities in the trade.[22] As at the beginning of these two centuries so at the end. Gerzina recounts the fuss that could still occur if non-slave Africans were stolen. The case of Prince William Ansah Sessaroko who instead of being taken to London to be educated was sold into slavery had international repercussions in the 1740s. His father, rightly annoyed, was prepared to favour French over British interests and was only placated when his son was freed, and feted in London.[23] Balancing the growing weight of the slave trade was the continued importance of African power at the point of sale. Referring to the 18th century Peter Wood remarks 'Most colonists would have marvelled at the ignorance of their descendants, who asserted blindly that all Africans looked the same.'[24] Europeans in dealing with Africans in Africa and with purchasing Africans had good reasons to make distinctions. The power relations on the African coasts also explain why the early accounts collected by Hakluyt show Africans as such ordinary human beings after the original extravagant descriptions. One trades with humans, not monsters or mythical creatures.

With these modifications to the usually presented picture of Africans in Britain we can now look at the cases which did involve the legality of slavery in Britain in this period. Right at the beginning of the period, in 1569, there was a case involving a Russian slave brought to England where the famous statement appears to have been made that 'England was too pure an Air for slaves to breathe in'. A hundred years later we appear to have the first case involving an African slave where those ringing words went unheeded. In Butts versus Penny it was decided that the slave status did exist in England since merchants bought and sold them 'and also being infidels, there might be a property in them . . . ' In 1694 this was reaffirmed in Gelly versus Cleve. Those were contradicted by Chief Justice Holt who in 1698 and 1701 decided that slavery as a status was not recognized in English law (Chamberlain versus Harvey and Smith versus Brown and Cooper). In 1706 Holt ruled that 'By the common law no man can have property in another'.[25] Shyllon rightly points out that these cases left the law in confusion, but fails to note the source of the confusion. What we have here is the Caribbean and American owners of slaves trying to assert rights derived from a legal status which existed in the colonies but not in England. The opinion in 1729 of the Attorney and Solicitor Generals, Yorke and Talbot, in 1729, is seen by Shyllon and others as produced by the West India interest wanting to impose this status in England. He describes it as a charter for slave hunters.[26] He does note that Mansfield described its status accurately as given in Lincoln's Inn Hall after dinner and therefore not to be taken seriously. Yorke, however, when he had become Lord Chancellor Hardwicke in 1749, reaffirmed his position in a more authoritative fashion in Pearne versus Lisle.[27] Yet a year later Baron Thompson in Galway versus Cadee declared that a man became free on setting foot in England. In 1762, before Mansfield's less straightforward judgement, Lord Chancellor Northington ruled similarly in Shanley versus Harvey.[28] Thus the legal opinions on the status of Africans in England remained an unsettled one throughout the period. The weight, however, of judicial opinion appears to be against the legality of slavery in Britain. Even the early 18th century swing in favour of it, coinciding as it does with the expansion of the New World slave colonies and involvement in the slave trade, is not decisive.

What we seem to have for understanding the status of Africans in England before 1750 is this. The economic relations between West Africa and England (indeed with Europe in general) had more to do with gold and ivory than slaves until the end of the 17th century. The power relations at the African end of the slave trade were firmly in favour of Africans right until the end of the trade. Across the Atlantic the number of Africans shipped into British (to use the wider term, following Eltis) possessions was small until the mid-17th century, rose dramatically from then on but grew even more quickly in the first half of the 18th century. To sum up then: in defining the relationship between Africans and Europeans the weight of West Atlantic slavery did not really tell until the end of the 17th century. The status of Africans in the Americas, though seemingly different from the beginnings of the transatlantic trade, is not in the English/British colonies firmly defined everywhere as being entirely different in kind from those of Europeans until Virginian decisions at the end of the 17th century. Thus the pressure from the American colonists to define the status of Africans in Britain is not unequivocally in favour of the distinctive slave status until the end of the 17th century. If we examine the evidence adduced about the status of Africans in Britain we see clearly confusion continuing throughout the period until in mid-century the nascent pro- and anti-slavery forces bring into being clearer definitions.

An examination of the Africans mentioned in most of the histories presents an equally mixed picture. Plainly the people mentioned in the legal cases and the advertisements for runaways were perceived as slaves by their owners, who would have had no problems in the colonies asserting those rights (if they were able to recapture and return home with them). In 1690 the interesting case of Katherine Auker reflected that dual status. She had been 'a servant to one Robert Rich, a planter in Barbadoes, and ... about six years since she came to England with her master and mistress; she was baptised ... after which her said master and mistress tortured and turned her out: her said master refusing to give her a discharge, she could not be entertained in service elsewhere. The said Rich caused her to be arrested and imprisoned ... Prays to be discharged from the said master, he being in Barbadoes.' The court ruled that she 'shall be at liberty to serve any person until such time as the said Rich shall return from Barbadoes'. Shyllon seems to see this case as an instance of judicial indecisiveness.[29] But what it does seems perfectly clear. Katherine Auker is treated like a servant in England – though slaves could be and were hired out, they could not hire themselves out without their master's permission even during their owner's absence. In her master's presence in England their contract remains in force – if returned to Barbados she would presumably revert to slave status. As English law overrode colonial law English judges could have ruled that slavery did not exist in the colonies but they were never confronted with a case of that nature.

All the histories describe black people who live in Britain performing a variety of different roles, though these are on the whole among the poor and powerless of society. Most are in domestic service, though some were servants in very grand homes. If we examine two attempts to locate, chiefly in parish records, all Africans in two London boroughs we find the same ambiguity of status. Of the 14 people baptised or buried at the churches of All Saints, Fulham and St Paul's, Hammersmith, between 1679 and 1750, two are described as servants (one of whom may not be African but is named

John Niger) and the others are described by their colour.[30] Hammersmith and Fulham were small districts of London well to the west of Greenwich, which not surprisingly with its maritime connections, boasts many more. Between 1593 and 1750 Joan Anim-Addo discovered 38 people, mainly in the parish records of churches in Greenwich, Woolwich, Lee and Charlton. Most of these were male – 26 (the same holds true of the Hammersmith and Fulham records), and a few are described as servants – the rest are described by colour.[31] A few children, including the two sons and a daughter of a black sailor, John Pady, appear in the baptismal records. What these records do not allow us to do is to resolve the issue of their status.

The conclusions cannot be definite. Until the records of Africans in Britain in these two centuries are slowly assembled (from parish records, newspapers, private papers and visual evidence) and analysed it would be foolish to come to hasty conclusions. What this paper has tried to do is to look again at the evidence for the slave status of Africans in Britain offered by previous writers and suggest that it is not as firm as it would appear. Who these Africans were, residing in Britain, temporarily or permanently, cannot be easily discovered nor can their legal status easily be determined.

NOTES

My thanks to Professor Ken Parker for prodding me and helping by his own work to change my thinking on the issue.

1   Edward Scobie, *Black Britannia: a history of blacks in Britain* (Chicago, 1972), vii. It should be noted that the same assumption is made in the work cited in note 30.
2   James Walvin, *Black and white: the Negro and English society, 1555–1945* (London, 1973), 1–2.
3   F. O. Shyllon, *Black slaves in Britain* (London, 1974), 2.
4   Folarin Shyllon, *Black people in Britain, 1555–1833* (London, 1977), 6–8.
5   Peter Fryer, *Staying power: the history of black people in Britain* (London, 1984), 1–10.
6   *Ibid.*, 14–19.
7   Ron Ramdin, *The making of the black working class in Britain* (Aldershot, 1987), 1–18.
8   Gretchen Gerzina, *Black England: life before emancipation* (London, 1995), 3–6.
9   Winthrop D. Jordan, *White over black: American attitudes toward the Negro, 1550–1812* (Chapel Hill, NC, 1968).
10   Richard Hakluyt, *Voyages of the Elizabethan seamen to America* (8 vols., London, 1907), vol. 4, 57–8. See 54–5 for the gold and ivory.
11   *Ibid.*, 63.
12   Hakluyt, vol. 5, 44–52.
13   Betty Wood, *The origins of American slavery: freedom and bondage in the English colonies* (New York, 1997), 42–55. For more detailed accounts of American slavery see Ira Berlin, *Many thousands gone: the first two centuries of slavery in North America* (Cambridge, MA, 1998) and Peter Kolchin, *American slavery, 1619–1877* (London, 1933). For Caribbean slavery see P. C. Emmer (ed.), *General history of the Caribbean, vol. 2: New societies: the Caribbean in the long sixteenth century* (London, 1999) and Franklin W. Knight (ed.), *General history of the Caribbean, vol. 3: The slave societies of the Caribbean* (London, 1997).
14   Renal Williams, *African Americans and colonial legislation in the Middle Colonies* (New York, 1998), 20.
15   Herbert S. Klein, *The Atlantic slave trade* (Cambridge, 1999), 76.

16 David Eltis, *The rise of African slavery in the Americas* (Cambridge, 2000), 9, Table 1–1.

17 Colin A. Palmer, 'The slave trade, African slaves and the demography of the Caribbean to 1750' in *General history of the Caribbean*, 16.

18 David Eltis, Stephen D. Behrendt, David Richardson and Herbert S. Klein, *The transatlantic slave trade: a database on CD-Rom* (Cambridge, 1999).

19 Eltis, 150.

20 See also Klein, 77.

21 Klein, 103; see also John Thornton, *Africa and Africans in the making of the Atlantic world, 1400–1800* (2nd edn., Cambridge, 1998) for the status of Africans in their dealings with Europeans.

22 Shyllon, *Black slaves*, 2.

23 Gerzina, 11–12.

24 Quoted in Daniel C. Littlefield, *Rice and slaves: ethnicity and the slave trade in colonial South Carolina* (Baton Rouge, 1981), 8.

25 Shyllon, *Black people*, 17. The 1569 case concerned a man called Cartwright. Shyllon's reference is to John Rushworth, *Historical collections of private passages of state* (London, 1680–1722), vol. 2, 468.

26 Shyllon, *Black people*, 20; *Black slaves*, 27.

27 Shyllon, *Black slaves*, 26.

28 *Ibid.*, 25.

29 *Ibid.*, 10–11.

30 Peter Fraser, *Before* Windrush: *the early black presence in Hammersmith and Fulham* (London, 2000), 3–4.

31 Joan Anim-Addo, *Sugar, spices and human cargo: an early black history of Greenwich* (London, 1996), 65–8.

The first Turks and Moors in England

Nabil Matar

Muslims were the first non-Christian and non-European people to have extensive relations with England. From the early modern period during Elizabeth's reign, Arab Maghribis traveled from Tunisia, Algeria and the independent kingdom of Morocco, as did Turks from the far reaches of the Ottoman Empire, to English and Welsh coastal towns, and to the royal centre in London. Ambassadors came with exotic gifts and with diplomatic and commercial treaties, while merchants brought with them mineral and food resources in exchange for industrial products, chiefly textiles. These Muslim visitors came to trade, negotiate, learn, observe and return with information about the *nasara*, i.e. the Christians of the north. Many of them were so curious about this new land and asked so many questions that they were suspected of being spies for their ruler – as was the Moroccan ambassador in 1600.[1] There was curiosity as well as espionage in the Muslim experience of England.

This paper will examine the earliest Muslims who came to England and left their mark on English life and society. First, there were the Turks and Moors who converted to Christianity: very few in number in the early modern period (1558–1685), these converts ceased to be Muslim although they continued to be designated as 'Turks' by their new co-religionists. Like the New Christians in Iberia, these converts were tested and investigated before they were, if ever, accepted as equal to 'true-born Englishmen'. Secondly, there were groups of captives who were brought to England in the 1620s and after: their records provide a unique source of social and regional information about the earliest Muslims in Britain.

Converts

The very first Muslim about whom some information has survived arrived in England in the mid 1580s. A Turk, born in Negropont, aged 45, was captured by William Hawkins aboard a Spanish ship and was brought to England. After a while, Chinano, which is the name given to him, probably from Sinan, grew to admire the virtuous life of the English Protestants, in contrast of course with the Spanish Papists, and decided to convert to Anglicanism and settle in England. The conversion took place in October 1586 and was conducted by the minister, Meredith Hanmer, at the Hospital of St

Katherine. The Turk confessed his new faith in Spanish, was baptized, and was given the Christian name of William.[2] Around two decades later another Muslim, converted to Anglicanism, was given the name John Baptista, after which he started receiving an allowance of 6 pence per diem to sustain himself.[3] Baptista, 'Horatio', who was baptized on 12 July 1606 in Mevagissey, Cornwall, and possibly other converts, raised English hopes about the conversion of the Muslims to Anglican Christianity.[4] In Thomas Middleton's *The Triumphs of Truth*, the poet presented a Moor and many of his people who had converted to Christianity as a result of the missionary effort of the English:

> My queen and people all, at one time won
> By the religious conversation
> Of English merchants, factors, travellers,
> Whose Truth did with our spirits hold commerce,
> As their affairs with us: following their path,
> We all were brought to the true Christian faith:
> Such benefit in good example dwells,
> It oft hath power to convert infidels.[5]

In 1624, one Salleman Alexander was baptized in London, and two others, 'Richard a poore Turke' and an unnamed Turk, in 1628.[6] But the most famous Muslim convert was Iusuf 'the Turkish Chaous' who was baptized on 30 January 1658. Although the official account of his conversion was published in that year,[7] there was another account that added significant details about the man and his background.

BM Harley 7575, fos. 19–23 present an overview of the conversion. Born in Constantinople, Isuf (Yusuf/Joseph) served the sultan as ambassador. He travelled to Venice, Muscovy and Vienna where, on one occasion, he resided for 18 months. One of his Christian slaves began preaching to him about Christ and, despite being beaten and silenced, the slave was so relentless in his evangelism that he finally prevailed and Isuf was convinced of the truth of Christianity. Apprehensive of the punishment he would receive were he to declare his new faith, Isuf decided to leave his family and country. After two years he was able to get to Smyrna and from there to Leghorn, Marseilles and Paris where he was put in the hands of priests who were to instruct him in the Catholic faith. The priests failed, however, to convince him of certain tenets of Catholicism (veneration of saints and the actual presence in the host), as a result of which he was left alone, 'troubled to find himself yoked with men of such a belief'.

Two Arabs who had been converted to Protestantism and who were living in Paris told him about another Christianity which was free of 'superstition, whereupon he resolved to be brought unto the Protestants of Paris'. Evidently Protestants in Paris had international connections that reached as far as the Levant, and were active in proselytizing even in the midst of Catholic society. Isuf succeeded in escaping from the priests and was taken by the two Arabs to a 'Protestant house, & became acquainted with the Ministers of Paris'. He embraced Protestantism but was soon pursued by the priests, so it was decided that he should escape to England, which he did in March 1657. Upon reaching London, he went for an audience with the Lord Protector who appointed him 'a livelihood' and put him under the care of Dr John Durie.

The converted but not yet baptized Isuf filled his time by mixing with merchants of the Turkey Company and with some French men. Dr Durie spied on him and quizzed those acquaintances on the Turk's faith. Upon being assured of Isuf's sincerity, he recommended, first, that he be

> boarded and lodged with some understanding honest Christian, who would at a reasonable rate provide one to teach him to read, write, & speak English at certain hours of the day.
> Secondly he should be made accquainted with Mr. Calandorne the Dutch Minister who speaks Italian, & with the Minister of the Italian Church who should with Mr. Despagne & my self be obliged to take some turns to converse with him till we judge it fit that he should be publickly baptized.

The Turk was baptized on Sunday, 3 January 'in the Afternoon Mr. Dury preached a Sermon concerning the Nature & Institution of Baptism, the Text was Acts 10.47'.

The account of the conversion of Isuf not only shows the range of experiences which a Muslim of a high social rank had in England – not all would be boarded or given audience with the ruler – but demonstrated the vitality of the Stranger Churches in the city during the Cromwellian period. London was crowded with Continental Protestants who were all members of linguistic/national churches: the French, the Italian, the Dutch, and if the two 'Arabians' accompanied Isuf to England, even an 'Arabian' Protestant church. Those churches were interassociated and came together with their theological and possibly financial resources when they met a common cause – as in this case of winning the soul of a Turk to Christ. To Isuf, London must have appeared quite an international and hospitable city since it had so many different ethnic communities with their own national, Protestant churches.

Captives

On 12 February 1625, a list was made of 'The names of the Turks & Moors taken by the English and demanded by the king and Diwans of Argeir'. It is the first *list* of Muslims in England, containing information on more than single individuals. The names, as far as they can be deciphered from the poor Spanish text, are the following:

> Haj Hamed bin haj Ibrahim Valentiano, from Candia/ Crete, 30 years old, who had been captured by a Genoan ship;
> Mustafa Cullogli;
> Hamed a Shareef Bin Hamad;
> Hamed of Cordoba, 25 years old, who was captured near Malaga;
> Hamed bin Gambora who was a slave in Gibraltar;
> Abdullah bin Renolt;
> A negress, Masouta, who was with Thomas Button;
> Ibrahim Tlemsani;
> Ali Tagarimo in Alacante;
> Yusuf Tollogly, a Tunisian, who was seized in Calais.
> There were also nine more 'Turkes & mores in Barnett Seames Custody Dwelling in devonshir neare totnas'.[8]

These 19 men (and one woman) came from all over the Islamic Mediterranean: from the Andalus to Tunis, and from Tlemsan to Crete; there were also Turks, such as Mustafa Cullogli and Arabs/Moors, such as the shareef Bin Hamed.

A day later, and in the west of England, in Exeter, a group of Muslim prisoners was tried before Sir John Eliot at the Admiralty Sessions. In a letter to Lord Admiral Buckingham, Eliot explained that there were 'Turkes & Renegadoes' some of whom 'this yeare came in at Plymouth' and others who had been in prison, two of them for eight years. They were 23 in number, four of whom he had reprieved along with a boy 'young, and not capable of the knowledge or reason of doing good or ill'; the rest were 'all sentenc'd, and if they cannott hereafter meritt Mercie . . . [will be] putt to death'.[9] The list attached to the letter, which refers to 'piratis apud Castrum de Exon', identifies the place of origin of the prisoners: a few were from Constantinople, including 'Mahomet minor', the majority were from Algiers and the rest were European renegades and pirates.[10]

Two months later, the list of captives 'demanded' by Algiers was copied again since King Charles I, who had just acceded to the throne, began negotiating about them with an Algerian messenger to whom he gave audience on 23 April 1625. On 25 April, only three or four 'Turkes or Moores' had been left in Exeter – those whom Eliot had reprieved; the rest must have been executed in accordance with the sentence passed on them. Elsewhere in the country, there were 30 Muslims in Plymouth, three or four in Bristol and 10 in the custody of the Devon baronet, Sir Edward Seymour.[11] Within a year, the numbers had grown, and by June 1626, Sir Francis Basset, vice-admiral of Cornwall, requested directions from the Commissioners of the Navy how to proceed with the 42 Turkish prisoners in his custody.[12]

In a letter to the Duke of Buckingham of 17 June 1626, Bassett had described how the Muslims in his custody were completely ostracized. 'I cannot finde any man so madd as to meddle wth them', he wrote; they were also 'so old as they are unfitt for any service;' still, he was afraid of 'dispos[ing] of them in the Countrey' lest they 'lye so neere the see, as it may be easie for them to steale a Bote, or take a Barque out and escape'.[13] As British captives were dispersed around the country in North Africa, so were Muslim captives dispersed around the country; and as some Britons managed to escape by makeshift boats, so it was feared, would these Moors and Turks. A month later, July, the captives in Plymouth, despairing of their conditions, and obviously unable to escape, resorted to a petition which they addressed to the King. They explained that they had been in 'great distress at Sea' and 'presuming uppon the late league made by his Maj[es]ties Ambassador' and the ruler of Algiers 'put into his Ma[jes]tis port of Plymouth' where they were 'detayned and questioned . . . uppon supposition that they were of Salley'.[14] Despite the translation from Arabic, it is possible to hear the desperate voice of 'Jeffera Reys Captayne Jeffer Ballu basha & 36 more Turkes and Moores in a shippe of Argeir now at Plymouth'.

Upon setting foot in England or Wales, captives and converts, prisoners and boys, would have found themselves strangers in a foreign land. Elizabethan and Jacobean England had no place for the non-Christian at a time when there was barely a place for the non-Anglican. The Act of Supremacy (I Eliz. cap. 1, sect. 15) had aimed at all non-Trinitarians within the Christian spectrum; the Act of Uniformity (cap. 2) had sought to ensure that all subjects attended 'parish church or chapel'. It also included a clause that emphasized that every person who took the oath did so 'upon the true faith of a Christian'. In light of these acts, the compendium for Justices of the Peace in England confirmed that neither 'an Infidell, Pagan, or Iew [could] get any thing within this realme, nor maintaine any action at all'. Muslims in England were thus in an environment that could not accommodate them legally. There was neither a religious nor an administrative framework within which they could be situated.[15]

How Muslims survived in the cold climate of the north, among a society that was used to images of the cruel and bloody 'Turk', is difficult to gauge. Only some of their voices have survived in petitions which they presented to monarchs. In March 1630, a petition was presented to King Charles I from a captive/prisoner from the southern part of Barbary. The petition is in an Englishman's pen to which 'Barkebesha a moore' added his signature in Arabic, of which his first name, Mabrook, is decipherable. The Moor hailed from the territory of Sus in southern Morocco, 'where all the gold commeth' and with whose ruler the king had 'a great and rich trade' – a trade that went back to 'the daies of Queen Elizabeth'. An English ship had been wrecked at Cape Blanco whereupon he, the petitioner, had

> released of late manye of yor suiects ... paying for them chardges of 300 ducatts ... out of his owne purse and sent them home free. Notwithstanding your petitioner is brought here prisoner by some of your marchants, upon bargaines and accounts betright[?] them and one of Sallie in that countrie, with whom your petitioner never made any bargayne or contract.
>
> Yo[u]r peitioner being a straunger thought it his duty to give yo[u]r Ma[jes]ty an account of his coming into your countrie, only desiring to have the honour to kisse yo[u]r Ma[jes]tys hands and knowe if it please your Ma[jes]tie to commaund him any service backe to his Lord and maister.[16]

Evidently, this 'straunger' had been entrapped by some English merchants one of whom was able to bring about his imprisonment.

Clearly, in the 1620s, Muslims were intruding on English life. Scores of Turks and Moors were being captured by British seamen as indiscriminately as Britons were captured by Barbary seamen. It was not always clear to the captors who among the Muslims was the pirate and who was the innocent traveller. That is why in two lists of captured Algerians and Moroccans who were taken on 21 June 1627, there is consistent reference to the professional and social background of the captives. The Algerian captives were the following:

The Names of Turkes & Moores belonging to Algeir taken the 21 of June 1627:
1. Solyman sonne of Mahamet Tailor
2. Mahamet sonne of Achmet, scriuan
3. Hagem Hamet sonne of Zeyn Tailor
4. Causim sonne of Garib shoemaker
5. Solyman sonne of Ally: Button maker
6. Mahamet sonne of Ally mender
7. Ebraim [Ibrahim] sonne of Useph shoemaker
8. Ally sonne of Usyn [Yaseen] Tailor
9. Sayid sonne of Caussim mender
10. Useph sonne of Abdalla soldier
11. Velly [Wali] soldier of Algeir
12. Shaban soldier —
13. Ragep of Algeir soldier
14. Omer sonne of Achmet Tailor
15. Hadgy musud [Maso'od] of Algeir sailor.[17]

The list explains a little about the captives: 1–13 had been away from Algeria for over a year, and while sailing near the English coast, were run ashore by Captain Hart of Dartmouth who had then taken their ship and imprisoned them. Since the capture, 13 others had died, 11–13 had been slaves at Madwill in Spain and had come to Flushing; the last two had come ashore in a tartan at Saltash with five more who were dead. Although there were three soldiers among the captives, the rest belonged to 'small' professions: buttonmaker, tailor, mender, shoemaker, sailor. These men were clearly not dangerous which may explain why they were permitted to go 'wandering and begging about the city of London'. As captives in North Africa often begged money for their ransom, so did these captives. The other list belonged to Moroccans:

> The Names of the Turkes and Moores belonging to Tutuan and Sally in barbery taken the 21 of June 1627:
> 1. Hamet Reys sonne of Yaah [Yahya] of Tutuan seaman
> 2. Mahamet sonne of Usin of Tutuan sailor
> 3. Mahamet sonne of Hussin of Tutuan sailor
> 4. Mahomet Hogy of Sally scriuan
> 5. Mahamet sonne of Achmet of Sally Tailor
> 6. Mussud sonne of Mahamet saylor
> 7. Abdaraman sonne of Ally Lasis sailor
> 8. Mahamet sonne of Mahmout: a boye
> 9. sa sonne of Ally cooke
> 10. Abderhaman sonne of Syd sailor
> 11. Mahamet sonne of Hassan sailor
> 12. Abdalla sonne of Hassan shoemaker
> 13. Ally sonne of Mahamet sailor
> 14. Causin [Qassim] sonne of Hamet: buttin maker
> 15. Umbarac sonne of Ally shippboye
> 16. Mahamet sonne of Achmet shipboye
> 17. Casamuch sonne of Useph [Yusef] shipp boye:
> 18. Hamet sonne of Hussin of Tutuan soldier
> He was a slave at Inn – & was one of those that stole awaye a galley from course & came to flushing.[18]

The first 17 captives had been holding captives in their ship, who, 'taking their opportunitie surprised them, and brought them into Cornwall, where they were imprisoned'. They were kept there for six months. These captives were not permitted to beg because they were viewed as dangerous. But the list interestingly shows a number of boys, a common feature of shipping in the early modern period. Their likely fate would have been the same as that of British ship boys who were seized by Barbary seamen: conversion and integration. Many Muslim boys, captured by Christian seamen, were converted: in a letter from Winchester on 31 October 1636, Dr Robert Mason explained that there were 'two young Moores not above 13 or 14 yeares of age who some think here in regard to the tenderness of their yeares may be made good Christians'. Otherwise, they would be condemned along with the other Moors with whom they had been captured, some to be executed in Portsmouth, and the rest in the Isle of Wight 'in regard to the fear and allarmes they haue given to these parts'.[19]

The early Turks and Moors in England were either converts to Christianity or captives. While the converts could hope to settle in the land, the captives, even those who were innocent buttonmakers and boys, could never become citizens while retaining their Muslim faith. This Christian exclusivity militated against any long-term Muslim-qua-Muslim presence in the British Isles.

A curious exception was the case of a famous Algerian corsair, as he was described in *La Gazette de France* in 1680.[20] Known as Canari, a Christian convert to Islam, he set himself up on the Isle of Wight and attacked Dutch ships, much to the satisfaction of the British Crown. In June 1686, it was reported from Portsmouth that he had seized a Dutch ship, 'laden with wine and brandy' and anchored 'her at St Helen's off the Isle of Wight'; in August, he seized 26 Dutch ships on their way to Algiers.[21] In France, it was reported that he sold his booty in London but that under pressure from the Orangists, merchants refused to buy his goods.[22] Canari protested on the ground that the 1682 treaty between England and Algiers stipulated that the English could sell their wares in Algiers. He demanded reciprocity, which he eventually obtained. He finally left the Isle of Wight and returned to Algiers where he died in 1688.[23] Canari thus may well have been the first Muslim off-shore entrepreneur in Britain.

NOTES

1 For a survey of Muslim ambassadorial visitors to England, see ch. 1 in N. Matar, *Turks, Moors, and Englishmen in the Age of Discovery* (New York, 1999).
2 See my discussion in N. Matar, *Islam in Britain, 1558–1685* (Cambridge, 1998), 126–9.
3 *CSPD, 1603–1610*, 216.
4 I am grateful to conference participant Kathy Chater for this reference.
5 *The Works of Thomas Middleton*, ed. A. H. Bullen (New York, 1964), 243.
6 I owe this information to Dr Claire S. Schen who kindly gave me a copy of her paper, 'England in a Turkish mirror: forming identity c. 1600', presented to the Renaissance Society of America, Florence, March 2000.
7 Thomas White, *A True Relation of the Conversion and Baptism of Isuf the Turkish Chaous, named Richard Christophilus in the presence of a full congregation, Jan. 30 1658 in Covent-Garden where Mr. Manton is Minister* (1658).
8 PRO, SP 71/1/53.
9 PRO, SP 14/183/51.
10 PRO, SP 15/183/51 I.
11 *Acts of the Privy Council, 1625–26*, 31.
12 PRO, SP 16/30/17.
13 PRO, SP 16/30/37.
14 PRO, SP 16/31/104.
15 See my discussion in N. Matar, 'The toleration of Muslims in Renaissance England: practice and theory', in John Christian Laursen (ed.), *Religious toleration: 'the variety of rites' from Cyrus to Defoe* (New York, 1999), 127–8.
16 PRO, SP 71/12/267.
17 PRO, SP 71/1/123.
18 PRO, SP 71/1/124.
19 PRO, SP 16/334/50.
20 *La Gazette de France* (1680), 325.
21 *CSPD, January 1686–May 1687*, 191, 234.
22 *La Gazette de France* (1688), 381.
23 *Ibid.*, 548.

29

Greeks and 'Grecians' in London: the 'other' strangers

CLAIRE S. SCHEN

London's Protestant émigré communities of the 16th and 17th centuries have long drawn historians' attention, but these strangers were not the only refugees or immigrants resident in the increasingly cosmopolitan city. 'Grecians', an indiscriminately labelled group that may have included Greeks, Armenians, Macedonians, 'Assyrians', and others, never attained the size or the status of the French and Dutch Protestant communities in early modern London, or in the history of the city in that period. Laura Hunt Yungblut has estimated that four to five thousand aliens lived in London in the late 16th century, drawing on surviving subsidy counts, but she did not note non-Western Europeans. Yungblut and Andrew Pettegree show an early high in immigration during the Elizabethan period, but the later 17th-century flood of refugees analysed by John Hintermaier eclipsed the 16th-century figures.[1] Many non-Western European refugees, however, appeared in the early 17th century, after the subsidy counts had been made on which Yungblut relies and between these distinct periods of European Protestant immigration. Parochial and civic records after 1600 reveal a group of men (I have found no evidence of women), from parts of the world affected by imperial expansion, war, and piracy, and more diverse than the immigrants often studied by historians.

For my first foray into this project I have analysed churchwardens' accounts, the records of the Court of Aldermen, and the State Papers Domestic. London had 108 parishes (110 including two precincts), but only 62 have extant churchwardens' accounts predating c.1620. Only 15 sets of accounts lack at least one mention of a Greek requesting charity. Greeks and others, including Turks and 'Barbarians', sought charity from parishes. Their claims were buttressed by certificates or letters from the King, the Duke of Buckingham, bishops, or the Lord Admiral or founded on narratives of great suffering under various 'tyrants' – Turks, pirates, Roman Catholics. Briefs describe named refugees, making it possible for the historian to trace supplicants through the city. Personalized details conveyed to churchwardens allow some tracing of unnamed men as well. Many unnamed individuals cannot be easily followed in their perambulations through London, however, because 17th-century churchwardens used imprecise racial and ethnic categories and did not consistently record names. Whether all or any of these men became permanent residents, or were only transient visitors or refugees, has been difficult to determine using parochial records. Perhaps guild records might reveal whether any of these men settled into working lives in the city.

Why did these 'other' refugees come to England? The remarkable expansion of the Ottoman Empire set refugees in motion from parts of the world that had not previously sent many immigrants to England. The fall of Constantinople, for instance, caused Greeks to flee that city. Jonathan Harris has shown that in medieval London, Byzantine wire-drawers were some of the first Greek immigrants, bringing coveted skills with them.[2] Mehmed II, however, brought conquered Greeks back to 'colonize' Istanbul.[3] By the late 16th century, the Ottoman Empire made a frightening and appealing example of imperial and economic power in parishioners' views of the world. Lecturers and ministers read prayers for thanksgiving, to mark the siege of Malta (1565) and the Christian victory over the Ottomans at the Battle of Lepanto (1571). Preachers offered sermons to collect ransoms for captives and to facilitate the penance of apostates.[4] John Awdeley reprinted a Viennese account of the siege of 'Jula' [the fort Gyula] in Hungary that included the prayer of thanksgiving 'for the defense of the Christians agaynst the cruel Turke', Suleiman I, the 'Magnificent' (1520–66), who died during the siege.[5] The English, however, also negotiated trade treaties with the Turks to bypass other European countries trading in the Mediterranean and in the East.[6] The English responded to Spanish, French, and Venetian trade by facilitating piracy in the Mediterranean and supplying goods, including tin and lead for munitions, to the Ottoman Empire. The Ottomans welcomed the addition of the English navy to Spain's distractions in the Mediterranean. Acknowledgement of the chaos on the seas deepened in the early 1620s, when parishes in London hired ringers to proclaim Prince Charles's safe arrival in Spain, through the dangerous seas beset by European, Barbary, and Moorish pirates, on his mission to marry the Spanish infanta.[7]

The Thirty Years War, and more broadly the antagonism between Protestant and Catholic countries, also led western and central European immigrants and refugees to travel or immigrate to London. European Christians played out wars of religion in physical and verbal battle, first having set themselves apart from Judaism and Islam in the model of medieval, united Christianity. Protestant and Catholic reform, however, had shaken this traditional unity. Stories of conversion from Judaism, Islam, and 'papacy' won their tellers small sums and may have evangelized among doubters or excited firm believers who heard the year-end reading of accounts in parishes.[8] The schism in Christianity shaped English responses to these strangers, particularly if they needed Protestant protection.[9] The English curried favour with Greek Orthodox believers, and even the Ottoman Turks, as spiritual allies against Catholics. England sent a Greek printing press to Istanbul in 1627 to publish Protestant tracts, which the Jesuits tried to suppress. The Ottomans temporarily banned the Jesuits from the city in response to the English ambassador's outcry.[10]

Parochial and civic records suggest a variety of refugee and immigrant experiences, with some arriving in London seemingly to stay, and others coming only to solicit aid to return home or to ransom family members from slavery. Marcus Abraham came to the Court of Aldermen in 1608 to ask for relief, but solicited relief in at least five parishes in 1613/14, suggesting that he had remained in the city for five years. The aldermen described him as a 'pore Christian merchant borne in Armenia under the

Dominion of the Turk', but some churchwardens called him a 'Captyve'.[11] 'Marke Abraham an armedian' collected 5s from the churchwardens of St Benet Gracechurch, during John Donne's tenure as rector.[12] Abraham appeared in the accounts of five parishes in 1613/14, with the churchwardens of St Stephen Walbrook calling him 'Greek' rather than Armenian.[13] He may have been religiously Greek Orthodox, but ethnically Armenian, modern distinctions not recognized by 16th- and 17th-century churchwardens. The records of St Mary Magdalene Milk Street suggest a lack of parochial consensus on helping strangers like Abraham: twice in 1613/14 the church-wardens granted him a few shillings, once calling him Armenian and once Greek, but the auditors refused these and other payments.[14] Five other parishes in the same year mentioned an 'Armenian' – including one 'that laye bedred' in St Benet Paul's Wharf.[15] Abraham may not have been the only Armenian in London, however, as St Helen gave 12d to him, a 'poore man', and 18d to an Armenian.[16] Allhallows Staining church-wardens gave 1s to a 'poore Armenian who had lycence to begge for his father and mother whome were taken by the Turks', reinforcing the impression that Abraham may have been a captive.[17]

The variants of Abraham's story – his profession, his captivity, his poverty – echoed the motifs of other Greeks' narratives in London parishes. Londoners knew the risks of overseas trade, as merchants and inhabitants in the city became increasingly cognizant of and dependent upon commerce and a nascent commercial empire.[18] Many parishes regularly granted relief to men and women carrying certificates and briefs, describing their losses by fire and at sea.[19] Even the cityscape reflected this maritime merchant experience and its inherent danger: William Fortune, the churchwarden of Allhallows Staining, recorded spending 8s for the vestrymen's dinner at a nearby tavern called the 'Shipwreck'.[20] Emrys Jones's analysis of rents in 1638 identifies Fortune's parish as one in the lowest category of average rents, less than £5, but despite apparent poverty the parish helped poor merchant strangers who had suffered losses.[21] Allhallows Staining and St Stephen Coleman Street granted small benevolences (1s or a little more) to Theodore Polomby, or Theodore Polun, a Greek who claimed to have lost £3000 at sea.[22] Another Greek merchant, Angelo Jacobus, or Angell Jacob, who 'had all his goods taken by the Turkes', collected a few shillings in 1626/7 in the same two parishes.[23] A Hungarian merchant claimed to have lost three ships to the Turks, worth £10,000.[24]

The motif of captivity coloured strangers' renditions of their suffering, whether fabricated or real.[25] Greeks, and others, who told of captivity in Turkish galleys, or capture by European pirates, produced certificates alleging their suffering or showed infirmities (like missing tongues or other mutilations) to portray the depth of their losses in the face of Turkish cruelty. Many of the refugees in London had come to redeem themselves and their families from captivity, usually in the North African outposts of the Ottoman Empire, Tunis and Algiers, or in Sallee. Although redeeming captives was a surviving Catholic act of mercy in Reformation England, the practice remained an important form of Protestant charity. The collections made at the round of sermons at Paul's Cross and St Mary's Spital, on the subject of Christ's Passion and Resurrection at Easter time, and their 'rehearsal' in a fifth sermon at Paul's, could be earmarked 'for the Redeeminge of Captives'.[26] In the early 1630s, St Mary Somerset's churchwardens paid 5s to a Greek 'that had a Certificate under the kinges hand of England that he was a Noble man in his countrye and was taken by the Turks hee and his foure brethren'.[27] That gift to a Greek nobleman was surrounded in the accounts by disbursements to a Greek minister who had been captured by the Turks and to another man who had lost his tongue to them.[28]

The narratives of loss or captivity, sometimes reinforced by official briefs and certificates, moved parishioners, but, more importantly, moved ministers and rectors to 'command' churchwardens to help strangers. Some gifts in St Benet Gracechurch were made 'by Consente', but at least one Greek received 2s 6d 'by Mr Donnes apoyntment'.[29] Although the careful notation of ministers' orders could convey lay hostility to the notion of helping the stranger poor, even 'deserving' stranger ministers, churchwardens in general explained their outlays in anticipation of a year-end audit. Pastors' special affinity for ministers, strangers and native poor ones, testified to their self-identification with professional brothers, but also exemplified a mission to further Protestantism, or at least 'non-Catholicism'. Protestants, especially Puritans, may not have understood or even known the iconographic elements of Orthodox worship, given their support for Greek ministers and bishops. Holy Trinity the Less readily relieved poor Greek and Moravian ministers, as well as people carrying passports or briefs, often at the request of 'Mr Doctor Dee' or the later rector Mr Harrison.[30] The minister in St Alphage ordered that the churchwardens give 3s 6d to a Greek minister in 1617/18, as did the rector in St Bartholomew's in 1627/8.[31]

The laudable practice of succouring poor captives and stranger ministers, however, challenged the discrimination inherent in relief and charity in the early 17th century, when the 'deserving' were in part identified as the resident poor. Not all parishes desired, or could afford, to help stranger poor, and some auditors disallowed their churchwardens' payments to strangers at the audit. In St Mary Magdalene Milk Street, where payments to Abraham had been negated, the churchwardens had a hard time meeting the rector's directives to help poor ministers and strangers and satisfying the auditors' oversight. The parishioners tried to restrict payments upon certificates, although they contributed to pensions and relief for the poor of the parish and helped poor ministers.[32] The churchwardens in St Mary's protected their funds (as all parishes did as the demands of poor relief stretched resources thin) and sought to force others to provide for their 'own' poor. They pursued a case in the Court of Aldermen, for example, to force the churchwardens of St Giles to provide for three small children brought from that parish to their own.[33]

Churchwardens and parishioners sensed that the problem of poverty had only worsened in London, even without considering the influx of poor and miserable refugees and immigrants. The elements of believability in Greeks' narratives – like Abraham's experience as a merchant and as a 'subject' of the Ottomans – and in the stories recounted by English-born veterans of piracy and foreign war persuaded many parishioners to help them. Churchwardens also knew, however, that the 'truth' could be forged. The case of George Alexander and John Nuello (or Millos) began with their captivity and a letter in Latin from the King, directed to foreign princes for their relief, in 1624. Alexander and Millos found George Jackson of St Sepulchre's in London to translate the letter and alter it, to read that the King directed the English to relieve the Macedonian and the Syrian (Assyrian in parochial sources). They were apprehended and brought to the Wells Sessions of the Peace, though the charges were unclear. The men had gathered money in St Michael Bassishaw and Holy Trinity the Less before the abuse/forgery was uncovered.[34]

Suspicion of Greek refugees' accounts and their letters continued, as seen in the case of the minister 'Gregory Argeropulus', who came before an alderman of London and the Justice of the Peace for London and Middlesex in 1634. An interpreter, a weaver named James Skelson of Shoe Lane, accompanied him to help answer questions about how the minister had obtained the King's letters of conduct and of collection. His explanation gives an indication of how well-connected Greeks made their way in London: with letters from the Patriarch of Constantinople addressed to the King, Argyropulus sought the help of another Greek named Andreas Paleologus and Skelson. The three visited Patrick Younge, keeper of the King's Library at Whitehall, '(who is a gent verye respective to the Greekish nation in regard of the knowledge that he hath in that Language)', for help in obtaining the King's letters. Younge prepared a draft that reached the King, who signed and sealed it, before a printer in Foster Lane made 300 briefs. Argyropulus distributed fifty in London, collecting £48 of which the interpreter was entitled to £12.[35]

Argyropulus's experience points to the existence of a small circle of Greeks and sympathetic Londoners upon which a new immigrant or refugee could rely. Some learned men in London indeed knew the Greek language, at least in its classical form. The minister also knew at least one Greek, already in London, whom he could approach for help. Many men like the minister and the 'Grecians' who asked for parochial charity carried briefs or passports, suggesting that they were only passing through the city on their way home. In St Martin Coney Street parish in York, the churchwardens gave five Greeks a couple of shillings, three of them carrying briefs as they made their way through England.[36] The case of Abraham, the man named Paleologus contacted by the minister Argyropulus, and the late medieval Byzantine wire-drawers studied by Harris, however, suggest that at least some Greeks did settle in the city more permanently.

I see no clear pattern in the geography of potential settlement or migration of Greeks in London, based on the evidence in parochial records and the Court of Aldermen. Using Jones's study of rents in 1638, the Greeks visited wealthy and poor parishes: six parishes with rents exceeding £20, eight parishes in the £11–20 range, six in the £5–10 range, eight with average rents of less than £5, and four parishes without data. Or, at least, these parishes recorded having helped Greek supplicants. By contrast, St Mary Woolnoth and St Michael Cornhill lumped together the 'stranger poor', leaving the impression to the modern historian that they did not help 'Greeks' in particular. On the other hand, Yungblut's study of aliens showed a low concentration of aliens in some wealthy inner city parishes. The eastern and western parishes and suburbs showed a high concentration of aliens in the 16th century, but the Greeks seemed to have stayed largely toward the eastern suburbs, in some central parishes, and just to the west of an imaginary central line in the city.

The chronicler John Stow offers a few clues about these patterns of settlement or migration. Harris noted the affinity between Greek and Italian immigrants in medieval London, but many of the parishes with Italian connections or communities (Tower Street Ward, St Edmund Lombard Street) unfortunately lack extant records.[37] In St Katherine Coleman Street, however, where Stow noted the presence of basket-makers, wire-drawers, and other foreigners in the time of Edward IV, the churchwardens did help Greeks in the 17th century.[38] In describing Bishopsgate Ward, Stow described many 'fair houses for merchants and artificers, and many fair inns for travellers'.[39] The wealthy St Helen's parish, in the ward close to Leadenhall where Stow described these inns and houses, showed a marked inclination to give charity to strangers, including Greeks. Of St Botolph's Billingsgate, Stow said 'divers strangers are there harboured', but the parish did not identify any of the 'poor strangers' as Greeks.[40] Stow claimed that collecting charity was hard among the 'Netherlanders', 'for the stranger will not contribute to such charges as other citizens do'.[41] He often lamented the apparent decline in charity, to put the remark into perspective, and perhaps he revealed his own distrust of the loyalties of the alien communities to London and its inhabitants' needs.

Perhaps the relatively few Greeks who remained tended to assimilate into 'English' life more quickly than did the larger Calvinist communities from Holland and France. Without a stranger Orthodox church in the early 17th century, perhaps Greeks who settled in England became Anglican parishioners. These Greek men may also have married English women. Harris identified two brothers, Andronicus and Alexius Effamate (Effomatos), who were gold wire-drawers living in London since the mid-15th century. Harris noted that Everard Effamat lived in Westminster, but was not identified as Greek.[42] One of the witnesses to the merchant tailor John Heres's will of 1521 was a man named Everard Effamat.[43] In another will from 1534, 'Edwarde Effamatt' is identified as the scrivener, perhaps related to the medieval wire-drawers.[44] Without marriage registers for confirmation, however, one cannot know with certainty whether the original Effomatos had children.

For the inhabitants of London, the Greek refugees could be ciphers to fill in with their particular imagined concerns. Churchwardens and ministers conflated modern categories of ethnicity and race, perplexed by the newness and foreignness of these refugees. Greeks had often been the victims of Turkish cruelty, whether as individuals or families who suffered in slave galleys or were 'despoiled' of their goods by the Ottomans or pirates. Londoners' acceptance of the facts and meaning of Greek suffering often cast the Greek refugees as 'deserving' poor, but not without controversy in some parishes and neighbourhoods, burdened by the demands on their resources and collections. London ministers and lay people could also identify the Greeks as being not Catholic, although they may have been ignorant of the finer points of Orthodox worship that violated prevailing anti-iconographic theology. The English, therefore, could see the Greeks as allies against Ottoman and Catholic foes in the wider struggles against 'papacy' and against Ottoman or Spanish attempts to construct a Universal Monarchy.[45]

NOTES

1 Laura Hunt Yungblut, *Strangers settled here amongst us: policies, perceptions and the presence of aliens in Elizabethan England* (London, 1996), 12–13; Andrew Pettegree, *Foreign Protestant communities in sixteenth-century London* (Oxford, 1986); John Hintermaier, 'The first modern refugees? Charity, entitlement, and persuasion in the Huguenot immigration of the 1680s', *Albion* (forthcoming).

2 Jonathan Harris, *Greek émigrés in the West, 1400–1520* (Camberley, 1995) and 'Two Byzantine craftsmen in fifteenth-century London', *Journal of Medieval History* 21 (1995), 387–403.

3 Halil Inalcik and Donald Quataert (eds.), *An economic and social history of the Ottoman Empire, 1300–1914* (Cambridge, 1994), 32.

4   Prayers for thanksgiving: STC 16508, 16508.3, 16508.9, 16509, 16510; Fiona Kisby, 'Books in London parish churches, c.1400–c.1603', paper delivered at the Harlaxton Symposium on 'The Church and learning', Harlaxton, Grantham, July 1999; to be published in C. Barron and J. Stratford (eds.), *The Church and learning in late medieval society: essays in honour of Barrie Dobson* (Grantham, 2000); Margo Todd, 'A captive's story: Puritans, pirates, and the drama of reconciliation', *Seventeenth Century* 12:1 (1997), 37–56; N. I. Matar, 'Muslims in seventeenth-century England', *Journal of Islamic Studies* 8:1 (Jan. 1997), 63–82; Matar, *Islam in Britain, 1558–1685* (Cambridge, 1998); P. M. Holt, 'The study of Islam in seventeenth- and eighteenth-century England', *Journal of Early Modern History*, 2:2, 113–23; Holt, 'Edward Pococke (1604–91), the first Laudian Professor of Arabic at Oxford', *Oxoniensia* 56 (1991), 119–30.

5   *Newes from Vienna the .5. day of August .1566. of the strong towne and Castell of Jula in Hungary* (London, 1566) [STC 24716]; Ferenc Szakály, 'The early Ottoman period, including Royal Hungary, 1526–1606,' in Peter F. Sugar, Péter Hanák, and Tibor Frank (eds.), *A history of Hungary* (Bloomington, IN, 1990), 86–7.

6   *New Cambridge Modern History*, vol. 4, 226–38; vol. 3, 252, 347–76; 'Northerners in the Mediterranean', in Inalcik and Quataert (eds.), *An economic and social history*, 364–79. See also, Azmi Ozcan, *Pan-Islamism: Indian Muslims, the Ottomans and Britain, 1877–1924* (Leiden, 1997), 1–5.

7   For example, GL, MS 4956/2, fo. 315v.

8   Converted Barbarian: GL, MS 1046/1, fo. 71v; converted Turk(s): CLRO, Repertory 39, fo. 147 and GL, MS 4383/1, fo. 16; reformed Spaniard: GL, MS 959/1, fo. 169v; converted Jew: GL, MS 66, fo. 44.

9   Sympathy for Bohemian or Moravian ministers: GL, MSS 4835/1, fo. 173; 1432/3, fo. 144v; 1303/1, fo. 44.

10 V. J. Parry, 'The period of Murad IV, 1617–48', in V. J. Parry, H. Inalcik, A. N. Kurat, J. S. Bromley (eds.), *A history of the Ottoman Empire to 1730* (Cambridge, 1976), 151.

11 CLRO, Rep. 28, fo. 208; GL, MS 4409/1, fo. 99.

12 GL, MS 1568, Part 2, fo. 458.

13 GL, MS 593/2, fo. 120v. See also: GL, MSS 6836, fo. 84v; 577/1, fo. 32v; 2596/2, fo. 15; 4409/1, fo. 99.

14 GL, MS 2596/2, fo. 15.

15 GL, MS 878/1, fo. 71.

16 GL, MS 6836, fo. 84v.

17 GL, MS 4956/2, fo. 247.

18 Anthony Pagden, *Lords of all the world: ideologies of empire in Spain, Britain and France c.1500–c.1800* (New Haven, CT, 1995), 67.

19 GL, MSS 4051/1, fo. 6; 5090/2, fo. 194v; 4956/2, fo. 313.

20 GL, MS 4956/2, fos. 327v, 313.

21 Emrys Jones, 'London in the early seventeenth century: an ecological approach', *The London Journal*, 6:2 (Winter 1980), 124 (map).

22 GL, MSS 4956/2, fo. 308; 4457/2, fo. 213v.

23 GL, MSS 4457/2, fo. 259; 4956/2, fo. 308.

24 GL, MS 2968/2, fo. 134v.

25 Roslyn L. Knutson, 'Elizabethan documents, captivity narratives, and the market for foreign history plays', *English Literary Renaissance* 26 (1996), 75–110; Schen, 'Constructing the poor in early seventeenth-century London', *Albion* (forthcoming).

26 CLRO, Rep. 40, fos. 103–30v. On sermons, see John Stow, *A Survey of London (London under Elizabeth: a survey)*, ed. Henry Morley (London, 1890), 182.

27 GL, MS 5714/1, fo. 83.

28 GL, MS 5714/1, fos. 83v, 89v.

29 GL, MS 1568, Part 2, fos. 468, 475.
30 GL, MS 4835/1, fos. 130, 131, 155, 173, 200v.
31 GL, MSS 1432/3, fo. 122; 4383/1, fo. 281
32 GL, MS 2596/2, fo. 20v.
33 GL, MS 2596/2, fos. 36v, 53.
34 *CSPD* vol. 158, 29; PRO, SP 14/158, fo. 37; GL, MSS 4835/1, fo. 151; 2601/1, Part 1, fo. 49v.
35 PRO, SP 16/259, fos. 32r-v; *CSPD* vol. 259, 13 (423), signed by Argeropulus [Argyropulus], James Skelsonn, Hugh Hamersley, George Longe.
36 Borthwick Institute, PRY/MCS 17, fo. 75.
37 Harris, 'Two Byzantine craftsmen', 398–9.
38 Stow, 168.
39 *Ibid.*, 188.
40 *Ibid.*, 214.
41 *Ibid.*, 215.
42 Harris, 'Two Byzantine craftsmen', 401.
43 PRO, PROB 11/21, fo. 171R.
44 PRO, PROB 11/25, fo. 128L.
45 Pagden, 4.

30

Irish Jewry in the 17th and 18th centuries

GORDON M. WEINER

(To the tune of *When Irish eyes are smiling*)

> Three Jews, they were a'talkin
>   'Bout the day when they would die
> And where they would be buried
>   Beneath God's glorious sky
> Lewinsky said Jerusalem
>   New York said Rubinstein
> But, when it came to Cohen he said:
> The Irish isles are mine.
>
> 'Sure, I long to lay my weary head
>   Beneath those leafy boughs
> In an Irish cemetery
>   Where the three-leafed shamrock grows
> For the devil he'll be lookin
> For to find me I suppose
> And he'd never think to look for me
> Where the River Shannon flows.

This ditty from the Lower East Side in New York City, composed in 1879, when the Jews and the Irish were competing for who was at the bottom rung of the social ladder, is false. The first recorded mention of a Jewish presence in Ireland occurs in 1079. In that year the *Annals of Inishfallen* state, 'Year 1079: Five Jews came over the sea with gifts to Tairdelbach and they were sent back again over the sea'.[1] This was a delegation from Rouen, and while they were refused permission to settle, documents after the Norman invasion of Ireland in 1171 affirm that a few Jews were indeed present on the island.[2] What is fascinating is that in both the 12th and 17th centuries, Jews helped finance the English invasions of Ireland, without any negative reaction on the part of the indigenous Irish population. For the Normans, a Rabbi Josce of Bristol supplied funds for the invasion between 1169–71. He was fined for lending money without the King's permission. Indeed, a debate exists among Jewish historians regarding the extent to which Jews provided 'the' major funding for the expedition.[3] In the 17th century, the Dutch firm of Machado-Pereira, along with individual Dutch and English Sephardim (Spanish and Portuguese Jews), were instrumental in financing the invasions of England and Ireland by William of Orange. A great deal of Jewish money was raised, of which Isaac Pereira contributed £36,000 and Abraham Lopes Suasso is said to have given William two million guilders and refused any security.[4] In both cases one would reasonably expect the Irish to react negatively to these Jewish practices. However, there is no documented anti-Semitism or indeed any hostile reaction towards the Jews, probably because the impact of the invasions was so drastic and the indigenous Irish population so hard pressed, that the Jewish role was simply ignored or unknown. Perhaps thankfully, no Irish work of history mentions the Jewish involvement in these invasions, and I remain somewhat anxious about even raising the point.

Jonathan Israel has documented that the Dutch Sephardim went through a major shift in economic focus in the second half of the 17th century, when their involvement in the Spanish/Portuguese trade fell off sharply.[5] What has not been fully documented was the attempt by the Sephardim to continue in this very lucrative trade by shifting their bases of operation. During the first half of the 17th century, when there were temporary trade disruptions, the Sephardim established bases of operation in Hamburg, other Hanseatic towns, and elsewhere to circumvent anti-Dutch restrictions. The Sephardim even employed English, French and Hanseatic ships to hide the Dutch origin of their trade. As the year 1650 approached, a number of factors coincided to reinforce these earlier trends, and to result eventually in the Jewish settlement of Ireland. Firstly, the Portuguese re-conquest of Brazil meant that *conversos* who had returned to Judaism there under a tolerant Dutch regime would now be subject to automatic conviction by the Inquisition as *relapsos*. Secondly, the separation of Portugal from the Spanish Crown in 1640 resulted in Portuguese *conversos* resident in Spain migrating to Amsterdam when their home economic base now became inaccessible. Thirdly, the onset of large-scale Cossack uprisings in the 1640s in Russia and Poland resulted in vastly increased Ashkenazic (Central and East European Jews) migration westward. And fourthly, the growth of the Anglo-Dutch colonial rivalry, which led to some Sephardic merchants migrating to England and eventually to Ireland to continue their participation in the lucrative trans-Atlantic trade. While the Dutch Sephardic Rabbi Menasseh ben Israel appealed to Cromwell in the 1650s to readmit the Jews to England using theological arguments, we know that the rabbi's son-in-law and possibly he himself had unsuccessfully tried to enter the trans-Atlantic trade in Amsterdam. His arguments about the economic utility of the Jews to England might in fact conceal his recognition of England's growing economic utility to the Jews. Indeed, we may see here a hitherto de-emphasized motive for Menasseh's mission to Oliver Cromwell.

As in the English case, there was no formal admission, or re-admission of the Jews to Ireland. A number of Sephardim settled as Jews, and not as *conversos*, in Dublin around 1660. Most of them came from Amsterdam, via London. Many of them were younger brothers and cousins of the international trading and banking firms. The Inquisition of the Canary Islands even commissioned a spy report on Sephardic Jews based in Ireland.[6] Inquisitorial testimony implicated Manuel and Francisco Lopes

Pereira and Jacob Faro of Dublin as *conversos* or *relapsos* resident there before 1665 and involved in the Spanish trade.

There was a suggestion that *converso* refugees from Portugal established a small synagogue in Dublin in 1660; but, until these Inquisition documents were consulted, no one had any idea who they were.[7] As was the case with Sephardim involved in international trade elsewhere, these Irish Sephardim employed numerous aliases to hide their true identities from the Iberian authorities.[8] Indeed, the two Pereira brothers were admitted as 'foreign Protestants' in Dublin in 1662.[9] In testimony presented to the Inquisition on 2 September 1665 Captain Juan Ramon repeated accusations he heard that the Pereira brothers and Jacob Faro were Irish Judaizers, relatives of convicted *relapsos*, and the secret consignees of ships that were involved in the Spanish colonial trade.[10] Obviously, there were major advantages for participation in the Spanish and Portuguese trades in being positioned in Catholic Ireland as opposed to Protestant London or Amsterdam. This Sephardic presence in Ireland only increased after the Glorious Revolution. William of Orange was beholden to Dutch and English Jews for war loans and contributions, and he gave Isaac Pereira the lucrative post of 'Commissary General of the Bread for their Majesty's forces in Ireland'. From at least 1674, the Dutch firm of Machado and Pereira was the chief provisioner for William of Orange's land forces.[11] The Sephardim constructed special prayers for William's English and then Irish victories and wrote Spanish poems dedicated to his triumph. Isaac Pereira brought a number of Dutch Sephardim to Ireland to aid him in carrying out his mission. Many of them stayed after the Boyne campaign in 1690 and formed the nucleus of the Sephardic communities in Dublin and Cork.[12]

In addition to the Sephardic merchants who first settled in Ireland, a stream of Ashkenazic immigrants soon followed. They too were connected to Amsterdam and London, but in a far different way. Yosef Kaplan and Miriam Bodian have documented the exclusionary aspects of the Dutch Sephardim *vis-à-vis* their Ashkenazic co-religionists.[13] I have gone a step further and have labelled this 'Jewish anti-Semitism', arguing elsewhere that the discrimination practised in both Amsterdam and London was based on Sephardic concepts of biological differences in blood and physiognomy.[14] The Ashkenazim were subjected to a series of discriminatory practices that made them an essentially different group from their Sephardic co-religionists. They could not pray together, intermarry, be buried together, or use the same physician. The Ashkenazim were excluded from the *Dotar* (the dowry society for poor girls), and the Sephardim were even forbidden to buy kosher meat from an Ashkenazic *shochet*. Two Sephardim in Amsterdam were even subjected to a *Cherem* (decree of excommunication) when caught patronizing an Ashkenazic butcher. What is important for this paper is that Sephardim in both Amsterdam and London decided that the best way to deal with the Ashkenazic immigrants was to earmark their *Tsedakkah* (poor relief) for getting rid of them. Case after case exists in the Dutch records showing the Sephardim sending hundreds and perhaps thousands of Ashkenazim back to the Germanic lands to face uncertain fates; and, after the English readmission, many were shipped there as well. However, the English Sephardim, younger brothers and cousins of their Dutch relations, now had to deal with the identical problem. They complained to the government in London about the swarms of poor Ashkenazim that were entering the country and they received permission to order all indigent Jews (i.e.

Ashkenazim) out of the country within five days. *Ascamah* 46 of the London synagogue reads:

> In the Name of the Blessed God.
> The Senores of the Mahamad ordered announcement to be made in the Synagogue that all foreigners [i.e. Ashkenazim] who were in this city and those who should come in the future in expectation that Ceddacka [poor relief] would support them, should within five days depart from the country; and in case they should not do so, that they should not come to the Synagogue; and for their passage the Ceddacka will aid them with what may be possible. And this was so ordained for the benefit of all this Kaal Kados [holy congregation] which God prosper.[15]

Thus, there emerges an intriguing development where the wealthy English Sephardim begin sending the poorer Ashkenazim to Ireland (the cheapest ticket); here the Jewish situation begins to parallel Anglo-Irish Christian relations. It is alleged that after the imposition of the Navigation Acts and the heightening of colonial exploitation by the English, most of the wealthy Sephardic merchants left Ireland simply because their international trade was greatly restricted. Now there were wealthy and 'superior' Sephardim in England and poor, 'lower class' Ashkenazim in Ireland. It is ironic that when Cromwell summoned the readmission conference in December 1655, the English spokesmen for the chartered companies argued that if any Jews were to be admitted, they should be confined to the provincial ports and barred from foreign trade.[16] By the end of the 17th century, the 'superior' London Sephardim had done precisely this. They successfully removed many of the 'inferior' Ashkenazim to these same provincial ports and Ireland (perhaps the most provincial of all from the English perspective). Further, these individuals largely restricted their economic activities to local or regional retail trades.

However, during the period of Sephardic residence in Ireland, a unique situation emerged that became a model for Jewish settlements in the expanding trans-Atlantic frontier. The hostility towards Ashkenazim one sees in London, Amsterdam, Bordeaux, Hamburg or other areas of Sephardic residence is absent from Ireland. There, both groups used the same synagogue, burial grounds, and other communal resources. There were no restrictions on intermarriage between the two groups or any of the other aspects of hostility seen elsewhere. As in other new communities, appeals for aid were made to the wealthier Sephardic synagogues in London and Amsterdam. Unlike the later appeals, the Irish aid was given largely without conditions. There was no clause inserted insisting on the maintenance of the Sephardic *Minhag* (liturgy) or a Sephardic majority on the Board of Directors. Perhaps because the Irish community made one of the earliest requests for aid, the Dutch and English Sephardim had not yet realized the need to find a way to insure their dominance through their donations. Or perhaps the notion was that the Sephardic presence in Ireland was to be only transitory, and thus not worth the creation of two separate communities.

It has been suggested that the Sephardim left Ireland after heightened British exploitation and the bank failures of 1727.[17] I have been able to find a few remaining there throughout the 18th century, but the community was indeed largely Ashkenazic. While the Penal Laws resulted in increased Catholic conversions to Protestantism, one also sees an increase in Jewish conversions. Jewish sources simply write this off as economic opportunism. There are a number of conversion tracts written in Hebrew by new converts, and we are unsure about the exact number of conversions. Notwithstanding, the Jewish community survived and in 1717 they rented and then purchased land for their first cemetery in Ballybough, Co. Dublin. A new Synagogue was opened in Dublin *circa* 1762. A Jewish cemetery already existed in Cork in 1727, a ritual slaughterer was there in 1753, and we are unsure about the exact 18th-century date of the establishment of a synagogue. In 1781 30 Jewish families arrived in Galway, and individual Jews resided in Waterford. The north seems to have attracted few Jews in the 18th century.

Both Jews and Catholics were officially barred from guilds. However, here the inability to keep out the majority Catholics worked to the benefit of the Jews. Both groups simply evaded the unenforceable economic laws and by mid-century a few Jews were accepted as journeymen in the guilds.[18] While most 18th-century Jews in Dublin were wholesale jewellers, one also sees Jewish chocolate makers, actors, pencil makers, druggists, and teachers.

Irish Jewry was largely ignored until 1714 when John Toland wrote the first plea for naturalizing Jews in the British Isles. In 1710, the bill allowing for the naturalization of foreign Protestants was repealed, and Toland may have been using the Jews to set an extreme example for his case.[19] While a recent controversy has erupted over whether Toland may be properly classed as an Irish philosopher, or the 'Father of Irish Philosophy', his largely favourable treatment of the Jews was far in advance of his times. Notwithstanding, he did suggest that after the Jews' expulsion from England and Ireland in 1290, 'a great number of 'em fled to *Scotland*, which is the reason so many in that part of the Island, have such a remarkable Aversion to pork and black-puddings to this day . . . '.[20]

In 1743 a bill for 'naturalizing persons professing the Jewish religion in Ireland' passed the House of Commons in Dublin, but was defeated in the Upper House by two votes, anticipating by a decade the English controversy over the Jew Bill. In the next five years three additional bills were blocked by the Irish peers.[21] Whereas David Katz and others argue convincingly that the English 'Jew Bill' controversy was a matter of party politics and had little to do with religion, this was not the case in Ireland.[22] There an anti-Semitic edge appeared in the debates and press accounts.[23] After the third Irish failure, the London-based Sephardim determined that they had not done enough, and appointed in 1746 a 'Committee of Diligence' which became today's Board of Deputies of British Jews.[24] In the late 19th century Michael Davitt suggested that the introduction of the bills was a protest against Jewish persecution on the continent and in England.[25] Others suggested this was a Protestant ploy to further Jewish immigration to Ireland and further dispossess the native Irish population.[26] Myriam Yardeni's economic interpretation of Harrington's *Commonwealth of Oceana* (1656) was negatively echoed by John Philpot Curran in the Irish Commons in 1792: 'We should become a wretched colony, perhaps leased out to a company of Jews, as was formerly in contemplation, and governed by a few tax gatherers and excisemen'.[27] In 1783 the Irish Naturalization Act specifically excluded Jews. This was only repealed in 1816. It has been suggested that this action reinvigorated the Dublin community and sparked immigration of Jews from Russia and Poland in the 1820s. Thereafter, the community was composed almost exclusively of Ashkenazim.

By the end of the 18th century, the Jews had become a recognized segment of Irish society. They continued to suffer from various disabilities alongside the native

Catholic population. This common experience sparked a number of comparisons between the Jews and Irish which found their way into print. More importantly, it temporarily forged bonds which linked both Jewish and Catholic emancipation, which was to come in the 19th century. Interestingly, the arena for this linkage tended to be in England, and was constructed largely between highly-placed English Jews and Irish politicians. The Jewish community residing in Ireland, while increasing in numbers throughout the 19th century, remained a community clearly set apart and setting itself apart by its differences. Thus, they became neither fully strangers nor fully citizens, but the continuation of this story goes beyond the chronological interests of this book.

NOTES

1 Séan MacAirt (ed.), *The Annals of Inishfallen* (Dublin, 1951), 235.

2 A. F. O'Brien, 'Commercial relations between Aquitaine and Ireland *c.* 1000 to *c.* 1550', in Jean-Michel Picard (ed.), *Aquitaine and Ireland in the Middle Ages* (Blackrock, 1995), 31–6; Robert Chazan, *Medieval Jewry in northern France: a political and social history* (Baltimore, MD, 1973), 15–19. Also see Louis Hyman, *The Jews of Ireland from earliest times to the year 1919* (Shannon, 1972), 1–10.

3 Joseph Jacobs, *The Jews of Angevin England* (London, 1893), 51 argues that Josce financed Strongbow's invasions, with the clear implication that he provided a major portion of the funds. This notion was accepted by Cecil Roth, *History of the Jews of England* (Oxford, 1941), 109, although he does not overtly suggest that the Jews supplied the major part of the funding. Salo Baron, *A social and religious history of the Jews* (New York, 1957), vol. 4, 82 repeats and amplifies Jacobs's claim. For an opposite view see Lionel Abrahams, *Transactions of the Jewish Historical Society of England* (hereafter *TJHSE*) 8 (1917), 173.

4 David Katz, *The Jews in the history of England, 1485–1850* (Oxford, 1994), 156–60; Daniel Swetschinki, 'The Portuguese Jewish merchants of 17th century Amsterdam: a social profile' (Brandeis University, Ph.D. thesis, 1979).

5 Jonathan Israel, *Empires and entrepôts: the Dutch, the Spanish monarch and the Jews, 1585–1713* (London, 1990), especially chs 7, 9, 14 and 15. Also see his 'The Dutch Republic and its Jews during the conflict over the Spanish Succession', in J. Michman (ed.), *Dutch Jewish history, vol. 2: proceedings of the fourth Symposium on the History of the Jews of the Netherlands* (Assen, 1989).

6 Lucien Wolf, *Jews in the Canary Islands, being a calendar of Jewish cases extracted from the records of the Canariote Inquisition in the collection of the Marquess of Bute* (London, 1926), xxxiv.

7 A controversy exists on this point between Hyman, *Jews of Ireland*, 12 and Bernard Shillman, *A short history of the Jews of Ireland* (Dublin, 1972), 13–17.

8 Hyman, 184.

9 HSQS 18, 338. Jews and Catholics were excluded from the freedom of Dublin by a decree in 1652. In 1678, a decree was passed that required a freeman to take the oaths of allegiance and supremacy. Only Jacob Nunes, a professing Jew, was admitted to the freedom of Waterford in 1702. See Hyman, 43.

10 Wolf, 197–8.

11 Katz, 157.

12 *Ibid.*, 160–1.

13 Yosef Kaplan, 'The Portuguese community in 17th-century Amsterdam and the Ashkenazi world', in Michman (ed.); also see his 'The attitude of the Spanish and Portuguese Jews to the Ashkenazi Jews in 17th-century Amsterdam', in J. Michman (ed.), *Transition and change in modern Jewish history: essays in honor of Shmuel Ettinger* (in Hebrew)

(Jerusalem, 1987); Miriam Bodian, *Hebrews of the Portuguese nation: conversos and community in early modern Amsterdam* (Bloomington, IN, 1997).

14 An early analysis of the Sephardim in Amsterdam, London, and Ireland is contained in my 'The settlement of the Sephardic Jews in Ireland', in B. Touhill (ed.), *Varieties of Ireland* (St Louis, MO, 1976). Also see my 'Sephardic philo- and anti-Semitism in the early modern era: the Jewish adoption of Christian attitudes', in R. H. Popkin and G. M. Weiner (eds.), *Jewish Christians and Christian Jews: from the Renaissance to the Enlightenment* (Dordrecht, 1994).

15 Lionel D. Barnett, *El Libro de los Acuerdos* (Oxford, 1931), 28.

16 Marcus Arkin, *Aspects of Jewish economic history* (Philadelphia, 1975), 107.

17 Cecil Roth, *A history of the Jews in England* (Oxford, 1964).

18 George Clune, *The medieval guild system* (Dublin, 1943), 161.

19 Katz, 234–5.

20 John Toland, *Reasons for Naturalizing the Jews in Great Britain and Ireland, on the same foot with all other nations* (London, 1714), 37–8. A notion of substantial Jewish migration to Scotland after 1290 and increasing concern with Jews has been recently reintroduced in the work of Arthur H. Williamson, 'British Israel and Roman Britain: the Jews and Scottish models of polity from George Buchanan to Samuel Rutherford', in Popkin and Weiner, *Jewish Christians*, 97–118; 'The Jewish dimension of the Scottish Apocalypse: climate, Covenant and world revewal', in Y. Kaplan *et al.* (eds.), *Menasseh ben Israel and his world* (Leiden, 1989), 7–30; and Marcia Keith Schuchard, *Emanuel Swedenborg and the Scottish rite of Freemasonry* (unpublished manuscript accessible through the Dept. of English, Emory University, Atlanta, GA).

21 *Journal of the House of Lords* (Dublin, 1779), vol. 3, 458, 544, 569, 572, 587; *Journal of the House of Commons of the Kingdom of Ireland* (Dublin, 1782), vol. 7, 974, 1037, 1039, 1138, 1145.

22 Katz, 240–83; H. S. Q. Henriques, *The Jews and English law* (Oxford, 1908), 154–7, 170–1, 198–201, 230–41; R. A. Routledge, 'The legal status of Jews in England 1190–1790', *Journal of Legal History* 3 (1982), 91–124; Robert Liberles, 'The Jews and their Bill: Jewish motivations in the controversy of 1753', *Jewish History* 2 (1987), 29–36; T. W. Perry, *Public opinion, propaganda, and politics in eighteenth-century England: a study of the Jew Bill of 1753* (Cambridge, MA, 1962); Albert M. Hyamson, 'The Jew Bill of 1753', *TJHSE* 6 (1912): 156–88.

23 Hyman, 46–50.

24 Albert M. Hyamson, *The Sephardim of England* (London, 1951), 124–5.

25 *Jewish Chronicle*, 18 July 1893, 7.

26 John Curry, *An Historical and Critical Review of the Civil Wars in Ireland, from the reign of Queen Elizabeth, to the Settlement of King William* (London, 1775), 262–3. Also see Huhner, 'The Jews of Ireland', *TJHSE* 5 (1902–5), 237.

27 Myriam Yardeni, *Anti-Jewish mentalities in early modern Europe* (Lanham, 1990), 229–31; J. T. Gilbert, *History of the City of Dublin* (Dublin, 1854–9), vol. 3, 139.

Part VI

Non-British settlers in the British American colonies

31

Sephardic settlement in the British colonies of the Americas in the 17th and 18th centuries

Yitzchak Kerem

While British colonial rule allowed the Sephardim and *conversos* returning to Judaism free settlement – as opposed to nearby Spanish colonies that officially viewed them as heretics or fleeing apostates – the Jews under the British in the Caribbean and North America still had to strive for religious freedom. In 1654 when the Jews were compelled to leave Recife in Brazil when the Portuguese reconquered the territory from the Dutch, most went to the other settlements in the Caribbean. These Jews —mostly, but not exclusively, Sephardic – brought with them to the Caribbean islands knowledge and experience in growing sugar cane, and in the production and trade of sugar. Their speciality was in refining sugar, but they would also become experts in the preparation of vanilla, cocoa, indigo, and other tropical crops.[1] The Jews exhibited a great proficiency in shipping and commerce,[2] which under the British in the colonies often became a source of jealousy and hatred.

The Jews chose locations of settlement in the Caribbean much more for economic, familial, and Jewish communal reasons than for considerations of which occupying power was there. These settlers were part of the elite Portuguese 'Nacion' network of former Portuguese crypto-Jews who returned to Judaism and established communal networks with Western Europe, and their establishment in the Americas was an extension of their desire to set up economic trading posts and practise Judaism quietly and as far away as possible from the Spanish and Portuguese Inquisition. Since the Jews had been well established in Holland since the 1580s and were only officially welcomed back to England in 1654, the communal base of the Portuguese and Spanish Jewish Congregation in Amsterdam and their integral ties with the Dutch West India Company served as an impetus for Sephardic settlement in the Dutch colonies of Surinam, Curaçao, St Eustatius and others. Nonetheless, even before Jews could officially come back to England itself, the Sephardim were settling in the English colony of Barbados as early as the 1620s,[3] and in Nevis by the 1640s.

Surinam

In 1652 a small group of Jews arrived in Surinam from England under the sponsorship of the English Governor, Lord Willoughby. Due to his efforts, a permanent settlement was founded in the interior of Surinam. Willoughby's achievements also include ceding 'some remarkable rights to the Jews to encourage settlement in this tropical wilderness. They were permitted religious freedom, including the right to construct their own house of worship, as well as political autonomy, the right to self-defence and ownership of agricultural tracts along the Cassipora creek by the Surinam River. A rich agricultural community flourished called Joden Savanna (Savannah of the Jews)'.[4] The Jews even formed their own militia which, led by Captain Isaac Pinto, combated pirates, slave uprisings, Indians, and invasions by French marauders from the nearby colony of French Guinea. By 1665 their first synagogue, Beracha Ve Shalom (Blessing and Peace), was established. English rule ended in 1667, when the Treaty of Breda between the English and the Dutch exchanged Surinam and New Amsterdam.

Jamaica

The largest Jewish settlement in the British Caribbean was in Jamaica. Shortly after the English captured the island in 1655 – and according to legend the conquering English navy was led by the Marrano navigator Campoe Sabbatha towards Kingston harbour before surrounding the Spanish men-of-war,[5] – poor Jewish mining prospectors or traders successfully petitioned the English to go to the island. Jews were admitted to Jamaica by the English officials as part of official policy to encourage commerce on the young colonial island.[6]

Efforts were made to attract Jewish planters to settle in Jamaica. They were assured that slaves could be brought, that they would receive double the amount of land usually permitted to other planters, and that provisions and other necessaries would be supplied. Families from Surinam came, as well as from Barbados and Nevis. By the end of the 17th century, there were 80 families on the island, but only a few were planters and there were only five Jewish-owned plantations. In Jamaica, and in the British Caribbean in general, the Jews in fact could not own slaves, as they were non-Christians, and could not use them in sugar growing and production. The Jews traded freely with Negroes, however, to the dismay of elements of white Christian British society on the island, and several prominent Jews took black women as wives.[7]

The Jews preferred trading and commerce. In 1668 the traveller Richard Blome noted that in Port Royal there was a 'Jews street' with a synagogue.[8] Port Royal was the main port for the buccaneers, who plundered the Spanish and Dutch in their cities or at sea, and the Jews turned the city into a commercial centre. The Jews, and other merchants, rushed to the island to capitalize on the low prices of the booty such as gold and silver-embroidered heavy cloths, silks, and laces.[9] But the Jews primarily profited from refining sugar and exporting it to Europe or by importing European goods to the island where they could be sold throughout the Americas.

The Jews knew Spanish and extended their trade to the Spanish and West Indian colonies, which increased the wealth of the island. The Jews were money-changers and the chief importers of bullion, and provided credit to planters who could not get loans from English mercantile houses, charging them 6 per cent over the regular interest rate.[10] They also capitalized by purchasing 'dollars with ryals of old plate' or accepted dollars from 'soldiers and indentured tradesmen' in exchange for the purchase of necessities. Naturally, their profits from loans were sources of resentment on occasion by both the colonial nobility and the poor segments of society.

Wright notes that 'In December 1670 the Governor, Sir Thomas Lynch, was instructed to give all possible encouragement to persons of different opinions of religion. When the English merchants of Port Royal protested against unfair and allegedly illegal competition from the Jews, Lynch asserted that all but 16 of the Jews in Jamaica had acquired denization papers entitling them to engage in retail trade, and that "the King cannot have more profitable subjects than they and the Hollanders"'.[11] Aubrey Newman notes that 'There was a steady trickle of applications from Jews for endenization', and that as the process of endenization 'involved costs of over £100', it suggests that a number of Jewish inhabitnts of the island 'had already achieved a fairly substantial status.'[12] Between 1665 and 1700, in addition, 93 Jews took out patents of naturalization and/or patents of land.[13]

While a good proportion of the Jews were indeed poor, some were substantial traders. Jealousy of the latter by Gentile traders led to unsuccessful attempts to expel them from the island. Fortunately, the governors of the island and the government in London ignored such attempts and praised the Jewish merchants for their devotion and willingness to supply goods that no one else wanted to.[14] When expulsion failed, the island's Assembly tried to tax the Jewish merchants heavily, and as Jewish opposition to this increased, so did the taxes.

Since 1655, 21 separate Jewish communities functioned on the island.[15] The Jewish cemetery at Hunt's Bay in the parish of St Andrew's has tombs which date back as far as 1672, but there may be a few which are even earlier.[16] The fatal earthquake of 1692 destroyed the Jewish synagogue along with the city of Port Royal. Most of the Jews in the aftermath resided in Kingston, but Spanish Town also had a sizeable Jewish population. In 1730 there were some 900 Jews on the island out of a total white population of 7148. By the early 19th century, the Jewish population of the island approached 2000.[17]

Despite the religious freedom which they appreciated, and their frequent service in the island's militia, the Jews still had to pay the 'Jew's tribute', a special government tax enforced from 1698 to 1739, and they could not hold public office, work for the government, or vote in public elections. Nor could they sit on juries, or exercise the franchise. Only in 1831 were these civil disabilities against the Jews repealed, 27 years before the Jews would enjoy the same freedoms in England.[18]

In 1740, imperial legislation permitted foreign-born Protestants and Jews to attain naturalization without having to adhere to the Established Church or take an oath of allegiance 'on the true faith of a Christian'.[19] Foreign Jews who had resided for seven years could receive naturalization and between 1740 and 1753, 185 Jews in the Americas took out naturalization. Amongst these were 140 Jews who resided in Jamaica.

Barbados

Barbados was the second largest Jewish Sephardic community in the British colonies of the Caribbean. A group of Jews from Recife was given permission to settle there in 1654.[20] Other newcomers came from the Jewish Spanish-Portuguese communities of Hamburg, Altona, and Gluckstadt from 1668 to 1677. 'In 1661 licences had been given to certain named Jews to continue their residence in Barbados, and certificates of endenization had been given to others, but opposition to their presence was expressed in part by attempts in 1665 to secure the expulsion from the island of Jews who had failed, as promised, to find gold mines on the island, and later by attempts to refuse to allow Jews to give testimony in the courts of law'.[21] After endenizened Jews were denied the right to testify in court in Barbados and their trade consequently suffered, an act of the Council passed in 1674 stated that Jews could testify in court, but only concerning matters of trade.

Regarding Jewish ownership of slaves and plantations, Aubrey Newman notes:

> There were restrictions upon the right of Jews to own slaves; non-natural born and non-naturalised Jews were forbidden to own more than one slave on pain of having the excess confiscated, and there were in Barbados, as elsewhere, restrictions upon the employment by them of 'indentured' non-Jewish labour. This was of course a great restriction on the possibility of Jews becoming plantation owners, the economy of these estates being to a very great extent dependent on the existence of such labour. None the less there were by the 1680s four Jewish planters owning quite considerable estates, and further evidence of Jewish involvement in the sugar industry – which was at that time beginning to take over as the sole crop of the island – is afforded by the patenting of a new sugar mill invented by a Jewish immigrant from Recife who was given the financial backing and political patronage of a group of English noblemen, including the Governor of Barbados.[22]

Another obstacle to the Jews in the sugar trade was that the British forbade them to hire Christians, or even freed blacks. The Jews usually freed the slaves they had, and those in the cities were limited to one slave per family. They also were excluded from the slave trade, which was in the hands of British and Dutch merchants. However, their speciality was converting sugar into molasses, and this was sent to Newport and elsewhere throughout the world and sold, enabling Sephardic merchants to fit out empty ships for Africa where they purchased slaves. In this 'triangular trade', slaves were sold in Barbados for molasses and other goods.

David de Mercado developed a new type of sugar mill and Barbados became a world leader in the production of sugar and rum. Resented by English planters, the near monopoly of Spanish and Portuguese Jews in the sugar trade was offset by the Council of Barbados, which levied taxes on them to create a parity between them, the English planters and other participants in the trade.[23] Gentile merchants in Barbados in general resented the Jews for their economic success in smuggling, importing and trading Dutch goods despite British bans, and in retailing sugar. Petitions called for the expulsion of the Jews from Barbados and accused them of the killing of Christ. Nonetheless, the Jews were protected by the governor and by royal legislation.

In 1678, the Jews of Bridgetown were affluent enough to hire a rabbi, Eliau Lopez, a former Marrano from Malaga, Spain. At that point the Jews already numbered 300 people. In 1710, though, there were only 240 Jews in Bridgetown and 20 in Speightstown. There must have been a decline due to older communal members moving to Amsterdam or New York and dying there.[24]

The majority of the Bridgetown Jews lived in the vicinity of Swan Street, often nicknamed Jew Street and it was there that they had their synagogue. In Speightstown, at the other end of the island, there was a smaller synagogue, which was dismantled in 1779 and never rebuilt. In Speightstown there was a tragic incident when Governor Burnet, after being invited to the wedding of a Jew, Lopes, was accused by the groom of stealing money. The groom and several of the Jews assaulted the Governor, and a riot ensued. In court Lopes had to pay £10,000. The episode agitated the local population against the Jews, and they were incited to expel them and to destroy the synagogue. In August 1753, the Mahamad of Bevis Marks (the 'Central Committee' of the Sephardic congregation) in London was called to remedy a dispute between the two Jewish communities, which it viewed as insoluble, but the issue could not go to court on the island as the *ascamot*, the decisions by Bevis Marks, were not incorporated by royal charter.[25]

In 1692 the Jewish community paid taxes totalling £750 while the Christians of the island paid only £675. As early as 1670 the Jews of Bridgetown complained that they were unfairly taxed. By 1704, the Christians paid £1500 and the Jews £750, and in 1709 the Christians paid £6000 while the Jews only paid £1500. By the mid-18th century, their financial status had eroded and in 1756 an attempt to compel the Jews to pay a special tax failed. Nonetheless, Jewish civic generosity continued. In 1786, in the hospital building fund campaign, the impoverished Jewish community gave more than one tenth of the money while in numbers they were less than one twentieth of the total population of the island and owned less than one per cent of the property.[26]

In addition, the Barbados community gave as much as it could to Jewish charity and helped the Jews of St Eustatius tortured and exiled by the British Navy commander Admiral Rodney, who was retaliating against the Jews for their active role in providing military ships to the American revolutionary insurgents.[27] The Barbados Jewish community also donated to the Terra Santa (Holy Land) fund sponsored by the Bevis Marks congregation.[28]

Eventually, by the latter part of the 18th century, the Jews of Barbados received full rights in court, could take oaths on the Torah (instead of being excluded for not swearing on the Christian Bible), and served in the army, which was compulsory for all white men who were not exempted. Some of the island's prominent rabbis included Eliahu Lopez, Meir Hacohen Belinfante and Raphael Haim Yitzhak Carigal. Noteworthy also was the poet Haim Refael de Mercado. By the 1790s, due to retail competition from Liverpool, and the Irish fabric trade, the wealthy Jews began to leave for London, but the major Jewish migratory wave headed toward Philadelphia and Nevis.

Nevis

There are only a little more than a handful of Jewish families in Nevis in the census lists of 1678 and 1707. Jews left Barbados because of high taxation and came to Nevis, but the migration of Jews from Nevis to the larger Jewish community of Barbados was also common. Indeed, many Jews of Barbados preferred to reside on that island, but travelled frequently to Nevis. The Amsterdam poet Daniel Levi de Barrios, who was familiar with the Caribbean and also temporarily resided in Tobago, noted in 1688:

> Already in six English cities it is known about the light of the six holy congregations of Israel, three in Nieves, London, Jamaica, the fourth and fifth in two parts of Barbados, the sixth exists in Madras-Patan.[29]

In 1671, the island was put under the separate administration of the Leeward Islands, independent of the Government of Barbados. There was a Jewish cemetery, and from it a path called 'Jews' Walk' which led to an old house known as the 'Jews' School'. The oldest grave in the cemetery is from 1679. The Jews' School was actually a synagogue with a women's gallery, judging by early 18th century accounts.[30]

An account written in 1724 about the Jews in Charlestown, the main town of the island, notes:

> There were then seventy households . . . near 300 whites, where of one quarter are Jews, who have a synagogue there, and are said to be very acceptable to the country part of the island, but far from being so to the Town.[31]

In the city the Jews were resented by the Gentile traders for undercutting prices. They were resented for being transient and seen as 'unfair competition' in trade. Ezratty writes:

> The Jewish traders of Nevis sailed all over the Caribbean, engaging in commerce with St Eustatius, Barbados, Curacao, Surinam, St Thomas and St Croix. Nevis Jews journeyed to Newport, Rhode Island, Holland, and England. All these destinations had well established Sephardic communities, and indeed, many Sephardim were related by birth or marriage to Nevis families.[32]

There were also Jewish slave-owners, but they did not occupy central roles on the island. The mineral springs of the island, an 18th-century tourist 'attraction', were not known to have been exceptionally beneficial to Jewish prosperity on the island. In 1701 their introduction of sugar planting and trading in Nevis prompted a repeal of the 1694 'Act against the Jews ingrossing commodities imported in the Leeward Islands, and trading with the slaves belonging to the inhabitants of the same.'[33] Salomon Israel served as a jury foreman and witness of wills for Christian friends and appears in documentation in c.1724,[34] and in 1769, indicating that 'Jews enjoyed the same civil status and responsibilities as their Christian neighbours'.[35]

The 1689 epidemic of fever and the 1706 French attack reduced the population of the island by a third.[36] After being about 70 souls and making up a fourth of the white population of New Charlestown, the Jewish population declined in the second half of the 18th century as the sugar trade declined. The latest grave in the Jewish cemetery is from 1768. Most Nevis Jews relocated to Sephardic Jewish congregations in the British colonies in North America.

New York

In 1654 a group of 23 Sephardim left Recife in Brazil after the Portuguese reconquered the colony there from the Dutch, and voyaged to Dutch New Amsterdam, from where Governor Stuyvesant wanted to deport them as they could not pay for their journey. While they were waiting for a judgment from the Dutch West India Company, which eventually did not support their deportation, a group of 15 settled in Newport. The New England Puritans there,who had fled persecution from the Anglican Church and sought religious freedom in accordance with Old Testament doctrine, Sabbath observance, and high priest rituals, treated the Jews as strangers and denied them the right to vote or hold office, but did not prevent them from settling. In 1658 the Jews established their religious and social life in the home of Mordechai Campanall, where they had a prayer *minyan* and 'masonry' meetings. However, in accordance with the Navigation Acts, enacted in England in 1651, 1660, and 1663, strangers and non-citizens were not permitted to trade within the colonies, and the New England Jewish communities did not grow.[37]

When the English captured New Amsterdam in 1664 and the colony became New York, the struggle to obtain religious freedom continued. Whereas in the home country in England, where Sephardic Jews were indicted for holding public worship and non-attendance at church in the 1670s and 1680s, in the territories of colonial America the Jews were allowed to practise their religion as long as the peace was not upset. In 1677 the Jews purchased their own cemetery.[38] In 1682 in New York it was reported that Jews held separate meetings and in the same year a second cemetery was acquired. However, even in 1685 the petition of the Jews to the English Governor Dongon requesting the right to exercise their religion publicly was refused by the local council. Public worship was only tolerated for those that professed faith in Christ. Despite positive gestures like Dongon's 1686 statement permitting all to exercise their religion openly as long as the peace was not disturbed and his annulment of the restrictive city charter at the orders of the King, in 1691 the General Assembly relapsed by 'limiting the liberty of worship to those professing faith in God by Jesus Christ'.[39] Nonetheless, in about 1686 public Jewish services were already being held and in 1695 it was reported that there was a synagogue.[40] Thus, the Jews of New York fought to create religious freedom and assisted in defining this practice. They contributed to the increase of religious liberty and helped in its attainment.

The Naturalization Act of 1740 enabled every Jew in the colonies to become naturalized, but there were two noteworthy exceptions. When Newport residents Aaron Lopez and Isaac Elizar applied in 1761 to the legislature of the Rhode Island Colony, which referred them to the courts, they were refused by the Superior Court of the Judicature in the County of Newport on the claim that, in accordance with a law made and passed in 1663, 'No person who does not profess the Christian Religion can be admitted free into the Colony'.[41] Thus Lopez moved to Swansey, Massachusetts, where after a two-month residence, he submitted a petition for naturalization to the Bristol County Superior Court of Judicature. After showing compliance with the 1740 Act and adhering to three necessary oaths, he became naturalized in 1762. His fellow Jewish petitioner, Isaac Elizar, was naturalized a year later in New York.

The southern colonies: Maryland, Virginia, Carolina, Georgia

Maryland and North Carolina were noted for their legislation infringing upon full rights for those of the Jewish faith. Maryland's famous 1649 Act of Toleration provided toleration and religious freedom for Roman Catholics and Protestants, but not for Jews. The South Carolina State Constitution of 1776 required the chief executive of the colony to take an oath to 'Maintain and defend the law by G-d, and the Protestant religion and the Liberties of America'. The Sephardic Jewish member of the Provisional Congresses of 1775 and 1776, Francis Salvador, saw no reason to record his objection to this provision. As the law was aimed against the Catholics, the Jews found no reason to be overly concerned.[42] Salvador was an exception as a Jewish politician. The South Carolina election law of 1721 excluded the Jews since it only enabled 'every free white man . . . professing the Christian religion' to vote, and each candidate elected to the assembly had to give an oath 'on the holy evangelists', which no Jew could perform.[43]

Anglican Virginia refrained from encouraging Jewish settlement within its borders. Although the Sephardic Isaiah Isaacs was the first known Jew to settle in Richmond in 1769, not very many Jews settled there before the Revolution. There is no evidence that the Jews had previously used the Naturalization Act of 1740 to settle in Virginia. Earlier laws were designed to oppose all those that 'failed to embrace or could not be embraced by the Anglican faith.'[44] Eakin points out that two and a half years before the Declaration of Independence, in Virginia, Baptist ministers were victims of violence and jailed for 'disturbing the peace', in other words for 'preaching the word of God as they understood it'. After the War of Independence and the Statute for Religious Freedom, Jews became more positively influenced to settle in Virginia. Virginian statesmen encouraged the promotion of religious freedom, as well as of self-determination.

Test oaths effectively barred Jews from public office in colonial Georgia. James Oglethorpe, member of the British Parliament and founder of the Georgia colony, overruled and ignored objections of the colony's Trustees in England, and permitted the Jews to settle in Savannah, after consulting lawyers in Charleston, who saw no legal constraint to their presence since the Georgia Charter only excluded 'papists' and 'slaves'. The original group of 42 Jewish settlers sent by the London Bevis Marks Spanish and Portuguese community to Georgia in 1733 were all Sephardim except for eight, and were led by Dr Samuel Nunes Ribeiro, former chief physician to the Grand Inquisitor in Lisbon, who treated an epidemic on the ship *William and Sarah* which carried the arriving Jewish immigrants up the Savannah River. The medical services of Ribeiro to the Jews and to the general Savannah community at the time of the fatal continuing plagues made a strong impression upon Oglethorpe. The admiration of Colonel Oglethorpe toward Dr Ribeiro, and his high regard for the Jews, were factors in his outflanking the opposition of the Georgia Trustees in England to Jewish settlement.[45]

In the War of Jenkins' Ear (1739–48), while the Spanish advanced northward from Florida in 1740–1, the Sephardim of Savannah fled to Charleston in Carolina in order to avoid falling prisoner to the Spanish, for, as former *conversos* who had fled Portugal in the 1720s, they risked being charged with apostasy and being burned at the stake.[46]

Many of the Sephardic settlers remained in Charleston or stayed north and chose not to return to Savannah after the end of the war, and the Savannah Sephardic Spanish and Portuguese community remained very small. In 1771, the Savannah Jewish community had only 49 Jews. In Savannah the Jews obtained religious freedom in practice, even though they were ostracized on paper and alienated politically.

By the time the struggle of the American Revolution was in full force, most of the Jews in the British colonies sided with the revolutionaries seeking independence, but there were Jews who were on the side of the Tories. In order to compel adherence to the revolutionary cause, the Rhode Island Assembly, in June and July 1776, passed legislation requiring loyalty oaths from all suspected Tories. Two Jewish leaders in Newport, Isaac Touro and Myer Pollock, refused to take the oath of loyalty on the grounds that it was against their religious principles as Jews.[47] Isaac Hart, who with Pollock, was commended by Edmund Burke for being committed to the British cause, had his property seized and was expelled from Newport in 1780. When taking refuge in a Long Island fort, he was shot, bayoneted, and beaten to death by members of the Continental Army. A fourth Newport Jew, Moses M. Hays, the third Sephardi out of the four Jews listed in a total of 77 suspected Newport residents, was actually a revolutionary. He refused to take the oath on grounds that he resented his loyalty being questioned. To his accusers, that were brought before him when he demanded it, he noted that, as a Jew it 'made it all the more unjust for the authorities to demand an oath of loyalty from him because these authorities were denying him the rights and opportunities of citizenship to which he was constitutionally entitled. They were demanding the responsibilities of citizenship without conferring the privilege.'[48] He also noted that 'Rhode Island was not alone in this slight, but other colonial legislatures and even the Continental Congress had failed to make provision for the rights of Jews'. In the end, he willingly signed the oath.

On face value, British treatment of the Jews as non-Christians may seem initially harsh, but it was the norm for the Jews worldwide who lacked civil and political rights while frequently suffering persecution. The short-lived British rule in 17th-century Surinam was at first exemplary and Jews were sceptical that its replacement, Dutch rule, would follow in its footsteps. On the other hand, war could have adverse effects for the Jews when it was the British attacking. When the British attacked Pomeroon (which became British Guyana), the Jewish settlement under the Dutch dispersed, its buildings were destroyed, and it never re-established itself. In St Eustatius, the Jews, as affluent merchants deeply involved in commerce under the auspices of the Dutch Republic and supplying ships and arms to the American revolutionaries, bore the brunt of the British military forces during their short-lived conquest. Even with the arrival of French rule, most Jews eventually went to St Thomas and the Jewish settlement dwindled.

Jewish commerce, and Sephardic Portuguese spiritual life prospered under the British, but by the late 18th and 19th centuries it drastically declined. The change in the means of production, the end of slavery, and natural disasters like earthquakes dismantled these affluent Portuguese merchant communities. Jewish poverty in Britain was farmed out to the colonies in North America, Australia, and elsewhere by the decisions of the Bevis Marks leaders in London. The Sephardic communities of Amsterdam, London, and even Salonika supplied rabbinical leaders to their fellow communities in the Caribbean and North America. Eventually the Jews of the Caribbean region migrated towards North America, but by the end of the 18th century they had not assimilated into British colonial or local society as did Sephardic Jewry on the North American continent. The Sephardic communities of North America forcefully paved the way for religious freedom for themselves and other minorities under the British, but did not themselves grow significantly.

NOTES

1 Mordechai Arbell, 'Genealogical research on Portuguese Jews in the Caribbeans and Guineas: facilities and difficulties', *Sharsheret Hadorot*, 11:1 (February 1997), 4–6.

2 Mordechai Arbell, 'The failure of the Jewish settlement in Tobago' in Margalit Bejarano and Efraim Zuroff (eds.), *Judaica Latinoamericana, estudios historicos-sociales III* (Jerusalem, 1997), 9–21.

3 Aubrey Newman, 'The Sephardim of the Caribbean' in R. D. Barnett and W. M. Schwab (eds.), *The Sephardi heritage*, vol. 2 (Grendon, Northants, 1989), 445–73; Mordechai Arbell, 'The Sephardim of the Island of Nevis', *Los Muestros* 35 (June 1999), 36–8.

4 Harry A. Ezratty, *500 years in the Caribbean: the Spanish and Portuguese Jews in the West Indies* (Baltimore, 1997), 14–15.

5 *Ibid.*, 40.

6 Richard D. Barnett and Philip Wright, *The Jews of Jamaica: tombstone inscriptions 1663–1880* (Jerusalem, 1997), xvii.

7 'Culture-Jamaica: shedding new light on the Jews', Inter Press Service, CNN, 21 December 1998.

8 Samuel J. Hurwitz and Edith F. Hurwitz, *Jamaica, a historical portrait* (New York, 1971), 14.

9 *Ibid.*, 14.

10 *Ibid.*, 42–3.

11 Barnett and Wright, xvii.

12 Newman, 451.

13 *Ibid.*

14 *Ibid.*, 452–3.

15 Ezratty, 40.

16 *Ibid.*, 3.

17 Hurwitz, 57.

18 Ezratty, 41; Hurwitz, 143.

19 Newman, 455.

20 Ezratty, 50.

21 Newman, 447.

22 *Ibid.*, 447–8.

23 Ezratty, 50–1.

24 Newman, 448.

25 *Ibid.*

26 *Ibid.*, 449.

27 Mordechai Arbell, 'The Jewish community of St Eustastius', *Pe'amim* 51 (1992), 124–34 [in Hebrew]; J. Hartog, *History of St Eustatius* (Aruba, 1976), and J. Hartog, *The Jews and St Eustatius* (St Maarten, 1976).

28 Newman, 450.

29 Mordechai Arbell, 'The Sephardim of the Island of Nevis', *Los Muestros* 35 (June 1999), 36–8.

30 Ezratty, 46.
31 Newman, 446.
32 *Ibid.*
33 Arbell, 37.
34 *Ibid.*
35 Ezratty, 45.
36 *Ibid.*, 36.
37 *Ibid.*, 12.
38 *Ibid.*, 12.
39 David and Tamar De Sola Pool, *An old faith in the New World: portraits of Shearith Israel 1654–1954* (New York, 1955), 32–5; Yitzchak Kerem, 'The impact of Sephardic migration in the Americas,' *Conference papers of the second Bereshit Conference, 8–12 October 1992, Villanova University* (Toledo, in press).
40 'Jews in colonial America', American Jewish Historical Society, 2. Jacob Rader Marcus noted that the 1695 synagogue was located on Beaver Street (Jacob Rader Marcus, *Early American Jewry: the Jews of New York, New England and Canada 1649–1794*, vol. 1 (Philadelphia, 1951), 48.
41 'Jews in Colonial America', 8–9.
42 *Since 1749: the story of K.K. Beth Elohim of Charleston, South Carolina* (Charleston, 1991), 2; Deborah Pessin, *History of the Jews in America* (New York, 1957), 47.
43 Charles Reznikoff, *The Jews of Charleston: a history of an American Jewish community* (Philadelphia, 1950), 6–7.
44 Frank E. Eakin Jr., *Richmond Jewry: fulfilling the promise* (Charleston, 1986), 2–3.
45 Malcolm Stern, 'The Sheftall Diaries: vital records of Savannah Jewry (1733–1808)', *American Jewish Historical Quarterly* 54, 246–7; and 'New light on the Jewish settlement of Savannah', I (New York, 1969), 174–9.
46 Yitzchak Kerem, 'Religious conflicts between Sephardic and Christian settlers in seventeenth- and eighteenth-century North America', in Bryan F. Le Beau and Menahem Mor (eds.), *Religion in the age of exploration: the case of Spain and New Spain* (Omaha, 1996), 149–61.
47 Jacob Rader Marcus, *Early American Jewry*, vol. 1, 154–7.
48 *Ibid.*, 156.

32

Dutch merchants and colonists in the English Chesapeake: trade, migration and nationality in 17th-century Maryland and Virginia

APRIL LEE HATFIELD

Historians of early America have long recognized the importance of Dutch trade with the 17th-century Chesapeake. Colonists themselves acknowledged their reliance on Dutch ships, protesting against England's Navigation Acts on the grounds that the exclusion of Dutch traders would ruin Virginia economically. Although John Pagan and others have emphasized the close financial relationships between Chesapeake tobacco producers and Dutch merchants, these merchants heretofore have been considered outsiders in the Chesapeake, by virtue of their nationality.[1]

Many Dutch merchants' involvement in Virginia and Maryland was deeper and more complicated than the historiography suggests. Several Dutch merchant families and many more individual mariners migrated from the Netherlands or New Netherland to the Chesapeake, settling permanently and becoming English denizens. These Dutch colonists fit into 17th-century Virginia and Maryland easily, sometimes marrying English colonists and sometimes acquiring positions of local importance. They were often virtually indistinguishable from English colonists in colonial and county court records, their Dutch background only infrequently apparent. The difficulty of identifying Dutch settlers in these records suggests that English colonists accepted Dutch merchants' settlement in the Chesapeake and perhaps suggests as well that Dutch immigrants consciously adapted themselves to English society as an economic strategy. The extent of Dutch colonists' involvement in local, colonial, inter-colonial, and transatlantic networks strengthens this perception.

Economic Importance

Dutch prominence in 17th-century Atlantic shipping, Dutch markets for tobacco, and Dutch sources for dry goods made Dutch traders crucial to Chesapeake planters.

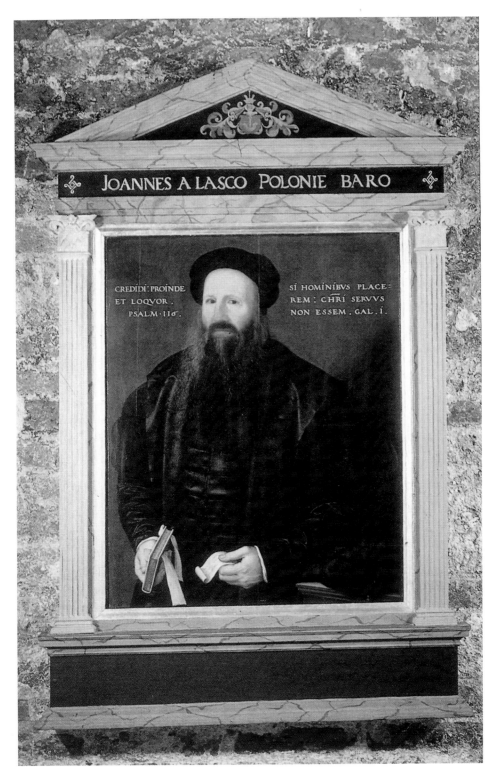

PLATE 1   John a Lasco (Johannes a Lasco Bibliothek, Emden)

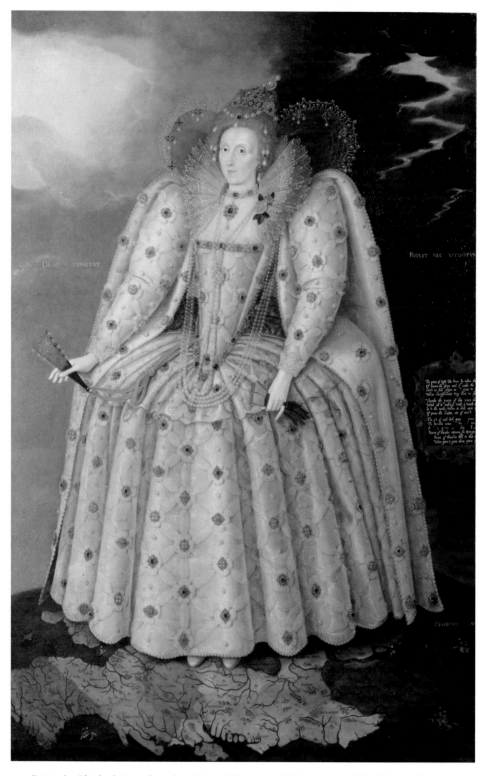

PLATE 4   Elizabeth I, attributed to Marcus Gheeraerts II (By courtesy of the National Portrait Gallery, London)

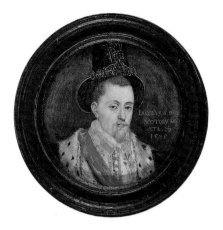
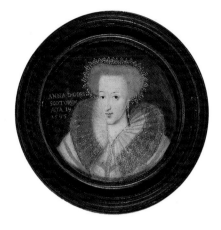

PLATE 5   James I and VI and Anne of Denmark by Adrian Vanson (Scottish National Portrait Gallery)

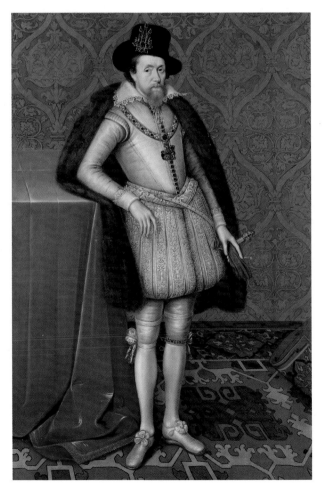

PLATE 6   James I, attributed to John de Critz I (By permission of the Trustees of the Dulwich Picture Gallery)

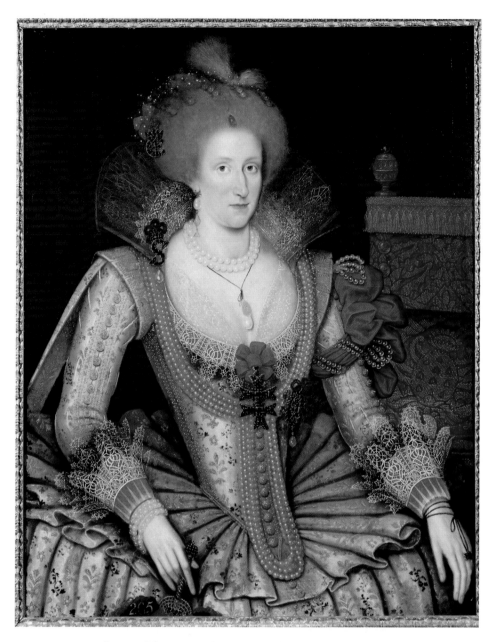

PLATE 7   Anne of Denmark by Marcus Gheeraerts II (The Royal Collection © 2001, Her Majesty
Queen Elizabeth II)

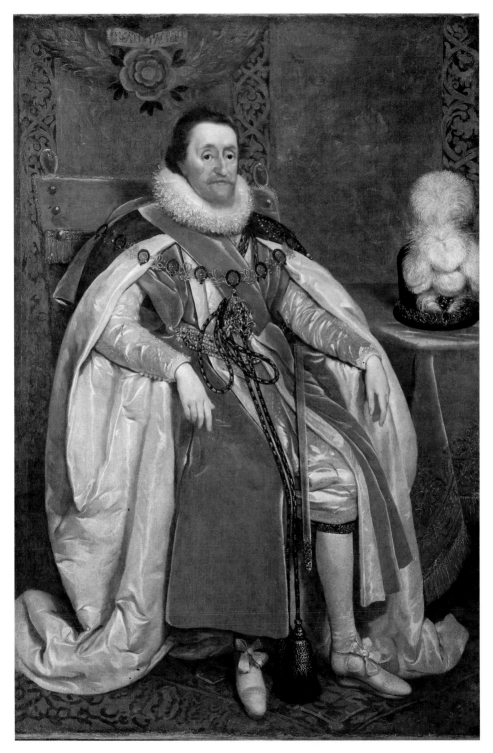

PLATE 8   James I by Daniel Mytens (By courtesy of the National Portrait Gallery, London)

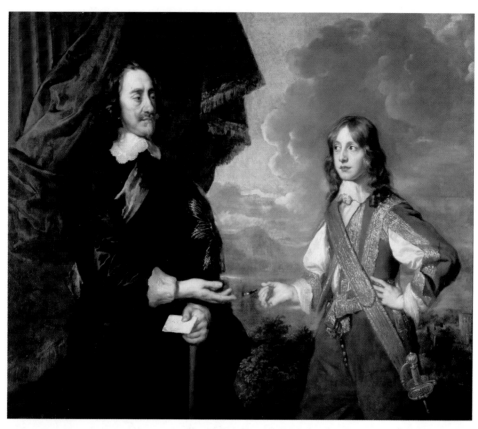

PLATE 9   Charles I and the Duke of York by Sir Peter Lely (Collection of the Duke of
Northumberland)

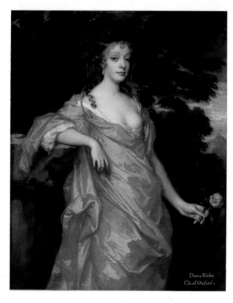

PLATE 10   Diana Kirke, later Countess of
Oxford, by Sir Peter Lely (Yale Center for
British Art, Paul Mellon Collection)

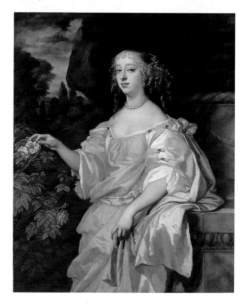

PLATE 11   Henrietta Boyle, later Countess of
Rochester, by Sir Peter Lely (The Royal
Collection © 2001, Her Majesty Queen
Elizabeth II)

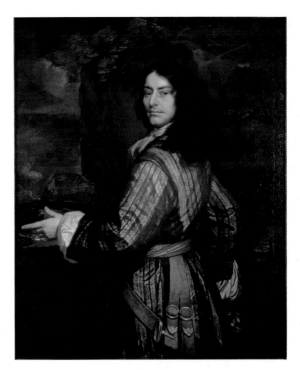

PLATE 12   Admiral Sir John Harman by Sir Peter Lely
(National Maritime Museum, London)

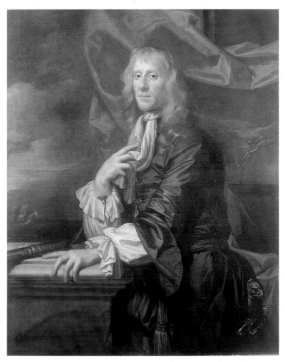

PLATE 13   Admiral Sir Jeremiah Smith by Sir Peter Lely
(National Maritime Museum, London)

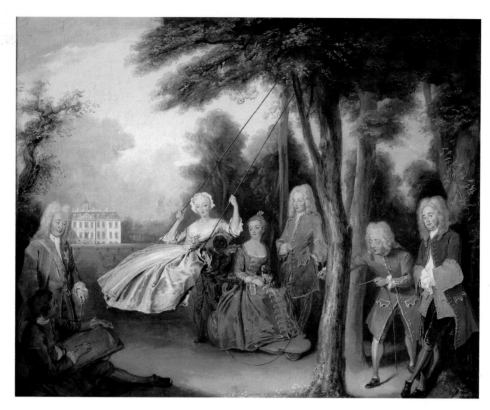

PLATE 16   Viscount Tyrconnel and his family by Philippe Mercier (© National Trust Photographic Library/John Hammond)

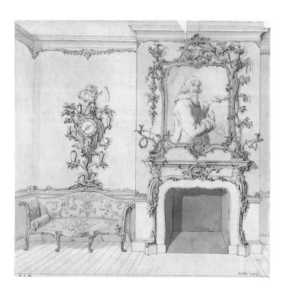

PLATE 18   Design for the side of a room by John Linnell (By courtesy of the V&A Museum)

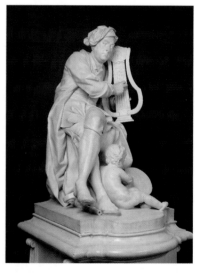

PLATE 19   George Frederick Handel by Louis François Roubiliac (V&A Picture Library)

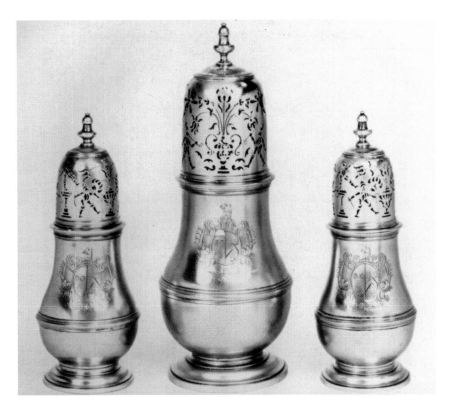

PLATE 20   Three sugar casters by David Willaume (Photograph in author's collection)

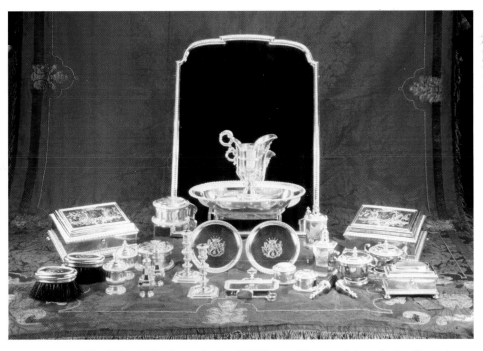

PLATE 21   The Kildare Toilet Service by David Willaume (Photograph in author's collection)

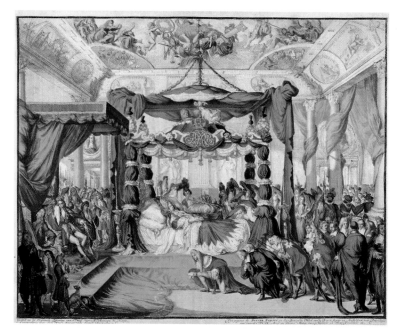

PLATE 22   Mary II on her deathbed (Atlas Van Stolk)

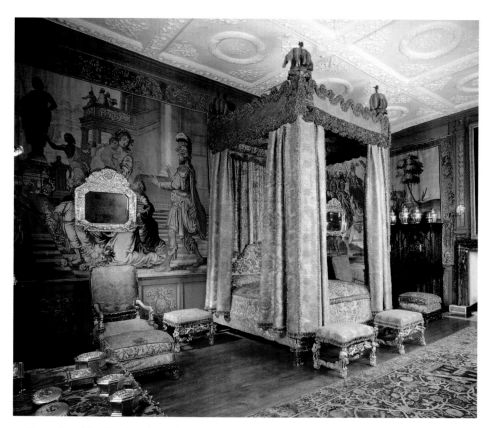

PLATE 23   The King's Bed, Knole (National Trust Photographic Library/Andreas van Einsiedel)

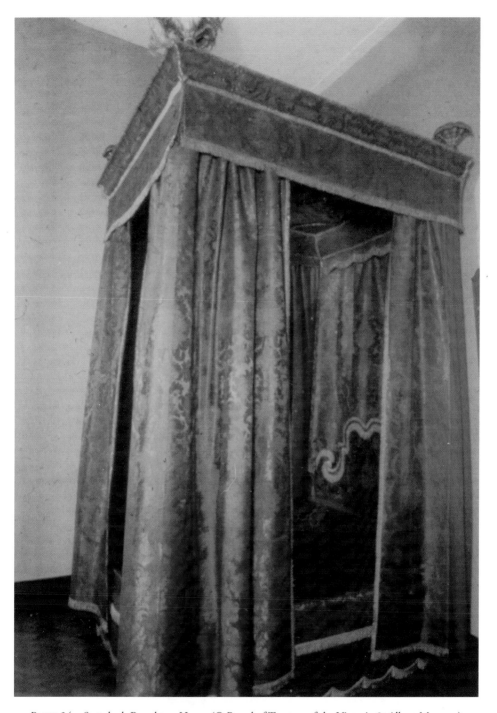

PLATE 24   State bed, Boughton House (© Board of Trustees of the Victoria & Albert Museum)

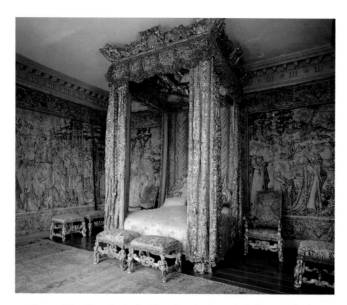

PLATE 25   State bed, the Venetian Ambassador's Room, Knole
(© National Trust Photographic Library/Andreas van Einsiedel)

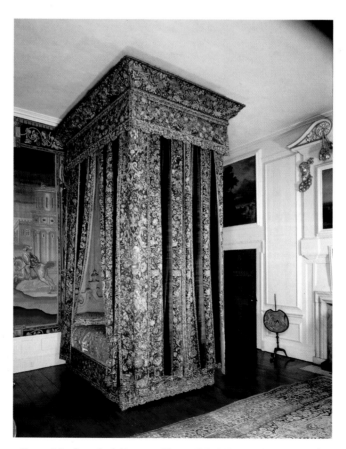

PLATE 26   State bed, Drayton House (Mark Fiennes/Country Life
Picture Library)

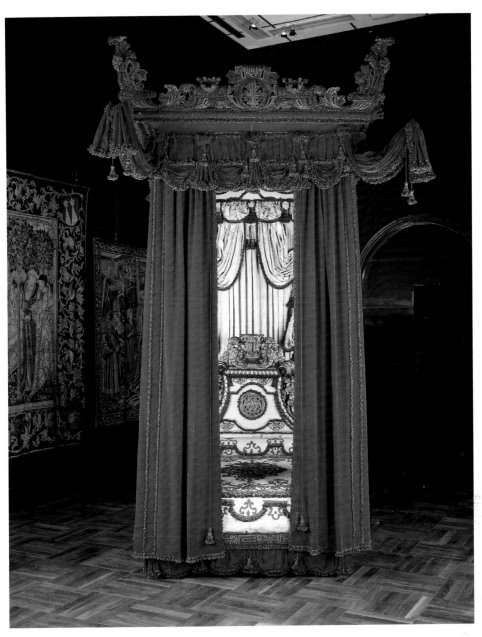

PLATE 27   State bed, Melville House (V&A Picture Library)

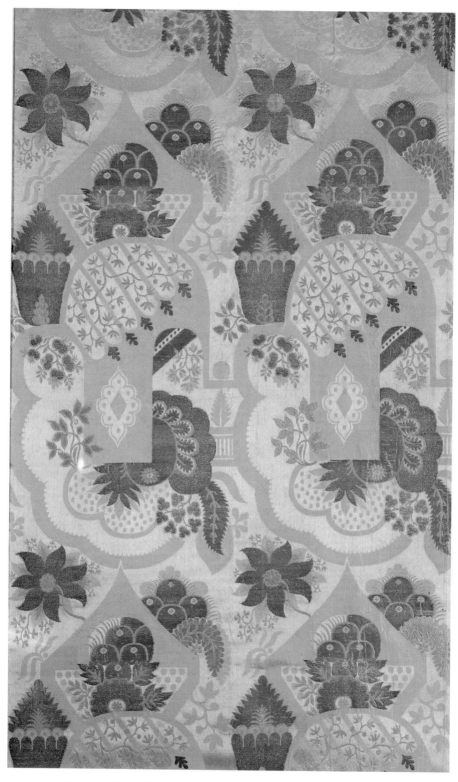

PLATE 28   Dress fabric by James Leman (Art Gallery of South Australia)

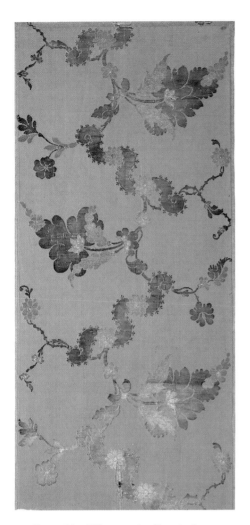

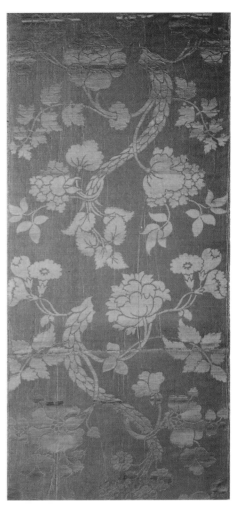

PLATE 29   Silk woven by Captain Peter
Lekeux's journeymen (Courtesy of the Trustees
of the V&A/J. Stevenson)

PLATE 30   Damask woven by Simon Julins's
journeymen (V&A Picture Library)

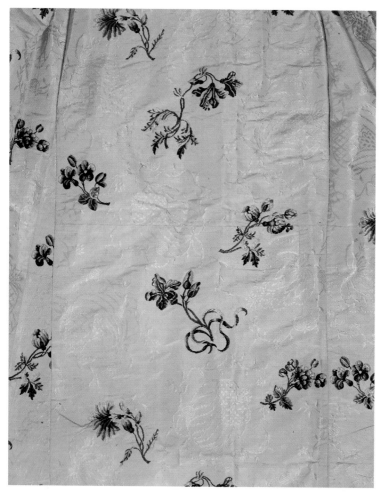

PLATE 31　Silk woven by Simon Julins's journeymen (Victoria & Albert Museum)

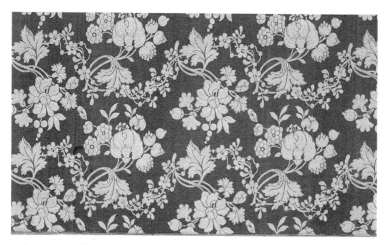

PLATE 32　Silk woven by John Sabatier's journeymen (Abegg-Stiftung, 3132 Riggisberg)

Dutch traders were important to Virginians and Marylanders from the outset of Chesapeake colonization. Given the central place of the Dutch in 17th-century Atlantic shipping this fact is not surprising.[2] Within the Chesapeake colonies, there were regional patterns to Dutch involvement. Transatlantic Dutch merchants traded tobacco from all parts of the Chesapeake to Europe, but intercolonial trade between Virginia and New Netherland (and via Dutch traders to other mainland and Caribbean colonies) was most important to the Maryland and Virginia Eastern Shore and to Virginia's Southside counties (south of the James River). The Dutch may have carried a larger percentage of the tobacco from these regions than from other parts of the Chesapeake. New Amsterdam was also a popular entrepôt for English traders, not only because it afforded cloth and other goods not easily available elsewhere but also because traders there could sometimes avoid English duties on trade goods bound for Europe.[3]

Dutch merchants' role in Chesapeake trade increased dramatically during the 1640s when the English Civil War disrupted English shipping. During the second half of the 17th century, the English Navigation Acts and the Anglo-Dutch wars complicated and made Virginia's trade with the Netherlands and with New Amsterdam illegal, but did not stop it.[4] The importance of Dutch commerce for Chesapeake planters led them to defend that commerce as part of their right to 'free trade' when Parliament implemented restrictive Navigation Acts during the Interregnum and Charles II reinforced them at the Restoration.[5] Individual traders found ways to skirt the restrictions against foreign ships and seamen. Ships whose Chesapeake voyages were recorded only because they had problems with the Navigation Acts make it clear that even ships trading between the Chesapeake and another English port often had non-English crews and captains.[6] Merchants of Dutch descent who had settled in the Chesapeake colonies remained there and maintained their positions in Dutch-English trade networks. After the English conquered New Netherland in 1664 many Dutch merchants there remained as New Yorkers and continued to trade as before, able to do so legally because Manhattan burghers were allowed 'free denizen' status by English authorities.[7] Illegal trade continued as well, though it is impossible to measure its extent.

Chesapeake colonists' favour toward Dutch traders also recognized that Dutch merchants and ships provided access to African labour sources at a time when the Dutch dominated the transatlantic slave trade. When Virginia and New Netherland signed a commerce and peace agreement in 1660, Virginia charged higher tobacco export duties for Dutch shippers than English, *unless* the Dutch brought slaves into the colony.[8] Access to slave trade through New Netherland or the Dutch Caribbean, or simply through contacts with Dutch merchants, may have provided advantages to Dutch merchant immigrants to the Chesapeake that would help explain their easy acceptance in the region, where English colonists would have valued anyone's ability to procure labour.

It seems likely as well that in addition to economic importance in general and access to African labour in particular, a sense of shared religious identity and history (especially among Puritan Virginians and Marylanders who were concentrated on the Southside and the Eastern Shore) made the transnational connections between English Chesapeake colonists and Dutch merchants and immigrants easier, especially when such connections were illegal. In 1653 during the first Anglo-Dutch War, when the

Puritan Richard Bennett was Governor of Virginia, New Netherland Governor Peter Stuyvesant sent Dutch Reformed minister Dominie Samuel Drisius to negotiate a commercial alliance between the two colonies. Drisius not only negotiated but also preached to English Puritans on the Eastern Shore while in Virginia. Stuyvesant recognized the degree to which religious and economic worlds were intertwined and attempted to use a sense of shared religious identity during the Interregnum to further New Netherland's economic goals. The prominence in intercolonial trade of individuals who had both Puritan and Dutch ties may have originated in the communities of English religious exiles in the Netherlands. In addition, the importance of Puritan New England and New Netherland in intercolonial trade networks may have given Puritan and Dutch Virginians an advantage in their business dealings.[9] Though Virginia's loudest defender of the right to free trade (and the one who finally signed the New Netherland trade agreement in 1660) was the Anglican Governor William Berkeley, many of those English Virginians with close Dutch connections were not only Protestant but Puritan.[10]

The dispersed nature of settlement and trade in the 17th-century Chesapeake meant that a large percentage of colonists interacted with Dutch merchants and mariners and recognized their economic importance to the region. David Ormrod and Dwyrydd Jones have described England's mercantile community at the end of the 17th century as 'thoroughly cosmopolitanized', as reflected by 'willing co-operation' with foreign merchants, actions they see as resulting from the convergence of British and Dutch economic and political interests.[11] In Virginia, Maryland, and New Netherland, colonists and officials displayed such willingness to see past ethnicity where trade was concerned by the mid-17th century. Dutch merchants in the Chesapeake enjoyed easy communication and socialization with Virginia planters and officials. The experiences of Dutch merchant David Pietersz de Vries illustrate the kind of socializing that accompanied 17th-century Chesapeake trade. Such socializing facilitated a familiarity that made Dutch merchants and mariners far from foreign to English Chesapeake colonists. When de Vries spent the winter of 1642–3 in Virginia, Governor Berkeley asked him for his company as he was 'in need of society'. De Vries spent several four- to five-day visits with Berkeley over the winter, and was grateful 'for the friendship which had been shown me by him throughout the winter'. That winter de Vries, another Dutch trader, and the ship's crew spent the winter going 'daily from one plantation to the other, until the ships were ready, and had their cargoes of tobacco', as Chesapeake trading required, interacting with colonists as they did business.[12]

Friendships formed during such stays were cultivated for both their economic and social value and could be long-lasting. On de Vries's way out of the Chesapeake that spring he spent the night with merchant and Councillor Samuel Matthews, whom he described as a 'good friend', an acquaintance made during de Vries's earlier visits to the region. Such relationships were not limited to ships' captains and wealthy colonists but included ordinary sailors and colonists, and even servants.[13] References to interactions on board ship and on land in accounts like de Vries's and in court cases suggest a relatively intense level of interaction between residents and mariners, and make no reference to any difficulties of language or ethnicity.

The largest presence of Dutch immigrants was on the Eastern Shore and Southside counties, where intercolonial trade was most important, and almost all the intercolonial traders in these regions have some recorded Dutch connection or experience.[14]

Maintaining a relationship with family in Amsterdam could be as valuable for a Chesapeake merchant as were ties with family in England.

Dutch immigrants in Virginia

When de Vries wrote about his experiences in the Chesapeake, he noted the need for Dutch (or any other) merchants to have factors in Virginia.[15] Whether or not they were following his advice, many Dutch merchants trading to the Chesapeake did either move there or encourage family members or trading partners to resettle. In Maryland more than half of the 17th-century naturalizations and denizations were for immigrants with obviously Dutch names or who had come to the Chesapeake from the Netherlands or New Netherland.[16] Some naturalizations, such as those for Eastern Shore merchant John Custis and Middlesex, Virginia, resident Nicholas Cock, were for people of English descent who had been born in the Netherlands.[17]

Even those immigrants coming directly from Holland often arrived with an eye on intercolonial as well as transatlantic trade. In 1650, for example, Lower Norfolk County, Virginia, merchant William Moseley, 'late of Rotterdam in holland', sold emerald, diamond, gold, ruby, and sapphire jewellery worth 612 guilders to Francis Yeardley for nine head of neat cattle, two draught oxen, two steers, and five cows. In July, before the sale of the jewellery, Moseley's wife, Susan, wrote to Francis Yeardley, agreeing to the terms of the sale and explaining that the decision to sell was because of *her* 'great wante of Cattle'. She assured Yeardley that she herself had gone from Rotterdam to The Hague to confirm the value of the jewellery with goldsmiths there.[18] The Moseleys sold the jewellery soon after they arrived in Virginia, when cattle were much more important than jewellery to their economic establishment and ability to develop a niche in an intercolonial trade network.[19]

The most clearly documented example of New Netherland-Chesapeake family ties is that centred around the Varlett family. Casper Varlett and his wife Judith Tentenier were merchants who moved from the Netherlands to Manhattan in the 1630s. Their names indicate Huguenot descent, strengthening J. F. Bosher's and David Ormrod's arguments that many early modern merchants operated in a 'Protestant International' world rather than one bounded by nationality.[20] Their only son, Nicholas, married Anna Stuyvesant, the sister of New Netherland Governor Peter Stuyvesant. Nicholas Varlett, also a merchant, traded to Curaçao and imported tobacco to New Amsterdam from Virginia.[21]

Two of Casper Varlett and Judith Tentenier's five daughters (the sisters of Nicholas) moved to the Chesapeake.[22] The first was Anna. She and her husband the surgeon George (Joris) Hack traded Chesapeake tobacco for Dutch cloth, white indentured servants, and enslaved Africans.[23] Anna Varlett Hack travelled to New Amsterdam several times between 1651 and 1661, apparently without her husband, in order to take care of their business there and undoubtedly also to visit her family.[24] Because George Hack was repeatedly referred to as a surgeon, and not a merchant, and because Anna did all of the recorded commercial travelling to New Amsterdam and came from a merchant family, the impulse to trade in the family probably came more from her than from her husband. In a New Netherland lawsuit she claimed a shipment of tobacco sent to her from Virginia by her husband as her private property. Once in the Chesapeake, George and Anna were responsible at least in part for the migration of other Dutch settlers from New Netherland to Virginia and Maryland. Additionally, they received headrights for Africans who may have come from New Netherland.[25]

Augustine Hermann was Anna Varlett Hack's trading partner and one of the Hacks' Virginia headrights. He had moved from Prague to New Amsterdam in 1643. In December 1650 or 1651, Hermann married Anna's sister Jannetje Varlett in the Dutch Reformed Church of New Amsterdam. They moved to the Eastern Shore at the end of the decade. Hermann traded extensively in Virginia before he moved to the Chesapeake, and was well known on the Eastern Shore. The Varlett/Hack and Varlett/Hermann families worked together, and both served as merchants to other colonists on the Eastern Shore, trading tobacco in their ships to New Netherland for Dutch cloth and for slaves.[26] A 1657 lawsuit illustrates the depth of Hermann's involvement in the Eastern shore economy and his importance (and that of other Dutch merchants like him) to the region. The case further reveals the often invisible network of personal communications necessary to conduct trade in the Chesapeake (a region without ports) and the ways in which the whole community was involved in maritime trade. Dutch merchants living in the Chesapeake, such as Hermann, connected English colonists to New Netherland and Dutch markets that they may not otherwise have had access to. Hermann, with the help of Netherlands-born Englishman John Custis, consolidated and carried the tobacco of multiple Eastern Shore residents to New Netherland, and a Dutch store owner kept it as it was being collected. Hermann's New Netherland crew members spent as much time as Hermann did on the Eastern Shore during the drawn-out tobacco collection process, interacting with colonists on their plantations as they picked up the crops, and thereby further exposing Eastern Shore residents to Dutch influence.[27]

The Hermanns, like the Hacks, lived and traded in both Virginia and Maryland.[28] The two families patented land near one another in both Maryland and Virginia. Only three days after Hermann received a grant for 4000 acres in Cecil County, Maryland, George Hack received a grant of 800 acres in the same county.

During 1665 George Hack and Jannetje Varlett died. George Hack's will, written 5 March 1665 and proved 17 April 1665, stipulated that half of his estate was to go to Anna and that his three children were to divide the other half, a property distribution more reflective of Dutch inheritance patterns than English, particularly if one of the three children was female (only two sons are listed in later records).[29] Anna Varlett Hack and Augustine Hermann remained economic partners and friends and applied for denizenship in Maryland at the same time in 1666.[30] They both, however, continued to spend time in both colonies, and though Anna had received Maryland denizenship, she apparently moved back to Virginia later that year and continued trading. In 1667, Anna Varlett Hack married Nicholas Boot, another merchant who had moved to Virginia from New Netherland several years before and had been naturalized by the Virginia Assembly in 1660.[31] He died only a year after his marriage to Anna Varlett Hack and she continued to trade.[32]

Not only did Anna Varlett trade independently, she engaged in the kinds of political activity commonly used by merchants to protect their economic interests. When unsatisfied with the judgment of an Eastern Shore county court in one of her business lawsuits, she requested an appeal to the General Court of Virginia, which intervened on her behalf.[33] Anna Varlett's willingness to appeal to the General Court reflects her comfort with the workings of Virginia's colonial government that she may have gained during similar activity in New Netherland.[34] Her success in the appeal indicates the ability of Dutch merchants to act effectively in the public sphere in various colonies.

Anna Varlett Hack Boot also continued to increase her landholdings through head-rights. In some of these, she was responsible for continuing the migration from New Netherland to the Eastern Shore.[35] The trade and migrations of the Varlett-Hermann-Hack-Boot family indicates the relationship between intercolonial economic and social ties. Intercolonial trade preceded the migrations that created an intercolonial family. Marriages and migrations strengthened the trade relationships and created webs that were not solely social or economic, but both.

In particular, the lives of merchants Anna Varlett Hack Boot and Augustine Hermann illustrate the ease with which Dutch-connected merchants operated in Virginia and Maryland. (Though Hermann was Czech rather than Dutch, he came to Virginia from New Netherland and is identified in the Chesapeake primarily by those ties.) Both were immigrants from New Netherland whose financial success in Chesapeake-New Netherland trade and ability to use Virginia's county and colonial courts to their advantage suggest they held recognizably important positions in the colony. Violet Barbour and Alice Clark have argued that Dutch women in early modern Europe more commonly engaged in long-distance trade than did other European women, and Dennis Maika and Martha Shattuck note that in New Netherland as well, women acted as merchants and were commonly considered their husband's business partners.[36] That Anna Varlett Hack Boot was so active as a merchant even after moving to Maryland and Virginia suggests that Dutch women's participation in such trade extended across the Atlantic not only to New Netherland but also to parts of English America. Susan Moseley's descriptions of her decision (discussed above) to sell her jewellery for cattle shortly after arriving in the Chesapeake from Rotterdam, provides further evidence that Dutch trading practices affected those women and men with Dutch heritage, even after they moved to English colonies where they were surrounded by English settlers whose expectations of women's commercial roles were quite different. The lack of any objection or even any remarks in English Chesapeake records might suggest that women traders may well have been familiar to English colonists for whom Dutch trade was so important economically. At least one Dutch-connected woman in the Chesapeake continued to follow Dutch rather than English naming practices, using her surname Barbarah DeBarette rather than her husband's (Garrett Vanswaringen's) after they moved to Maryland from New Amstel. More notably, the Maryland court recorded her surname following Dutch practices, even as she was being naturalized in the English colony in 1669.[37]

One of the only other examples of a Chesapeake woman independently engaged in long-distance trade also involves Dutch contacts. Ann Taft [or Toft], a spinster living in the Pungoteage region of the Eastern Shore (where Anna Varlett Hack Boot had her plantation), did business and made personal and economic contacts from New England to Jamaica, providing further evidence that in this Chesapeake region with significant Dutch presence gender conventions may have been different from what they were elsewhere in English colonial America. In 1666 Taft traded between New England and Virginia using a ketch belonging to Dutch Virginia merchant Simon

Overzee.[38] Three years later Ann Taft was still shipping goods with Overzee. This time, she was trading between the Eastern Shore and Nevis.[39] She and Eastern Shore merchant Edmund Scarborough (who was an important trader to New Netherland) were involved together in a 4000–acre Jamaican estate.[40] Taft's residence in a county with Dutch settlers, her repeated use of a ship owned by Dutch immigrant Simon Overzee, and her trade with Scarborough and others familiar with New Netherland and the Netherlands may have eased her entry into a long-distance commercial world not commonly the domain of English colonial women.

Dutch merchants and settlers provided important economic contacts for many English colonists in the 17th-century Chesapeake. Financial concerns weakened ethnic prejudices and significantly reduced any Chesapeake commitment to English metropolitan mercantilist visions. Such easy incorporation of Dutch merchant activity and settlement in the Chesapeake did not occur without Dutch co-operation. The apparently conscious effort some Dutch merchants made to fit in, by anglicizing their names, anglicizing their boats' names, speaking English, and seeking out co-religionists, contributed to their easy acceptance in Virginia and Maryland that may have provided leeway for Dutch women to maintain independent economic activity. In the 17th century, Virginians' frequent dependence on Dutch merchants and seamen for sufficient access to European goods and markets and African slaves, particularly during the English Civil War, affected English colonists' perspectives on international rivalries and on national and individual goals of colonization in ways that facilitated significant Dutch involvement in local Chesapeake society.

NOTES

1   John R. Pagan, 'Dutch maritime and commercial activity in mid-seventeenth-century Virginia', *Virginia Magazine of History and Biography* 90 (1982), 485–501; Susie M. Ames, *Studies of the Virginia Eastern Shore in the seventeenth century* (Richmond, 1940), 8–9, 45–67; Philip Alexander Bruce, *Economic history of Virginia in the seventeenth century* (New York, 1896). This tendency to regard Dutch residents as outsiders is true even for regions such as the Southside counties and the Eastern Shore, where immigrants from Holland and from Dutch New Netherland settled disproportionately. Douglas Deal has noted that the Eastern Shore 'had more than its share of wealthy Dutch residents, who expanded the already existing commercial network that linked several prominent merchant-planters on the Shore with Dutch traders and ships' captains on both sides of the Atlantic'; but he argues that 'that network dissolved abruptly after the first of the Anglo-Dutch wars'. J. Douglas Deal, *Race and class in colonial Virginia: Indians, Englishmen, and Africans on the Eastern Shore during the seventeenth century* (New York, 1993).

2   C. R. Boxer, *The Dutch seaborne empire, 1600–1800* (1965, reprinted London, 1990). Because of its location, New Amsterdam was a common stopping point between New England and Virginia, and so Virginians' Dutch and New England trades overlapped. For examples see David Peterson [Pietersz] de Vries, *Voyages from Holland to America, AD 1632–1644*, trans. Henry C. Murphy (New York, 1853), 63–4; Susie M. Ames (ed.), *County Court records of Accomack-Northampton, Virginia, 1632–1640* (Washington, D.C., 1954), xxxvii, 22–3.

3   For examples of Virginians involved in Dutch trade, see Ames, *Studies*, 47, citing Northampton Wills and Deeds, 1657–66, 33. Eastern Shore planter and merchant Colonel Argoll Yeardley also traded tobacco to Peter Jacobson at Manhattan. When Yeardley died,

his wife Ann and her second husband John Wilcox maintained the relationship with him at least long enough to clear the accounts. Northampton Order Book 1657–64, 3.

4 In 1655 Edmund Scarborough purchased slaves in Manhattan and had to petition the Dutch Council for permission to return to Virginia. The Council decided that 'the opinion of every one having been asked, to grant the request', provided that Scarborough give £5000 bail that he and his mariners would not enter the Delaware Bay. Ames, *Studies*, 49, citing Berthold Fernow (ed.), *Documents relative to the colonial history of the state of New York*, vol. 12 (Albany, 1877), 94.

5 Pagan, 498–9; Ames, *Studies*, 49–50.

6 For example, on 25 April 1655, Richard Hincksman petitioned Oliver Cromwell that his ship *Rose of London* be allowed to proceed to Barbados with stranger mariners because he was unable to hire enough English seamen for the voyage. *CSPC 1574–1660* (London, 1860), 423, no. 42.

7 Dennis J. Maika, 'Jacob Leisler's Chesapeake trade', *De Halve Maen* 67 (1994), 11. According to Maika, 'Trade between Manhattan and the Chesapeake continued uninterrupted after the English imperial government's intrusion into New York in 1664', though Cathy Matson argues that by that time the 1660 Navigation Act had already altered tobacco trade routes so that less Chesapeake tobacco went through New Netherland en route to Europe. Cathy Matson, *Merchants and empire: trading in colonial New York* (Baltimore, 1998), 18.

8 English shippers normally paid two shillings per hogshead tobacco, foreign shippers ten shillings per hogshead. The Dutch (or other Christian nations in amity with England) would pay two shillings per hogshead only for the amount of tobacco they received as payment for African slaves. William Waller Hening (ed.), *The Statutes at large; being a collection of all the laws of Virginia, from the first session of the legislature, in the year 1619*, vol. 1 (Richmond, 1809), 540; Pagan, 497.

9 Ames, *Studies*, 48–9; Edward D. Neill, *The Virginia Company of London* (Washington, D.C., 1868), 234–5; Northampton County Court Order Books, 1654–61, typescript by Susie May Ames, Virginia Historical Society MSS 3N8125a, folder 1, 36–7; Babette M. Levy, 'Early Puritanism in the southern and island colonies', *American Antiquarian Society Proceedings* 70 (1960), 144.

10 For a discussion of the importance of shared Puritanism to 17th-century Atlantic commerce, see David Ormrod, 'The Atlantic economy and the "Protestant Capitalist International", 1651–1775' *Historical Research* 66 (1993), 197–208; J. F. Bosher, 'Huguenot merchants and the Protestant International in the seventeenth century', *William and Mary Quarterly* 3rd ser., 52 (1995), 77–102. For the concentration of Puritans on the Virginia and Maryland Eastern Shores see Levy, 107–12 and James Horn, *Adapting to a new world: English society in the seventeenth-century Chesapeake* (Chapel Hill, 1994), 388–99.

11 Ormrod, 204–5 citing Dwyrydd W. Jones, *War and economy in the age of William III and Marlborough* (Oxford, 1988), 256.

12 de Vries, 183–4.

13 *Ibid.*, 187–9.

14 Two of the wealthiest Eastern Shore merchants, Stephen Charleton and Edmund Scarborough, traded extensively to both New Netherland and New England. Susie M. Ames (ed.), *County court records of Accomack-Northampton, Virginia, 1640–1645* (Charlottesville, 1973), xiii; Ames, *Studies*, 47.

15 de Vries, 112–3.

16 For a list of those 17th-century Marylanders receiving denization and naturalization certificates, see Jeffrey Wyand and Florence L. Wyand (eds.), *Colonial Maryland naturalizations* (Baltimore, 1986), 1–9. The denizations and naturalizations were expensive and probably only pursued by those for whom the trading advantages provided by such status mattered.

Denization and naturalization records therefore represent only a portion of the actual Dutch settlers in Maryland and Virginia.

17 For Cocke, see P. W. Hiden, 'Smiths of Middlesex County, Virginia', *William and Mary Quarterly* 2nd ser., 10 (1930), 215. For Custis see 'Proceedings of the House of Burgesses', *Virginia Magazine of History and Biography* 8 (1901), 391. Chesapeake immigrants of English descent who identified themselves as coming from the Netherlands had probably moved there for religious or commercial reasons. Because many Dutch immigrants to Virginia and Maryland anglicized their names, it is not always possible to tell whether someone moving from Holland was of Dutch or English descent. In either case, their presence strengthened Chesapeake-Dutch ties and weakened any sense of ethnic difference.

18 Emphasis added. Library of Virginia (Richmond), Norfolk County Wills and Deeds C, 1651–6, 24–25a, recorded 10 November 1652.

19 *Ibid.*, 8, 9a, 24.

20 See Ormrod and Bosher (as in note 10). The Dutch merchants and colonists I have identified in this article clearly were at home in this world, but some of the culture they brought to the Chesapeake was clearly based on their residence in the Netherlands or New Netherland as well.

21 In 1660 and 1661 he went to Virginia as a representative of New Netherland to help negotiate the commerce treaty between the two colonies. Casper Varlett was a merchant with ties to the Dutch West India Company. Edwin R. Purple, 'Contributions to the history of the ancient families of New York, Varleth—Varlet—Varleet—Verlet—Verleth', *New York Genealogical and Biographical Record* 9 (1878), 53–62, 113–25; 10 (1879), 35–8. For this and other citations on the Varlett family, I am indebted to Brent Tartar and Daphne Gentry for unpublished research notes on the life of Anna Varlett Hack Boot, compiled for the Library of Virginia.

22 Purple, 54, 60. The three daughters who did not move to Virginia were Maria, Catherine, who married François de Bruyn of New Amsterdam, and Judith, who married Nicholas Bayard (the son of Samuel Bayard and Anna Stuyvesant Bayard Varleet). Judith was accused of witchcraft in 1666 but lived until after 1707.

23 Nell M. Nugent (ed.), *Cavaliers and pioneers: abstracts of Virginia land patents and grants, 1623–1800* vol. 1: *1623–1666* (1934, reprinted Richmond, 1992), 265, 285, 412.

24 The last New Amsterdam record with her name was in January 1661: Purple, 54. Though when she was in New Netherland, Anna Varlett followed Dutch naming practices and did not use her husband's name, in English records she frequently appeared with the name of her first or second husband.

25 In April 1659 George Hack was granted a certificate for 1350 acres for 27 headrights, including people of English, Dutch, and African descent. The headrights included: George Nicholas Hack; Sepherin Hack; An[n] Kathrine Hack; Domingo, a Negro; George, a Negro; Kathrine, a Negro; Ann, a Negro; Hendrick Volkerts; R'nick Gerrits; Bermon Nephrinninge; Giltielmus Varlee (Varlett?); Augustine Hermons; Barnard Rams'; Augustine Rieters; Adrian Rams'; Claus Gisbert; Brigitta Williams; and Cornelis Hendrickson. Library of Virginia, Northampton County Court Order Book, 1654–61, folder 4, 32–4 (5 April 1659).

26 Purple, 54–7.

27 See Library of Virginia, Northampton County Court Order Books, 1654–61, folder 3, 10–15, 35–6.

28 On 19 June 1662, Augustine Hermann received a grant of 4000 acres in Cecil County, Maryland, for a plantation they named Bohemia Manor. In 1655[65?] he moved servants and goods to Northampton County, Virginia, to establish a plantation there. Ames, *Studies*, 66. He held on to Bohemia Manor and spent time in both Chesapeake colonies, as well as in New Netherland.

29 Library of Virginia, Accomack County Deeds and Wills, 1664–71, 11; Nugent, vol. 1, 525.

30 *Archives of Maryland*, vol. 2: *Proceedings and acts of the General Assembly of Maryland, April 1666–June 1676*, ed. William Hand Browne (Baltimore, 1884), 144–5. This is confusing, however, because there is also a Maryland denizenship for Hermann 'late of Manhatans Merchant' recorded on 14 January 1660. *Archives of Maryland*, vol. 3: *Proceedings of the Council of Maryland, 1636–1667*, ed. William Hand Browne (Baltimore, 1885), 398.

31 Boot settled in Gloucester County during the 1650s. See H. R. McIlwaine (ed.), *Journals of the House of Burgesses of Virginia 1659/60 – 1693* (Richmond, 1914), 10. Nicholas's name was sometimes rendered as Claus, while Boot also appears Boodt, Bout, Boat, Bootsen.

32 Library of Virginia, Accomack County Deeds and Wills, 1664–71, 68. Anna probably died in 1685, when her two sons qualified as administrators of her estate and referred to her in a deed as 'Ann our mother lately deceased'. *Archives of Maryland*, vol. 2, 144–5

33 Library of Virginia, Accomack County Orders and Wills, 1671–3, 134. H. R. McIlwaine (ed.), *Minutes of the Council and General Court of colonial Virginia 1622–32, 1670–1676* (Richmond, 1924), 320.

34 For reference to the New Netherland lawsuits, see Purple, 54.

35 In January 1672 she was granted certificate for 1250 acres due for headrights, including a Sarah Varlett. Library of Virginia, Accomack County Orders and Wills, 1671–3, 48. In September 1674 she received a certificate for 450 acres for nine headrights, including William and Kath Varlett. Accomack County Orders and Wills, 1673–6, 180. The following month (on 8 October) Anna Boot patented 1350 acres in Accomack, 900 being part of 1000 granted her under the name of Ann Hack, widow, 450 for nine persons including William Varlett and Kath Varlett. Nugent, vol. 2: *1666–1695* (Richmond, 1977), 158.

36 Maika, 'Jacob Leisler's Chesapeake trade', 206; Martha Dickinson Shattuck, 'A civil society: court and community in Beverwyck, New Netherland, 1652–1664' (Ph.D. dissertation, Boston University, 1993), 164.

37 The naturalization record lists entries for Garrett Vanswaringen, born in Reensterdwan, Holland; Barbarah DeBarette, born in Valenciennes in the Low Countries when under Spanish rule; Elizabeth Vanswaringen, daughter of Garrett and Barbarah born in New Amstel; and Zacharias Vanswaringen, son of Garrett and Barbarah born in New Amstel. Wyand and Wyand, 1–9.

38 Endorsed 28 June 1666, 'Mrs Ann Taft To the Hono[ura]ble John Wintropp Esq[ui]re Gov[e]rnor of the Southern parts of New England'. Massachusetts Historical Society (Boston), Winthrop Papers, n.p., microfilm reel 8.

39 Ann Taft indicated to the Northampton court members that she knew James Russell, Lieutenant-Governor of Nevis, and that he was trustworthy and qualified to carry out their requests. Library of Virginia, Accomack County Order Book, 1666–70, 94–5, 261–2.

40 St Jago, Minutes of the Council of Jamaica, 1672, in *CSPC 1669–1674*, 382, no. 881.

33

The Dutch in 17th-century New York City: minority or majority?

Joyce D. Goodfriend

In 1664, during the second Anglo-Dutch War, England captured the territory known as New Netherland from the Netherlands and renamed it New York. The consequences of this transfer of sovereignty for world history were far-reaching, but in this paper I propose to examine just one question that bears on the theme of this conference. Did the imposition of English rule on New Netherland transform the Dutch who had lived in New Amsterdam from a majority to a minority?

On the face of it, the answer to this question appears to be a simple yes. Once English governance commenced, the Dutch inhabitants of the small settlement at the tip of Manhattan Island lost both legal rights and customary privileges and were relegated to a subordinate status. This is not to say that the Dutch colonists were reduced to the condition of a conquered people. As white Protestant subjects of a culturally advanced western European country, 17th-century Dutch men and women were not about to be treated as would the indigenous people of a non-Christian society. In recognition of the similarities between the Dutch and English peoples, as well as the political uncertainties associated with the protracted Anglo-Dutch conflict, the Articles of Capitulation were conciliatory and the 'conquered' Dutch were given a variety of concessions.

Those Dutch who stayed in New York were allowed to keep their property, maintain their inheritance customs, and practise their religion without interference. Their contracts were declared valid. They were designated denizens of the British empire and allowed to trade with England and its colonies.[1] Although the form of municipal government was soon changed, no legal impediments were placed in the way of Dutch participation in civic life. As long as they swore an oath to England, the men of New Amsterdam were eligible to hold positions on New York City's Common Council.

Neverthless, the city's long-term residents lost rights and privileges as the new English rulers altered the status of Dutch institutions and reversed the policies of the Dutch West India Company government. Roman law, which had authority in the Dutch Republic and its colonies, gave way to English common law. Direct trade with the Netherlands, though permitted during the early years of transition, became more and more difficult as newly transplanted English merchants insisted on enforcement of the Acts of Trade.[2] Although the Dutch were guaranteed freedom of religion, the Dutch Reformed Church was disestablished in New York. Public money was no longer set aside to support the Church's ministers. When Domine Johannes Megapolensis approached the Governor in 1669 and requested funds for his salary, he was told 'if the Dutch will have divine service their own way, then let them also take care of and support their own preachers'.[3]

Not only did the Dutch Reformed Church lose its privileged status, but the intolerant religious policy of the New Netherland government was overturned by the Duke of York. Lutherans, Quakers and Jews, groups which had been denied the right to hold services in public under Dutch West India Company rule, were now permitted to worship openly.[4] By 1669 the Lutheran congregation was conducting services in New York City.[5] The religious uniformity championed by Director-General Petrus Stuyvesant and the Dutch Reformed clergymen was a thing of the past.

In a fundamental sense, then, the Dutch were transformed from a majority to a minority in English New York. Associated with the losing side in the latest round of the wars for empire, they had become subject to English power. Even though the Dutch briefly regained dominion over New York during the final Anglo-Dutch war in 1673–4, the city soon returned to English hands, leaving the residents to come to grips with a future that lay within the British empire. The rights and privileges the Dutch had enjoyed as the dominant group in a colony ruled by men of their own nation were curtailed and the pathway to wealth and power, though by no means foreclosed, was now no longer smooth.

Yet, this is not the whole story. If one adopts a sociological perspective, it becomes apparent that New York City's Dutch inhabitants, despite their obligation to submit to English governance and to follow English regulations, retained a number of the characteristics of a majority.[6] If this was the case, then the corollary to this proposition must also be true. English New Yorkers, while officially privileged, in certain respects resembled a minority group in the small 17th-century city. The anomalous aspects of the situation of the English in New York did not escape the notice of contemporaries. A group of local Anglican leaders, writing in 1699, reflected that until the Church of England was established in 1697, New York had been 'like a conquered Foreign Province held by the terrour of a Garrison, rather than an English Colony, possessed and settled by people of our own Nation'.[7]

New York City's ethnic demography supplies the cornerstone of the argument that the Dutch exhibited many attributes of a majority group. The Dutch outnumbered the English in the city by a considerable margin throughout the 17th century. As late as 1699, the English constituted only about a third of New York City's white population and it was not until the early decades of the 18th century that the English population drew close to the Dutch in size.[8] The less than impressive English presence in New York is, in part, due to the insufficiency of immigration to the province from the British Isles. Although a substantial number of English men entered the city in the years immediately after the conquest, many soon departed. Turnover was a major feature of the city's English population during the 17th century. Of 110 English men enumerated on the city's tax rolls in 1676–7, only 15 (or 14 per cent) were present on the 1695 tax list.[9] In the 1680s, British immigration slowed to a trickle, Governor Thomas Dongan remarking in 1687 that 'for these 7 yeares last past, there has not come over into this province twenty English Scotch or Irish familys'.[10]

Equally important in explaining the numerical superiority of the Dutch in 17th-century New York City is the fact that the great majority of New Amsterdam's Dutch residents opted to remain in the city after the conquest, rather than return to the Netherlands. Their decision was influenced by the lenient terms of surrender offered by the English as well as by the fact that many had lived in the city for over a decade, were married and had children, and were established in business. Well-entrenched in New York City, Dutch families had little inclination to uproot themselves. A sizeable portion of the population had been born in America and knew no other home.

Not only were the Dutch more numerous than the English in 17th-century New York City, they were bound together by intergenerational kinship networks as well as long standing ties to the Dutch Reformed Church, the nucleus of the city's Dutch community. English community development, by comparison, was stunted. Family formation among English immigrants was strikingly slow. Those English who came to New York City were predominantly young single men, many of whom remained in the city only a short while. Of those who did stay, some married into local Dutch families and were absorbed into Dutch family circles.

It was not only the weakness of English family networks, but the lack of an institutional centre that hindered the forging of an English community in 17th-century New York City. At the heart of the problem was the inordinately long time it took to establish the Church of England in the city. Despite the fact that New York City was nominally an English city after 1664, Trinity Church did not open its doors until 1697, more than thirty years after the English first claimed the colony. Until then, Anglican worship was held in the Dutch church and the number attending was small. A visitor to the city in 1679 reported that 'there were not above twenty five or thirty people in the church' when the English minister conducted Anglican services.[11] Nearly two decades later, the great majority of New Yorkers still were connected to the Dutch Reformed Church, which had erected a new place of worship – the Garden Street Church – in 1693. In 1698, the congregation boasted 650 members, not to mention many others who attended worship regularly or on occasion.[12] By contrast, as late as 1724, the rector of Trinity Church could only claim that 'the usual number of Communicants is one hundred and upwards'.[13]

Given their numbers, their solid communal base in the Dutch Reformed Church, and their secure economic position (which I have documented elsewhere),[14] the Dutch in 17th-century New York City surely had the hallmarks of a majority group. The case for the ascendancy of Dutch culture in the city is less clear-cut, since public discourse was controlled by the English.[15] But there is sufficient evidence to suggest that the city's popular culture, which, for the most part, was transmitted orally, was still largely shaped by Dutch values. The pervasiveness of the Dutch language in daily life and the perpetuation of Dutch dietary preferences, architectural styles, fashions, holidays and inheritance customs attest to the vitality of the local Dutch culture which existed alongside the official English culture.[16]

New York City's English residents, though privileged by virtue of their connection to the ruling power, were, in practice, often at a disadvantage in everyday affairs. Surrounded by Dutch men and women in the streets, in the taverns, and in the marketplace, they may, at times, have been psychologically overwhelmed by those who were, in theory, a vanquished people.

But the social and cultural dominance of the Dutch in New York City could not be perpetuated indefinitely. Several developments in the late 17th century served to loosen the sway of the Dutch in New York City.

In the 1680s, Protestant refugees from religious persecution in Louis XIV's France began to emigrate to New York.[17] In the space of two decades, the city's ethnic demography was appreciably altered, as scores of Huguenots established homes in the city. These exiled Protestants rapidly coalesced into a cohesive community centred round the Eglise Françoise à la Nouvelle York founded in 1688. By the end of the 17th century, when the city had a little more than 4200 white inhabitants, Huguenots formed nearly 10 per cent of the population.[18]

The Huguenot immigrants elicited the sympathies of New York's Dutch, since there were long standing historical ties between Dutch and French adherents of the Reformed faith. New York City's Dutch Reformed minister, Henricus Selyns, who witnessed the arrival of the widening stream of refugees, heaped praise on a newly arrived French preacher in a 1683 letter to the Classis of Amsterdam. 'Domine Peter Daille, formerly Professor at Salmurs [Saumur] has become my colleague. He exercises his ministry in the French church here. He is full of zeal, learning and piety. Exiled for the sake of his religion, he now devotes himself here to the cause of Christ with untiring energy'.[19] Selyns's congregants also perceived an affinity with their persecuted brethren. Bonds between the Dutch and French Reformed in New York were not confined to an ecclesiastical context. Business partnerships and marriages connected Dutch and French families.

Those affiliated with the Dutch Reformed Church viewed the Huguenots as potential confederates in their efforts to curb Anglican power in the city. During the early years of the Huguenot migration to New York, the position of the Dutch Reformed Church was not protected by law and the Dutch were wary of English officials and their local supporters who were planning to establish the Church of England in the city. Only in 1696 did the New York City Dutch Reformed Church receive a charter that placed it on a secure legal foundation. At the height of the Huguenot immigration, then, the Dutch were eager to persuade the French newcomers, fellow Reformed Protestants, to make common cause against the Anglicans.

Though the Dutch envisioned the Huguenots as religious and political allies, they were aware that Huguenot settlement in New York City created a competing ethnic bloc. Under Dutch rule, immigrants from a variety of cultural backgrounds took up residence in New Amsterdam and gradually were woven into the fabric of Dutch society as a result of exposure to the Dutch language, attendance at the Dutch Reformed Church, and intermarriage. At the time the English conquered New Netherland in 1664, the city's population included substantial numbers of Germans, English, Norwegians and French, many of whom were well along in the process of becoming culturally Dutch.

But the French immigrants who arrived in the 1680s and 1690s had no intention of being integrated into the Dutch community and instead formed an independent constituency. More significantly, they had compelling reasons for siding with the English in New York. Their circumstances as refugees and their dependence on the for a place of sanctuary placed them in the debt of the English. They had been promised personal security and the freedom to worship in their own fashion in return for loyalty to the Crown. By casting their lot with the English rather than the Dutch in New York

City, the Huguenots could anticipate future benefits in the form of preferment. The English, in turn, were disposed to look favourably on the French immigrants, if for no other reason than that they added to the numbers of non-Dutch in the city.

The expansion of New York City's non-Dutch population took place at a time when local Dutch culture was gradually becoming divorced from its metropolitan roots. New York's Dutch residents received virtually no reinforcement from the Netherlands, especially after 1674. Though immigration from the Netherlands was permitted by the 1664 articles of surrender, relatively few Dutch men and women journeyed from their homeland to New York, certainly not enough to keep local people abreast of changes in metropolitan culture.

New York City's Dutch population grew almost entirely through natural increase and, as the years passed, American-born Dutch came to predominate in the Dutch community. These second- and third-generation members of Dutch families experienced not only an attentuation of personal ties to kinfolk in the Netherlands but a gradual detachment from contemporary Dutch culture. Largely cut off from the wellsprings of Dutch culture, they were poised to absorb elements of Anglo-American culture.

The deracination of the American-born Dutch was accelerated among a small but important segment of New York City's Dutch population consisting primarily of wealthy merchants. Power-hungry men with ambitions to succeed in this English-controlled society, they voluntarily embraced English ways and deliberately curried the favour of English officials in order to garner a share of the rewards available to men loyal to the Crown. The willingness of members of the Dutch elite to distance themselves from their ancestral culture fractured New York City's Dutch community and weakened its influence.

The Dutch community was further divided by clashing opinions on religious styles. Some remained committed to Reformed orthodoxy, while others expressed sympathy for the Pietist point of view. Those who held to orthodox beliefs emphasized faithfulness to doctrine and performance of the liturgy as the crucial aspects of Reformed religion. Pietists denounced orthodoxy as formalistic and lacking in spirit, opting for an experiential form of religion that focused on spiritual truths transmitted to the heart rather than the mind.[20] Pietist sympathizers played a prominent role in the largely Dutch movement led by Jacob Leisler in 1689 in sympathy with the Glorious Revolution in England. The disastrous outcome of Leisler's Rebellion and the consequent decline in status of Leisler's Dutch supporters undermined Dutch power in New York City.

The fissures in the Dutch community, especially when seen against the backdrop of a flourishing French community, threatened the pre-eminent position of the Dutch in the city. But it was initiatives by the English around the turn of the century that ultimately negated any claim New York City's Dutch could make to majority status. The founding of three institutions with far-reaching cultural influence – William Bradford's press, Trinity Church, and the Charity School sponsored by the Society for the Propagation of the Gospel in Foreign Parts (SPG) – gave the English a decisive advantage in their contest with the Dutch for primacy in New York City's cultural arena.

Printer William Bradford's decision to move his printing business to New York City in 1693 inaugurated a new era in the city's communications history.[21] Prior to this date, the primary method of circulating ideas, for both the Dutch and the English, was word of mouth. Access to books imported from Europe or Boston other than the Bible or devotional works was largely limited to the elite. Oral communication was the rule for average men and women.

The opening of Bradford's press had profound consequences for the Dutch residents of the city, since the new printer confined his output almost exclusively to works in English.[22] English New Yorkers could now use the medium of print to mould popular opinion, while their Dutch neighbours lacked this means of disseminating their views in their native tongue. Domine Henricus Selyns, the Dutch Reformed minister, voiced his frustration at the absence of an outlet for Dutch publications in the city to a friend in the Netherlands in 1696: 'One has no occasion here to publish and to make anything known in print as our printer understands nothing but the English language'.[23] Bradford's press gave the English a communications monopoly that placed them on a different level from the Dutch.

New York City soon boasted another forum for broadcasting English views. Trinity Church, which opened in 1697, became the centre of New York City's English community and its rector, Willam Vesey, became the spokesman for Anglican interests. The religious balance in New York City shifted perceptibly as the Dutch no longer had the advantage of dominating religious discourse in the city.

Shortly after 1700, the triad of new English cultural institutions was completed with the commencement of the SPG mission to New York City. The SPG promoted the Anglican cause as well as the English language through its educational enterprises such as the charity school.[24] Aimed at spreading Anglican principles and, more generally, English values among New York City's diverse population, the SPG successfully introduced English culture to poor New Yorkers of diverse backgrounds.

It would be another generation before the English reached demographic parity with the Dutch in New York City. But in the interim, they had taken crucial steps toward ensuring their cultural dominance. By effectively wielding three key instruments of cultural power – the press, the pulpit and the classroom – they were able to define the standards for New Yorkers. They had assumed the role of a majority.

The Dutch, despite their numbers, saw the cultural authority they had enjoyed since the conquest eroding. As English culture became more pervasive in New York City, Dutch residents were increasingly occupied with devising ways to preserve what they deemed most essential to their way of life. By the early 18th century, New York City had become an English domain and the descendants of the early Dutch colonists were performing the classic role of a minority group.

NOTES

1   Robert C. Ritchie, *The Duke's province: a study of New York politics and society, 1664–1691* (Chapel Hill, 1977), 22.
2   *Ibid.*, 58–9, 109; Cathy Matson, 'The "Hollander Interest" and ideas about free trade in colonial New York: persistent influences of the Dutch, 1664–1764', in Nancy Anne McClure Zeller (ed.), *A beautiful and fruitful place: selected Rensselaerswijck seminar papers* (Albany, 1991), 251–68.
3   Rev. John Megapolensis to the Classis of Amsterdam, 17/27 April 1669: *Ecclesiastical*

records of the state of New York, ed. Edward T. Corwin, 7 vols. (Albany, 1901–16), vol. 1, 602.

4   Joyce D. Goodfriend, *Before the melting pot: society and culture in colonial New York City, 1664–1730* (Princeton, 1992), 84.

5   Megapolensis to the Classis of Amsterdam, 17/27 April 1669: *Ecclesiastical records*, vol. 1, 602.

6   The argument in this paper is based on evidence presented in Goodfriend, *Before the melting pot*. Citations are only provided for specific facts.

7   'Churchwardens and Vestry of Trinity Church, New York, to Archbishop Tenison, New York, 22 May 1699', in *Documents relative to the colonial history of the state of New York*, ed. E. B. O'Callaghan, 15 vols. (Albany, 1856–87), vol. 4, 526.

8   Goodfriend, 62, 155.

9   *Ibid.*, 53.

10 'Governor Dongan's report to the Committee of Trade on the Province of New-York', 22 February 1687, in *The documentary history of the state of New York*, ed. E. B. O'Callaghan, 4 vols. (Albany, 1850–1), vol. 1, 103.

11 Bartlett Burleigh James and J. Franklin Jameson (eds.), *Journal of Jasper Danckaerts 1679–1680* (New York, 1913), 75–6.

12 Goodfriend, 89.

13 *Ibid.*, 205.

14 *Ibid.*, 61–110.

15 For important insights into the cultural consequences of the English conquest of New Netherland, see Donna Merwick, *Death of a notary: conquest and change in colonial New York* (Ithaca, 1999).

16 For further discussion of the issue of Dutch cultural persistence and references to relevant recent scholarship, see Joyce D. Goodfriend, 'Writing/Righting Dutch colonial history', *New York History* 80 (January 1999), 5–28.

17 The fullest account of the New York City Huguenot community is found in Jon Butler, *The Huguenots in America: a refugee people in New World society* (Cambridge, MA, 1983). The French background of Huguenots who settled in New York is discussed in Charles W. Baird, *History of the Huguenot emigration to America*, 2 vols. (New York, 1885).

18 Goodfriend, *Before the melting pot*, 62.

19 Henricus Selyns to the Classis of Amsterdam, 21/31 October 1683: *Ecclesiastical records*, vol. 2, 866–7.

20 On Dutch Pietism, see James Tanis, 'Reformed Pietism in colonial America', in F. Ernest Stoeffler (ed.), *Continental Pietism and early American Christianity* (Grand Rapids, 1976), 34–73 and *idem, Dutch Calvinistic Pietism in the Middle Colonies: a study of the life and theology of Theodorus J. Frelinghuysen* (The Hague, 1967).

21 On William Bradford, see Alexander Wall, Jr., 'William Bradford, colonial printer: a tercentenary review', *Proceedings of the American Antiquarian Society* 73 (1963), 361–84.

22 Bradford's Dutch language publications are listed in Hendrick Edelman, *Dutch-American bibliography 1693–1794* (Nieuwkoop, 1974). Of 1100 Bradford imprints between 1693 and 1744, only ten were in Dutch. Goodfriend, *Before the melting pot*, 276, n. 14.

23 Henricus Selijns to Theodorus Janssonius Almeloveen, New York, 30 October 1696: Manuscript letter, Special Collections, University of Utrecht Library, MS 996 (6k4), vol. 2, fo. 133r. I am grateful to Jaap Jacobs for showing me this letter and to Jos van der Linde for translating it.

24 On the work of the SPG in New York, see William Webb Kemp, *The support of schools in colonial New York by the Society for the Propagation of the Gospel in Foreign Parts* (New York, 1969; originally published 1913).

34

Anglican conformity and nonconformity among the Huguenots of colonial New York

Paula Wheeler Carlo

Many students of the Huguenot experience in British North America have argued that the refugees rapidly conformed to Anglicanism. For example, in his article 'Why did the Huguenot refugees in the American colonies become Episcopalians?' Robert M. Kingdon explored the reasons for this transfer of religious affiliation by the Huguenots.[1] Although he did not insist that they all flocked to Anglicanism, Jon Butler argued that the distinctive characteristics of the Huguenots quickly vanished once they reached the Americas.[2] My examination of three communities in colonial New York that attracted significant numbers of Huguenots calls for a reassessment of these arguments. I have found three divergent examples of the Huguenot religious experience in this colony: a French Reformed congregation that remained independent until the beginning of the 19th century; a French Reformed church that became Dutch Reformed during the 18th century; and a French Reformed church that conformed to Anglicanism in 1709.

Some of the first Europeans to settle the Dutch colony of New Amsterdam in the 1620s were French-speaking 'Walloons'. Among their ranks were French Protestants who had fled to the Netherlands during the French Wars of Religion (1562–98) and during the renewed persecutions under Louis XIII and Cardinal Richelieu after 1620. The French and Dutch Reformed Protestants of New Amsterdam shared a church building at several different locations and conducted services in their respective languages both before and after the English conquest of the colony in 1664. The French finally built a church of their own in 1688 when their numbers were swelled by the influx of new refugees following the Revocation of the Edict of Nantes. The French Church of New York continued to exist as an independent Reformed Protestant congregation for most of the 18th century. Church records were written in French and services were conducted in French and then in both English and French in the second half of the century. However, a host of problems and controversies assailed this congregation until its doors were closed in 1776 during the disruptions of the American War for Independence. The church reopened in 1796, but in 1802, after much soul-searching and debate about finances, members voted to join the Episcopal fold in order to avail the church of a financial bequest that was dependent upon such conformity. To this day, weekly services are conducted in French at l'Eglise Française du Saint-Esprit on East 61st Street in New York City.

The village of New Paltz, situated about 70 miles north of New York City, was founded in 1677 by 12 Huguenot men and their families. Prior to their arrival in North America between 1660 and 1675, the founders of New Paltz had left France for the German Palatinate where free exercise of Reformed Protestantism was guaranteed under the 1648 Treaty of Westphalia. Scholars disagree as to whether or not, and for how long, the New Paltz church remained independent, but here the issue does not involve conformity to the Church of England, but rather to the Dutch Reformed Classis of Amsterdam. Kingdon argues that the French church may have joined with the Dutch as early as 1727, while Gilbert Chinard, in *Les réfugiés huguenots en Amèrique*, believes the church remained independent.[3] Based on the sources I have examined, neither explanation appears to be entirely accurate. French continued to be spoken in New Paltz until about 1750. However, from the mid-1720s on, many documents, including church records, were interspersed with Dutch or written entirely in Dutch. Around 1750 Dutch became the main language until it was supplanted by English *c.*1800.[4] Although the predominant language of the New Paltz church became Dutch, this does not necessarily mean that the congregation was under the authority of the Classis of Amsterdam. Indeed, by mid-century Dutch Reformed churches were embroiled in a controversy over whether or not their ministers should be educated in Europe and ordained by the Classis of Amsterdam or if a Dutch Reformed school of theology should be founded in the colonies. Ultimately the latter faction won out. Chinard thus may be correct in saying that the New Paltz church remained independent, of the Classis of Amsterdam that is, but not independent of the Dutch Reformed Church in America.[5] As in other Huguenot settlements, the major problem for New Paltz lay in finding and affording a French Reformed pastor, a task made increasingly complex by the lack of French Reformed schools of theology. Due to its relatively isolated rural location, New Paltz afforded its inhabitants fewer religious options than did New York City. Because of this factor, New Paltz managed to resist Anglicization for a longer time than the other communities I have examined. On the other hand, because of its isolation, New Paltz did not attract significant numbers of Huguenot settlers, unlike New York City, which offered more opportunites for commercial enterprise. By the third generation, the founding families of New Paltz had to look outside their limited ranks for marriage partners in nearby communities which were predominantly Dutch. Moreover, the influences of Anglo-American culture made no significant impact in the New Paltz area until the end of the 18th century, after the colonies had become independent. So the ultimate fate of French Protestantism here was absorption into the Dutch Reformed Church in America which was closer in doctrine and governance to the French Reformed Churches than was the Church of England. This move enabled the Huguenots of New Paltz to preserve much of their religious heritage, but at the price of sacrificing their use of the French language.

The town of New Rochelle, which is located south of New Paltz and north of New York City, was founded by and for Huguenot refugees in 1687. Most of the original settlers were from the Atlantic coast of France and had left in the years immediately surrounding the Revocation of the Edict of Nantes. After a brief respite in England, they had chosen to uproot themselves once again. Others had fled from the French West Indies after the Revocation. Because of their comparatively large numbers and the initial homogeneity of New Rochelle, Huguenots in this community were able to have their own French church and pastor almost immediately. Nevertheless, pressure from British officials seems to have caused this congregation to accept Anglican conformity in 1709. Several families objected to this move and broke away in protest, forming a separate congregation which they felt better preserved the tenets of their faith. In 1728 there were about a hundred of these nonconformists in the town.[6] Unfortunately few primary sources, other than some sporadic records, are available for this church in the 18th century.[7] Around the time of the American War for Independence it was closed for several decades, then reopened as a Presbyterian church in 1812. Meanwhile, until 1760, the Anglican congregation had ministers who conducted services in French, kept church records in French, and with financial assistance from the Society for the Propagation of the Gospel in Foreign Parts (SPG), supported a boarding school where French language and culture were part of the bilingual curriculum.

On the surface, New Rochelle appears to be the most 'French' of the three settlements. At the outset it was ethnically and religiously homogeneous, in contrast to heterogeneous New York City or the predominantly Dutch Hudson River Valley area where New Paltz was situated. Its settlers were among the last to leave France, unlike the founders of New Paltz, who had left well in advance of the Revocation, spending several years in the German Palatinate before emigrating to North America and naming their new home in honour of *Die Pfalz*. Moreover, even its name was French, commemorating the Huguenot stronghold of La Rochelle. In view of these facts, it is quite surprising that this community was the first to abandon Huguenot beliefs and practices in order to conform to the Church of England. But just how 'Anglican' in belief and practice was the conforming church in New Rochelle? We are able to answer this question for the second quarter of the 18th century based on the content of a variety of written sources, which include church records, letters between the church's ministers and the Secretary of the SPG., and sermons. The most salient evidence is contained in 73 manuscript sermons written and delivered in French between 1724 and 1741 by the Reverend Pierre Stouppe, who had been educated in Geneva and ordained in London before ministering to the New Rochelle church from 1724 until his death in 1760.[8]

The New Rochelle church records were kept in French by Stouppe until February 1757. They primarily document baptisms and each entry is signed by Stouppe and two or three *anciens*. They do not tell us how frequently Communion was offered and reveal little about actual doctrines. Subsequent entries through June 1765 are in the hand of Stouppe's successor, the Reverend Michel Houdin.[9] Before his conversion to Anglicanism in 1747, French-born Houdin had been a Franciscan missionary in Canada. After his conversion, Houdin was an itinerant missionary for the SPG and served as a guide for British troops during the Seven Years War.[10] When Stouppe died in 1760, the New Rochelle church requested a pastor who could preach in French as well as in English, so the SPG assigned Houdin to the post.[11] Like Stouppe, Houdin delivered messages in both English and French, but English was rapidly becoming the preferred language for religious services at that time. Because of his past as a French Roman Catholic, it is possible that Houdin felt a strong need to prove his loyalty to

Great Britain and it was during his ministry, which coincided with the final years of the Seven Years War and the beginning of protests against British government and taxation policies, that English replaced French as the predominant language of the New Rochelle church.

Correspondence with the SPG is largely a numerical recounting of numbers of communicants and baptisms. It informs us that Communion was offered four times per year. (The independent church in New York likewise offered Communion four times a year.) The correspondence also reveals problems with the rival nonconforming congregation, and details efforts to educate the young and to Christianize the slaves owned by members of the community. While Stouppe used English in his correspondence with the SPG, he wrote his sermons and kept church records in French. In contrast, all of Houdin's entries in the church records were in English.

Based on the content of the sermons that Stouppe delivered between 1724 and 1741, it appears that the 'conforming' church in New Rochelle was very much like the 'conforming' churches in Great Britain. To quote Robin Gwynn regarding the Huguenot experience in England, 'the evidence suggests that the conformists were Anglican in name rather than by deep conviction'.[12] Since there are over 900 pages of Stouppe's manuscript sermons, the following analysis will concentrate on beliefs that distinguish the Reformed Churches from the Church of England. These include the nature, number, and efficacy of the sacraments, the doctrine of election, the role of good works in salvation, perseverance of the saints, and use of images for religious purposes.[13]

In a series of sermons on Section 53 of the Catechism, Stouppe refuted the belief in the Real Presence of Christ in the Eucharist. He insisted that the bread and wine commemorate the sacrifice of Jesus Christ, and merely serve to augment pre-existing faith. It is the shed blood of Jesus Christ, not the sacrament, that is the remission for our sins and it is Jesus alone who sanctifies our hearts. Moreover, Stouppe warned that Communion should only be administered to those persons who have embraced the truth of the Gospel and who have given indication of their instruction, their faith, and repentance. Wicked persons who partake of this sacrament will not be justified since justification can only follow the 'calling' of God.

In several sermons on Section 52 of the Catechism, Stouppe attacked those five sacraments that were not used by the Apostles or the primitive church, calling them 'les cinqs prétendus sacrements'. Although he accorded sacramental status to baptism and Communion, he did not believe that they conveyed saving grace. They were merely commemorative acts of obedience that were instituted by Jesus Christ. According to Stouppe, the 'Romanish' church has misled the people by creating five additional sacraments. However, since the Church of England also acknowledged these rites, he could have been making an indirect criticism of that church for granting them sacramental status. Another 'Roman' (and Anglican) practice he did not condone was the sign of the cross. He repudiated this practice in a sermon on Section 48 of the Catechism, arguing that the Apostles of the early church did not use it .

Regarding Section 20 of the Catechism, Stouppe wrote: 'Our works do not merit us the Grace of Justification, also they do not merit us eternal life'. However, our works 'are necessary and useful with regard to God, to ourselves, and to others'. Our 'good works are a light before men' and reveal us to be 'a peculiar people'. They enable us to glorify God and to render obedience to him as he has commanded us. Good works keep us from stumbling and 'affirm our Election and Vocation'. True repentance is the source of good works and they must always accompany our faith. In another sermon on Section 20, that was preached in February 1732, Stouppe once again insisted that the only way to obtain justification is through faith in Jesus Christ. He emphasized that 'good works do not proceed the grace of justification and are not the cause of justification due to the imperfection of our good works'. Moreover, in a sermon on Section 19 of the Catechism, Stouppe placed his views on justification in direct opposition to those of the Roman Catholic Church, leaving no room for the Anglican *via media:* we are justified before God by our faith in Jesus Christ, not by our merits.

In a sermon on Section 19 of the Catechism, Stouppe unequivocally states that 'we are corrupt by nature' and backed up this statement with references from both the Old and New Testaments. 'Without grace we are incapable of having good thoughts... we can do nothing'. Although he identified several virtuous pagans, he nevertheless affirmed that our 'actions must not only conform to the Law of God, but from a heart filled with his love, purified by faith, and having no end but his glory'.

The Calvinist doctrine of perseverance of the saints is not a dominant theme in Stouppe's sermons, however, it is alluded to in several places. Referring to Section 16 of the Catechism, Stouppe wrote: 'If you repent and completely renounce sin . . . if you convert with all your heart . . . you will persevere constantly in holiness and virtue [and] you will live'. On 13 June 1725 he preached that 'Justification follows the calling and if God has called us we are justified for eternity'.

Stouppe was unequivocally opposed to the use of religious images in churches. In a sermon on Section 7 of the Petit Catechism, he argued that the second commandment expressly forbade all sorts of representations, including the use of painting and sculpture. While these were acceptable for historical purposes in the political and civil realm, they must not be employed for religious purposes. He further condemned the idolatry of the pagans and of the 'superstitious papists'. Might he be condemning as well Protestants who retain the use of religious imagery?

How did Stouppe's sermons compare with the 96 sermons preached by the Revd Louis Rou, pastor of the independent French congregation in New York from 1710 to 1750?[14] Stouppe's textual sources came from both the Scriptures and the Catechism. Rou, in contrast, rarely preached from the Catechism, preferring instead to make extensive use of Scriptural references, particularly the Psalms. There are only five existing sermons in which Rou mentioned the Catechism and all of them critiqued and even ridiculed the belief in Jesus Christ's literal descent into hell after his crucifixion. Rou refuted this notion with Scripture and extended explanations of ancient Greek and Hebrew texts. Stouppe also composed at least one sermon on the same topic. Similar to Rou, he argued that a 'veritable and real descent into hell is superstitious'. Stouppe, likewise, quoted Scriptures and analysed ancient Greek terminology to prove his point.[15] Although Rou rejected the notion of a literal descent into hell, he did not reject such miraculous feats as the resurrection of Jesus Christ or the bodily resurrection of the dead in Christ to their eternal reward in heaven.[16] Moreover, all of his messages closed with an exhortation to look forward to the promise of the next life for God's Elect. While Stouppe composed a number of sermons on the sacraments, Rou's manuscripts were remarkably absent of references to them. Instead he insisted that the 'Knowledge of God and of Jesus Christ are the only means to obtain eternal life'.[17] Like Stouppe, Rou argued that good works are not a means to salvation, but rather a result of it and that Christians should be 'lights unto the world'.

The central message of the sermons of Louis Rou is Calvinistic, not unlike that of his contemporary, Pierre Stouppe. But the Calvinism of both men was tempered by the toleration and rationalism of the Enlightenment, that is, unless they were railing against the 'iniquitous idolatry' of the 'Romanish' church, which both men deplored with venom. From Stouppe's point of view, those of the 'Romish' persuasion were far more in error than the Jews or 'Mahometans'.[18]

While Stouppe occasionally mentioned ancient Greek and Roman philosophers or the fathers of the primitive church, Rou did so regularly, possibly to showcase his erudition as well as to bolster his arguments. Both appeared to be sincere men who were conscientious and diligent in the preparation of their sermons. However, Rou's writings were often tinged with an arrogance or condescension that was not apparent in Stouppe's manuscripts. Stouppe's sermons invariably focused on the larger issues of faith and always ended with a practical application. In contrast, Rou's sermons occasionally delved into esoteric Biblical passages and were frequently weigheddown by hefty doses of pedantry – a characteristic that may have provoked some congregants to leave the French Church of New York during his ministry.

Despite financial exigency, difficulty in finding a French-speaking pastor after Rou's death, and the ongoing defections of members, particularly to Anglican and Dutch Reformed Churches, the French Church of New York managed to survive. It never became Anglican during the 18th century, although the issue of conformity arose a number of times. The suggestion was always laid to rest by members of the consistory who wished to retain independence 'out of respect for our forefathers'. Nevertheless, the church did become Episcopalian in 1802, but this decision was not an easy one. During the American War for Independence, the church had been seized by the British and used to store supplies, consequently it fell into disrepair. The remaining members began meeting once again in January 1796 in the German Reformed Church building until a new French church could be constructed. In December 1796 the Trustees of l'Eglise Reformée Protestant Française à la Nouvelle York wrote to the Reformed Church of the Canton of Berne in Switzerland, requesting a French-speaking ecclesiastic 'who preaches the word conforming to the Holy Scripture and the doctrines of Calvin'.[19] Six years later, they still had not secured a minister who met these criteria. In October 1802, 'with intense regret' the Trustees urged the congregation to vote in favour of conformity to Anglicanism (i.e. Episcopalianism) so that the church would be able to receive a legacy of £1000 that was contingent on conformity to the English liturgy. The Trustees pointed out that this move 'would increase both revenues and the number of members' and was 'absolutely indispensible to the future existence of the church'. They further argued that this 'innovation was but a pure and simple addition of ceremonies' and that 'the dogmas of religion would remain the same in all aspects'. Moreover, the church would retain its independence. In addition to this financial inducement, entering the Episcopal fold would facilitate their quest for a pastor. After the congregation unanimously consented to the change, it was decided that once they had received a new pastor, he would procure books containing the English liturgy in the French language.[20]

In conclusion, many Huguenots in colonial New York did not embrace

Anglicanism as fully and eagerly as Kingdon has argued. Neither did they 'vanish' as quickly and completely as Butler has claimed, at least not when religious dogmas and use of the French language for religious purposes are the evaluative criteria. On the other hand, they did not retain the visibility and distinctiveness of the New York Dutch who have been studied by Joyce Goodfriend.[21] The Huguenots, unlike the Dutch, had been tempered by the crucible of persecution. Before leaving France they had learned how to blend in in the public sphere, exercising their religious beliefs in the private sphere. Once they arrived in New York, this pattern was replicated: they continued to use the French language in the private religious sphere, while adopting English (or Dutch in the case of New Paltz) as their language in the public sphere and in communications with people who were not French. During the 18th century, modifications were made that enabled French Protestantism to survive in some form. Hence, the Huguenots of New York can be found at various points along the continuum between the aforementioned paradigms of Butler's vanishing Huguenots and Goodfriend's highly visible Dutch. Some Huguenots, like the DeLanceys, who left the New York French church to join the Anglican Trinity Church, totally embraced English culture – in marriage, in language, in religion, and in politics – to the extent that they became staunch Tories during the War for Independence. The inhabitants of New Paltz, out of necessity, gradually merged with the Dutch in marriage, language, and religion during the course of the 18th century and only began to use English at the close of that century. Meanwhile those at the conforming church in New Rochelle and at the independent French church in New York retained Calvinistic beliefs and used French for religious purposes until the latter half of the 18th century when disruptions from the Seven Years War and the War for Independence made this increasingly difficult. When these churches reopened in the 1790s, their members would join other inhabitants of the United States in becoming a new people – Americans.

NOTES

1   Robert M. Kingdon, 'Why did the Huguenot refugees in the American colonies become Episcopalians?' *Historical Magazine of the Protestant Episcopal Church* 49 (1980), 326.
2   Jon Butler, *The Huguenots in America: a refugee people in New World society* (Cambridge, MA, 1983), 199–215.
3   Gilbert Chinard, *Les réfugiés huguenots en Amérique* (Paris, 1925),183.
4   Use of language in New Paltz is a complex issue. Certainly the founders of New Paltz would have needed to learn some Dutch upon their arrival in New Netherland since they lived among the Dutch in Kingston and Hurley for several years before purchasing the land that would become New Paltz. Undoubtedly many of the Huguenot settlers and their descendants could speak, read, and possibly write in both French and Dutch, at the very least. For example, extant wills indicate that some households had Bibles and other religious books that were written in both languages. In addition, church records, records of town meetings, wills, deeds, receipts, and other written documents are recorded in either of these two languages, and occasionally in English, throughout the colonial period.
5   The available evidence concerning the New Paltz church's relation with the Dutch Reformed Classis of Amsterdam is difficult to interpret. Whenever the New Paltz church was without a regular pastor, which was quite frequent during the first half of the 18th

century, members would travel 15 miles to the Dutch Reformed church in Kingston for marriages and baptisms. Because of this occasional attendance and occasional monetary contributions, the Kingston church insisted that New Paltz was part of its congregation and became angry whenever New Paltz tried to assert its independence. Both churches appealed to the Classis of Amsterdam, which acted as a mediator in the dispute. In 1750, New Paltz consistory members wrote to the Classis that 'the Paltz, as a French Reformed Church, had always been accustomed to be provided with a minister and consistory of its own, but as they were now vacant, however, they were willing to promise to unite with Kingston for the support of a minister from Europe; but with this understanding that whenever they could have a minister of their own again, they might then consider themselves released from this promise'. In 1752 the Classis issued a decision somewhat more favourable to New Paltz than to Kingston, maintaining that because of its growing population and distance from Kingston, New Paltz should be independent. (Edward T. Corwin, *Ecclesiastical records of the state of New York* (Albany, 1901–16), vol. 4, 3141–3; vol. 5: 3209–10, 3269–70). From this it might appear that the New Paltz Church was under the authority of the Classis because it seemed willing to submit to its judgment in this dispute. However, it was not unheard of for different Reformed churches to look to unaffiliated Reformed bodies to arbitrate disputes if asked to do so. What is certain, however, is that the New Paltz church could not remain independent indefinitely since there were no more French Reformed clergymen. From the 1730s to the 1760s, the visiting and part-time pastors of the New Paltz church were all independent-minded Pietists who argued that a Reformed school of theology should be opened in the colonies and that ministers did not have to be ordained by the Classis of Amsterdam, but rather by a Coetus in New York. In 1766 a second church, that was subordinate to the Classis of Amsterdam, was founded in New Paltz. Nevertheless, the two churches were merged into one in 1775, after the Dutch Reformed churches in America had established a school of theology and broken ties with the Classis of Amsterdam.

6 Pierre Stouppe to the Secretary of the Society for the Propagation of the Gospel in Foreign Parts, July 1728: Society for the Propagation of the Gospel (hereafter SPG), 'Records', Series A, vol. 21, 349–57 (on microfilm) (Yorkshire, 1964).

7 New York Historical Society, MS Collection, French Church of New Rochelle, 'Records', 1756–64.

8 Library of the Huguenot Society of America, New York, Pierre Stouppe, 'Sermons', 1724–41. These unpublished manuscripts in French have been bound into one volume and are organized according to Sections of the Catechism and placed in descending order.

9 Trinity-St Paul Episcopal Church, New Rochelle, French Church of New Rochelle, 'Records', 1725–65.

10 Houdin is mentioned in a letter as being present at the capture of Quebec: SPG, 'Records', Series B, vol. 3, 178–92.

11 New York Historical Society, MS Collection, French Church of New Rochelle, 'Petition of Members of Church of England to the S.P.G. for Minister', 23 July 1760.

12 Robin Gwynn, *Huguenot heritage: the history and contribution of the Huguenots in Britain* (London, 1985), 57.

13 The following discussion is drawn from the one volume of Pierre Stouppe's Sermons, 1724–41, held at the Library of the Huguenot Society of America, New York. Individual folio references are not provided here but the location of the sermons can be easily found as they are organized according to the section of the Catechism they treat.

14 New York Public Library, MS Collection, Louis Rou, 'Sermons and other Writings', 1704–50, 3 vols. These unpublished manuscript sermons in French are available on microfilm.

15 Louis Rou, 'Sermon on the descent of Jesus Christ into Hell' (titles of sermons have been

translated by the author of this article). Rou composed five different versions of this sermon based on Section 10 of the Catechism which he preached at the French Church in New York on repeated occasions between 1720 and 1742. All five versions are in vol. 2 of his 'Sermons and other Writings'; however, they do not appear in sequence.

16 Rou, 'Sermon on the Resurrection of our Saviour Jesus Christ', 'Sermons', vol. 3 (two versions); 'Sermon on the immortality of the Soul', vol. 1 (two versions).

17 See sermon of same name in Rou, 'Sermons', vol. 2.

18 Comments such as these are interspersed throughout the sermons of Stouppe and Rou. For Stouppe see especially the sermons on Sections 46, 48, 49, 50, 51, 52, and 53 of the Grand Catechism, which concern the sacraments, and on Section 7 of the Petit Catechism, which concerns the use of painting and sculpture for religious purposes. For Rou see the five sermons 'On the descent of Jesus Christ into Hell' mentioned above and the three sermons entitled 'Against transubstantiation', all of which are in vol. 2 of his 'Sermons'.

19 New York Historical Society, MS Collection, 'Letter from l'Eglise Reformée Protestant Française à la Nouvelle York to the Rev. Pierre Antoine Samuel Albert de Lausanne, Suisse, 6 Dec. 1796'.

20 New York Historical Society, MS Collection, 'Proceedings of the Trustees of l'Eglise Reformée Protestant Française à la Nouvelle York, 1796–1802'.

21 Joyce Goodfriend, *Before the melting pot: society and culture in colonial New York City, 1664–1730* (Princeton, 1992).

35

Jacob Leisler and the Huguenot network in the English Atlantic world

David William Voorhees

In February 1650, the French Reformed pastor Jacob Victorian Leisler brought before the Reformed consistory of Frankfurt-am-Main, the petition of the two youngest daughters of the late Elias Chevalier. The two girls, 'who are of French ancestry', wished, he complained, to join the German Reformed congregation since 'they attend German sermons and receive Holy Communion in the same language'.[1] This was not the first, nor would it be the last, time that this Frankfurt French Reformed minister addressed the issue of the children of his communicants assimilating into the host German culture. For over a decade he had struggled to preserve his congregation's cultural identity during a period when relative religious calm in France, contrasting with the Thirty Years' War's utter devastation of the German countryside, had curtailed French Protestant immigration.[2]

The petitions of Elias Chevalier's daughters, as well as those of others, reveal that in 1650 the Reverend Leisler ministered to an increasingly aging resident alien mercantile community being eroded by assimilation. What connected the Frankfurt congregation to French Reformed congregations in France and elsewhere in exile were trade and kinship networks rather than a cohesive institutional structure.[3] Several decades later these international connections became the life line for a wave of Protestant refugees fleeing France in the wake of King Louis XIV's persecutions of the Reformed faith. The Huguenot merchants' 'peculiar combination of trade, religion, and family', John F. Bosher notes, 'were what sustained them in the face of cruel treatment by the French authorities and enabled them to join the Anglo-Dutch forces that were resisting French aggression'.[4] The career of the Reverend Leisler's son Jacob, who in 1689 led a New York rebellion on behalf of King Louis XIV's nemesis, William, Prince of Orange, sheds additional light on Huguenot trade and kinship networks and their role in the Huguenot diaspora into the Atlantic world, as well as on the influence of Huguenot political thought on the early development of English America.

Frankfurt, an imperial free city near the confluence of the Main and Rhine rivers, was ideally situated to be a link in the Huguenot émigré network. Its yearly trade fairs attracted French and Dutch merchants seeking to extend their markets, and both groups had in 1554 established Reformed congregations in the city. But the wealth of the Calvinist merchants created resentment among Frankfurt's Lutheran patrician magistrates and guildsmen of this 'foreign element', and in 1562 the city council banned the Reformed from publicly exercising their religion. The two communities subsequently held services in the nearby village of Bockenheim, then under the jurisdiction of the counts of Hanau.[5] Despite exclusion from public worship and political disenfranchisement, Frankfurt's French Reformed community included the city's most affluent merchants and bankers.[6] Samuel and Daniel Jordis, who traded by sea to Venice and Leghorn, Jacob de Famars, who traded in Dutch and French textiles, and Jean Du Fay, who imported English and French goods, exemplify the wealth and far-flung commercial connections of Frankfurt's French Reformed merchants by the mid-17th century.[7]

The Reverend Jacob Victorian Leisler's call to Frankfurt in 1638 reflected the Frankfurt French Reformed community's international connections. Leisler, a son of a former councilor to both the Counts of Oettingen and to Prince Christian of Anhalt, and a graduate of Altdorf, the Academy at Geneva, and Heidelberg, was ministering to the French-speaking community of Frankenthal when a Spanish purge of Protestants forced him to flee in 1637. Frankenthal's and Frankfurt's French churches were members of the Palatine Circle of Reformed churches, which was organized at a Reformed synod at Emden in 1571, and this synodal relationship helps to explain Frankfurt's call of Leisler.[8] His call was also undoubtedly aided by a family connection to Geneva Academy president Simon Goulart. It was Goulart's late son-in-law, the deceased Timothée Poterat, cousin to Leisler's mother-in-law, whom Leisler succeeded to the Frankfurt French Reformed pulpit.[9]

After the Reverend Leisler's death in 1653, French Reformed kin and trade contacts shaped the career of his eldest son Jacob, who was 12 years old at the time.[10] This was expedited through the Frankfurt congregation's correspondence with numerous Huguenot émigré communities throughout Europe. These included the French Church at Amsterdam, where Simon Goulart the Younger, second cousin of the Reverend Leisler's wife and brother-in-law of Timothée Poterat, had served as pastor until his death in 1628, and London's Threadneedle Street church, whose minister, Christopher Cisner, had a personal friendship with the Reverend Leisler.[11] Dutch connections also included a prominent West India Company shareholder, Godert van Rede, lord Nederhorst, patron of New Netherland patroon Cornelis Melyen, a Walloon from Antwerp with whose family Jacob Leisler would later have close associations, and the D'Orville and Rademaker families, whose relations included a Frankfurt church elder Daniel D'Orville.[12]

In April 1660, Jacob Leisler, barely aged 20, sailed aboard the *Gilded Otter* from Amsterdam as a junior military officer for the Dutch West India Company colony of New Netherland.[13] Perhaps one of the abovementioned connections helped him to obtain this minor command. The key figure, however, was probably the wealthy Frankfurt merchant Jacob de Famars the Elder, an elder in the Reverend Leisler's congregation, a shareholder in the West India Company, and godparent to Jacob's brother Hans.[14] De Famars, originally from Valenciennes, was in close contact with the Huguenot community in Leiden, and, as we shall see, Leiden's Huguenot community figures prominently in Leisler's early trade.[15]

Within a year of his arrival in New Netherland, Jacob Leisler abandoned a military career and entered into the fur and tobacco trade. A decade later he was among New

York's most prominent merchants, and by 1685 possibly the province's richest merchant.[16] His phenomenal rise to wealth can be traced in his traffic along Huguenot trade networks. In January 1663, for example, Guy Jacobsen, a 'Frenchman from Boston', received from the 22-year-old Leisler '244 heavy deer skins and 22 rolls of Spanish tobacco' consigned to Jacobsen's cousin, Artuy Le Brethon at The Hague, or, 'in his absence', Charles Barbou, a Huguenot merchant from Paris living in Amsterdam.[17]

As Leisler's trading network expanded, shared religious affiliation was often a factor. In 1662 he appears as a baptismal sponsor for a child of Nicholas de la Pleine, a merchant from Bresuire, France, and for a child of merchant Henri Couturier, a former member of Leiden's French [Walloon] congregation. Couturier's wife, Lizbeth Coppyn, was from Valenciennes and possibly a relation of Jacob de Famars.[18] Leisler's baptismal sponsorship, an unusual honour for a bachelor, shows that he was well known to these families. Marriage reinforced Leisler's relation to Couturier when the following year Jacob wed the widowed Elsie Thymens, sister-in-law of Couturier's brother Jacques.[19] Elsie, several years older than Jacob, who was then under the legal male age of 25 to marry without guardian's consent, had been left in considerable debt by her late husband, Pieter Cornelis van der Veen. That the marriage banns were proclaimed the day after the court applied pressure on Elsie to remarry suggests that the match was arranged, possibly by the Couturiers and Johannes de Peyster, guardian of Elsie's children.[20]

The Reverend Leisler's reputation as a French Reformed pastor and friend to the persecuted gained Jacob access to Walloon and Huguenot mercantile capital. By the 1680s Leisler was trafficking in metalwork and toys from Nuremburg, Hamburg linens, Dutch and Flemish linens, English woollens, and Swiss and French luxury goods, as well as in American tobacco and furs, grain products, horses, and whale oil, and in the African slave and European indentured servant markets.[21] The international French Reformed community provided the contacts that allied him with Huguenot merchants and their relations in North America, the West Indies, on the coasts of Africa, and in Europe – a network that John Bosher describes as 'Protestant International'.[22] Significantly, it was these international contacts that allowed Leisler to prosper after New Netherland was transferred to English sovereignty.

A 1677 bill of exchange provides insight into Leisler's trade network after the final English takeover of New Netherland in 1674. Mark Cordea, a Normandy merchant living in St Mary's County, Maryland, and acting as Leisler's Maryland factor, became indebted to Leisler for £58,882 of 'good and Merchantable tobacco and caske' as payment for 'Negroes received'. Cordea offered partial payment with a bill of exchange for the sum of £98 English sterling directed to Henri Couturier, now living in London as a factor for Leiden merchants and a member of the Threadneedle Street church. Leisler, upon reaching England, signed over this bill of exchange to John Dorville, London representative of the D'Orville family, who in turn signed it over to London notary Abraham DeSmith, a relative of Couturier's from Valenciennes.[23]

For Huguenot migration to America, an important trade connection occurred in the early 1670s when Gabriel Minvielle, a merchant from Bordeaux, became a business partner with Leisler.[24] In 1676 Leisler and Minvielle received a licence from the Dutch West India Company to purchase slaves from, and trade with, the Company's colony of Curaçao. Pierre D'Orville, brother the Frankfurt church elder Daniel

D'Orville, was a director in the reconstituted West India Company after 1674 and may have been influential in their obtaining this grant. Moreover, Pierre was from Hanau, where the widow Leisler moved with her children in 1658, and would later become related to the Leislers when in 1704 Jacob's brother Johann Adam married Charlotte Burckhardt, a step-daughter of Susanne D'Orville.[25] Leisler and Minvielle would become instrumental in establishing a Huguenot refugee colony in New York.

Plans for this Huguenot colony may date to 1683, when Leisler began to purchase lands in Westchester County. Plans became formalized in 1686, however, when, after King Louis XIV's revocation of the Edict of Nantes unleashed a torrent of official violence against Protestants, a large number of Huguenots fled to New York from French colonies on the Caribbean islands of St Christopher, Guadeloupe, Marie-Galante, and Martinique.[26] Many of the first wave of refugees had been substantial planters and slave holders in the West Indies and were familiar with Leisler and Minvielle through trade. André Thauvet, from the island of Marie-Galante, for example, was married to a sister of Benjamin Faneuil, a merchant of La Rochelle and Rotterdam, who was involved in trade with Leisler and Leisler's future son-in-law Jacob Milborne.[27] It was undoubtedly such connections that made New York an attractive refuge for these men.

Leisler, Minvielle, and refugees Isaac des Champs, Jean Boutellier, and André Thauvet formed a committee to find a suitable place for the colony, to be called New Rochelle after La Rochelle in France. The site they initially selected for the settlement was on Davenport Neck in Westchester County, a site that Leisler and six others purchased and divided into plots of six to 42 acres, Leisler securing the largest share.[28] On 2 July 1687, Leisler, acting on behalf of those already on the land and those who expected to take up lands, signed an agreement with John Pell to purchase another tract running from the Boston Road to the shore on land granted to Pell the previous year and known as Pelham Manor.[29] Before the purchase was complete, Leisler became the colony's sole agent and financier. On 20 September 1689, John and Rachell Pell conveyed to Leisler 6,000 acres, plus 100 acres for a 'French church erected or to be erected by the inhabitants', for the 'valuable consideration' of £1675 sterling provincial money.[30]

New Rochelle was but one Huguenot community to arise as refugees poured into the province. By 1688 six French congregations had been organized in New York: two in New York City, and one each at New Paltz, New Rochelle, on Staten Island, and on Long Island, and one in East Jersey at Hackensack.[31] This was New York's first mass alien immigration since the initial European settlement, and it generated compassion as well as suspicion and hostility in a region rapidly sliding into steep economic depression.[32] With New York City's Huguenot population approaching nine per cent, and with the Roman Catholic English King James II placing his co-religionists as commanders of the royal garrisons at Albany, New York City, and on Long Island, Louis XIV's persecutions of Protestants in France intensified fears that England's Catholic king had similar plans for the overwhelmingly Calvinist province.[33] The 'Sorrow and Fear of New Yorkers', a New York City Dutch Reformed church communicant later reflected, 'was unusually great and frightful, for hearing . . . what great success the Dragonnades in France had had, and seeing how the foundation was being laid to introducing the same here in every manner, we could well imagine what was in store for us'.[34]

When in Spring 1689 word spread that the Dutch Calvinist William, Prince of Orange, had replaced Louis XIV's Roman Catholic cousin, James II, on England's throne, disorders occurred throughout England's American colonies. On 31 May 1689, the New York militia seized the New York City fort from James II's regular soldiers and called for a representative provincial committee to oversee civil affairs until the arrival of the new rulers' representatives. On 28 June the committee appointed Jacob Leisler captain of the fort and on 16 August commander-in-chief of the province.[35] Two years later, on 16 May 1691, Leisler swung from the gallows till 'halfe dead', then was beheaded for treason.

Leisler's tragic end becomes more comprehensible when the ideological aspect of the Huguenot diaspora is considered. His grandfather, Dr Jacob Leisler, had in the mid-1590s attended the University of Basel, the then-centre of Huguenot political ferment from whence poured forth the 'flood of pamphlets' supporting the Navarrese party in France. These pamphlets articulated a theory of revolution that justified resistance against tyranny as a religious duty.[36] Leisler's father, a Geneva Academy graduate, was a disciple of the revolutionary theorist Theodore Beza, Calvin's successor as Geneva president.[37] Even more important is a family connection through Leisler's maternal grandmother to Simon Goulart, Beza's successor at Geneva.[38]

Goulart's 1576 three-volume *Memoirs of the State of France under Charles IX* contained a number of revolutionary Huguenot political tracts including Beza's *The Right of Magistrates* (1574), *The Politician* (1574) and *Political Discourses* (1574), and François Hotman's *Francogallia* (1576). Published in French, German, and Dutch editions, and frequently reprinted, this work was highly influential in popularizing the compact theory of government and justification for resistance as a means for religious reform. The *Memoirs* appears in the libraries of New Yorkers, and Leisler undoubtedly possessed a copy of this work by his relative.[39] Indeed, Leisler's declarations of June 1689 and his subsequent justifications for New York's revolt closely follow the construction of the arguments presented in the *Memoirs*.[40]

Huguenots in France in the 1680s rejected the *Memoirs*' radical ideas, fearing that doctrines of resistance based on an inalienable right to resist would provoke the French authorities. The most distinguished articulator of this stance was the Huguenot philosopher Pierre Bayle, who, in exile in Rotterdam, urged patience with Louis XIV. In contrast to Bayle, theologian Pierre Jurieu, also in Rotterdam exile, espoused a radical millenarianism. It was Jurieu's writings that revived theories of resistance among Huguenots in the diaspora. Leisler took these arguments a step further and gave them, as Jon Butler notes, an 'anti-aristocratic – if not democratic' cast.[41]

Leisler's 'murder', as they termed it, was due to a number of complicated factors that have fuelled arguments among historians for generations. Although four years later England's Parliament, at the King's direction, cleared Leisler's name and declared his government to have been a legitimate one, a Huguenot aspect to the affair should not be overlooked. Growing hostility toward foreigners in England in the wake of the 1688 Dutch invasion contributed to the failure of Leisler's London lobby. Petitions by the Huguenot pastor Pierre Reverdy in England to the Bishop of London 'to procure the Kings letter' for Leisler as interim governor were ignored.[42] Applications presented to the Lords of Trade and the Privy Council on Leisler's behalf by Charles Talbot, Earl of Shrewsbury, and Charles Mordaunt, Lord Monmouth – Whigs in political decline in 1689–90 – were altered precisely because Leisler was seen as a

'Walloon'.[43] To Englishmen, the revolution had to appear English whether at home or in the colonies.

Leisler is described in 18th-century sources as the organizer of Huguenot relief efforts in New York.[44] They illustrate this with a story that, when one refugee family landed at Manhattan so destitute that a city court ordered them sold into servitude to pay the ship charges, Leisler used his own funds to purchase their freedom.[45] They also cite him as a founder of, and an elder of, New York City's first French Reformed congregation established under the ministry of Pierre Daillé.[46] Leisler had been prominent in the Dutch Reformed church as a deacon, and it is known that he left the Dutch church after Daillé's arrival in New York in 1683.[47] Unfortunately, the records of Daillé's congregation are lost, and the origin of the story of the refugee family has eluded detection.

Nonetheless, Jacob Leisler's career provides another sturdy link in what John Bosher terms the 'elusive historical subject' of trans-Atlantic Huguenot mercantile networks. Moreover, Leisler's network suggests that the entrance of Huguenots fleeing Louis XIV's persecutions into the English Atlantic world was not through England alone, but via a number of routes. In addition, Leisler demonstrates that along such networks Huguenot political thought was also disseminated into English North America. Filtered through Dutch and German as well as English lenses, Huguenot political thought would form, to paraphrase Quentin Skinner, one of the foundations for modern American political development.

NOTES

Research for this paper was supported by the Huguenot Society of America.

1 Stadtarchiv, Frankfurt-am-Main, Archiv Franz Reformde Gemeinde [hereafter FRG] 14:28 (Rev. J. V. Leisler Notation, 1 Feb. 1650); FRG 30: 30r–30v (Frankfurt Consistory Minute, 1 Feb. 1650); transcriptions and translations, Papers of Jacob Leisler Project, New York University, nos. 0909, 1889 [hereafter JLP].

2 *Troisième Jubilé Séculaire de la fondation de l'Eglise Réformée Française de Francfort-sur-Mein* (Frankfurt am Main, 1854), 21–2, 54. On 11 Aug. 1641, Leisler wrote: 'In consideration that the Youth of our Church is extremely weak in the French language, even for the most part ignorant, it has been decided that after having recited their French Catechism, they will be instructed in German on the principal points of Christianity, and that for an Interim, until GOD gives them the grace to understand French better', FRG 38:153v (Rev. Leisler's Protocol Book), [JLP 0925:45].

3 Jon Butler, *The Huguenots in America: a refugee people in New World society* (Cambridge, MA, 1983), 17–19.

4 J. F. Bosher, 'Huguenot merchants and the Protestant International in the seventeenth century', *William and Mary Quarterly*, 3rd ser., 52 (Jan. 1995), 100.

5 JLP 0816. For a study of Frankfurt during this period see Gerald Lyman Soliday, *A community in conflict: Frankfurt society in the 17th and early 18th centuries* (Hanover, NH, 1974). *Troisième Jubilé Séculaire*, 16–22.

6 Friedrich Clemens Ebrard, *Die französisch-reformierte Gemeinde in Frankfurt am Main 1554–1904* (Frankfurt-am-Main, 1906), 110f; Alexander Dietz, *Frankfurter Handelsgeschichte* (5 vols., Frankfurt-am-Main, 1911–25), vol. 3, 217. In 1591, church members

Bastien and Robert de Neufville, Jean du Fay, Jean de Famars, Jean Lieven, and Antoine de Bary were among those who lent money to Henry IV of France.

7 Dietz, vol. 4, 30ff., 49ff., 52–5, 91–3, 110–12.

8 Toennies-Volhard, *Die Familie Leissler*, 4–5; David William Voorhees, 'The "fervent Zeale" of Jacob Leisler', *William and Mary Quarterly*, 3d ser., 51 (July 1994), 451–2. The 'Palatine Circle' included congregations at Schönau, Heidelberg, St Lambert, and the Walloon and Flemish congregations at Frankenthal and Frankfurt am Main. Ebrard, 106ff.

9 P. Cuno, 'Geschichte der wallonisch-reformierten Gemeinde zu Frankenthal', in *Geschichtsblättern des Deutschen Hugenotten-Vereins*, 3 (1894), vol. 3, 19; *Bulletin de la société de l'histoire du protestantisme français* 56 (1907), 79; FRG 4:1608–1645 (Actorum des Französischen und Niederlandischen Kirchen-Wessen). Leisler married in Geneva, 17 Aug. 1634, Susanne Adelheid Wissenbach, daughter of Catherine Aubert: St Pierre, Geneva, Marriage Registers and G. Brandes, 'Stammbaum der Familie Leisler 1475–1890', Staatsarchiv des Kantons Basel-Stadt, Basel. Catherine's first cousin Pierre Aubert, 'Imprimeur ordinaire de la Republique et Académie de Genève', married Jael Goulart, daughter of Simon Goulart. See A. Choisy, L. DuFour-Vernes, *Recueil généalogique suisse: Genève* (3 vols., Geneva, 1902–18), vol. 1, 277–82; Armand Garnier, *Agrippa d'Aubigné et la parti protestant* (3 vols., Paris, 1928), vol. 3, 156, 163–4, 175–6; Leonard Chester Jones, *Simon Goulart 1543–1628* (Geneva/Paris, 1917), 279.

10 Stadtarchiv, Frankfurt-am-Main, Bockenheimer Kirchenbuch 1630–44, Baptismal Record, 2:129a (31 March 1640); details of the Revd Leisler's death are found in FRG 31: 8v (Frankfurt French Reformed Protocol Book, 9 Feb. 1653).

11 Choisy and DuFour-Vernes, *Recueil généalogique suisse*, vol. 1, 277–82. FRG 60:6v-7 (Frankfurt Church to Christopher Cisner, 14/24 June 1651) [JLP 0841]; Hans Georg Wackernagel (ed.), *Die Matrikel der Universität Basel* (5 vols., 1951–63), vol. 3, 361. no. 63.

12 FRG 60:4v-5 [JLP 0836]. On 27 Mar. 1639, Leisler married Jean Rademaker, son of Jacob Rademaker, merchant of Amsterdam, to Catharina, daughter of Jacob de Walbourg of Frankfurt. FRG 38:143 (Leisler's Protokollbuch) [JLP 0925:7]. Although Nederhorst died in June 1648, it is possible that Jacob Leisler's connection with the Melyn family originated with this relationship. For the Frankfurt congregation's communication with Nederhorst as the Dutch delegate to Munster see FRG Hoft Schmal Folio, 4:22. For Nedershorst's relation with Melyn see Paul Gibson Burton, 'Cornelis Melyn, Patroon of Staten Island and some of his descendants', *The New York Genealogical and Biographical Record*, 67 (Jan. 1937), 1: 5–12 [hereafter *NYGB Record*]. The 'Letter Book of Jacob Melyen' [*sic*], son of Cornelis Melyn, American Antiquarian Society, Worcester, MA, reveals the close relation between Leisler and the Melyn family.

13 New York State Archives, Albany, NY, NY Col. MS 13:106.

14 Bockenheimer Kirchenbuch Taufregister, 1646–63, 1:np.

15 'A good friend wrote on January 10th of this present year, i.e. 1647, from Leiden to one of his friends here . . . the above-mentioned private person (namely Jacob de Famars the elder)', FRG 108: 187–9v (Relation on Osnabrück, March 1647), [JLP 0820].

16 Dennis J. Maika, 'Jacob Leisler's Chesapeake Trade', *de Halve Maen* 67 (Spring 1994), 9–14. For the evaluation of Leisler's estate see 'valuation of the best and most affluent inhabitants of this city', 4 March 1674, in Edmund B. O'Callaghan and Berthold Fernow (eds.), *Documents relative to the colonial history of the State of New York* (15 vols., Albany, NY, 1853–87), vol. 2, 699 [hereafter cited as *DRCNY*]. In addition to his own wealth, estimated in 1676 as at least £5000 sterling, the New York courts in 1684 gave Leisler control of the estates of his father-in-law, Govert Loockermans, and of his mother-in-law, Marritje Jans, whose combined estates were valued at the 'enormous sum' of £52,026 sterling in 1692. See Firth Haring Fabend, '"According to Holland Custome": Jacob Leisler and the Loockermans estate feud', *de Halve Maen* 67 (Spring 1994), 6–7.

17 Berthold Fernow (ed.), *The minutes of the Orphanmasters of New Amsterdam* (2 vols., New York, 1902–7), vol. 2, 47–8. For Le Breton see *De Nederlandsche Leeuw* 56 (Jan. 1938), 422–3; for Barbou see *ibid.*, 35 (July 1917), 171–4.

18 Baptisms in the New Amsterdam Dutch Reformed Church, 1662, *NYGB Record* 6 (July 1875), 150–1. De la Pleine was born in Bresiure, France, 1 July 1634; he married Susannah Cresson, daughter of Pierre Cresson of Picardy, France, on 1 September 1658. Marvin G. Delaplane, *The Delaplaines of America* (Utica, KY, 1998), 1–3. For Couturier see Charles X. Harris, 'Henri Couturier an artist of New Netherland', *New-York Historical Society Quarterly* (1927), 45–52, C. A. Weslager, *The Swedes and Dutch at New Castle* (New York, 1987), 223–30.

19 *Orphanmasters*, vol. 2, 48–9.

20 *Ibid.*, vol. 1, 233, 234, 235–7.

21 Voorhees, 'Fervent Zeale', 457. Leisler's shipments may be partially followed in the Plymouth/Penrys, Falmouth, and Dover, England, Port Books, PRO E 190/1047/12, E 190/666/8, 190/667/77, E 190/1052/3.

22 Bosher, 77.

23 William Hand Browne (ed.), *Archives of Maryland* (72 vols., Baltimore, MD, 1883–), vol. 66, 353–4; vol. 69, 19–23; Maika, 'Jacob Leisler's Chesapeake Trade', 13, note 18. Cordea's birthplace is found in Jeffrey A. Wyand and Florence L. Wyand (eds.), *Colonial Maryland naturalizations* (Baltimore, 1975), 6. Although Cordea died a Roman Catholic, it is believed that he was a convert from Calvinism: Historic St Mary's, Cordea file, courtesy of Lois Green Carr. Couturier joined the Threadneedle Street church on 25 Nov. 1674, HSQS 21; he and his wife Elizabeth Coppyn thereafter appear in the Canterbury French church records, HSQS 5, 288, 302, 305.

24 Bosher, 85–6; Charles W. Baird, *History of the Huguenot emigration to America* (2 vols., New York, 1885; reprinted Baltimore, MD, 1973), vol. 2, 140; On 13 Feb. 1674, Leisler sued Minvielle for 'dead freight of 5 hhds of tobacco, which deft should have shipped in Pieter van Essams ketch'. Berthold Fernow (ed.), *Records of New Amsterdam* (7 vols., New York, 1897), vol. 7, 53, 59. Van Essam is also called Pieter Meniet in these records, and is possibly of French origin, *ibid.*, 65.

25 West Indies Company passport to Jacob Leisler for Curaçao, 10 July 1676, and WIC Amsterdam Chamber to John Doncker, Director in Curaçao, 11 July 1676, WIC archives, The Hague. For Pierre D'Orville see Norbert H. Schneeloch, 'Die Bewindhebber der Westindischen Compagnie in der Kammer Amsterdam 1674–1700', in *Economisch- en sociaal-historisch jaarboek* (The Hague, 1971), 17, 39–40. For the D'Orville family see Johan E. Elias, *De Vroedschap van Amsterdam 1578–1795* (2 vols., Haarlem, 1905), vol. 2, 959–60; *De Nederlandsche Leeuw Maanblad van het Koninklijk Nederlandsch Genootschap voor Geslacht- en Wapenkunde*, 57 (January 1939), 15–16.

26 Baird, 1:229–33; *DRCNY*, vol. 9, 300, 312.

27 Georgana Klass Willets, 'The children of Andre Thauvet and Suzanne Faneuil', *NYGB Record* 117 (Apr. 1986), 87–9; Georgana Klass Willets, 'Faneuil family', *NYGB Record*, 116 (July 1985), 152–3, shows the relationship between Faneuil and Thauvet. For Faneuil's trade connections with Milborne and Leisler see Gemeentearchief, Rotterdam, ONA.

28 The other purchasers were Jean Bouteillier, Isaac Des Champs, Andre Thauvet, Daniel Streing, Etienne Lumprey, and M. Paquinet: Westchester County Archives, Records of Deeds, Liber B, 60; Morgan H. Seacord and William S. Hadaway (eds.), *Historical landmarks of New Rochelle* (New Rochelle, NY, 1938), 8–11, 9. In that year Alexander Allair from La Rochelle, France, by way of St Christopher, settled on these lands, followed the next year by Theolophelus Forestier. Glena See Hill, 'The Allaire family of La Rochelle, France', *NYGB Record* 125 (July 1994), 137–40.

29 Robert Bolton, *The history of the several towns, manors, and patents of the county of Westchester from the first settlement to the present time* (New York, 1881), 585–6. Morgan H. Seacord, 'Huguenot settlement of New Rochelle', *Quarterly Bulletin of the Westchester County Historical Society* 9 (July 1933), 62–6; Herbert B. Nicols, *History of New Rochelle* (New Rochelle, NY, 1938), 16–18. On 12 Nov. 1688, Leisler traded 400 acres, 'being his own proportion in the Great Lotts', for 'forty two acres of land upon the neck and fourteen by the mill' belonging to Thauvet, Leisler reserving his 'eight acres procento out of the four hundred acres'. Westchester County Archives, Record of Deeds, Liber C: 373.

30 Caryl Coleman, 'Introduction', in Jean Forbes (ed.), *Records of the Town of New Rochelle 1699–1828* (New Rochelle, NY, 1916), ix–x, xiii–xvi. The original deed is in the Huguenot-Thomas Paine Museum, New Rochelle. A map of Leisler's New Rochelle purchase may be found in New York State Archives, Albany, NY, Land Papers, 4:14.

31 William Warren Sweet, *Religion in colonial America* (New York, 1943), 207.

32 Robert C. Ritchie, *The Duke's province: a study of New York politics and society, 1664–1691* (Chapel Hill, NC, 1977), 190–5.

33 For Huguenot population figures see Joyce Goodfriend, *Before the melting pot: society and culture in colonial New York City, 1664–1730* (Princeton, NJ, 1992), 47–8. The Roman Catholic commanders were Jarvis Baxter at Albany, Bartholomew Russell at New York City, and Capt. Webb for Long Island and Staten Island. William Harper Bennett, *Catholic footsteps in old New York: a chronicle of Catholicity in the city of New York from 1524 to 1808* (New York, 1909), 82–111, 196.

34 Letter from Members of the Dutch Church of New York to the Classis of Amsterdam, 21 Oct. 1698, *New York Historical Society Collections* [hereafter *NYHS Collections*], 1:398. Also see 'Loyalty Vindicated' (1698) in Charles M. Andrews (ed.), *Narratives of the Insurrections* (New York, 1915), 375–6.

35 Commissions are in Edmund B. O'Callaghan (ed.), *The Documentary History of the State of New-York* (4 vols., Albany, NY, 1848–52) [hereafter *DHNY*], vol. 2, 5, 11.

36 *Die Matrikel der Universität Basel*, vol. 2, 411; Quentin Skinner points out that John Locke's writings, often credited as inspiring the development of American political thought, are to a 'remarkable extent' based on the 'same set of arguments'. Quentin Skinner, *The foundations of modern political thought* (2 vols., Cambridge, 1978), vol. 2, 239. Schloss Harburg, Germany, Oettingen-Oettingenshe archiv 1: 2766, 2790, 2853–54; 2: 1606, 1643a, 1664; Staatsarchiv Amberg, Germany, Amberg Stadt Nr. 510a-c.

37 Sven Stelling-Michaud (ed.), *Le Livre du Recteur de l'Académie de Genève (1559–1878)* (6 vols., Geneva, 1959–79), vol. 1, 170; vol. 4, 310; Voorhees, 'Fervent Zeale', 451–2.

38 Choisy, *Recueil généalogique suisse*, vol. 1, 277–82; FRG 157:11.

39 *Mémoires de l'estat de France sous Charles IX: contenans les choses plus notables, faites & publiées tant par les Catholiques que par ceux de la religion . . .* (3 vols., Geneva, 1578); Lord King's half of Locke's library cited in Herbert D. Foster, 'International Calvinism through Locke and the Revolution of 1688', in *American Historical Review* 32:3 (April 1927), 495 n.19; see also 492, 494–5. For discussion of Goulart's *Mémoires* see Skinner, *Foundations of modern political thought*, vol. 2, 304–9.

40 Voorhees, 'Fervent Zeale', 454 n. 31. Leisler's 'Declaration of the Inhabitants Soldjers', 31 May 1689, for example, follows in construction the Prince de Condé's *Declaration* of 1562, *DHNY* vol. 2, 10–11. For a discussion of the Huguenot theory of popular sovereignty, see Skinner, vol. 2, 228–9, 232–5, 312–13, 338–45. For Leisler's justification for the use of elections, see Leisler to Gilbert Burnet, 7 Jan. 1689/90, *DRCNY*, vol. 3, 654–7.

41 Butler, *Huguenots in America*, 19, 26, 154; Gerald Cerny, *Theology, politics and letters at the crossroads of European civilization: Jacques Basnage and the Baylean Huguenot refugees in the Dutch Republic* (Dordrecht, 1987); Guy Howard Dodge, *The political theory of the Huguenots of the dispersion* (New York, 1947).

42 Petition of Pierre Reverdy to the Bishop of London, 30 Dec. 1689, PRO, CO5/1081, 218–19.

43 Statement of Ensign Joost Stol, 23 May 1690, *NYHS Collections*, vol. 1, 297–8; Memorandum of the Lord President to the Board of Trade, 23 May 1690, PRO, CO5/1081, 310. For a discussion of the political climate in England, see Jonathan I. Israel, 'The Dutch role in the Glorious Revolution', in Jonathan Israel (ed.), *The Anglo-Dutch moment: essays on the Glorious Revolution and its world impact* (Cambridge, 1991), 142–3.

44 *NYHS Collections*, 1:424.

45 Charles Fenno Hoffman, 'Jacob Leisler', in Jared Sparks (ed.), *The Library of American Biography*, vol. 3 (Boston, Mass., 1844), 192; William Dunlap, *History of the New Netherland, Province of New York, and State of New York* (2 vols., New York, 1839–40), 153. Leisler's action inspired Emily C. Judson's short story, 'The French emigrants', in *Alderbrook: a collection of Fanny Forester's Village Sketches* (Boston, 1847), 198–205.

46 *NYHS Collections*, vol. 1, 424. See also Alfred V. Wittmeyer (ed.), *Register of the Births, Marriages, and Deaths of the 'Eglise Française à la Nouvelle York' from 1688 to 1804* (New York, 1886; repr. Baltimore, MD, 1968), xxvi, 45, 63.

47 Leisler was elected a deacon of the New York City Dutch Reformed church in 1670, 1674 and 1680. Collegiate Protestant Reformed Dutch church offices, 45 John Street, New York City. 'Register der Predicanten, Ouderlingen en Diaconen, 1668–1700'.

36

From ethnicity to assimilation: the Huguenots and the American immigration history paradigm

BERTRAND VAN RUYMBEKE

Anyone who has read a monograph on the Huguenot emigration to British North America knows that the French refugees rapidly and thoroughly assimilated.[1] Migrating during the 1670s and 1680s, they quickly sought naturalization, adapted to the economic conditions of the New World, conformed to Anglicanism or fused with other Calvinist denominations, intermarried with English or Dutch colonists, anglicized their names and lost the use of their native language so that by the mid-18th century they no longer existed as a distinctive 'national', religious and linguistic group. Thus, the first and second generation's thorough espousal of the dominant Anglo-American or, in New York, Anglo-Dutch, values and lifeways led the third generation Huguenots to become indistinguishable from their neighbours.

These conclusions, widely accepted by the academic community, raise, however, two challenging questions. First, since any description of the issue of assimilation rests on the implicit assumption that the Huguenots formed an ethnic group, to what extent can we speak of Huguenot ethnicity? Then, should the Huguenot experience in early America be described as integration, acculturation or assimilation, or do these terms correspond to successive phases of their absorption by the dominant group? After looking at how this post-migratory experience has been described by successive historians of the Huguenot Refuge in North America, this essay addresses these two questions.

All students of the Huguenot migration to America have stressed their rapid assimilation into the diverse host societies that they encountered but have done so using clearly distinct approaches that reflect the historiographical trends of their times and may not have been quite as objective as they have claimed.

Although Charles W. Baird, pioneer historian of the Huguenots in America, spent little time discussing their assimilation, briefly mentioning 'the value of [their] contribution to the American character and spirit' in the introduction of his voluminous *History of the Huguenot emigration to America*, he nonetheless established a historiographical tendency that endured for almost a century, until the 1970s.[2] To Baird and his successors, the Huguenot migrant, although not a White Anglo-Saxon Protestant, not only assimilated with success but also contributed to the building of an implicitly unique American identity.

In his wake, Arthur H. Hirsch, author of a monograph on the Carolina Huguenots, emphatically wrote about 'an influence on Carolina that cannot be erased'.[3] Although Hirsch claimed to have 'tried to get at the truth, regardless of current theories and traditions', his study is topically and interpretatively embedded in the resurgence of immigration studies that occurred among historians and sociologists in the 1920s under the leadership of the Harvard (historical) and Chicago (sociological) schools.[4] Apart from the Huguenot's beneficial contribution, Hirsch's thesis focuses on the issue of assimilation.[5] In his view, this 'successful' assimilation reflected a capacity to adapt and survive not as a distinct group but as an in-distinguishable element of American colonial society. The Huguenots, this southern European people who had the 'opportunity to absorb the refinements of English life before embarking for South Carolina', were a reassuring example of how thoroughly non-British migrants could adopt the lifeways and beliefs of the dominant Anglo-Protestant group.[6]

In contrast to Hirsch, Amy Friedlander, in her 1974 unpublished dissertation entitled 'Carolina Huguenots: a study in cultural pluralism in the Low Country', measured the Huguenot experience with methodological and interpretative tools borrowed from recent works in cultural anthropology, ethnology and sociology, especially those of Milton Gordon, Fredrik Barth, and E. K. Francis.[7] Her work was the first historiographical attempt to discuss the issue of Huguenot ethnicity and to define the Huguenot adaptation to their Carolina host society in terms of integration, acculturation and assimilation. Friedlander, whose meticulous study spanned four generations of Huguenots, reached an ambiguous conclusion, however, as she was unable to determine whether the Huguenots had integrated or assimilated into South Carolina society. In her view, and as the choice of the word 'pluralism' in her title implies, the Huguenots seem to have assimilated in espousing the dominant Anglo-American religious, political and cultural values while retaining a diffuse identity through the preservation of kinship ties and oral traditions.[8]

In his 1983 seminal study of the Huguenot emigration to British North America, Jon Butler further explored the dynamics of the Huguenot assimilation in three different early American host societies: New England, New York, and South Carolina. With Butler's book, the pendulum of historiographical interpretation swung far to the opposite side from the time of Baird and Hirsch, describing the Huguenot experience in unqualified terms. Butler, for example, wrote about the ' disintegration', the 'dis-appearance', and the 'failure to sustain religious and social cohesion', of the Huguenots, which illustrated the ' indelible pathology of 17th-century French Protestantism'.[9]

Ironically, although Butler's study shares little with Hirsch's in terms of method-ology and interpretation, they both emphasized the Huguenots' complete assimilation albeit from quite different perspectives. What was to Hirsch success and a sign of cultural vitality was to Butler failure and a sign of religious and ethnic decrepitude. Perhaps because he approached the Huguenot experience as a religious rather than an immigration historian, Butler tended to describe it in partially negative terms. An attentive and knowledgeable reader unequivocally feels that Butler must have been annoyed by the hagiographic literature that permeated Huguenot studies in the United States through the latter part of the 19th and most of the 20th century and that his book was a reaction to it.

Although greatly indebted to Butler's study, recent historiography has qualified his interpretations. John Bosher and R. C. Nash, for example, have argued that the Huguenots' economic success did not result from their assimilation into local host societies but was instead due to their ability to preserve a distinctive membership in a Huguenot familial and ethno-religious transatlantic trading culture, which was part of the famed 'Protestant International'.[10] In my work on the South Carolina Huguenots, I have emphasized the gradual aspect of the integration of the Huguenots into the political, cultural and socio-economic fabric of early Carolina.[11] While raw statistics and naturalization or ecclesiastical laws may indicate rapid and unchallenged assimilation, careful perusal of probate and family records reveals the existence of a practical compromise between adoption and adaptation. Thus, for example, several years after petitioning the Carolina assembly to become an Anglican parish, most likely to benefit from legislative funds, the newly elected Huguenot vestrymen still referred to themselves by the French Calvinist word of *anciens*.[12]

Addressing the issue of assimilation within the framework of American immigration history implies a retroactive perception of the Huguenots as a distinct ethnic group.[13] Yet, the inescapable methodological necessity of applying a conceptual paradigm elaborated by historians and sociologists who studied 19th- and 20th-century migration to a 17th-century phenomenon prevents us from taking the concept of ethnicity for granted. In other words, the historian of the Huguenot emigration to North America must address the fundamental, yet often-evaded, question of Huguenot ethnicity before trying to discuss their assimilation into the Anglo-American host society.

Beyond the acknowledged difficulty and anachronistic risk of using the concept of ethnicity in the pre-national period of European history, in order to address the question of Huguenot ethnicity, the historian must first define the term Huguenot and then delineate what the Huguenots in early America had in common to determine to what extent they belonged to a specific group. This clarification is all the more necessary as ethnicity, being anchored in specific time and place, is eminently contextual. To be ethnically French in the late 17th century does not imply the same characteristics as in the 19th and 20th centuries.

In Europe at the time of the Revocation of the Edict of Nantes, a Huguenot, strictly speaking, was a French Calvinist or French Reformed. He or she lived within the admittedly changing borders, but borders nonetheless, of 17th-century France and was a subject of Louis XIV. He or she also was Francophone although the mother tongue may not have been French but a dialect or *patois* of Celtic, Provençal or Germanic origins.[14] This restrictive definition allows us to differentiate Huguenots from Walloons, French-speaking Swiss Calvinists, and Alsatian Lutherans. This distinction must be made since it was recognized by the refugees themselves who were always very precise in identifying their regions or countries of origin.[15] Furthermore, this nuance is not only semantically appropriate but also indispensable for historical accuracy as few Walloons emigrated after 1650, Alsatians were not subject to the pre-Revocation persecutions, and in the 1680s the Swiss were in no way religious refugees but economic migrants.[16]

In France, the Huguenots had more in common with their Catholic counterparts than has usually been acknowledged. Like the rest of the French population, as Elisabeth Labrousse stressed, the Huguenots were undoubtedly 'proud to be French', and viewed foreigners with 'tacit condescension'.[17] They were also involved in their communities and shared many of the lifeways of their Catholic social peers as recent community studies have shown.[18] They were, however, as Labrousse wrote, 'French in a peculiar way' [*des Français particuliers*].[19] Except in some areas in Languedoc, Poitou and Normandy, they tended to be more urban, more artisanal, and more 'bourgeois' than Catholics. They followed a different religious calendar, attended *le temple* instead of *l'église*, participated in neither processions nor pilgrimages, and revered neither saints nor bishops. They constituted a minority group, or 'subnation' to use the terminology of the *Harvard encyclopedia of American ethnic groups*, which can be regarded as ethnic inasmuch as it was defined by religious and somewhat cultural criteria rather than linguistic and regional like the Basques or Bretons.[20] Furthermore, the Huguenots, whom the royal and ecclesiastical authorities referred to contemptuously by the generic term of Protestant, were resisting a process of forced assimilation into the dominant Catholic majority, which intensified in the decades preceding the Revocation.

In the diaspora, and particularly in America, the Huguenots ceased to be simply 'Protestant', became French Calvinists and lost their regional identities, which in France had been their primary identifying trait after religion. When they arrived in the new host society, the native population's identifying criteria took precedence over their own, giving them an ascriptive ethnic identity.[21] Within their own group, however, the Huguenots continued to use regional origin and congregational or kin membership (when they came from the same province) as the main criteria for identification.

The terms Calvinist and Reformed, although somewhat generic, were probably meaningful to all Huguenots. The use of the word French as the primary identifying trait, however, was new to most except the very few who had travelled beyond the borders of France for commercial or military reasons. Although, as French historians have shown, there was a true sentiment of peoplehood, *'une conscience nationale'*, in early modern France, apart from being born in the kingdom of France and being a subject of Louis XIV, to be 'French', at least nominally after the migration, essentially meant that they were *not* English, Irish, Swiss or Dutch.[22] Although, and especially in England, the term 'French' probably evoked a multitude of often unpleasant character-istics, in essence it carried linguistic and vaguely cultural (rather than national) connotations. In colonial South Carolina for example, the Huguenots were barred from legislative eligibility on the sole grounds that they were unaccustomed to British liberties because they hailed from a land ruled despotically, thus equating France with absolutism, and that they were not proficient enough in English.[23]

In the context of American immigration history it is quite appropriate to define the Huguenots as an ethnic group provided that the term be devoid of narrowly national connotations.[24] In British North America, the term Huguenot became synonymous with French, meaning Francophone Calvinists, as the group included significant proportions of Swiss and Walloons.[25] Thus, although the Huguenots are discussed in the *Harvard encyclopedia of American ethnic groups* under the rubric 'French', when historians refer to the Huguenots they usually mean French-speaking Protestant migrants.[26]

This usage led to the coinage of the redundant and somewhat characteristically American phrase of French Huguenot, while its logical counterparts, Swiss Huguenot and Belgian Huguenot, are, however, never used. The lexical association, 'French Huguenot', which is inappropriate in a European context – not only because a Huguenot is necessarily French and a non-French Calvinist is anything but a Huguenot but also because in post-Revocation France the French are at least nominally all Catholics (*nouveaux* and *anciens*) – makes sense, however, in America. Thus, whereas in France the interchangeable terms 'Huguenot' and 'Protestant' had carried religious, cultural, and even perhaps socio-economic, connotations, across the Atlantic the term 'French' adopted linguistic and broad cultural rather than strictly national connotations while the word 'Huguenot' took on a restrictive religious meaning, becoming the equivalent of Calvinist.[27]

In early America the three external distinctive features of the Huguenot group were their alien status, their language, and their brand of Calvinism. It is these characteristics that set the Huguenots apart from the rest of the settlers giving them the status of an ethnic group as an object of historical study. In this context assimilation therefore refers to the disappearance of these traits through the gradual erosion of the group boundaries.

Although very often used in a loose sense, the term assimilation refers in fact to an extraordinarily complex phenomenon which is difficult to describe, measure and explain, and this for three main reasons. First, assimilation is multidimensional. It operates at different levels and is of different natures. Thus, it can be collective or individual; socio-economic, religious, linguistic, or national; and also cultural or structural. Second, the process of assimilation can reach different stages depending on the group and period studied. Third, the conceptual tools that historians have borrowed from sociologists and cultural anthropologists to define and study assimilation are constantly evolving along with historiographical methods, objectives and interests.[28]

Therefore, before evaluating the Huguenot experience in early America through the prism of immigration history, one must first clear up the confusion caused by the interchangeable use by many historians of the three concepts of assimilation, integration, and acculturation. Assimilation, termed incorporation when the process is complete, refers to the total loss of ethnically distinctive characteristics of a minority group in its absorption by the host society through homogenization. Integration, also called amalgamation, describes a mutual adaptation process in which each group values the other's contribution to the establishment of a common culture. Finally, acculturation implies changes in both groups following their coming into contact. While acculturation and assimilation have sometimes been used interchangeably, it seems that historians and anthropologists now regard the former as an intermediary phase towards full assimilation, although both phenomena can exist independently.[29]

At first glance, the Huguenot transatlantic experience can be analysed in terms of assimilation or even incorporation. However, it remains difficult to measure how gradual and thorough this process actually was. Historians must also be particularly cautious in their use of the extant, and somewhat biased and incomplete, sources before reaching hasty conclusions. The fact that probate records, for example, indicate that most Huguenots recorded their wills in English early in the 18th century does not mean that they had lost the use of the French language. Private correspondence shows that the Huguenots actually used French among themselves and with relatives in the colonies and in Europe, while conducting official transactions in English. Furthermore, the Huguenots of the first and second generations certainly spoke French at home to their parents and grandparents. Thus, when we measure the degree of linguistic assimilation, a crucial distinction must be made between the public and private spheres, since a form of bilingualism persisted through most of the 18th century.

A similar observation can be made concerning the rate of exogamous marriages. An analysis of the marriage records by ethnicity (French/English and French/Dutch) undeniably shows that the Huguenots quickly married outside their community. However, the identification of the brides and grooms reveals a much more complex reality.[30] The Huguenots may actually have married outside their ethno-religious, but not social, group. This trend is particularly marked among the elite, who intermarried with wealthy members of the English or Dutch group to consolidate their estates or commercial networks.[31] In other words these unions were ethnically exogamous while socially endogamous. Significantly enough, this behaviour had actually started back in France before the migration, as Bosher has shown, when Huguenot merchant families were already intermarrying with English and Dutch Protestants who had settled in Bordeaux and La Rochelle.[32] This type of exogamous union should not be interpreted solely as a sign of assimilation but also, and perhaps chiefly, as the continuation of pre-migratory socio-economic and familial strategies. Furthermore, the matrimonial market being fairly small in early America, one can easily imagine the union of children of English-French marriages, who most likely perceived themselves as members of the dominant English majority. If statistically this type of marriage is regarded as English/English, it is doubtful, however, that these couples had lost all of the ethnic traits of their Huguenot grandparents.

Additionally, if the Huguenots can be described, from without, as a fairly homogeneous group, they actually constituted an intricately diverse community. The Huguenots, in the American use of the term, varied in their national (Swiss/French), regional (Atlantic/Northern/Southern France) and social origins (agricultural/artisanal/professional), their habitats (rural/urban), their languages (Normand, Occitan, Picard, etc.), their Calvinism (synodal/ congregational), and their cultural ways rooted in regional traditions. This diversity implies that before melting, so to speak, into the host societies, the Huguenots assimilated nationally, regionally, linguistically, religiously, culturally and, to a lesser extent, socially among themselves. This process of inner assimilation was a necessary preliminary phase towards assimilation into the dominant group. Thus, for example, the Huguenot socio-economic and pastoral elites, who tended to be more receptive to assimilation through which they could reinforce their dominant position within and outside the Huguenot community, served as a buffer between the English-Anglican provincial elite and the rest of the group. Intermarriage with the English elite brought stability to the group in the inevitably chaotic and divisive assimilation process. Unsurprisingly, where this elite was absent, as in St Denis Parish, South Carolina, turmoil and rebellion, not to say secession, soon followed Anglican conformity.[33]

It can also be argued that in the process of assimilation, the Huguenots did reach a stage of acculturation during which they influenced the dominant group. Ironically, the best illustration of this phenomenon is to be found in their critical and often-heralded religious assimilation. Records show that, in the South Carolina rural parishes, for example, in conforming to Anglicanism the Huguenots in fact contributed a decisive touch of Calvinism to the colony's Church of England that accentuated its low-church nature. To the dismay and anger of the Bishop of London's representative based in Charleston, Huguenot conformist vestrymen controlled the parishes in quasi-total independence like a Calvinist congregation. Pastors preached without surplices, parishioners had never heard of the Book of Common Prayer, and communicants refused to kneel.[34]

Sylvester Primer, a 19th-century linguist, even described in the South Carolina Low Country what could be called a process of linguistic acculturation through which the Francophone Huguenot settlers influenced a dominant but evolving English language cut off from its source. In two articles published in the 1880s and devoted to 'all peculiarities in the pronunciation of Charleston', Primer explained how geographical isolation, linguistic conservatism, the presence of an elite educated in Europe, and the absence of 'a large floating population of mixt nationality' created a favourable environment for the preservation of archaic language forms. Noting that 'many sounds in the daily speech of the Charlestonians were brought from England with the first colony in 1670', he also identified 'the Huguenot element in Charleston's pronunciation'. Thus, according to Primer, the importation and preservation of French sounds contributed to the peculiar nature of the English spoken in 19th-century Charleston. This linguistic influence, however, dwindled in the aftermath of the Civil War as Charleston, 'through her greater contact with the outer world', began to lose 'her older pronunciation and archaic forms and expressions' until they became no longer noticeable.[35]

This acculturation, which is a facet of the larger question of the adaptation of the European settlers to New World living conditions, suggests that instead of describing the Huguenot experience in America solely in terms of assimilation into a dominant group, one may also speak of parallel and interactive creolization. This creolization was religious, linguistic and economic. In South Carolina, Virginia, and, to some extent New York, for example, the Huguenots did not take up slavery in order to assimilate into the English or Anglo-Dutch dominant culture, but all these groups turned to slavery as a viable answer to the challenge of a new economic environment.[36] Similarly, the abandonment of the chimerical projects of viticulture, olive growing, and sericulture for cattle ranching and rice culture by the South Carolina Huguenots, which, in my view, represents the most thorough facet of their adaptation to the New World, was simultaneously undertaken by the British.

The multifaceted assimilation process of the Huguenots in British North America thus needs to be studied using a varied approach since each aspect requires specific analysis.

First, contrary to what some have written, I think, numbers did matter. The relatively low number of refugees who settled in British North America, less than 3000 before 1710, especially considering the dispersion of the coastal settlements, hastened the process even if it was not the most decisive factor of their assimilation.[37] Then, if Anglican conformity can be regarded as the loss of a distinctive trait of the group and fits the assimilation paradigm, it also involved an acculturation process through which the Huguenots influenced the nature of the colonial Anglican Church. The Huguenot loss of traditional economic activities, however, cannot be interpreted as a sign of assimilation since they did not adopt specific British ways but adjusted to new economic conditions. Furthermore, the economic success of the Huguenot merchants was not the consequence of any sort of assimilation but, conversely, resulted from their capacity to maintain predominantly Huguenot commercial networks that had been established before the dispersion. Then, the loss of nationality, perhaps the most visible indication of assimilation, is actually, in the short term, the least pertinent of all since after becoming naturalized British subjects the Huguenots were still regarded as French and, at times, discriminated against. Finally, only the loss of the French language can be truly interpreted as a manifestation of complete assimilation but the paucity of extant private correspondence and the obvious lack of oral sources make it particularly difficult to gauge.

To conclude, one may say that the Huguenots assimilated into early American host societies, in the sense that they adopted most of the Anglo-American, and in New York Anglo-Dutch, lifeways and intermarried with settlers of British and Dutch origins. However, this assimilation involved an acculturation process through which the Huguenots religiously, culturally and perhaps linguistically influenced the dominant group in the context of the establishment of creolized pluralistic societies.

NOTES

The author wishes to thank Jon Butler, Paula Carlo, Leslie Choquette, Bernard Cottret, Darlene Daehler-Wilking, Lou Roper, David W. Voorhees, and Meredith van Ruymbeke for their comments on earlier drafts of this essay.

1   The main works on the Huguenot emigration to North America are Charles W. Baird, *History of the Huguenot emigration to America*, 2 vols. (New York, 1885); Arthur H. Hirsch, *The Huguenots of colonial South Carolina* (Columbia, SC, 1999 [originally published 1928]); Amy E. Friedlander, 'Carolina Huguenots. A study in cultural pluralism in the Low Country, 1679–1768' (Unpublished Ph.D. dissertation, Emory University, 1979), and Jon Butler, *The Huguenots in America. A refugee people in New World society* (Cambridge, MA, 1983). See also Myriam Yardeni, *Le refuge protestant* (Paris, 1985), ch. 9.

2   Baird, *History*, iv.

3   Hirsch, *Huguenots*, 264.

4   François Weil, 'Migrations, migrants et ethnicité', in Jean Heffer and François Weil (eds.), *Chantiers d'histoire américaine* (Paris, 1994), 410–11; Rudolph J. Vecoli, 'Ethnicity: a neglected dimension of American history', in Herbert J. Bass (ed.), *The state of American history* (Chicago, 1970), 75–80; Russell A. Kazal, 'Revisiting assimilation: the rise, fall, and reappraisal of a concept in American ethnic history', *American Historical Review* 100 (1995), 442–8; Thomas J. Archdeacon, 'Melting pot or cultural pluralism: changing views on American ethnicity', *Revue Européenne des Migrations Internationales* 6 (1990), 14–17. An influence all the more predictable since Hirsch defended his dissertation on the Huguenots in Colonial South Carolina at the University of Chicago. Hirsch, *The Huguenots*, xxxii.

5   Hirsch, for example, has a chapter entitled 'The assimilation of the Huguenots', *The Huguenots*, 90–102.

6 *Ibid.*, 154.

7 Friedlander, 'Carolina Huguenots', 11–18; Weil, 'Migrations, migrants et ethnicité', 414–18; Milton M. Gordon, *Assimilation in American life: the role of race, religion, and national origins* (New York, 1964); Fredrik Barth (ed.), *Ethnic groups and boundaries: the social organization of culture difference* (London, 1969); E. K. Francis, *Interethnic relations: an essay in sociological theory* (New York, 1976).

8 Friedlander, 'Carolina Huguenots', 316–21.

9 Butler, *The Huguenots in America*, 199–215.

10 John. F. Bosher, 'Huguenot merchants and the Protestant International in the seventeenth century', *William & Mary Quarterly* 3rd series 52 (1995), 77–102; R. C. Nash, 'The Huguenot diaspora and the development of the Atlantic economy: Huguenots and the growth of the South Carolina economy, 1680–1775', paper read at the conference 'Out of New Babylon: the Huguenots and their diaspora', Charleston, SC, 1997.

11 Bertrand van Ruymbeke, 'L'émigration huguenote en Caroline du Sud sous le régime des Seigneurs Propriétaires: étude d'une communauté du Refuge dans une province de l'Amérique du Nord britannique, 1680–1720' (Thèse de doctorat, 2 vols., Sorbonne-Nouvelle, 1995).

12 *Ibid.*, vol. 2, 431.

13 Kathleen Neils Conzen, David A. Gerber, Ewa Morawska, George E. Pozzetta and Rudolph J. Vecoli, 'The invention of ethnicity: a perspective from the U.S.A.', *Journal of American Ethnic History* 12 (1992), 3–4.

14 For a captivating study of the linguistic diversity in early modern France, see Philippe Barbaud, *Le choc des patois en Nouvelle-France. Essai sur l'histoire de la francisation au Canada* (Sillery, Quebec, 1984).

15 The South Carolina naturalization list of 1697, for example, is unambigously entitled 'Liste des François et des Suisses'.

16 About the Walloons, see E. M. Braekman, *Le protestantisme belge au 16e siècle* (Carrières-sous-Poissy, 1999); the Alsatians, see Bernard Vogler, 'Les protestants alsaciens et les paix de religion (1555–1648)', in Michel Grandjean and Bernard Roussel (eds.), *Coexister dans l'Intolérance: l'Édit de Nantes (1598)*, special issue of the *Bulletin de la Société de l'Histoire du Protestantisme Français* 44 (1998), 465–9 and 'Louis XIV et les protestants alsaciens de 1680 à 1690', in Roger Zuber and Laurent Theis (eds.), *La Révocation de l'Édit de Nantes et le protestantisme français en 1685* (Paris, 1986), 173–86.

17 Elisabeth Labrousse, *Conscience et conviction. Etudes sur le XVIIe siècle* (Oxford, 1996), 71, and *La révocation de l'édit de Nantes. Une foi, une loi, un roi?* (Paris, 1990 [originally published 1985]), 63–4.

18 See for example, Gregory Hanlon, *Confession and community in 17th-century France: Catholic and Protestant coexistence in Aquitaine* (Philadelphia, 1993).

19 Labrousse, *La révocation*, 63–4.

20 William Petersen, 'Concepts of ethnicity', in Stephan Thernstrom, Ann Orlov, and Oscar Handlin (eds.), *Harvard encyclopedia of American ethnic groups* (Cambridge, MA, 1980), 235; *idem*, 'On the subnations of Western Europe', in Nathan Glazer and Daniel P. Moynihan (eds.), *Ethnicity: theory and experience* (Cambridge, MA, 1975), 179–82.

21 Donald L. Horowitz, 'Ethnic identity', in Glazer and Moynihan (eds.), *Ethnicity*, 118.

22 See for example Myriam Yardeni, *La conscience nationale en France pendant les guerres de religion, 1559–1598* (Paris, 1971).

23 'The Representation and Address of severall of the Members of this present assembly return'd for Colleton County, and other Inhabitants of this Province', quoted in Daniel Defoe, *Party-Tyranny, or an Occasional Bill in miniature; as now practised in Carolina. Humbly offered to the consideration of both Houses of Parliament* (London, 1705) in

Alexander S. Salley, Jr. (ed.), *Narratives of early Carolina, 1650–1708* (New York, 1911), 236–47.

24 Timothy L. Smith, 'Religion and ethnicity in America', *American Historical Review* 83 (1978), 1155–7; Frank Shuffelton (ed.), *A mixed race: ethnicity in early America* (New York, 1993), 3–16; Petersen, 'Concepts of Ethnicity', 234–5; Robert H. Winthrop, 'Ethnicity', in Robert H. Winthrop (ed.), *Dictionary of concepts in cultural anthropology* (Westport, CT, 1991), 94–8.

25 In 17th-century New England, 'French' even meant Jerseyans. David T. Konig, 'A new look at the Essex "French": ethnic frictions and community tensions in 17th-century Essex County, Massachusetts', *Essex Institute Historical Collections* 110 (1974), 168–9.

26 Patrice L. R. Higgonet, 'French', in *Harvard encyclopedia*, 379–88. Interestingly enough, in the *Harvard encyclopedia* the Walloons are under the rubric Belgian and the Alsatians have their own separate entry whereas in the *Dictionary of immigration history*, which was published ten years later, the Huguenots have an entry but not the French. Joan R. Gundersen, 'Huguenots', in Francesco Cordasco (ed.), *Dictionary of American immigration history* (Metuchen, NJ, 1990), 300–4.

27 In a non-academic use, however, the term French needs to be juxtaposed to the word Huguenot as a cognitive identifier since the latter is unknown to the layman.

28 Harold J. Abramson, 'Assimilation and pluralism', in *Harvard encyclopedia*, 150; Winthrop, 'Acculturation', in *Dictionary of concepts*, 3–6; Francis X. Femminella, 'Assimilation', in *Dictionary of American immigration*, 51–5.

29 Milton Gordon, *Assimilation*, 60–71, and *Human nature, class, and ethnicity* (New York, 1978), 166–80; Abramson, 'Assimilation and pluralism', 150–60; Horowitz, 'Ethnic identity', 115–19; Friedlander, 'Carolina Huguenots', 11–12 and Brenda F. Roth, 'The French Huguenots of colonial South Carolina: assimilation and acculturation' (M.A. thesis, University of Colorado, 1989), 7–15.

30 As Joyce Goodfriend points out, in order to interpret marriage patterns of successive generations 'it is essential to delve into the family histories of representative individuals'. *Before the melting pot: society and culture in colonial New York City, 1664–1730* (Princeton, 1992), 178.

31 Bertrand van Ruymbeke, 'The Huguenots of proprietary South Carolina: patterns of migration and settlement', in Jack P. Greene, Rosemary Brana-Shute, and Randy J. Sparks (eds.), *Money, trade and power: the evolution of South Carolina's plantation system* (Columbia, SC, 2000).

32 Bosher, 'Huguenot merchants', 81–8.

33 Butler, *Huguenots in America*, 117–20; van Ruymbeke, 'L'émigration huguenote', vol. 2, 436–9.

34 Amy Friedlander (ed.), 'Commissary Johnson's report, 1713', *The South Carolina Historical Magazine*, 83 (1982), 259–71; van Ruymbeke, 'L'émigration huguenote', vol. 2, 423–31.

35 Sylvester Primer, 'Charleston provincialisms', *Publications of the Modern Language Association of America*, 3 (1887–8), 227–43, and 'The Huguenot element in Charleston's pronunciation', *ibid.*, 4 (1888–9), 214–44.

36 There were, of course, Huguenots who came from the Caribbean with slaves, but they were few in number.

37 Butler, *Huguenots in America*, 210.

Creating order in the American wilderness: state-church Germans without the state

JEFFREY JAYNES

In 1729 the German Reformed pastor George Weiss wrote colonial North America's second German-language pamphlet: *Der in der Americanischen Wildnusz . . . - angefochtene Prediger.*[1] This tract expressed a fear common to German immigrant clergy, that the 'New World' lacked proper moral order. These religious leaders responded with an escalating commitment to establishing appropriate ecclesiastical institutions in the American colonies. In the pamphlet Weiss presents a hypothetical interchange between a pastor and a member of a sect he had encountered in the Pennsylvania frontier: a Newborner. Weiss used the interchange to ridicule the perfectionist tendencies of the sectarian and to chastise his seeming rejection of biblical and pastoral authority.[2] As one might expect, Weiss's pastor emerges victorious from this conversation and fellow German immigrants were warned of the dangers associated with the Newborn.

Although Weiss's pamphlet focuses on this theological battle, for my purpose the more revealing exchange occurs between the pastor and a colonial 'politician'. These two debate the question of liberty of conscience and its purported social benefits. The politician argues for the value of freedom stating that compulsion ought to be avoided, especially in matters of belief. The German pastor has a very different view and counters, 'In Germany, freedom is limited and one cannot believe and do just whatever one wills'.[3] Furthermore, he observes that in Pennsylvania people abuse this so-called freedom and act shamelessly. For Weiss and others Pennsylvania's environment of religious freedom and plurality conflicted with familiar state-church patterns of civil and moral authority and encouraged church leaders to emphasize the need for organization and discipline.

By the time Weiss died in 1761 the situation for German Lutheran and Reformed immigrants – the state-church Germans – had changed dramatically. In less than two decades dozens of churches had been organized, nearly 100 ministers had been added to the handful of initial clergy, and two bodies now provided networks for congregational oversight: the Lutheran Ministerium and the Reformed Coetus.[4] Personal writings and polemical tracts of these church leaders expose the motivation for this effort and the church orders (*Kirchenordnungen*) which they adopted as the constitutional basis for their churches reveal particular adaptations to the situation in Pennsylvania. For them, as for Weiss, there was a tension between Old World mentality and New World reality, or between state-church experience and a voluntary or free church environment, that determined the necessity for their efforts and the direction they would take.

Just as mid-16th-century England welcomed Reformed Protestant exiles through the benefits of King Edward's 1550 charter, so Pennsylvania, in the late 17th century, was heralded as a haven for a host of alienated religious groups. William Penn's charter offered religious sanctuary and numerous agents, or *Neuländer*, invaded the German Reich, especially the Rhineland, literally beating the drum (*Werbetrommel*) of New World opportunity.[5] Aaron Fogleman has identified three primary waves of German immigration to colonial North America prior to the War for Independence.[6] German sectarians – Mennonites, Quakers, Schwenkenfelders, and Dunkers (Weiss's 'Newborners') – were the clear majority during this initial wave of immigration and settlement. Historians of the Middle Colonies, Pennsylvania in particular, have traditionally paid the most attention to this varied group of first arrivals.[7] These sectarians were not only the first to arrive, but they were also the first to publish. Conrad Beissel, eventual leader of the Ephrata cloister, published his *Mystyrion Anomias* just a year before Weiss published his pamphlet.[8]

However, by the middle of the 18th century German immigrants with a state-church affiliation emerged as one of the largest segments of the colony's population. Fogleman notes that Reformed and Lutheran Germans dominated the third wave of migration (1717–75), with estimates ranging from 70,000 to 100,000, or roughly one third of Pennsylvania's population.[9] Recently, historians have paid significantly more attention to this German state-church contingency. Many of these studies have been completed in an attempt to determine how 'German ways' – using the phrase of A. Gregg Roeber, adapted from David Grayson Allen – remained in a New World environment.[10] Roeber himself has investigated how particular German notions of liberty and property informed the policies of Lutheran settlers in Pennsylvania, Georgia, and the Carolinas.[11] Fogleman, on the other hand, has demonstrated how the dynamics of Rhineland village life, especially their strong communal pressures and an interest in frustrating external hierarchies, re-emerged in the tensions of colonial German communities. Of particular importance for this study is Thomas Müller's work on the German Lutheran pastor, Heinrich Melchoir Mühlenberg, *Kirche Zwischen Zwei Welten*.[12] Müller describes how Mühlenberg's expectations of state support, established during his early years of ministry in Brandenburg-Prussia, evaporated as he carried out his ministry in Pennsylvania and New Jersey. All of these works have sought a trans-Atlantic perspective in an attempt to investigate the persistence of German cultural and religious patterns.

My interest here is to explore, in a similar fashion, how ideas of church structure and discipline survived this trans-Atlantic relocation. In order to clarify the problem, I will briefly analyse the sentiments expressed by church leaders in their personal writings, in reports, and in polemical treatises. Then, I will discuss insights gathered from my research on the church constitutions, or *Kirchenordnungen*, which structured the religious life of state-church immigrants. The writings of these early ecclesiastical leaders demonstrate their belief that a lack of moral restraint threatened the faith and virtue of their communities. Their emphasis on congregational oversight and the need to encourage church discipline was subsequently enacted in numerous *Kirchenordnungen,* which were drafted in the 1740s and 1750s. Thus, the organization of German state churches provides clear evidence of how Old World patterns conflicted with a New World environment and of how ecclesiastical structures were adapted to fit the new situation.

The organization of German state-church congregations occurred sporadically through the decades of the 1720s and 30s, but accelerated significantly in the 1740s. For the German Reformed Church, the pioneer work of Johann Boehm was critical. Boehm, a school teacher and not an ordained minister, arrived in 1720 and composed the first Reformed *Kirchenordnung* in 1725.[13] His organizational efforts eventually yielded to Michael Schlatter, an immigrant pastor from the Swiss canton of St Gall. Schlatter had been commissioned by the Amsterdam Classis to 'bring these churches into a proper ecclesiastical order and organization and to present the Reverend Synod a faithful report of their true condition'.[14] Schlatter consolidated congregations and was especially concerned for providing 'proper order and regulation by ordaining elders and deacons'. Beyond the local level Schlatter helped to establish Pennsylvania's first German Reformed Synod (Coetus) in 1748. At its initial meeting, the Coetus adopted Boehm's *Kirchenordnung* as its basic organizational document.[15]

The growth and consolidation of the German Lutheran Church in Pennsylvania was primarily the work of the previously mentioned Heinrich Melchior Mühlenberg. Mühlenberg arrived in 1742, sent by Gotthilf August Francke and the pietist Lutherans at Halle and commissioned by Friedrich Michael Ziegenhagen, the Royal Court Chaplain at St James in London. Like Schlatter, most of Mühlenberg's early ministry involved visiting a vast array of congregations. His initial concerns were preaching, administering the sacraments, and counselling, rather than church organization *per se.* Nevertheless, Mühlenberg played a pivotal role in the organization of the German Lutheran Ministerium in August 1748, shortly after the formation of the Reformed Coetus.[16]

Two issues, in particular, alarmed state-church clergy like Boehm, Schlatter, and Mühlenberg as they proceeded with the task of establishing churches. First, they feared that church members, or those formerly aligned with the state churches, would be enticed into a 'sect'. An anonymous letter to Germany dated January 1734 lamented, 'we live in a land full of heresy and sects. We are in the utmost want and poverty of soul'.[17] Mühlenberg, likewise, commented in a letter to a friend, 'there is no sect in the world that is not sheltered here'. Even the Moravian Brethren, temporarily led directly by Count Nicolaus von Zinzendorf, were regarded with deep suspicion. The Moravians (*Herrnhuttern*) were viewed as religious chameleons who could 'metamorphize themselves into Lutherans, sometimes Reformed, sometimes into all religions'.[18] Boehm vigorously attacked them charging that 'their doctrine is destructive of the soul and subversive of the conscience'.[19]

This concern for the sects, however, was symptomatic of a larger issue confronting the German state-church leaders. In this broadly tolerant and relatively free environment, they found no adequate basis for spiritual and moral authority. Weiss's dialogue between pastor and politician, which highlighted this tension between liberty and licence, identified the fundamental fears and reservations German Lutheran and Reformed leaders had about Pennsylvania.

Other German state-church pastors shared Weiss's concerns. As early as 1702, Justus Falkner, one of the first Lutheran clergymen in Pennsylvania, described German immigrants as 'destitute of altar and priest, [they] roam about this desert, a deplorable condition'.[20] In 1733, the Lutheran Revd Christopher Schulze returned to Germany to raise money for churches in the colony. Schulze warned his countrymen that children and future generations of immigrants would revert to heathenism if appropriate assistance were not provided.[21]

Mühlenberg also lamented the moral condition of this new land. When he requested new pastors from Germany, he insisted that they be firmly converted since, 'here one may be easily induced into carnal indulgence and dissolute habits'.[22] He contrasted Pennsylvania with the 'Fatherland' stating that 'there is more opportunity and freedom to sin here'.[23] Mühlenberg complained that the colony was a 'free un-bridled country' plagued with scoffers and that English laws were 'too lax in some instances'.

Reformed pastors Boehm and Schlatter had similar opinions. Boehm struggled with establishing proper channels of authority as he presented his *Kirchenordnung*. He chastised the Reformed church in Philadelphia for contesting the proper role of the sponsoring Dutch churches when the congregation argued that they were in a free country and did not have to take orders from anyone, especially the Dutch.[24] As Schlatter organized churches he was especially concerned with the proper instruction for the youth. He argued that without effective schools, children would have 'only their corrupt nature to guide them' and would thereby 'grow up as wild shoots'.[25]

Thus Mühlenberg, Boehm, Schlatter and other church leaders expressed a deeply felt concern for the social situation they encountered in Pennsylvania. They worried about the effects of a society whose freedoms were greater than those they were familiar with in Germany. More than merely the lack of pastors and churches contributed to their anxieties. Familiar institutions – the church, schools, and even the family – were threatened by a generally disordered society that overwhelmed the immigrants.

Further complicating the situation for state-church leaders was the lack of support from the secular government. Appeals made to civil authorities for aid in enforcing some aspect of church discipline almost always ended in disappointment for the pastors. Boehm stated clearly that in Pennsylvania one must act 'without the help of the secular authorities'.[26] When Boehm, like Weiss, had a confrontation with a member of the Newborn 'sect', he expected some form of intervention or censure. Instead he commented in frustration, 'there is no punishment in this country for such blasphemers'.

As Müller has argued convincingly in his analysis of Mühlenberg, this Lutheran clergyman clearly anticipated that the state would add its weight to sanctioning church standards of morality.[27] In his journals, Mühlenberg described an incident in which a man was banned from the church for sexually molesting his own daughter. The pastor was shocked that the offender was able to leave the city without any punishment by public authorities.[28] In another situation St Michael's Church in Philadelphia brought charges against a man who had attempted to rape his servant. According to Mühlenberg, the judge 'had a laugh over the affair' and set the man free without penalty. Moreover, Mühlenberg was infuriated by the offender's taunt that 'in Pennsylvania, neither the devil nor a parson could tell him what to do'.[29] Thus, German immigrant pastors were confronted not only with an unfamiliar environment, but with the realization that civil support for their concerns would be almost non-existent. This situation was not what they were accustomed to in the predominantly state-church territories of the German empire. Saxon Halle, Brandenburg-Prussia, Baden-Württemberg, and the Palatine duchies— the areas of heaviest emigration— all had differing but relatively effective consistories, which blended religious and secular authorities in the enforcement of public morality.[30]

Confronted with a society that seemed morally lax and with the awareness that the state would assume little responsibility for establishing Christian virtue, church leaders became even more committed to their organizational efforts. Not only were churches organized, but they were structured in such a way that they could respond to the deficiencies that seemed apparent in this society. The church orders (Kirchenordnungen) written during the middle of the 18th century reflect the same social concerns ecclesiastical leaders expressed in tracts and personal writings. In particular, matters of church discipline and moral oversight featured prominently in these documents. An analysis of several of these orders will clarify their concerns and demonstrate the efforts of the state-church pastors to resurrect a morally ordered society.

For the German Reformed churches, Boehm's Kirchenordnung which had been revised for the Coetus in 1748, served as a model for subsequent efforts. The issue of discipline and the need to restrain licence with ecclesiastical supervision were fundamental features of the document.

This church order emphasized, first of all, the need to assure proper conduct among the clergy members of the consistory. Article One stated that any member of the consistory whose conduct was offensive was 'to be admonished by the remaining members of the consistory'.[31] Failure to heed this warning would result in removal from office. The consistory would meet twice annually, and the minister was required to record all that transpired.

In addition to clerical leadership, the entire congregation was under the discipline outlined in the order. Article Ten stated, 'Should a member of the congregation, male or female, fall into any sin, he shall be placed under the supervision of the consistory until he promise and give evidence of amendment of life'.[32] Article Five, on baptism, limited sponsorship 'to those whose lives are blameless'. The mutual responsibility of moral oversight was affirmed in Article Thirteen,

> if anyone knows of any scandal concerning another, be that one an officer or member, he shall feel conscientiously bound to make known the same, not from envy or hatred, but to prevent all offence.[33]

The entire congregation, therefore, was obliged to duties of discipline.

In the foreword to the order, Boehm wrote that he had formulated it, 'as much as possible in accordance with the condition of the province of Pennsylvania'. The implication was clear: in a society of limited restraints, the church must assume a leading role in enforcing acceptable moral standards.

Mühlenberg drafted the most influential German Lutheran church order, which was adopted by St Michael's Church in Philadelphia in 1762.[34] While Roeber has analysed in detail the property concerns associated with this *Kirchenordnung*,[35] I am more interested in its disciplinary features. As with the Reformed order, the first sections focused on disciplining clergy, especially those whose teaching or lifestyle violated Biblical standards. The order stressed the need for corroborated testimony before proceedings could be instigated against a minister. However, it was also clear that any minister who failed to heed admonishments would be removed from office. Elders and trustees (*Vorsteher*) were also subject to the discipline of the council (*Kirchenrat*), but again, only when complaints could be substantiated.[36] Although keenly interested in discipline, Mühlenberg and others apparently were also concerned about abuses of church power and authority.

Chapter Three of the St Michael's order delineated the privileges and responsibilities of the church members. Matters of discipline dominated this discussion. After identifying the marks of a member in good standing, the order stated that stubborn members, those who violated proper conduct and authority, would not be tolerated. The church had no secular authorities to support its punishments, so it relied on the one power it did have – stripping errant members of congregational privileges. Communicant members who publicly violated God's commandments were to be admonished by the pastor then warned before the entire congregation. The repentant would be quietly restored to full participation; the unrepentant lost all voice in the church, but their names were not to be broadcast publicly.[37]

While Boehm's *Kirchenordnung* and the St Michael's order profoundly influenced their respective denominations, church orders also served a vital function at the congregational level. The *Kirchenordnung* of the Lutheran congregation in Heidelberg Township, Berks County, adopted in 1753, provides a clear illustration. The preamble to this *Kirchenordnung* identified the need for order and the lack of formal organization in the congregation as reasons for making the agreement.[38] Like the orders noted above, the document stressed the role of church leaders. Two deacons, elected annually, were charged with 'keeping a watchful eye on the congregation and admonishing such as lead disorderly lives'. Deacons were expected to be 'honest and free from coarse, prevailing sins and vices'. Church membership only included those recorded in the church book and they alone were allowed to participate in the sacraments. Article Eight stated, 'All members irregular in life and behaviour shall be dealt with according to the teachings and directions of the Lord Jesus – Matt. 18'.[39] The Lutheran church order of Heidelberg Township thus reveals that concerns for moral and social order were common to the frontier parish as well as to the larger church body.

A final example of these discipline-laden *Kirchenordnungen* is the 'Eight Articles' of the Lancaster Evangelical Lutheran Church, which was written by Mühlenberg's associate Johann Handschuh (1749). These articles are a simplified version of the orders already considered. Article Three stated, 'Everyone should promptly adhere to our Christian Church discipline and keep an eye on the others, and notify the pastor of anything of importance to him'.[40] The notion of mutual oversight remained, but the process of church discipline bypassed officers like deacons or trustees in favour of the pastor. Articles Four and Five addressed specific issues which evidently had plagued the congregation. Article Four instructed young people to avoid frivolous behaviour at catechism instruction, while Article Five forbade drinking at funerals. Thus, the

Lancaster church leaders attempted to govern areas of special concern by means of the discipline established in their church order.

As German state-church congregations, both Lutheran and Reformed, moved into the latter half of the 18th century, they did so with a renewed emphasis on organization and congregational discipline. George Weiss's image of the solitary German pastor, crying out and frustrated in a desolate society, no longer applied. Now this individual was part of a network of former state churches which were more numerous, more geographically diverse, more adequately staffed, and clearly committed to promoting their own moral authority in a pluralistic society. Not only the organizing efforts of the pastors, but the documents they produced, the *Kirchenordnungen*, reveal their attempts to reconcile this new world situation with familiar patterns of social and moral order. The state-church model, with its support of territorial consistories, had to yield to a free church, or even as Thomas Müller suggests, a *Volkskirche*, model. These state-church Germans had lost the protective umbrella of the state, but their church had adapted to life in the 'American wilderness'.

NOTES

1   George Michael Weiss, *Der in der Americanischen Wildnusz unter Menschen von verscheidenen Nationen und Religionen hin und wieder herum Wandelte und verschiedentlich angefochtene Prediger: Abgemahlet und vorgestellet in einem Gespraech mit einem Politico und Neugeborenen, verscheidene Stuck insonderheit die Neugeburt betreffende, verfertiget, und zu Beforderung der Ehr Jesu selbst aus eigener Erfahrung an das Licht gebracht* (Philadelphia, 1729). See also *The first century of German language printing in the United States of America*, vol. 1 (Publications of the Pennsylvania German Society, vol. 21, Göttingen, 1989), 1.

2   See the concluding comments in Weiss, 28–9.

3   The dialogue: 'Politicus: Ich denke, dass eine solche Freyheit sehr gut seye, wenn Sie nur nich wird mitzgebrauchet . . . Minister . . . ich sehe, dasz die Freyheit in Pennsylvania leyder'. Weiss, 2.

4   For a detailed analysis of the churches organized in Pennsylvania, see Charles Glatfelter, *Pastors and people: German Lutheran and Reformed Churches in the Pennsylvania field, 1717–1793*, 2 vols. (Breinigsville, PA, 1981).

5   William O'Reilly has surveyed numerous 18th-century editions of the *Karlsruhe Wochenblatt oder Nachrichten* discovering a variety of compelling advertising schemes. William O'Reilly, 'Conceptualizing America in early modern central Europe', *Pennsylvania History* 65 supplement (1998), 102–3.

6   Aaron Fogleman, *Hopeful journeys: German immigration, settlement, and political culture in colonial America, 1717–1775* (Philadelphia, 1996), 4–11. The Lutheran pastor Heinrich Mühlenberg, a participant/ observer in this German migration, identified five periods of German settlement in the region, beginning in 1680 and continuing until 1754. See Kurt Aland (ed.), *Die Korrespondenz Heinrich Melchior Mühlenbergs aus der Anfangszeit des deutschen Luthertums in Nordamerika*, vol. 2: *1753–62* (Berlin, 1987), 172–7.

7   A. Gregg Roeber, 'In German ways? problems and potentials of 18th-century German social and emigration history', *William and Mary Quarterly*, 3rd ser., 44:4 (October 1987), 763.

8   Conrad Beissel, *Mysterion Anomias. Das Geheimniss der Ungerechtigkeit oder der bosshaftige Widerchrist entdeckt und enthüllt bezeugend dass alle diejenigen zue dem*

Gottlosen Wider-Christ angehören, die bereitwillig die Gebothe Gottes verwerfen unter welchen ist sein heiliges, und vom selbst eingensetzter Sieben-Täger Sabbath . . . (Philadelphia, 1728); see also *The first century of German language printing*, vol. 1. For more on Beissel and his work at Epratha see, A Gregg Roeber, 'XVII. Der Pietismus in Nordamerika im 18. Jahrhundert' in Martin Brecht (ed.), *Geschichte der Pietismus*, vol. 2: *Der Pietismus im achtzehnten Jahrhundert* (Göttingen, 1995), 676–7.

9 Fogleman estimates conservatively, however. A. Gregg Roeber opts for a significantly larger representation of state-church Germans in Roeber, *Palatines, liberty, and property: German Lutherans in colonial America* (Baltimore, 1993), 95–101. For additional estimates and analysis see Marianne Wokeck, *Trade in strangers: the beginnings of mass migration to North America* (University Park, PA, 1999).

10 Roeber, 'In German Ways', 750–4, and the influential study of David Grayson Allen, *In English ways: the movement of society and the transferal of English local law and customs to Massachusetts Bay in the 17th century* (Chapel Hill, NC, 1981).

11 Roeber, *Palatines, liberty, and property*, 311–32

12 Thomas Müller, *Kirche zwischen zwei Welten. Die Obrigkeitsproblematic bei Heinrich Melchior Mühlenberg und die Kirchengründung der deutschen Lutheraner in Pennsylvania* (Stuttgart, 1994).

13 William Hinke, *Ministers of the German Reformed Congregations in Pennsylvania and the other colonies in the 18th century* (Lancaster, PA, 1951), 12.

14 Michael Schlatter, *A True History of the Real Condition of the Destitute Congregations in Pennsylvania* (1752), printed in Henry Harbaugh (ed.), *The life of Rev. Michael Schlatter* (Philadelphia, 1857), 135.

15 See the 'Vorrede' in Johann Philip Boehm, *Der Reformierten Kirchen in Pennsylvanien: Kirchen-Ordnung* (Philadelphia, 1748), ii.

16 Müller, 252–3. The obstacles encountered in organizing the Lutheran Ministerium are evident in concerns addressed to Mühlenberg and his associates from rural Pennsylvania congregations. See *Korrespondenz Mühlenbergs*, vol. 1: *1740–52* (Berlin, 1986), 313–17.

17 Theodore Schmauk, *History of the Lutheran Church in Pennsylvania, 1638–1820*, vol. 1 (Philadelphia, 1902), 225.

18 *A Protestation of the Members of the Protestant Lutheran and Reformed Religion in the City of Philadelphia jointly concerned in the Lease of their Meeting House in Arch Street* (Philadelphia, 1742).

19 William Hinke (ed.), *The life and letters of Rev. Jacob Philip Boehm* (Philadelphia, 1916), 348.

20 Justis Falkner, 'Curiose Nachricht', in Schmauk, *History of the Lutheran Church*, 129–30.

21 'Matricul of the Augustus Evangelical Lutheran Congregation of New Providence, usually called Old Trappe Church, 1729–1777', in Julius Sachse (ed.), *Pennsylvania German Society Proceedings and Addresses* vol. 6 (1896), 14–15.

22 Heinrich M. Mühlenberg, *The journals of Heinrich Melchior Mühlenberg*, trans. Theodore Tappert and John Doberstein, vol. 1 (Philadelphia, 1942), 101.

23 *Nachrichten von den Vereinigten deutschen evangelische-lutherischen Gemeinen in Nord-America*, ed. Johann Schulze (hereafter *Hallesche Nachrichten*), vol. 1 (Halle, 1787), 204.

24 *Life of Boehm*, 205.

25 *Life of Schlatter*, 203.

26 *Life of Boehm*, 202.

27 Müller, 201–16.

28 Mühlenberg, *Journals*, vol. 1, 265.

29 *Hallesche Nachrichten*, vol. 1, 907–8.

30 An important overview of the German consistorial system is presented in Karl Müller, 'Die Anfänge der Konsistorialverfassung in lutherischen Deutschland', *Historische Zeitschrift*

102 (1909), 1–21. For Halle and Brandenburg Prussia, see Hans-Walter Krumwiede, *Zur Entstehung des landesherrlichen Kirchenregiment in Kursachsen und Braunschweig-Wolfenbüttel* (Göttingen, 1967), and Emil Sehling, *Die evangelischen Kirchenordnungen des XVI. Jahrhunderts*, vol. 1 (Leipzig, 1902), 358–457. For Baden Württemberg, see Martin Brecht, *Kirchenordnung und Kirchenzucht in Württemberg vom 16. bis 18. Jahrhundert* (Stuttgart, 1967). Mühlenberg repeatedly mentioned his obligations to territorial consistories in Germany, e.g. Württemberg's consistory at Stuttgart (*Korrespondenz Mühlenbergs*, vol. 2, 56, 75), and the Hessian consistory at Darmstadt (*Korrespondenz Mühlenbergs*, vol. 1, 58). He believed that consistories played an especially important role in validating pastoral ministries; see *Korrespondenz Mühlenbergs*, vol. 2, 206.

31 Boehm, *Der Reformierten Kirchen*, 2.

32 *Ibid.*, 3.

33 *Ibid.*, 4–5.

34 St Michael's *Kirchenordnung* in *Hallesche Nachrichten*, vol. I, 962–72, 1237. Mühlenberg had worked with others to draft a *Kirchenordnung* for St Michael's in 1753. This order essentially reworked an earlier liturgical order (*Kirchen-Agenda*) adopted in 1748. However, Mühlenberg and his patrons still found the existing orders unsatisfactory. *Korrespondenz Mühlenbergs*, vol. 2, 5, 102, 127, 180, 276, 558.

35 Roeber, *Palatines, liberty and property*, 251–8.

36 *Hallesche Nachrichten*, vol. 1, 966. Mühlenberg had long hoped for an order that would effectively address both church leaders and members. In writing to Franke and Ziegenhagen he noted (1754), '... so erwarten wir gehorsamt (a) entweder die teutschen common prayers und liturgie (b) oder eine complete und zum besten der Gemeinen ausgefertigte Kirchen Ordnung, wornach sich die Prediger, Alteste, Vorsteher und Gemeins Glieder richten mussen, wie sie nicht schuldig werden wollen'. *Korrespondenz Mühlenbergs*, vol. 2, 127.

37 *Hallesche Nachrichten*, vol. 1, 970. Mühlenberg was also aware that any approach to church discipline would be much more congregational in Pennsylvania than was the case in Germany. He commented, 'Sie haben schon manches ipso usu eingeführt was zur Kirchenzucht gehöret, und in Teutschland von manchen vergeblich gewünscht wordern: soll dasselbe nun als ein beständig geltendes Gesetz vestgestellet und in dieser Kraft von den Gemeinen angenommen und erkannt werden'. *Korrespondenz Mühlenbergs*, vol. 2, 294.

38 'Declaration and Agreement (*Kirchenordnung*), Evangelical Lutheran Church in Heidelberg Township, 1753', reprinted in H. S. Kidd (ed.), *Lutherans in Berks County: two centuries of continuous church life* (Reading, PA, 1923), 491. In 1757 the church at Heidelberg became a 'Union Church', uniting the Lutheran and Reformed congregations in the community.

39 *Ibid.*, 492.

40 See the 'Eight Articles' in Schmauk, 310.

Part VII

The Huguenot immigration into England
of the late 17th century

Part VII

The Huguenot immigration into England of the late 17th century

38

Rewriting the Church of England: Jean Durel, foreign Protestants and the polemics of Restoration Conformity

JOHN McDONNELL HINTERMAIER

In several ways Jean Durel is an odd choice for a conference dedicated to examining the experience of immigrants and refugees. Durel was a man of the establishment, a hired pen ready to take up the causes of the state church. For his efforts he earned extensive preferment and royal favour. Thus, his life seems far removed from the many thousands of French Protestants and other refugees who made their home in England. Yet it would be too easy to dismiss Durel as an excessively ambitious creature of the Church of England. For in Durel's life and writing we catch a glimpse of the ethos that came to dominate in the Restoration and its profound effects on the vexed questions of toleration, comprehension and conformity. His was a renovated Laudianism that embraced the Reformed Churches of Europe as a useful ally in the struggle against Nonconformity in church and state. In this essay, we shall see how Durel's connections and friendships shaped his views, how his writings articulated a common ground for Conformity in and through the Book of Common Prayer, and how his astute sense for arguments that would resonate with Restoration culture helped to change the direction of Anglican polemics. In the end, we should see how Durel opens a useful window into the mental world of the second half of the 17th century and how refugees shaped that world.

Durel was born on the island of Jersey in 1625.[1] After taking his first degree at Merton College, Oxford, he studied in France with Amyrauld at Saumur. Evidently out of loyalty to Charles I, he left France in 1647 to help defend Jersey against Parliamentary forces. When the island fell in 1650, Durel joined the exiled Court in Paris. In the French capital, Durel was ordained, beginning his career as a member of the clergy.

The persons involved in his ordination give us important clues into Durel's ecclesiastical affinities and friendships. According to John Evelyn, Durel was ordained on Trinity Sunday, 1650.[2] Thomas Sydserf, the ousted Bishop of Galloway in Scotland, presided at the ordination and John Cosin (then Dean of Peterborough, later Bishop of Durham) preached the sermon. Since Durel would later write ardently in defence of the Book of Common Prayer, it seems more than coincidental that he was ordained by Bishop Sydserf, who had been a leading figure in the imposition of the Scottish Prayer Book, and presented by Cosin, whose influence on the 1662 Book of Common Prayer was profound.[3] While this evidence is only circumstantial, it is important to note that Durel travelled from the beginning in Laudian circles.

After his ordination he was chaplain to the duc de La Force. Durel next shows up as Charles II's appointee as minister of the French Church in the Savoy.[4] For his efforts there, Charles recommended him to the Bishop of Winchester for the sinecure held by Sydserf, since Durel had 'been the chief means of bringing the English liturgy' into the French Church.[5] In 1662, the king ordered that his French translation of the Prayer Book be used in all the churches of the Channel Islands as well as in the Savoy.[6] From 1662 onwards Durel advanced through the ranks of the Church of England. He moved from a prebend at St George's Chapel Windsor to a prebend at Durham to Dean of the Chapel at Windsor in a little more than ten years.[7] In 1669 Durel was made Doctor of Divinity at Oxford.[8] His rapid preferment caused Anthony Wood to argue that 'had he lived some years longer, there is no doubt but he would have been promoted to a bishopric'.[9] In Wood's view, Durel 'was a person of unbyassed and fixed principles, untainted and steady loyalty' to the Stuart kings. He 'dar[e]d with an unshaken and undaunted resolution to stand up and maintain the honour and dignity of the English church, when she was in her lowest and deplorable condition'. After the Restoration, Wood noted that 'no one of late years hath more plainly manifested, or with greater learning more successfully defended . . . the justness and reasonableness of the established constitutions' of the Church England 'against its most zealous modern opponents than he hath done'. So it would seem that Durel was of the same ilk as Peter du Moulin, whose spirited defence of the monarchy had won him great advancement.

Yet there is much more to Durel than simple categorizations as an arch-Conformist. For the very nature of what passed for Conformity had changed during the Interregnum. We also know that those who some historians are eager to call 'Anglicans' disagreed sharply amongst themselves about the best path to be taken at the Restoration.[10] Hardline Laudians like Peter Heylin continued to stress that the Church of England was a Catholic church, sharing everything but error with the Church of Rome. Heylin harboured a deep antipathy towards foreign Reformed Churches and was critical of the Reformed doctrine of the English Church as expressed in the Thirty-Nine Articles and the homilies.[11] Heylin's attempts to gloss over the obvious Calvinist theology of most Conformists often relied on appeals to the Prayer Book to show that the real stance of the church was Catholic.[12] His characterization of the Church of England did not go unchallenged by Conformists. Thomas Fuller and Robert Sanderson, among others, condemned Heylin for his deceptive reading of the history of the Reformation and for his sympathies toward Rome.

Durel became implicated in this conflict when he was asked by Charles II to review Heylin's *Aerius Redivivus, or the History of the Presbyterians.*[13] Durel had the sharpest criticism for Heylin's contention that the Huguenots of the 16th century were seditious tyrannicides and that the Guises were justified in suppressing them.[14] Durel responded that Heylin wrote 'as if he were hired by the house of Guise' and was carried by his passion 'beyond all the bounds of truth and raison, against those churches whom he calls Calvinists'.[15] Fred Trott argued that Durel's criticism was influential in delaying the publication of Heylin's book until 1672.[16] But Trott also contended that 'Durel's condemnation of Heylin shows that he was no Laudian'.[17] While Durel clearly detested Heylin's assertion that the community of Reformed Churches was complicit in the English Civil War, this alone does not make him a non-Laudian. No less a Laudian than John Cosin had experienced a change of heart about the French Reformed Church, so we must not associate a friendly stance toward foreign Protestants as an invalid position for a Laudian to hold in the 1660s.[18] Durel, John Bramhall, and Cosin saw the prudential advantages of presenting a kinder, gentler face for Laudianism and Conformity in general.[19] Durel's particular deployment of this strategy, and the criticism it engendered occupies the final portion of this essay.

Durel's first entry in the battle for the Book of Common Prayer was his sermon *The Liturgy of the Church of England asserted.*[20] Taking St Paul's instruction to the Corinthians, 'But if any man seem to be contentious, we have no such custom, neither The Churches of God' as his text, Durel proceeded to demonstrate that the Prayer Book was approved by all of the foreign Reformed Churches and was the pre-eminent guarantor of unity in the Church of England. Durel quickly identified Presbyterians with contention and castigated them for breaking the requirements of both religion and morality 'that men be of a mild, facile, and complying disposition, that they shun contests and disputations' in matters of things indifferent.[21] In his version of the history of the Civil Wars, Durel saw a logical connection between the critiques of the Bishops and liturgy in the early 1640s and the fact that 'some of them come to that pass as to reject all manner of Ministers, all manner of Liturgies, even to the Lord's Prayer, the Creed . . . Ten Commandments . . . Infant Baptism, and the Celebrating of the Lord's Supper'.[22] To counter the slide into Independency, Durel praised the first English Reformers for the sensitive reform of the Church which retained all that was good in Roman Catholicism, and reduced 'to their lawful use those things which had been abused', and abolished 'all that was either absolutely bad or altogether useless and superfluous'.[23] Durel's main departure from the vehement Laudianism of a Heylin was his criticism of the Pope for his corruptions 'which had defaced, sullied, and empoisoned that fair Liturgy of the ancient Church'.[24] The high regard Durel had for the Prayer Book's apostolic purity allowed him to lament 'that persons who profess Christianity, which is so reasonable, should upon so slender an account as is that of the use of a White Surpliss, dye the fields and scaffolds with the innocent Blood of their Brethren, and . . . with the Sacred Blood of their lawful Sovereign, in whose preservation they were bound to shed every drop of their own!'[25]

Once Durel had associated resistance to the liturgy with sedition and regicide, he moved to show that the Book of Common Prayer was the pre-eminent Protestant liturgy. To further his aim, he enlisted the help of the foreign Reformed Churches. He assured his audience 'that there is not any one of the things which these people condemn as evil in our Church, which is not practised in one or other of the Reformed Churches beyond the Seas: or which they do not either approve of as good and necessary, or at least bear with as indifferent'.[26] After citing brief examples of the Conformity of the Reformed Churches, he concluded with the claim that 'our liturgy is an admirable piece of Devotion and Instruction. It is the marrow and substance of all that the Piety and Experience of the first five centuries of Christianity, found most proper to Edification in the publick Assemblies'.[27] Durel ended his sermon with a refutation of the argument that the Prayer Book was really the Mass. He noted that this was an argument of 'weak and silly people' because 'all of us, Protestants, say of our own Doctrine, that it is all to be found in the *Belief* of the Church of *Rome*: for, we say, she believes all that we believe (and we say it with Truth) but we do not believe all that she believes'.[28] Moreover, those who made this argument had never seen a missal or breviary nor would be able to understand one if they had.[29] Durel, however, did not rest with his sermon.

His next contribution to the defence of liturgical Conformity was the loquacious *A View of the Government and Publick Worship of God in the Reformed Churches beyond the Seas.*[30] In this work Durel expanded on his treatment of the foreign Reformed Churches to entice Nonconformists back into the English Church. In his dedication to the Earl of Clarendon, he explained that his book was intended 'to contribute something towards the bringing of those that stand yet at a distance from our Church, to a better understanding of her, so to full communion with her'.[31] But Durel's conciliatory message was only aimed at those who had been deceived into thinking that the foreign churches supported English Nonconformity. Taking full advantage of his status as a Frenchman and as one who had served as a chaplain to Huguenot nobles, Durel proceeded to inundate his reader with 300 plus pages of quotations from various Reformed leaders (both dead and alive) to support his case.[32] Animated by his skilled hand, foreign divines as diverse as Calvin, Melanchthon, Bucer, and Amyrauld spoke with a unified voice – that there was nothing in the government, doctrine, or, especially, the liturgy of the Church of England that warranted Nonconformity.[33] Durel also showed his reader that, given the chance, the foreign churches would embrace episcopacy and the Book of Common Prayer. He claimed in several places that the Prayer Book was, when judged by the standard of conformity to the early Church and compared to the other Protestant liturgies, 'the best and most perfect of them all, as coming nearest unto it'.[34] He ended his treatise by calling for peace and conformity. He argued that those who would not conform would have to 'grant in the next place, that of all those that profess the Reformed Religion, you are a sect by your selves, having not your like anywhere under Heaven'.[35]

Fred Trott has noted that 'the fact that [Durel's] arguments would appear plausible even to a liberal like [Thomas] Fuller meant that the Puritans were being marginalized in a much more effective way than any of Heylin's diatribes could accomplish'.[36] Even though it was clear that Durel had taken liberties with some of his sources, his argument had more cultural capital than those of his critics.[37] The King certainly valued Durel's brand of Conformity, and it appears to have resonated with the majority of the clergy. Durel and other Conformists sought to remove contentious issues of doctrine and ceremony by asserting the practical unity of the church around the government of bishops and the use of the Book of Common Prayer. Opponents of this coalition, like Henry Hickman, tried to use the publication of Heylin's *Aerius Redivivus* (in 1672) to smear Durel as a bigoted Laudian and a bad historian.[38] But by the time Heylin's book was published, the unification of Conformists was all but complete (if short-lived).

Jean Durel helps us to see that the Restoration and the experience of the Interregnum helped to cement the identity of those loyal to the English Church. Durel and others used the general weariness with sectarian rule to push a programme of reconciliation between Laudians and Conformists. This creative synthesis set the groundwork for a revitalized Church of England. In the process, the vehemence of the debate between Dissenters and 'Anglicans' increased sharply. The intractability of the debate encouraged the growth of a 'latitudinarian' movement in the Church and the search for a new ground for comprehension and toleration. Yet it also encouraged a hardening of positions that ensured that the Church of England would never again be a comprehensive church. Thus, Durel and his compatriots highlight the complexity of the Restoration church settlement and encourage us to find new categories to describe how Conformity and Nonconformity were imagined after 1660.

NOTES

1   These details are drawn from the *DNB* and from Charles and William Marshall (eds.), *The Latin Prayer Book of Charles II* (Oxford, 1882), 1–3.

2   John Evelyn, *Diary of John Evelyn*, vol. 3: *1650–72*, ed. E. de Beer (Oxford, 1955), 8–9.

3   G. J. Cumming, *The Durham Book* (Durham, 1962).

4   *CSPD, Charles II (1660–1)* (London, 1860), 529.

5   *CSPD, Charles II (1661–2)* (London, 1861), 124.

6   *Ibid.*, 508.

7   *CSPD, Charles II (1664–5)* (London, 1863), 301; *CSPD, Charles II (1666–7)* (London, 1864), 452; *CSPD, Charles II (1678)* (London, 1870), 428.

8   Anthony Wood, *Fasti Oxonienses* Part 2: *1641–91* (London, 1820), 317.

9   Anthony Wood, *Athenae Oxonienses*, vol. 4 (London, 1820), 89.

10 Fred J. Trott, 'Prelude to Restoration: Laudians, Conformists and the struggle for "Anglicanism" in the 1650s' (Ph.D. thesis, University of London, 1992).

11 From Anthony Milton, *Catholic and Reformed: the Roman and Protestant churches in English Protestant thought, 1600–1640* (Cambridge, 1995) we know that Heylin's prejudices were typical of Laudian thinking of the 1620s and '30s.

12 Detailed in Trott, 163–232.

13 *Ibid.*, 349–75. Durel's comments can be found in Bodleian Add. MS C. 304b, fos. 74–9.

14 P. Heylin, *Aerius Redivivus: or the History of the Presbyterians* (Oxford, 1670), 41–68, 416–23.

15 Bodleian Add. MS C. 304b, fo. 74.

16 Trott, 363.

17 *Ibid.*, 366.

18 G. J. Cumming *The Godly Order* (London, 1983), 130–1, 136–8.

19 The use of Laudianism in the post-Restoration period can be problematic. Scholars have tended to see Laudianism as a spent force – seeing the ideas of the latitude-men as the avant-garde of the next large- scale movement in the Church of England. This argument certainly has its merits, but tends to overlook the creative re-configuration of Conformists and Laudians as they united around a defence of the Prayer Book and episcopacy.

20 John Durel, *The Liturgy of the Church of England asserted in a sermon. Preached at the Chapel of the Savoy, before the French Congregation upon the first day that Divine Service was there celebrated according to the Liturgy of the Church of England*, 2nd edn. (London, 1688). I am using the second edition because it elucidates the interpretation of Durel in the later 17th century.

21 *Ibid.*, 4.

22 *Ibid.*, 9.

23 *Ibid.*, 12.

24 It must be remembered that Laudians found errors in the Catholic Church, e.g. Cosin's attack on transubstantiation and Laud's conference with Fisher. Durel echoed the Laudian notion that the Church had one universal liturgy during its primitive age.

25 Durel, *Liturgy of the Church of England*, 16.

26 *Ibid.*, 17.

27 *Ibid.* The Laudians' insistence on the purity of the Patristic church is graphically illustrated by Brian Duppa's annotated Book of Common Prayer in the Bodleian Library [C.P. 1639 d. 3(1)]. Duppa focuses all his attention on the first five centuries of the Church to prove the antiquity and validity of the Laudian interpretation of the Prayer Book and its rubrics.

28 Durel, *Liturgy of the Church of England*, 28.

29 *Ibid.*, 29. The key text that made the connection between the Prayer Book and the Mass was Robert Baillie, *A parallel between the Mass and the Service Book* (London, 1641). Baillie had based his analysis on his reading of both the missal and the breviary so Durel is indulging his petulance towards Baillie's book here.

30 John Durel, *A View of the Government and Publick Worship of God in the Reformed Churches beyond the Seas. Wherein is shewed their conformity and agreement with the Church of England, as it is established by the Act of Uniformity* (London, 1662).

31 *Ibid.*, A3v.

32 *Ibid.*, 13.

33 *Ibid.*, 15, 113, 118, 196, 220–36, 280–3.

34 *Ibid.*, 16.

35 *Ibid.*, 312.

36 Trott, 369.

37 [Henry Hickman], *The Nonconformists vindicated from the abuses put upon them by Mr. Durel and Scrivener* (London, 1679).

38 *Ibid.*, 6–9.

39

Henry Compton,
Bishop of London (1676–1713)
and foreign Protestants

SUGIKO NISHIKAWA

Henry Compton, Bishop of London from 1676 to 1713, was born in 1632, a younger son of the Royalist Earl of Northampton. He was ordained in 1666 and, later, his brilliant and also turbulent career as Bishop of London began in 1676. Indeed his life as a churchman was stormy because he was actively engaged in the politics of Restoration England. To anyone who reads about the Huguenot refugees who fled from the persecution of Louis XIV into England in the 1680s, he appears first and foremost as a most devoted friend and protector of the refugees.

Faced with the influx of Huguenot refugees throughout the 1680s, Compton spared no effort to help them settle in England. After the Revocation of the Edict of Nantes, in April 1686, Compton made an ardent appeal to the clergy of his diocese to help the Huguenots:

> You have such an object of charity before you, as it may be, no case could more deserve your pity. It is not a flight to save their lives, but what is ten thousand times more dear, their conscience. They are not fled by permission, (except the ministers, who are banished), but with the greatest difficulty and hardship imaginable. And therefore it will be an act of the highest compassion to comfort and relieve them, as being performed to persons whose afflictions it is hard to say, whether of mind or body are the greater.[1]

It is remarkable that in this oft-quoted appeal, Compton neither took into account the question of the Huguenots' nonconformity to the Church of England, nor did he hesitate to help Protestant refugees whoever they were. Conformity to the Church was of the utmost importance to many churchmen in Restoration England, so Compton's message was in open defiance of the reluctance of some prelates to accept non-Anglican Protestants. For example, in the same year, William Sancroft, then Archbishop of Canterbury, could not help complaining that the conformity of the Huguenot congregation in the Savoy Church, London, was not satisfactory, and he insisted that they should conform in every respect to the Church of England. Compton replied to Sancroft that the Huguenots already conformed sufficiently, according to the usages required by Charles II, and thus evaded the issue.[2] Even more remarkable in Compton's appeal of 1686 is that, in his sympathy towards the persecuted brethren, Compton did not hide his antagonism towards the Roman Catholic religion. As James II regarded open criticism of his religion as an insult to himself, Anglican prelates came under increasing pressure from him when they joined in the relief activities for the Huguenots. Some prelates avoided mentioning the persecution in France in their official circular letters for the fund-raising campaign for the Huguenots, though they privately gave financial help available to them. Compton's attitude incurred the King's displeasure. Yet Compton allowed the clergy of his diocese to preach anti-Roman Catholic sermons. Soon, the Vicar of St Giles, John Sharp, subsequently Archbishop of York, provoked the King's anger because of an anti-Roman Catholic sermon; and while public attention was aroused, this issue culminated on 6 September 1686 with Compton himself, who had been protecting Sharp, being suspended from the exercise of all episcopal functions.[3] Later, in 1688, Compton was the only prelate who signed the invitation to William of Orange, subsequently taking up arms and joining the Glorious Revolution.

Compton's devotion to persecuted Continental Protestants and his hatred of popery seem to have been unparalleled especially in the 1680s. As Bishop of London, who was in charge of churches overseas,[4] from the outset he keenly monitored the Protestant situation on the Continent. He received news and stories of his foreign brethren's sufferings,[5] and also corresponded not only with the Huguenots in France but also with the Protestants in Denmark, Poland, Germany and the Swiss cantons.[6] From the foreign Protestants' point of view, it was he after all whom they asked for help in case of need. The French Church of London and the Vaudois churches in the valleys of Piedmont alike always paid deep respects to Compton.[7] Knowing the Bishop had a passion for gardening, those Protestants sent Compton new flowering plants and seeds from various places such as the Cape of Good Hope, Bermuda and Paris.[8] In 1702, Abel Boyer, himself a Huguenot refugee, wrote of Compton that 'this prelate, by his dissuasive charity, and wise conduct, had gained the love and esteem of all the Protestant Churches both at home and abroad.'[9] Again in 1722 Boyer recalled the life of the Bishop very affectionately:

> He was always easy to access, and ready to do good offices . . . *He was, in a particular manner, charitable and bountiful to the poor French refugees, who by his death sustained an irreparable loss* [original italics].[10]

The 19th-century historian Leopold von Ranke regarded Compton as an example of a renewed 'consciousness of its Protestant character' in the Church of England, awakened by the Huguenot sufferings, adding that 'the exiles stood far nearer to the nonconformists in creed and ritual than to the high-church party, but no regard was paid to this. Henry Compton, Bishop of London, devoted to the unhappy strangers an attention which they could ordinarily have expected only from one who was in complete agreement with them.'[11] It is something of a mystery that the Huguenot refugees flocked to the Church of England when they had fled from France to preserve their Calvinist faith. There were, of course some exceptions like Jaques Fontaine who refused to conform to the Church of England,[12] but the great majority – clerical and lay – seem to have had no problem with accepting Anglican doctrine and liturgy. Perhaps Compton's attitude was partly responsible for this.

His commitment to foreign Protestants leads us, however, to the complex question of his own religious and political proclivities. In particular, what was his view of those Protestant churches that had a church order and ministerial commission different from that of the Church of England? Partly because he never wrote any theological works dealing with this matter (he was apparently a man of action), little attention has been given to the point. Or worse, a one-sided view of him has produced a number of inconsistent impressions. For example, Compton recently has even been called 'a Whig and broad churchman' since he 'hoped to protect the Huguenots from Tory attack' around 1707.[13] On the other hand, taking into account his political associates during the reign of Queen Anne, one cannot help noticing that Compton ended up as a Tory bishop: he expressed opposition to the practice of occasional conformity, which helped non-Anglican Protestants to hold civic or state offices by 'occasionally' taking Anglican Communion. He also become a supporter of Henry Sacheverell and Francis Atterbury, both staunch High Churchmen and strong opponents of toleration toward Dissenters and Presbyterians.[14] Atterbury notoriously expressed anti-foreigner remarks.[15] Moreover Compton consistently tried to influence clergymen in favour of Tory candidates in parliamentary elections.[16] Among modern historians, Edward Carpenter describes Compton as a practical man who responded to circumstances as they arose, though, referring to Compton's support for a bill against occasional conformity, the author adds that 'it is not easy to see how different circumstances could justify this reversal of a former attitude towards dissenters'.[17] On this view, Compton was counted as a High Church bishop, yet personally a man of moderate convictions.

For a High Churchman the episcopacy and liturgy of the Church of England would normally have carried most weight.[18] But given the impact of the persecution of the Huguenots and the Catholic threat in the 1680s, it may be understandable that a not very bigoted High Church bishop such as Compton would overlook the issue of foreign Protestants' conformity to the Church of England. Moreover, as Carpenter has also implied, Compton increasingly became associated with staunch High Churchmen like Sacheverell and Atterbury only after the Revolution. Carpenter added that after the Revolution, because Tenison, the Low Church Archbishop of Canterbury, was deeply concerned about the fate of the Protestants on the Continent, Compton's role as their guardian was accordingly diminished.[19]

Nevertheless, it cannot be emphasized too strongly that Compton's concern for the Protestant religion abroad did not disappear until the very end of his life. In pursuit of his responsibility for the Church of England overseas, he kept in touch with religious affairs outside England, and continued to voice concern about the sufferings of foreign Protestants after the Glorious Revolution. Compton was a High Church bishop and at the same time a supporter of distressed foreign Protestants; i.e. both positions were quite compatible.

Without dwelling here on the matter of High Church and Low Church, I shall only point out that a fear of the aggressive Catholic policy of Louis XIV caused a wide spectrum of Protestants across Europe to welcome the idea of strengthening Protestant unity. Among High Churchmen, Compton and some prelates such as John Sharp, Archbishop of York, John Robinson, and John Smalridge were keen promoters of the rapprochement policy with non-episcopal Protestants abroad.[20] In fact, in the 1700s, the High Church become more enthusiastic than the Low Church about pursuing

Protestant unity because for High Church bishops the underlying agenda was the expansion of the episcopal order to which Low Church bishops such as Thomas Tenison and Gilbert Burnet were opposed.[21]

This High Church policy can be called 'ecclesiastical imperialism' but Continental divines, trying to keep up correspondence with leading Protestant clergy in Britain, responded favourably to High Churchmen with a view to creating a Protestant union. Some Huguenots, such as Samuel de l'Angle, Jean Claude, and Claude Groteste de la Mothe, welcomed the English leadership for Protestant solidarity against popery. Daniel Ernst Jablonski, the court preacher at Berlin, having studied at Oxford in his youth, sought to reconcile the hostile divisions between Lutherans and Calvinists in Brandenburg by introducing the Anglican episcopal order and the Book of Common Prayer. Swiss divines, such as Anton Klingler, Jean-Frédéric Ostervald, and Jean Alphonse Turrettini, had long been worried about the Counter-Reformation and looked to the Church of England as the head of the Protestant interest and potential mediator in the conflict between the Lutheran and Reformed Churches.[22] The Continental Protestants, appealing to the Church of England as a pillar of the Reformed religion in Europe, willingly showed deference to the episcopal order. By the time of the Hanoverians, if foreign Protestants wanted to have the support of England, they would claim that they were episcopalians: a Calvinist educational institute in Nagyenyad in Transylvania, Hungary, called itself 'the episcopal university and college of Enyed' and the Protestants in Lissa in Poland claimed the validity of the episcopacy of the Bohemian Brethren, when their representatives visited London around 1714. A contemporary English divine spoke ill of them as 'episcopal beggars'.[23] These Continental Protestants continued to regard Compton as their primary mediator. Though Compton extricated himself from any actual negotiations for union with foreign Protestants during the decade preceding his own death, leaving them to other High Churchmen, he still carried on a correspondence with foreign Protestant churches, and 'endeavoured to promote in them a good opinion concerning the doctrine and discipline of the Church of England, and her moderate sentiments of them.'[24]

After all, High Churchmanship hardly implies lack of interest or sympathy in the situation of foreign Protestants. True, after the Glorious Revolution, Bishop Compton's participation in relief activities for foreign Protestant refugees appeared less prominently than before. But this can be partly explained by the fact that several institutions were founded involving the foreign Protestants. They must have reduced Compton's work dramatically. For example, as far as the Huguenot refugees at home were concerned, they came to rely on a more consistent form of aid, in the shape of the 'Royal Bounty'. Two official organizations, the French Committee, representing the refugees, and its supervisor, the English Committee, both appointed by the sovereign, became responsible for distribution of the Bounty.[25] Although on occasion accused of putting money in members' own pockets, and of maladministration,[26] the committee, nevertheless, operated tolerably well until the 19th century.

Compton's encounter with Thomas Bray, and the subsequent foundation of the Society for the Propagation of the Gospel in Foreign Parts (SPG) as well as that of the Society for Promoting Christian Knowledge (SPCK), also came as a great relief to the overworked Bishop. Thomas Bray was Rector of Sheldon in the diocese of Coventry. The Bishop was initially so impressed by Bray's writing and work as a parish priest, that he chose him as his Commissary for Maryland in 1695. Bray shared the anxiety of the Bishop about the activities of the Roman Catholic *Congregatio pro propaganda fide*. Thus Compton gave him his full support when Bray suggested plans for a counter organization, 'the intended Congregatio pro propaganda fide et morbus Christianis', which later grew into the SPCK in 1699 and the SPG in 1701. Both societies greatly helped Compton to propagate 'Protestantism' at home and abroad; the SPG in particular officially took over many of his duties in the plantations of America.[27] Yet the activities of the SPG were firmly limited to the orbit of the Church of England. On the other hand, the SPCK became vigorously involved with relief activities for foreign Protestants.[28] Sporadic as they may have been, the SPCK made great efforts to keep up co-operation with the Protestants on the Continent to promote Protestant reformation against Rome. Their correspondence network, beginning with the Halle Pietists and the Swiss divines, soon expanded from Danzig to the Waldensian valleys of Piedmont.[29] The information they obtained through the network was diligently reported to Compton.

Despite his advanced age and fragile health,[30] Compton remained actively involved in foreign Protestant affairs. The records of the SPG suggest, however, that in his last decade the interest of the Bishop in Protestants abroad was increasingly confined to the members of his own church. When it supported the dispersal to New York of the Palatines who had recently immigrated to England, Compton made efforts to provide a chaplain who could 'read the common prayer in High Dutch.'[31] He also assisted with a plan to establish Anglican churches in Rotterdam and Amsterdam.[32] Compton also took a particular interest in foreign students and scholars. Again, he was increasingly inclined to educate them on Anglican lines.

It is clear, in conclusion, that Compton had opted for the propagation of the Church of England rather than Protestant internationalism by the 1700s, though he continued to take a sincere interest in the fate of Protestantism abroad. He remained ambitious to perform good works both at home and abroad in order to achieve completion of the Protestant Reformation in the face of the Catholic threat. But with the foundation of the SPCK and of the SPG, his evangelistic concerns and energies became confined to matters concerning the Church of England and his concept of Protestant Reformation turned more strictly to a reformation on Anglican lines.

In short, there is in the late Stuart Church of England an element of what might be called ecclesiastical imperialism. Yet, as the case of Compton has shown, High Churchmen actively kept up correspondence with leading Protestant clergy on the Continent and were well informed about Continental affairs: accordingly, in the event of Protestant crisis they could respond swiftly. The most significant example of such a response can be seen in Compton's actions in the events surrounding the Revocation of the Edict of Nantes. His reception of the Huguenots in the 1680s may be regarded as an example of pragmatism in the face of an international Protestant crisis – an exceptional concession made at a time when the Catholic threat of Louis XIV loomed largest. As such, it was not incompatible with what Ranke called a consciousness of the 'Protestant character' of the Church of England.

The diminishing role of High Churchmen partly explains why the Church of England became insular and less concerned about the welfare of Continental Protestants after the Hanoverian Succession. Compton's death was soon followed by that of John Sharp. Added to the deaths in the 1710s of those High Church bishops, the ascendancy of the Low Church under the Hanoverian kings led to a loss of interest within the Church of England in the fate of Continental Protestants. In spite of the fact that Archbishop Wake was a keen promoter of the alliance of Protestants, he found no bishop to share his sense of responsibility to their Continental brethren.

NOTES

1 Bodl., Tanner MSS, 30, fo. 10.
2 Bodl., Rawlinson MSS, C. 983, fo. 120.
3 Abel Boyer, *The History of King William III* (London, 1702–3), vol. 2 (1702), 76–83; Nathaniel Salmon, *The Life of the Right Honourable and Right Reverend Dr Henry Compton* (London, 1715), 17–39; Edward Carpenter, *The Protestant Bishop: being the life of Henry Compton, 1632–1713, Bishop of London* (London, 1956), chap. 6.
4 For the origins of the Bishop of London's jurisdiction overseas, see Geoffrey Yeo, 'A case without parallel: the Bishops of London and the Anglican Church overseas, 1660–1748', *Journal of Ecclesiastical History*, 44 (1993), 450–75. At the time of the Reformation, no provision was made for episcopal control over the English abroad. According to Yeo, although it cannot be established why he was given it, in the course of the 17th century the Bishop of London was assumed to have responsibility for churches overseas, and Compton confidently accepted the task.
5 Bodl., Rawlinson MSS, 982 C. fos. 17–23, 25, 31, 147; 984 C. fos. 17, 25, 27, 62, 68.
6 Sugiko Nishikawa, 'English attitudes toward Continental Protestants with particular reference to church briefs *c.*1680–1740' (Ph.D. thesis, University of London, 1998), chap. 3.
7 *Ibid.*, 131–2, 238–50; HSQS 58, 4.
8 Bodl., Rawlinson MSS, C. 982, fos. 7, 13, 27. Cf. Sandra Morris, 'Legacy of a bishop: the trees and shrubs of Fulham Palace Gardens, introduced 1675–1713', *The Journal of the Garden History Society* 19 (1991), and 'Legacy of a bishop (Part 2): the flowers of Fulham Palace Gardens introduced 1675–1713', *ibid.*, 21 (1993).
9 Boyer, vol. 2, 76.
10 Abel Boyer, *The History of the Life and Reign of Queen Anne* (London, 1722), Appendix, 62–3.
11 Leopold von Ranke, *History of England*, vol. 4, 267–8, quoted in R. L. Poole, *A history of the Huguenots of the dispersion at the recall of the Edict of Nantes* (London, 1880), 105.
12 For Jaques Fontaine, see D. W. Ressinger (ed.), *Memoirs of the Reverend Jaques Fontaine 1658–1728*, Huguenot Society New Series 2 (London, 1992).
13 Hillel Schwartz, *The French Prophets: the history of a millenarian group in eighteenth-century England* (Berkeley, 1980), 56.
14 Carpenter, chap. 11.
15 Francis Atterbury, *English Advice to the Freeholders of England* (London, 1714), quoted in Anon., *The State-Anatomy of Great Britain* (London, 1717), 15.
16 Nishikawa, 134–5.
17 Carpenter, 193.
18 *Ibid.*, chap. 10; G. V. Bennett, 'King William III and the episcopate', in G. V. Bennett and J. D. Walsh (eds.), *Essays in modern English church history: in memory of Norman Sykes* (London, 1966), 124–31; John Spurr, *The Restoration Church of England 1646–1689* (London, 1991), 380; Mark Goldie, 'John Locke, John Proast and religious toleration 1688–1692', in John Walsh, Colin Haydon and Stephen Taylor (eds.), *The Church of England, c. 1689–c. 1833: from toleration to Tractarianism* (Cambridge, 1993), 163–4.
19 Carpenter, chap. 10, 342–3.

20 Nishikawa, chap. 3. Cf. George Every, *The High Church party 1688–1718* (London, 1956), chap. 5.

21 Frederick Bonet, the Prussian representative in London, who had many friends among High Churchmen, observed in 1711: ' . . . the conformity to be wished for beyond the sea relates more to Church government than to any change in the ritual or liturgy. The clergy here are for episcopacy, and look upon it, at least, as of apostolical institution, and are possessed with the opinion, that it has continued in an uninterrupted succession from the Apostles to this present time; and upon this supposition, they allege there can be no true ecclesiastical government but under bishops of this order; nor true ministers of the gospel, but such as have been ordained by bishops; and if there be others that do not go so far, yet they all make a great difference between the ministers that have received imposition of hands by bishops, and those that have been ordained by a synod of presbyters.' Quoted in Thomas Sharp, *The life of John Sharp, D. D. Lord Archbishop of York*, 2 vols. (London, 1825), vol. 1, 428–9.

22 Nishikawa, chap. 3.

23 *Ibid.*, 107–17.

24 William Innys *et al.* (eds.), *Biographia Britannica: or, the Lives of the most eminent persons who have flourished in Great Britain and Ireland*, 6 vols. (London, 1747–66), vol. 2 (1748), 1430.

25 W. A. Shaw, 'English government and the relief of Protestant refugees' *English Historical Review* 9 (1894); R. A. Sundstrom, 'The Huguenots in England 1680–1876: a study in alien assimilation' (Huguenot Library, London, unpublished revised version, 1978, of Ph.D. dissertation originally submitted at Kent State University, 1972), chap. 2; Raymond Smith, 'Financial aid to French Protestant refugees 1681–1727: briefs and the Royal Bounty,' *HSP* 22 (1970–6).

26 PRO, SP 34/24/27.

27 For the difference between the SPCK and the SPG, see Nishikawa, chap. 4. The SPG obtained a royal charter on 16 June 1701.

28 Nishikawa, chaps 2 and 4.

29 For example, two Danzigers were introduced as corresponding members in 1709, and two Vaudois were admitted as corresponding members in 1706. SPCK Archive, London, Abstract Letter Books, Received, nos. 1580, 1654, 1671, 1923; SPCK, Minute Book, vol. 2–4, fo. 340.

30 Rhodes House, Oxford, USPG Archive, SPG Calendar, 7A16, 36, 42; William Whitfield, *A sermon on the death of the late Lord Bishop of London, preach'd, Aug. 11. 1713* (London, 1713), 22–3.

31 SPG Calendar, 6A157, 158.

32 SPG Journal, 1701–7, 91, 93–4, 97; SPG Committee, 1702–10, 37; Henry Compton, *Good Brother* (London, 1706) in Christ Church, Wake MSS, Epist. 18, fo. 446; Bodl., Rawlinson MSS, 982 C, fo. 162.

40

'An unruly and presumptuous rabble': the reaction of the Spitalfields weaving community to the settlement of the Huguenots, 1660–90

CATHERINE SWINDLEHURST

In the summer of 1683 rising tensions amongst the Spitalfields weavers concerning the mass arrival of Huguenots in the eastern metropolitan parishes sparked a series of complaints about disorderly behaviour within the weaving community. The weavers were described as riotous, and there were fears of violent disturbances: 'the factious party thereabouts has been very bold and presumptuous this last week: and . . . they do cabal together oftner than has been usual'.[1] Although it was not uncommon for the weavers to socialize in certain public houses, during August 1683 these meetings took on a more ominous tone, as the weavers gathered 'in opposition to the French weavers in their neighbourhood'.[2] Anxieties over weaver uprisings were rife as warnings were made that, if the weavers 'can get a sufficient number together, they will rise and knock them [i.e. the French] on the head'.[3]

Despite the potential for violence, these tensions subsided by the end of the summer, but lay just below the surface throughout much of the 1680s. The reasons behind these frustrations has often been attributed simply to English xenophobia in an age of developing national identity. But such a view ignores the impact of immigration on the street level, and how the influx of a new community changed economic, social, political, and cultural structures within a burgeoning urban setting.

In the years between 1660 and 1690, the redefinition of Spitalfields, from a semi-rural out-parish of London to part of the City's suburban landscape, had profound effects in the creation of a distinct community ethos. After the Great Fire, the population of Spitalfields boomed, as people relocated en masse to the cheaper, cleaner and, often, safer suburbs. The physical environment of the eastern suburbs changed dramatically with the construction of new neighbourhoods, as did the social context of the area.[4] While the western suburbs became populated with those engaged in luxury trades and persons of higher status, the eastern parishes attracted manufacturing groups.[5]

Spitalfields did have listed among its residents some members of polite society; how-ever, the area was primarily defined by its tradesmen and mariners. Despite the influx of new residents, the population of the area became and remained, at least in social structure, fairly homogeneous: Spitalfields, like its neighbouring suburbs, was a manufacturing district.

Throughout the period, the area became increasingly identified with weaving. The burgeoning population of weavers in Spitalfields resulted in a growing proportion of the community being influenced by the fortunes of the weaving trade. This effect was magnified by the pervasiveness of the trade in other sections of the community. Even householders who were not themselves weavers were often reliant on the income derived from family members employed by some branch of the weaving trade, either as assistants or as out-workers.[6] The entrenchment of the weaving trade within Spitalfields' community structure meant that the social and trade aspects of com-munity life were intrinsically linked. Threats to trade, therefore, were significant economically, but were also noticeable more generally in family and neighbourhood life.

As the eastern metropolitan suburbs became more settled, Spitalfields residents had a vested interest in creating and maintaining some sort of social and economic status quo; and increasingly this community foundation was based upon the weaving trade. The concentration of similar trades and ranks within the Spitalfields community inevitably led to the development of social perceptions that defined the norms and codes of conduct of its members. These rules of trade were based on the concept of fair competition within the manufacturing community. Success was based on the ideals of hard work, skill, enterprise, opportunity, and above all, honesty. Practices that upset the balance of trade were regarded with suspicion and resentment. And those who did not operate within the socially accepted parameters of 'fair trade' were subject to universal disapproval, and/or punishment.[7]

Newcomers to the area and to the trade were expected to live and work by these communally established rules, and were generally assimilated into the local social and economic structure. There was a tendency to blame economic instabilities on the more immediate effects of the influx of new weavers to the trade and their perceived unfair trading practices, rather than the larger economic issues affecting the London weaving trade; a trade which, in the mid- to late-17th century, was particularly precarious.

The population shift from the City parishes out to the suburbs throughout the mid-17th century was accompanied by the mass arrival of Huguenots and other Continental Protestants, which dramatically altered the structure and dynamic of the Spitalfields community.[8] Although European Protestants had been immigrating to London and other parts of southern England since the late 1500s, the number of new arrivals, especially Huguenots, rose dramatically in the second half of the 17th century, as French Protestants found it increasingly difficult to cope with the growing hostility in France under Louis XIV.[9] The majority of Huguenots probably arrived in the years immediately following the Revocation of the Edict of Nantes in 1685; however, research has shown that a large number of refugees arrived in England in the 1670s and early 1680s.[10] These foreign weavers, who were easily identifiable as outsiders, were often held to a higher standard of trade and social conduct by established residents. Threats to the balance of trade and therefore, to the composition and precepts of the community, were often associated with foreign interlopers in Spitalfields and other developing metropolitan suburbs in this period.

This massive influx of people of a distinct culture and language, as well as different trade skills, had a huge influence on the metropolitan communities in which they settled; an influence which has been scarcely addressed by historians. Although much is known about the Huguenots' influence on various luxury trades within the metropolis, such as jewelry and fine metal trades, and the silk trade, little is known about how they interacted with established trade communities.[11] Some work has been done on specific families; however, how these families fit into the wider metropolitan community, and the more general English society, is still a mystery. The Huguenots, by their sheer numbers, changed the social and cultural dynamic of the neighbourhoods in which they lived. Their effect on the established communal structure was amplified by the fact that the majority of Huguenots settling in the eastern out-parishes were weavers by trade. The mass arrival of the Huguenots over such a small period upset local trade and social balances of the developing suburbs. In the eyes of established residents, the settlement of the Huguenots posed several threats to their livelihoods, including the potential for foreign or unfair trading practices and standards; the introduction of new and trade-altering skills; and the imposition of too many craftsmen and assistants in the trade. These worries were manifested in fears of foreign influence; that English weavers would be left out of new skills; and that underemployment would, with the large numbers of new workers, become endemic to the trade.

The large number of Huguenots was seen as threatening to local economies, both in the increasing size of the population, and the fact that they were not English.[12] However, a certain amount of sympathy was felt for the Huguenots, given that they were Protestant immigrants from a Popish nation: they were largely regarded as refugees of conscience, having left their homes and their families in the face of Catholic persecution. But, Protestant victims or not, the Huguenots were still French, and therefore foreign, which made their intentions, especially given their relatively sudden and dramatic appearance in London manufacturing circles, somewhat suspicious.

On the other hand, the arrival of French immigrants also represented the potential for the assimilation of French weaving techniques and fashions into the English weaving trade. France and the French silk industry were both the nemesis and the spur towards development of the English silkweaving trade in the late 17th century. For many London weavers, the French trade was something to be both revered and copied, as well as to be scorned and protected against. France was popularly viewed as a sort of vortex of Popish evil, but at the same time, it was respected as an economic power and a fashion centre. The arrival of the Huguenots in England represented new hope in the competition with France in the quality and design of various luxury goods.[13]

The introduction of new skills and methods dramatically altered the defining features of the London weaving trade by shifting its focus away from ribbon weaving and towards broadloom silkweaving. The Huguenot weavers brought new fabric designs as well as new weaving and finishing techniques to the London trade. In 1684, for example, John Larguier of Nimes was granted the status of master when he proved that he was 'fully inabled to weave and perfect lutestrings, alamodes and other fine silks as well for service and beauty in all respects as they are perfected in France'.[14] His freedom was granted on the 'condition that he imploy himself, and others of the English nation, in making the said alamode and lutestring silks for one year from this day'.[15] The influx of new ideas was generally perceived as a positive contribution from the foreign weavers, but it was not without its concerns.

Amongst the most significant anxieties expressed by English weavers was that the Huguenot craftsmen would keep their new technologies to themselves by only working with other French weavers. Throughout the 17th century, complaints to the Weavers' Company that 'foreign member[s] employ more French journeymen then English', were common.[16] These concerns were not without some basis, as they reflected how the Huguenots interacted socially in their new-found London communities. In France, the Huguenots had been systematically isolated from the rest of Catholic society over several decades preceding the end of official toleration in 1685. Those who immigrated to London were faced with a different sort of isolation: one based on culture and language. It is not surprising then, that French refugees operated, socially and economically, within a distinct sub-community.

In London society, the Huguenots were socially defined in terms of language and religion. Their use of French aurally demarcated them as different from others in their neighbourhoods; but language also had broader social implications. Although the Spitalfields Huguenots were essentially Calvinists, language barriers meant that they had to form their own churches; thereby segregating themselves from an important social institution within the parish community. Spitalfields and other eastern out-parishes had a strong tradition of Nonconformity, with substantial Quaker and, later in the 18th century, Methodist congregations, operating within the communal dynamic.[17] But French nonconformity had the unfortunate tendency to be labelled as 'Popish' by frustrated English manufacturers, especially in times of economic uncertainty.

The language and cultural barriers faced by Huguenots in London society were intensified by their tendency to group together geographically. In the eastern suburbs, Spitalfields was one area that attracted large numbers of French refugees. An examination of the Four Shillings in the Pound Aid assessment for 1693 shows some grouping of French householders in certain streets.[18] Generally speaking, French names arise on every street listed in the assessment. However, a large number of French names appear in alleys and courts, rather than on the main streets, which may reflect their poorer financial situations as newly established residents: households with street frontages were generally more expensive than other properties.[19]

Given the Huguenots' social and physical segregation, which was both internally and externally imposed, it is not surprising that they often became scapegoats during economic downturns. The large influx of French weavers, especially in the late 1670s and 1680s, led to accusations of French masters only hiring French weavers; or worse, hiring untrained journeymen: 'boyes of fifteene, sixteene or eighteene yeares of age that come over from all parts of [foreign] countreys and here are sett at worke by many of your [foreign] congregation whether they can doe the tenth parte of their trade, yea or no'.[20] French weavers were also accused of accepting lower wages than the standard paid to English weavers, thereby causing underemployment among those journeymen established in the London trade:

> Our weaving trade is grown so dead,
> We scarcely can get us bread . . .
> Because the French are grown so ill,

> In selling their work at under price,
> Which makes tears run from our eyes
> And weavers all may curse their fates
> Because the French work under rates . . . [21]

The frustration of the resident weavers only increased with the rise in the number of French weavers settling in London. The Weavers' Company had traditionally been the outlet for the weavers' complaints; but, as the 17th century progressed, the guild became less able to deal effectively with the weavers' concerns; especially as the Huguenots tended to settle in areas like Spitalfields, which were beyond the legal jurisdiction of the Weavers' Company. The expense and relative ineffectiveness of prosecution against renegade French weavers meant that increasingly, the Company's only option was to petition the Huguenot churches to ask for their co-operation in controlling the weavers. In 1683, the French Church of London, noted that:

> The Company complains that there are those who violate the regulations for strangers ordained by the King and Council some years ago, employing people who have not served their apprenticeship as weavers or been received by the Company, refusing to employ English weavers, and speaking disrespectfully and offensively about the governors of the Company. After giving this warning, the Company intends to exact from offenders every fine and advantage given it by law. The Consistory, acknowledging that the King had given strangers only limited freedom, urges Church members to submit willingly to the Weavers' Company's regulations.[22]

With no official recourse available to address their growing frustrations, the weavers turned to their own community of workers to deal with their situation.

As the decade progressed, it appeared to many established weavers that the floodgates to immigration had been opened. The complaints to the Weavers' Company about the unfair trading practices of foreign weavers increased throughout the early 1680s. And hostility to French refugees in general became more pronounced. In 1681, James Jeffries expressed his fears of an uprising in Spitalfields: he noted that an increased number of weapons and armour were found amongst Spitalfields residents.

> that some of those that have them say that those weapons are to defend themselves against the Papists and a Popish successor . . . [a] Cooper [who] is much employd in making iron capps . . . believes that much the greater quantity hee makes is for the malcontents and not for the more loyall.[23]

By August 1683, frustration levels amongst the weavers, concerning the alleged trade abuses by the French weavers, had reached a peak. There were increased reports of weavers meeting in alehouses to discuss the problems associated with French weavers. One informant reported that he had ' . . . found out the three houses of their meetings viz at the sign of the Poor Robin in Bishopgate Street, at the sign of the Town of Hackney in the same street, and at the Cock in Whitegate Alley near the Feilds . . . '.Tis expected on Thursday or Friday they will meet together again'.[24] The weavers met to discuss, among other things, trade concerns and different manners of solving them: 'some of the weavers, the most sober and rationull, discoursed of petitioning the Company that French masters might imploy as many Englishmen as French'.[25] Others were reported to have put together 'a petition to his Majesty the purpose of which is in opposition to the French weavers'.[26] However, it was the potential for violence posed by those weavers who were not so 'sober and rationull' that caused concern amongst the ruling order.

In response to the increased agitation and apparent organization amongst the weavers, on 9 August, Charles II ordered that horse guards be 'quartered about Islington, Hackney or Mile End to keep the weavers in order'.[27] Throughout the month, the weavers threatened to riot. On 25 August, an informant reported that 'he was desiered by two jorneymen weavers (severally) to meet in Swan Feilds one Monday morning and he doth conclude is in order to some bad designe, it being the same method they took when they burnt the ingin loombs'.[28] And on the Monday in question, 'the Trained Bands weare kept at Devon sheare Square that day, expecting the weavers would rise'.[29] By early September, however, the movement seems to have lost momentum, and in the months following the turbulent summer, there are no further official reports of weaver disaffection.[30] It is quite possible that the increased presence of troops in the metropolis was enough to quell the raucous activities of the weavers. This was certainly the popular conception: 'the loyal men there concur in the opinion that, if a troop of horse be quartered at Whitechapel, near them, it will be a means to awe the rabble'.[31] Whatever the case, the tensions within the weaving community certainly caused concern among both the French weavers, and regional and Court officials, who feared a disturbance as violent and prolonged as the engine loom riots that had gripped Spitalfields in 1675. Despite the increasing tensions, it is significant that no rioting took place, especially in light of the violence that occurred in other parts of the country.

In Norwich, only a week after the tensions in London had been quelled, large-scale rioting took place against the French:

> The French, who are established here, have been the innocent cause of certain troubles. The English have imagined that our nation here are only a troop of Papists masquerading as Protestants and would ruin their trade. Thereupon the rabble of this town made a regular riot and thronged all the streets, dragging the French about, sacking their houses and actually killing a woman.[32]

The Norwich disturbances indicate that anti-French sentiment was not just limited to Spitalfields and the other metropolitan weaving districts. It was a problem wherever there were large concentrations of the refugee population, especially in areas where there was little trade differentiation. Norwich, like Spitalfields, contained a high concentration of weavers; but for some reason, the riots never came to fruition in the capital. Perhaps, it is an indication of the organization and control exercised by the London weavers; or it could just be indicative of more effective government information and intervention within the metropolis. Regardless of the outcome of the tensions in each city, the Norwich disturbances provide a grim reminder of the scale and intensity of popular disaffection felt for the French weavers.

Although there were no further large-scale disturbances in London against the French weavers in the years following 1683, tensions remained just below the surface. There were many complaints to the Weavers' Company and to Parliament about the unfair trading practices of the Huguenot weavers in the 1680s and early 1690s. In 1686, the Weavers' Company petitioned Parliament, stating that 'they find that the trades are become very numerous by the late prohibition of French [raw and thrown] silks and the admitting of great numbers of Frenchmen and other aliens'.[33] The minutes of the French Church of London also reflect complaints about the French weavers, but from a social perspective, rather than for trade infractions. In the early 1690s, 'Mr de Primrose reported that a Spitalfields constable complained about the unruly behaviour of some French people in that area. Debauchery will be preached against strongly, and a notice will be given in a week's time'.[34] And two years later, 'it was reported that there were tavern-keepers in Spitalfields who had been caught by the J.P. with people indulging themselves in their houses during the sermon. Tavern keepers of this church are to be warned by elders . . . to avoid such disorder in future'.[35] Through the years, the complaints against the French immigrants became less frequent and certainly less threatening, as the Huguenots were accepted and assimilated into their respective London communities.

Despite their eventual disappearance as a distinct linguistic and cultural group within the London landscape, the Huguenots had a huge influence on the communities in which they settled. Their language is reflected in some of the street names, such as 'French Alley', and 'Flower de Luce Street', in Spitalfields. Their Calvinism helped to shape the nonconformist religious atmosphere of the eastern out-parishes, which prompted Queen Anne to include Spitalfields among the choices for the '50 New Churches Act' in the early 18th century.[36] And perhaps most obvious, was their introduction of new weaving techniques and designs into the London fashion scene, which revitalized and re-defined the London weaving trade. Despite these contributions, or maybe because of them, it took several years before the French weavers were accepted into the burgeoning London weaving community.

The disturbances of 1683 reflect the turbulence found in these developing metropolitan trade communities. The influx of French weavers posed an immediate and obvious threat to the established weavers. The Huguenots' dramatic impact on the weaving trade caused suspicion and resentment amongst their English counterparts, who feared that the French weavers would upset the balance of trade within the London weaving community. As Huguenot immigration slowed in the 1690s, Spitalfields and surrounding communities began to maintain a more settled population, and therefore, a more consistent and secure communal identity. Despite the fact that this ethos was still largely defined in terms of the weaving trade, the concept of 'neighbourhood' and the social community of Spitalfields became increasingly important. Community networks, especially those between French and English weavers, grew much stronger. Although there were still occasional social and trade disputes between French and English weavers, these appear to have become less important towards the end of the 17th century, as a more united weaving community looked to outside forces to blame for trade difficulties.

NOTES

1   PRO, SP 29/431/21.
2   *Ibid.*
3   *Ibid.*
4   For more detail on the expansion of the eastern parishes, see M. Power, 'East London

housing in the 17th century', in Clark and Slack (eds.), *Crisis and order in English towns, 1500–1700* (London, 1972), 237–62.

5   For more detail of the contrast between London's eastern and western parishes, see M. Power, 'The east and west in early-modern London', in E. W. Ives, R. J. Knecht and J. J. Scarisbrick (eds.), *Wealth and power in Tudor England: essays presented to S.T. Bindoff* (London, 1978), 167–85.

6   Journeymen and smaller master weavers have become the economic indicators for the historian of how trade is faring because they tended to be the first recognizable casualties of a downturn. Their assistants and those involved in other subsidiary trades were probably in a much more precarious employment situation, as a slump in trade would result in the termination of less essential assistants in order to economize. However, as these people were rarely household heads, or even, for that matter, of the age of apprenticeship, it is difficult to track their ebb and flow within the trade. In any case, for both journeymen and the sub-trades, there was a fine line between steady employment and relative prosperity, and underemployment and financial hardship. As the families of smaller masters and journeymen were often involved in different facets of the same trade, small ripples in the trade could have dramatic effects on the overall family income.

7   This ideal of a community culture that defined the norms and rights of its members has been used by historians, particularly E. P. Thompson, to describe community relations primarily amongst groups of rural labourers, within the context of a 'moral economy'. See for example, 'The moral economy of the English crowd in the 18th century', *Past and Present* 50 (1971), 78–9; A. Charlesworth and A. Randall, 'Morals, markets and the English crowd in 1766', *Past and Present* 114 (1986), 200–13; and A. Randall, 'The Gloucestershire food riots of 1766', *Midland History* 10 (1985), 72–93.

8   For an indication of the migration of people into London and its effect on occupational networks, see S. R. Smith, 'The social and geographical origins of the London apprentices, 1630–1660', *Guildhall Miscellany* 4:4 (1973), 195–206.

9   For more on the influence of Protestant refugees on the metropolitan silk trade in earlier periods, see Lien B. Luu, 'French-speaking refugees and the foundation of the London silk industry in the 16th century', *HSP* 26:5 (1997), 564–76.

10 The peak years of Huguenot influx in this period were 1681–2, due to the billeting of the *dragonnades* in Protestant households in France; and 1686–8, as a result of the revocation. See R. Gwynn, 'The arrival of the Huguenot refugees in England, 1680–1705', *HSP* 21:5 (1969), 373.

11 See for example, J. Evans, 'Huguenot goldsmiths in London and Ireland', *HSP* 14:4 (1932), 496–554; J. Shears, 'Huguenot connections with the clockmaking trade in England', *HSP* 20:2 (1960), 158–76; H. Tait, 'Huguenot silver', in I. Scouloudi (ed.), *Huguenots in Britain and their French background, 1550–1800* (London, 1987), 89–112; and D. C. Coleman, *Courtaulds: an economic and social history* (Oxford, 1969), 1–8.

12 For more on the xenophobia of the London weavers see J. Ward, *Metropolitan communities: trade guilds, identity, and change in early modern London* (Stanford, CA, 1997), 138–42; T. Harris, *London crowds in the reign of Charles II: propaganda and politics from the Restoration until the exclusion crisis* (Cambridge, 1987), 199–204. This sort of economic and cultural xenophobia continued into the 18th century; see L. Colley, *Britons: forging the nation, 1707–1837* (London, 1992), 85–100.

13 Despite the fact that Huguenots were often prohibited from living within several miles of these silkweaving centres. For example, Paul de la Vau was made free of the London Weavers' Company after proving he had 'served at Tours and was banished thence for religion'. See Guildhall Library (hereafter GL), MS 4655/9, fo. 33.

14 *Ibid.*, fo. 12.

15 *Ibid.*, fos. 37–8. In 1688, three other weavers, Paul Clowdesly, William Sherrard and Peter

Ducleu received a patent 'for the sole making of certain silks called alamodes, ranforcees and lutestrings, heretofore only made at Lyons, for fourteen years'. See PRO, SP 44/71/394.

16   GL, MS 4655/9, fos. 3, 29.

17   For evidence of Nonconformist communities, see: the Quaker memoirs found in T. Compton, *Recollections of Spitalfield: an honest man and his employers, the recollections of a Baptist, turned Congregational, minister*, in A. Peel, 'The diary of a deacon at White Row Chapel, Spitalfields', *Transactions of the Congregational Historical Society* 15 (1946), 177–85; and the presence of independent and Quaker churches in Stepney and Spitalfields in G. L. Turner, 'The religious condition of London in 1672 as reported to King and Court', *Transactions of the Congregational Historical Society* 3 (1908), 192–205.

18   CLRO, Assessment Box 40.12.

19   For an explanation of the wealth differentials that existed between those inhabiting street frontages and those in alleys and courts, see J. Boulton, *Neighbourhood and society: a London suburb in the 17th century* (Cambridge, 1987), 166–95.

20   GL, MS 4647, fo. 296.

21   *The valiant weaver* (London, 1681).

22   HSQS 58, 113–14.

23   PRO, SP29/417/78.

24   PRO, SP29/431/21.

25   PRO, SP29/431/20.

26   PRO, SP29/431/21.

27   PRO, SP29/430/79.

28   PRO, SP29/431/3.

29   PRO, SP29/431/20.

30   At least not amongst the State Papers where much of this information was discovered.

31   PRO, SP29/431/21.

32   As translated in *CSPD 1683*, 363. The original letter, found in PRO, SP29/431/88, is in French.

33   PRO, SP31/5/40.

34   *Minutes of the Consistory*, 274.

35   *Ibid.*, 348.

36   Robin Gwynn, *Huguenot heritage: the history and contribution of the Huguenots in Britain* (London, 1985), 101.

41

Huguenot integration in late 17th- and 18th-century London: insights from records of the French Church and some relief agencies

Eileen Barrett

Integration is rarely a smooth continuum. Rather, it is made up of several phases, lasting longer or shorter periods, some of which may overlap, or happen simultaneously.

Initially, there needs to be the development of a basic two-way toleration which enables host society and migrant to co-exist – this might be termed *accommodation*. It is usually followed by *acculturation* and *economic absorption*, where the migrant gradually acquires aspects of the language, dress, diet, and so on, of the new society, and becomes able to contribute to the economic life of the community. Sometimes this can even be a two-way process, with the host population acquiring new skills, knowledge, or cultural traits from the migrant – like the Huguenot introduction to England of silk-weaving skills and, apparently, oxtail soup.

Later on, there develops much fuller *integration*, with each group having adjusted so that they respect and value the contribution of the other. Finally – but usually only with intermarriage and the consequent blending of ethnic characteristics in the next (and succeeding) generations – there comes *amalgamation*.[1]

Closely interwoven with this process is the concept of changing identity, and how the migrant perceives him- or herself, (although it also involves how the migrant is perceived by the host community). Identity is a slippery concept because it is complex and multifaceted. It is not fixed. In different situations, people will emphasize different dimensions of their individual and collective memories to construct who they are.[2] A person may even find that he or she has a number of available positions and that some of them are in competition. There are constant choices to be made about how one perceives oneself and how one presents oneself. The *process* of constructing an identity is no different for the migrant than it is for anyone else. However, the *choices* involved are often more numerous.

All this suggests that the process or processes of integration are not linear. That is to say, the migrant does not move from being 'stranger' to 'citizen' in straightforward progression. Rather, there may be oscillation backwards and forwards between old and new and, gradually, a synthesis of both. Migration, it has been suggested, is 'a long-term if not life-long process of negotiating identity, difference and the right to fully exist and flourish in the new context'.[3]

This is certainly borne out by what can be gleaned from Huguenot records relating to refugees who arrived in London in the late 17th century and the first half of the 18th century. While I have not yet been able to go further, and examine, for example, English parish records, which would shed further light from the angle of the host population, it is nevertheless obvious that there were conflicting forces at work, throughout the integration process, on this migrant population in early modern London.

Of significance was the *size* of the migration, particularly in the late 17th century. These were not just a handful of Protestants fleeing persecution. As we know, there were thousands of them – probably over 20,000 in the London area alone – so that, as Robin Gwynn has calculated, at the turn of the 18th century some 5 per cent of Londoners were probably Huguenot.[4] This generated both positive and negative effects.

On the negative side, a population of this size could not go unnoticed, and it is evident that there was hostility towards the newcomers at various times. The 'Pest House', for example – used for a while as temporary accommodation for the refugees – was at one point the proposed target of a group of Whig apprentices who, labelling the refugees as papist spies, were planning to attack the building and pull it down, until the Mayor discovered what was afoot and intervened.[5]

However, the records of the consistory of the French Church of London are dotted with references to efforts by the church officials to manage the behaviour of their 'flock', so as not to attract adverse attention from the English. The congregation is warned against eating in church between services, because it is offensive to some 'et surtout à ceux de la Nation'.[6] They are asked to stop their children from making a noise in the street,[7] and they are reprimanded for leaving church early. One notice specifies that such behaviour 'ne scandalise pas seulement les ames pieuses de ce Troupeau, mais aussi les peuples parmi lesquels nous vivons'.[8] There is an obvious concern here about English opinion, and it suggests that the aim of church discipline at this particular time went beyond the usual efforts to improve the moral conduct of the membership. Rather, it had acquired a more urgent and specific goal – to minimize hostility from the local populace.[9]

And efforts against attracting adverse attention to the Huguenot community were not limited to what went on in and around the church building itself. There were attempts to curtail drinking and drunkenness among the Huguenot popu-lation, by such means as exhortations to the congregation, direct approaches to inn-keepers, and instructions to the elders to keep a close eye on what went on in their *quartiers*.[10]

Similarly, it was obviously seen as desirable to keep people out of the civil courts, because the church officers warned the congregation against having their neighbours arrested and put in prison.[11] This suggests that an overall positive image was recog-nized as an important factor in gaining acceptance for the French-speaking community.

But apart from creating problems for the newly-arrived refugees, it is likely that the 'spotlight effect' engendered by the huge influx spilled over on to longer-established migrants. Certainly, one or two more well-to-do citizens involved in political activity seem to have come in for special scrutiny. For example, in 1681, the Grand Jury of the City of London decided *not* to support a bill presented against a Whig accused of high treason, and the inflential Bishop of London, no doubt casting around for ammunition to use against the members of the said Jury, lit upon the fact that one of them, Guillaume Carbonnel, was also an elder of the French Church of London. This prompted an effective demand by the Bishop for Carbonnel to resign from the church's consistory, deeming it 'inappropriate' that he serve on both bodies. The consistory, however, stood firm and replied that, although it would much prefer that members of the church did *not* get involved in public affairs, it was often impossible given that some of them were naturalized or denizens – a valid point – and it noted that 'Others before Carbonnel have served on the City Jury, and we would be in an awkward position if we could not make use of members eligible for such business'.[12] We can gather from this that it was not unusual for migrants to want to maintain their French links over a period of many years, and to be a part of *both* societies and cultures, but we have a clear example here of their being pressured by English authorities to drop their 'stranger' connections and identity.

However, while there was hostility from certain quarters, there is also evidence of considerable sympathy – a sympathy that was probably only magnified by the size of the migration, underlining, as it did, the desperation of the French Protestants and the severity of their persecution. A positive result of this was the generous contribution to public collections, which permitted such practical and immediate assistance as the provision of temporary lodgings – ranging from the previously-mentioned refugee centre at the Pest House through to the provision of rented housing for them and the payment of board with individual landlords.[13]

Fortunately, the French churches in London, both at Threadneedle Street and the Savoy, with their Calvinist tradition of caring for the needy, were well-organized to provide relief to these masses of newcomers (though one must not underestimate the burden of extra work), and they could call upon the services of a sizeable, well-integrated, and often influential, membership. A number of these long-term residents served turns as officers of the church, and through their tireless efforts large numbers of the refugees – many of whom had fled with nothing – were provided with food, shelter and clothing, and given tools so that they could begin to earn a living.

However, it was not always easy to absorb the refugees into the economic life of their new country, especially in such large numbers. In particular, many guilds seem to have been reluctant to accept foreigners, which somewhat hindered the newcomers in becoming established. The Feltmakers' Company, for example, tried at one point to limit the number of licensed French hatmakers to five.[14] On the other hand, guild influence was less strong in the suburbs, and it was there that numerous Huguenots settled – especially around Spitalfields. Many were able to set up in business on their own there, or were found employment with already-established French craftsmen or merchants, and younger ones were often bound as apprentices to French masters. As Natalie Rothstein has also shown, in her work on silk weavers and their insurance policies, Huguenots tended to deal with other Huguenots, and to help each other when in difficulty.[15]

Women on their own (and research indicates that this was a group of not-inconsiderable size)[16] would nevertheless have had particular problems and, although the evidence is circumstantial, it seems likely that many managed on a mixed economy of whatever they could earn, from work that was nearly always low-paid, and some-times intermittent or seasonal, too – supplemented by relief whenever and wherever they could obtain it, often from more than one source at a time.[17]

Another way in which the size of the migration would have affected the speed and ease of integration was in the sense of community it doubtless gave. Despite dislocation and hardship, there was the comfort and reassurance of belonging to a large group of people who had shared the same troubles – people who had a common religion and a common language. The consistory records, for example, show that hundreds of people made *reconnaissances* in church for having betrayed their faith under duress.[18] This generally involved confessing their fault before the assembled congregation. Doubtless there was an element of shame attached to this, but I suspect it may also have been very therapeutic given the terrible persecution some of them had suffered, and it probably served to strengthen the bonds of community.

However, a strong sense of community is likely to have had both positive and negative effects on the *ongoing* process of assimilation. In the short-term, it would have been extremely beneficial. The basic mechanics of daily existence – finding one's way around, obtaining the necessities of life, and so on – would have been greatly helped by being able to share information in a common language, not to mention by having the assistance of the already-settled French-speaking population. Church records show, for example, that there were French-speaking medical workers on hand to tend to the injured and sick, which must have been particularly welcome at such a stressful time.[19]

Long-term, though, I suspect it may have slowed the process of total integration. From the end of the 17th century, for instance, numerous friendly societies sprang up. These societies were designed to maintain links and to foster self-help among people from particular regions – and in fact they were among the earliest mutual benefit societies to be founded anywhere in England.[20] One of the first was apparently the *Société des Parisiens*, founded in 1687, but numerous others followed, and such societies were still being formed into the middle of the 18th century.[21] This suggests that many migrants were not simply retaining loose French links but that there was a widespread keenness to maintain a specific identity. Of course, this may just have been dictated by practical self-interest, because the English poor relief system was often difficult to tap into, and aid from 'establishment' bodies such as the French Church of London was perceived, by some at least, as being directed towards certain favoured groups. Pierre Bonnel, for one, having been denied assistance by the deacons of the French Church, retorted that he would have certainly received something if he had been Gascon.[22] But the fact that members gathered regularly and frequently – usually about once a fortnight – and that they met in places such as taverns, suggests that the social aspect was at least as important as the financial one, and probably not least because of language. While one of course needs to be wary of modern comparisons, it is perhaps not without significance that present-day *foreign-language* migrants to New Zealand, for example – be they Serb or Samoan – seem to feel much more need to form clubs than do, say, British, North American or Australian migrants.

The number of new French churches formed again suggests that many migrants wanted to retain their specifically French identity. Of course, one must allow that, in many cases, this may have been secondary to maintaining a form of worship for which they had sacrificed so much, but we must not ignore the fact that at least half of these churches were Conformist – that is, they used the Anglican liturgy translated into French. This rather suggests that, for a good number of people, it was the French language and the sense of community that were the important factors – more, perhaps, than the form of worship. In fact, it has been suggested that some of the churches may have been founded on specific regional links, with the ministers gathering around them members of their own French *pays*.[23] By the end of the 17th century some 28 French congregations existed in and around London. There were still 20 of them in 1730, and even 50 years later this number had only dropped to 15. It is not till 1800 that we can see a significant falling-off, with just eight churches surviving till that date.[24] For the people attending those churches, a specific French identity and sense of community obviously remained important for a considerable time.

But apart from the size of the migration, there were other factors that may have influenced how easily the migrants integrated. A very important element, if purely in terms of economic survival, was the availability or otherwise of some sort of ongoing welfare provision. Even supposing a successful settling-in period and the finding of some sort of gainful employment, the migrant was just as vulnerable as the host population to periods of ill-health, occasional unemployment, and, eventually of course, old age. But English poor relief was available only if one had settlement in a parish, and parishes were generally reluctant to give settlement to people they saw as being a potential drain on parish funds – so it is highly unlikely they would have welcomed refugees. *Some* female migrants may of course have gained access to English poor relief by marrying English men – just as there were English women who received assistance from Huguenot sources by virtue of their French husbands[25] – but there is little evidence, at least in the records I have studied so far, that English relief was commonly available to French migrants. Indeed, I have found only one reference to a poor migrant receiving relief from an English parish – that particular case involving a father and son who had been placed in a parish workhouse for a time.[26]

Similarly, the reluctance of guilds to accept foreigners would have cut the Huguenot migrants off from another potential source of assistance: that is, guild pensions that were provided for members in old age or times of illness. A search of the Weavers' Company records for the period 1735–50, for example, reveals scarcely any French names among its lists of pensioners.[27] Of course one cannot discount the possibility of names having been Anglicized, but it does suggest that skilled French migrants were at an ongoing disadvantage in their access to relief in times of need.

For this reason, the welfare assistance available from the French churches, the benefit societies, and other French-run agencies such as the soup kitchens, the Pest House, and then (from 1718 onwards) the new French Protestant Hospital, was of considerable importance to the Huguenot community. Yet at the same time it risked promoting separatism. People seeking assistance from these sources (as also from the Royal Bounty funding for the refugees) needed to retain their French links in order to be eligible. What is more, they often needed to be recommended by a respected member of the French community.[28] This implies an active fostering of those links, and not merely passive knowledge of family tree and geographic origin.

There is evidence, too, that paupers receiving regular assistance from the French

Church may have been given distinctive clothing to wear, because the poor relief records mention white bodices which were to be taken from the hospital storeroom and dyed 'in the colour which our poor wear'.[29] This may perhaps have been somewhat akin to the English practice, introduced in 1697, of requiring those receiving poor relief to wear a badge indicating the parish from which they were drawing their assistance.[30] It would, however, have marked the Huguenot poor quite distinctly as belonging to the French community and thus being 'different'.

There were also separate French charity schools, one for the girls and one for the boys, and, again, the pupils had a special uniform – although there are indications here that it was more like that of their English counterparts since there is reference to the boys being given caps 'like the children in English charity schools wear'.[31]

In addition, there is little evidence of regular co-operation between French and English relief agencies. Certainly the Royal Bounty funds were administered by joint French and English committees, but there seems to have been little interaction between, for example, the French Church of London and English parishes operating in the same area. There are a few entries concerning some houses in Kingsland Road which seem, for a time, to have been jointly owned with the parish of St Leonard's, Shoreditch,[32] but, apart from that, there are, in FCL poor relief records for the period 1735–50, only three references to the deacons being in direct contact with English parish authorities over matters of poor relief (although I exclude here any contact involved in organizing pauper burials, since nearly all Huguenot burials took place in Anglican churchyards, the French churches not having their own cemeteries).[33]

On the other hand, successful integration of migrants must eventually have occurred because the records show that the names of families receiving poor relief in the 1680s are substantially different from those receiving assistance 50 or 60 years later.[34] This suggests that the earlier group either succeeded in establishing themselves economically, or else that they became integrated into English society sufficiently to be eligible for English poor relief.

Also, in arguing for a degree of (partially imposed) separatism, I do not wish to imply that the Huguenot community was isolationist. Indeed some migrants were only too enthusiastic in their adoption of English customs – including newer habits such as gin-drinking (itself recently imported from Holland). Apart from women, who were prominent in the gin trade both as vendors and consumers, one of the main groups of consumers were men involved in more sedentary trades such as weaving[35] – so it is not surprising that there were those in the Huguenot community who succumbed to the habit. Even the fairly well supervised inhabitants of 'La Providence' (the French Hospital) were apparently not immune, because the records mention one or two of them trying to smuggle in gin, or being found in a drunken condition. One widow, Jeanne Debuze, was punished on four separate occasions between 1752 and 1755, and she was even threatened with expulsion in 1753 – although the threat was evidently not carried out because two years later she was still there and still offending.[36]

A particularly positive force for integration, however, was that the Huguenot community had much to contribute to English society. In the area of poor relief alone, there appear to have been several practices which came to be emulated by the host community. La Providence, for instance, was not only the earliest known subscription hospital in England, but seems to have set an example in the standard of care it gave to inmates (and especially to mental patients)[37] – and mention has already been made of the laudable example in self-help as represented by the numerous Huguenot benefit societies. Another positive example set by the Huguenots was in the careful administration of their poor relief funds. Expenditure was scrupulously recorded in the accounts and any surplus income (such as bequests and legacies) was regularly invested at interest – the latter a practice that seems to have been rare in English parishes at that time.[38] Similarly, the organization of the French charity schools attracted interest and positive comment from the host community, with William Maitland noting that 'This is a Management so laudable, that it well deserves to be copied after by the Trustees of our Parochial and other Charity Schools'.[39]

To summarize, then, what do Huguenot documents relating to discipline and poor relief tell us about the integration of French migrants in early modern London? Firstly, I suggest, there was a great sense of community among the immigrants and, for a long time, many of them identified themselves very strongly as French. The size of the migration may have posed particular problems, but assistance was well-organized, and the discipline exercised by the French churches (and, in particular, the French Church of London) sought to keep friction to a minimum between migrant and host population. Economic absorption may have been difficult for many, but Huguenot sources of poor relief provided a long-term, reliable, safety net until such time as the migrant had become part of the English community. The Huguenots were a well-organized, coherent community who relied to a large extent on their own resources. This, and the wealth of ideas and skills they brought to their new country, no doubt earned them respect and acceptance, and eased their passage from 'stranger' to 'citizen'.

NOTES

1   The phases identified here, and the names given them, have been taken from Andrew Trlin, *Now respected, once despised: Yugoslavs in New Zealand* (Palmerston North, 1979), 184.
2   Rina Benmayor and Andor Skotnes, *Migration and identity*, International Yearbook of Oral History and Life Stories, vol. 3 (Oxford, 1994), 11.
3   *Ibid.*, 8.
4   Robin Gwynn, *Huguenot heritage: the history and contribution of the Huguenots in Britain* (London, 1985), 36.
5   Tim Harris, *London crowds in the reign of Charles II: propaganda and politics from the Restoration until the Exclusion Crisis* (Cambridge, 1987), 204.
6   Library of the French Church of London, Soho Square (hereafter FCL), MS 7 (Livre d'actes de 1679 à 1692), 26 February 1682.
7   *Ibid.*, 27 June 1682.
8   *Ibid.*, 26 April 1685.
9   See also Myriam Yardeni, *Le Refuge protestant* (Paris, 1985), 64.
10 MS 7, 22 July 1683, 23 July 1684, 29 April 1688, 8 July 1688.
11 A warning was issued that 'ceux qui font arrêter leurs prochains pour les constituer prisonniers' would be publicly suspended from communion. *Ibid.*, 14 August 1687.
12 HSQS 58, 65.
13 In December 1681, for example, a Mr Smythies was paid £10 'pour la subsistance de 65 personnes en Golding Lane pour une semaine': *Ibid.*, 10. See also HSQS 49, 12.
14 Norman G. Brett-James, *The growth of Stuart London* (London, 1935), 490–2.
15 Natalie Rothstein, 'The sucessful and the unsuccessful Huguenot: another look at the London silk industry in the 18th and early 19th centuries', *HSP* 25:5 (1993) 439–50.
16 Eileen Barrett, 'An examination of the disciplinary treatment of men and women in the

French Church of London in the 1680s as evidenced by the *Actes* of the consistory for that period' (unpublished Dip.Hum. research exercise, Massey University, 1994), 29–30; Eileen Barrett, 'Huguenot poor relief in Hanoverian London: assistance to widows in the period 1735–1750' (unpublished MA thesis, Massey University, 1997), 8–9.

17 Barrett, 'Huguenot poor relief', 39–44.

18 Barrett, 'An examination of the disciplinary treatment', 29.

19 Eileen Barrett, 'Poor relief provided to Huguenot widows, 1681–1695, through the French Church of London: a preliminary study' (unpublished BA (Hons) research essay, Massey University, 1996), 36.

20 Barrett, 'Huguenot poor relief', 74.

21 William C. Waller, 'Early Huguenot friendly societies', *HSP* 6 (1898–1901), 204; HSQS 56, 90; C. F. A. Marmoy, 'L'entraide des réfugiés français en Angleterre', *Bulletin de la Société de l'Histoire du Protestantisme Français* 115 (1969), 600–2.

22 FCL, MS 81 (Chronological register of poor with particulars of relief afforded 1740–51), fo. 318.

23 Robin Gwynn, 'Disorder and innovation: the reshaping of the French churches of London after the Glorious Revolution' in O. P. Grell, J. I. Israel, N. Tyacke (eds.), *From persecution to toleration: the Glorious Revolution and religion in England* (Oxford, 1991), 262.

24 Robin D. Gwynn, 'The distribution of Huguenot refugees in England, II: London and its environs', *HSP* 22: 6 (1976), 561–7.

25 Barrett, 'Huguenot poor relief', 51.

26 FCL, MS 83 (Chronological register of poor with particulars of poor relief afforded 1729–1739), fo. 298; FCL, MS 111 (*Livre des réfugiés fevrier 1735/36:* Day-book of monies disbursed to poor refugees and names of recipients, 18 February 1736–25 February 1741), [e.g.] 8 March 1738; HSQS 55.

27 Personal communication from John Chapman, London.

28 Barrett, 'Huguenot poor relief', 95.

29 FCL, MS 58 (*Livre des délibérations 1733):* 17 Aug 1737.

30 Stephen Macfarlane, 'Studies in poverty and poor relief in London at the end of the seventeenth century' (D.Phil thesis, Oxford University, 1982), 157, 189; Dorothy Marshall, *The English poor in the eighteenth century: a study in social and administrative history* (London, 1926), 103.

31 Ms 58, 17 Feb. 1745.

32 *Ibid.*, 31 July 1737 and 1 March 1738.

33 *Ibid.*, 8 Nov. 1738, 14 May 1740 and 15 May 1745.

34 Barrett, 'Huguenot poor relief', 97.

35 G. E. Mingay, *Georgian London* (London, 1975), 134–5.

36 HSQS 52, vol. 1, entries under Debuze, Jeanne.

37 Barrett, 'Huguenot poor relief', 54–5.

38 *Ibid.*, 31–2.

39 From William Maitland's *History of London* (1739), quoted in 'The churches, chapels, schools, and other charitable foundations of London in 1739', *HSP* 3 (1888–91), 573.

42

Huguenot thought after the Revocation of the Edict of Nantes: toleration, 'Socinianism', integration and Locke

JOHN MARSHALL

In August 1690 34 Huguenot ministers in England wrote to their colleagues in the Netherlands about the need for concerted Huguenot efforts to maintain the 'capital points' of their faith against 'Arian' and 'Pelagian' views. They then attempted to obtain condemnation by Huguenot ministers in London of the 'false, pernicious and scandalous' propositions related to 'Socinianism', 'the matter of tolerating' and 'internal grace' which had already been condemned by the Walloon synods. In March 1691 96 Huguenot ministers subscribed to their maintenance of the 'constant doctrine of the French Protestants', including anti-Socinian belief in the orthodox doctrine of the Trinity of three equal, co-eternal and consubstantial Persons, the Incarnation, and Christ's satisfaction, and anti-Pajonist belief in the necessity of regeneration by the internal operation of the Holy Ghost. They declared that they 'detest[ed]' the 'Opinions of Socinus' as 'Heresies which absolutely overturn the Foundations of the Christian Faith' with whose followers or teachers 'we can have no Religious Communion'. These Huguenot ministers exhorted their fellow ministers to attack Socinianism in private and in public. Such orthodox commitments and actions were then further publicized in just such an attack, Claude Groteste de Lamothe's Trinitarian 1693 *Discourses Concerning the Divinity of our Saviour*.[1]

These Huguenot ministers attempted to silence several ministers in the conformist French churches in London whom they viewed as 'heretical' or 'heterodox', including André de l'Ortie, minister at the Savoy. When he protested that he had been falsely accused of Socinianism, they supplied a lengthy double-columned account setting his views against the impeccably orthodox Calvinist Trinitarian views of Testas of Threadneedle Street, with whom he had privately debated on the eternal generation and divinity of Christ.[2] In the early 1690s, several Huguenot ministers were forced from their pulpits, including the 'Socinian' Matthieu Souverain, a popular preacher at the new conformist church at Le Carré, Soho, and his colleague Daniel Du Temps, whose burial expenses were allegedly refused in 1693 by orthodox Huguenot ministers on the grounds that he was a 'dog of a Socinian'. When Theodore Maimbourg died in 1692 as a widely reputed Socinian, orthodox Huguenot ministers commenced an investigation of four ministers who had attended him: Souverain, de L'Ortie, Du Temps, and Du Temps's son-in-law.[3] When in the mid-1690s there were disputes leading to a significant schism over Socinianism in the large Huguenot community at Canterbury, further proceedings against 'Socinian' Huguenot ministers, again including Souverain, were called for by orthodox Huguenot ministers.[4] In October 1692, orthodox Huguenot ministers framed 13 articles for subscription which stated strongly their commitment to the French confession of faith, to the orthodox doctrine of the Trinity, satisfaction, and to the anti-Pajonist 'internal and immediate operation of the Holy Ghost' as 'necessary' for 'our conversion'. The articles registered 'detestation' of Socinianism, and rejected several Socinian doctrines (sleep of the soul after death; denial of the identity of bodies at the resurrection; denial of eternity of torments in hell) and the allegedly Socinian tenet that reason was to be 'judge' of the 'articles' of faith. They equally and equally significantly condemned the 'dishonesty' of those who said they personally believed in the doctrine of the Trinity, but could not find 'certain proofs' of it in Scripture and thought it legitimate to maintain communion with those who rejected it. In their eyes there was thus no significant distinction between tolerant 'Arminians', 'Pajonists', and 'Socinians'.[5] Huguenot refugee ministers who were probably Christologically Socinian and also significantly 'Arminian' or 'Pajonist' and tolerant, such as Charles Le Cène, or Trinitarian but 'Pajonist' and tolerant of those who did not accept the orthodox doctrine of the Trinity, such as Isaac Papin, were unable to gain ministerial posts in England in the 1680s and 1690s.[6]

These measures were in very significant part a direct continuation in England of theological battles that had been fought within the Huguenot community in France over previous decades, including anti-Socinian condemnations and the 1677 condemnation of Pajonism for its support for the hypothetically universal offer of salvation, defence of free will, and support for mediate rather than immediate operations of grace, positions which opponents identified with Socinianism.[7] For such views, various pastors had lost their posts in France in the 1670s and early 1680s. These included Souverain, synodically condemned by the synod of Poitou in 1682 for views variously described as 'Pajonist', 'Arminian' and 'Socinian', Noël Aubert de Versé, synodically deposed as 'infected' with Socinianism in 1669; and Le Cène, accused of expressing 'Pelagian' and 'Arian' views in sermons and unable to gain a post at Orléans in the early 1680s.[8] Theological students who had had their degrees issued with qualifications included Papin, Pajon's nephew and Le Cène's fellow student at Saumur.[9] The English measures were thus in part direct continuations of these actions, and even involved some of the same people.[10] They were also imitative of measures taken in the Netherlands in the 1680s by synods under the influence of Pierre Jurieu, dominant and domineering theologian of the Huguenot refugees, and formerly a stout defender of Huguenot orthodoxy in France.[11]

The story so far, then, is a story of the maintenance by the majority of orthodox Huguenots of a distinct, essentially Calvinist Huguenot identity in England and in the Netherlands, with Huguenots attempting to maintain in exile the orthodox faith for which they had gone into exile and attempting to police the beliefs of their fellow ministers as a separate religious community in England and internationally. Lamothe's

Discourses affirmed that the articles to which French ministers had subscribed were those of the Confession of Faith of the Reformed Churches in France, and that he was giving written proofs of 'the constancy of our faith'. Focusing on Huguenot identity, constancy, and solidarity, he held that such a declaration would carry weight because of the great number of refugees and since it was on account of religion that they had been banished from their own country. Huguenot ministers of conformist and nonconformist congregations and various lay Huguenot leaders attempted at various moments to co-ordinate the refugee community as one community in England, as through a General Assembly from 1697.[12]

Yet Lamothe, himself a conformist minister, held that it was the duty of French ministers to give public support to the 'best persons' in the Church of England who had defended the orthodox doctrine of the Trinity, and had his *Discourses* published in an English translation. He argued that Huguenot ministers were testifying to their orthodoxy because they had been questioned on this matter by the Bishop of London, Compton. And he indicated that the articles to which they had subscribed were agreeable to the articles of the Church of England. The 13 articles proposed in 1692 were similarly declared agreeable to those of the Church of England. Conformist French churches used the Church of England liturgy, translated into French, and the General Assembly, as only advisory, was permitted by the Bishop of London and Archbishop of Canterbury.[13]

It should be recalled that the 'Toleration Act' of 1689 provided indulgence from the penalties of the law for worship outside of the Church of England only to Trinitarian Protestants. English Socinians who publicly and repeatedly denied the doctrine of the Trinity faced penalties, Socinianism was still depicted in this period by many of its English opponents as an heretical 'poison', and over the next thirty years it was repeatedly made clear that published anti-Trinitarianism was unacceptable in England, for instance through passage of the 1697 Blasphemy Act and through the loss of posts or preferment by Anglicans who questioned the doctrine of the Trinity, such as William Whiston.[14] It was to the Bishop of London, Compton, that orthodox Huguenots appealed against Souverain and Du Temps in 1689, and Compton who pressed Souverain to stop preaching. It was Compton who requested proofs of Huguenot orthodoxy in 1691.[15]

Orthodox Huguenots such as Jean Armand Dubourdieu and Jean Graverol contributed works in support of intolerance explicitly aimed at both the French refugee community and at the English nation in the Bangorian Controversy, a controversy over toleration involving hundreds of works attacking the extensive tolerationism of Bishop Benjamin Hoadly.[16] Many of the attacks on Hoadly's tolerationism were by English Anglicans, including no less than 17 editions in 1717 of *A Letter to the Bishop of Bangor* by Andrew Snape, Chaplain to George I. William Wake, Archbishop of Canterbury, informed the House of Lords that Socinians, Arians and Deists were 'not so much as tolerated' and defended 'confessions of faith' and 'fundamental articles'.[17] When François Parrain de Durette published (in French) *A Treatise Concerning the Abuse of Confessions of Faith*, a book which declared creed makers anti-Christian, the Bishop of London branded it an 'infamous book' in a circular letter to the French churches. Jean de La Motte added further defences to the utility and necessity of confessions of faith, in French and surely primarily for the Huguenot community, in which he cited Bishop Edward Stillingfleet on viewing the Anglican articles as articles of peace requiring that one not oppose positions taken by the church.[18] Opponents of toleration of Socinianism among Huguenot refugees therefore had very considerable reasons to view their anti-Socinianism as not merely maintaining their distinct faith and identity, but also as showing themselves, at English episcopal request, acceptable as not being heretical refugees, and as integrating them into the English church and polity in identifying with a significant body within the Church of England in their orthodox commitments.[19]

Yet some of the Anglican hierarchy after 1689 were supporters not merely of the toleration granted in 1689, but also thought allowable at least the private expression of anti-Trinitarianism, and more generally read the Anglican articles as allowing significant disagreements about belief on matters such as the operation of God's grace. The most 'latitudinarian' of these, Bishop Hoadly, was to urge those 'who had found a shelter here from Persecution' to avoid persecuting others.[20] Thus the orthodox Huguenots' desires for integration and identification with many Anglicans and with much of Anglicanism involved a desire to influence the Anglican church away from a feared 'latitudinarian Anglican' acceptance of heterodoxy and heresy. An early 1690s petition of some French ministers to the personally orthodox Calvinist but tolerant William and Mary thus expressed simultaneously their own identification with the Church of England and their fear that some of its leaders might support toleration. It asked William and Mary not to prefer those 'infected' by the 'spirit' of toleration, to appoint court preachers of impeccable orthodoxy, and to forbid the preaching or printing of works defending Socinianism or toleration. Aligning Arminianism with Socinianism, it also attacked the Oxford and Cambridge teaching of Episcopius's Arminianism, branding him a 'demi-Socinian' devoted to rendering Trinitarianism unnecessary. The petition both thanked God that there were 'not too many Socinians in England' and noted that some in the Church of England wrongly did not think that Socinianism was a 'damnable heresy', and wholly 'antichristian'.[21]

While orthodox Huguenots' actions were in part dictated by desire to integrate into a significantly intolerant host culture, then, supporters of Anglican 'moderation' could attack these orthodox Huguenots first as failing to integrate with actual Anglican 'moderation' in practices of tolerance for private anti-Trinitarianism, and second for attempting to usurp Anglican authority over its communicants. The set of articles which Lamothe printed had been subscribed to by large numbers of French ministers, and their meetings in 1693 produced a further list of articles for subscription by all ministers. Some Huguenot ministers themselves refused to subscribe, however, alleging the lack of appropriate Anglican authority, a point apparently then backed up by archiepiscopal command to desist. This was still being pointed out over twenty years later, in a tolerationist work which recorded a Huguenot minister as having questioned the Huguenot council held in London against Socinianism: 'I want to know by what authority we Refugees do all this; whilst there are bishops and other Ecclesiastical Superiors'.[22] An anonymous critic of the proposed 1693 articles complained about imposing not only 'those Doctrines which have been held fundamental in all the times of Christianity but also controverted points wherein very good and learned men differ among themselves'; he hoped that French ministers could 'learn in their exile to be as moderate as are many learned Divines of the Church of England' who suffered judgments to vary in 'those difficult points wherein good Christians did never yet agree'.[23]

Devoted tolerationists moreover represented orthodox Huguenots' actions as testifying that they were failing to integrate into English religious liberty. In *Reflections on two Discourses Concerning the Divinity of our Saviour* in 1695, published anonymously (with a postscript signed by 'EE'), Lamothe was attacked as an 'eminent demagogue of the French nation'. For this author, the council of French churches was under English law 'a riot' since 'it assembled by no legal Authority, and the Assistants at it are punishable by our Laws'. Escalating the rhetoric of denunciation, this condemned their ministers as 'Peepers, Lurchers, and trapans' who 'skulk about the Presses, Booksellers shops, and even at private houses, to get informations about unlicensed books, and heterodox Opinions and Persons' and to inform against people to the civil and ecclesiastical courts, to the 'Danger of the Persons whom they illegally inform against, and prosecute for matters of mere Conscience and Religion'. The author said that they had given 'an insufferable provocation, there being nothing so intolerable as that Refugees for Conscience, should turn Informers and Persecutors for Matters purely conscientious, for mere dissent in Points of Faith'. The proceedings attempted against André de L'Ortie on the basis of his privately debating the orthodox doctrine of the Trinity were described by 'EE' in the postscript as 'contrary to the express words of the Statute' of toleration, since this allowed toleration even for Socinians if they 'content themselves to hold their opinions, or to reason or discourse of them in familiar Talk' (The 'Toleration Act' specified only that 'any person that shall deny in his preaching or writing the doctrine of the blessed Trinity' was not to be tolerated). 'EE' even suggested that a 'publick spirited person who loves liberties' should prosecute de L'Ortie's opponents. The final note driving home the attack on intolerance as a failure to integrate was the declaration that ''tis not for refugees to trample upon the laws of the Country where they are received and protected'.[24]

Protest about Huguenot intolerance as inappropriate in a land alleged to be that of religious liberty came not merely from outside the Huguenot community, but also from within it. Claude Rey was a Huguenot tradesman who engaged in a dispute in the mid-1710s with his minister, La Chappelle, in his account because he could not accept the minister's accounts of baptism and of the precise degree of torment and glory of souls after death. He therefore issued in 1718 – and thus partly as another contribution to the Bangorian controversy – what he explicitly called 'an appeal to the English nation', *An Account of the Cruel Persecutions, raised by the French clergy since their taking sanctuary here against several worthy ministers, gentlemen, gentlewomen, and tradesmen, dissenting from their Calvinistical scheme.* Discussing every instance detailed already and many others, Rey pilloried the French ministers for inappropriate intolerance, for having excommunicated opponents and attempted to deprive them of the means of subsistence, caused several to be pressed, and for having 'stoned others in the streets, calling them Dogs of Hereticks . . . saying they would willingly pay for so much Rope as would hang them, or so much wood as would burn them'. According to Rey, they had said to his customers and 'workmen' that he was himself 'a Jesuit, a Socinian . . . [and] an atheist'.[25]

This cruelty was for Rey 'aggravated' because done by people who had lost their estates by persecution; and even more because done 'in a free country wherein they are themselves protected'. For Rey, 'our french people; jacobites and papists are the only persecutors in their kingdom' the 'high-church mob is not better taught in this new kind of Christianity, than our People'. Issuing his work to appeal to the 'English nation', Rey declared that that nation was 'the bulwark of Protestantism against Popery i.e. of Christian liberty against Church Tyranny'. He was hoping that they would interpose between the actions taken against those who had 'dared to shake off the yoak of your Calvinisticall scheme'. Defending a defender of Hoadly, La Pillonière – a Catholic turned Protestant whose former confession was used in debate against both him and Hoadly – Rey declared him a steady friend to 'the Revolution Principles and to the Prostestant Religion'. Here it is crucial to underline that Rey is making a case for the Huguenots failing to integrate into English society and polity by defining English values as lying at one radical tolerationist or Hoadlian point on the political and religious spectrum.[26]

Entered in the lists in the Bangorian Controversy in English translation in support of Hoadly's tolerationism by Hoadly's tutor François La Pillonière, who added much of his own argument, Parrain de Durette's *A Treatise Concerning the Abuse of Confessions of Faith* (1718) argued that one had to have communion with all Christians and to condemn those who opposed this requirement. It declared that Graverol's *Defence of the Reformed Synods and Pastors* had set up a 'Protestant Popery' in which 'the Church hath a Right to determine, which is the true sense of the controverted texts of Scripture; and to oblige the People to submit to its decisions'.[27] Either texts were plain and all Protestants agreed or they were 'obscure'; if there was obscurity then it 'contains no such Doctrine as is necessary'. It argued that some truths were fundamental to one Christian and not to others, and declared that the foundation for all was that Jesus was the Messiah. The 'whole bible' was said to contain 'nothing but this great truth'. Turning the two sins of heresy and schism back on the accusers, it declared that those who cut others off 'under pretence of rejecting some controverted points' not 'clearly revealed' made 'a Schism' and that 'the most damnable of all Heresies', is non 'Toleration, and Want of Charity'. Depicting toleration as promoting Anglican integration, for La Pillonière it was English toleration that had made most French refugees conformists by choice.[28]

La Pillonière cited Bayle's *Philosophical Commentary* approvingly as arguing for toleration (as well as Locke's *Letter Concerning Toleration*). Rey cited Bayle's *Philosophical Commentary* in defence of toleration, and claimed that even his ministerial opponent La Chappelle in private had warmly praised this work. One of the accusations made against de L'Ortie was that he approved Bayle's *Philosophical Commentary*; de L'Ortie had replied that it was a 'very good book'.[29] Tolerationist Huguenots in England and their associates were thus citing the leading Huguenot theorist of toleration, Bayle, and attempting to identify England as a land of religious liberty; Bayle's *Philosophical Commentary* had been initially published pseudonymously as translated from the English and as allegedly published at Canterbury with suggestion that excellent tolerationist arguments had a long history in England. It was probably the work favouring 'universal toleration' that the orthodox Huguenot ministers in England condemned in 1690.[30]

Space permits only a sketch of the barest outlines of some of the tolerationist Huguenots' arguments here; I pursue extended analysis of this case elsewhere.[31] For Bayle, toleration was all or nothing: 'there can be no solid reason for tolerating any one sect, which does not equally hold for every other'. Bayle was explicit: Pagans, Jews, Turks, and Socinians deserved toleration. Magistrates were to leave to God the task of punishing heretics who 'disturb not the public peace'. Moreover, for Bayle, those did not blaspheme who did not speak against the divinity they acknowledged. For Bayle, God requires 'no more of us than to examine and search after [truth] diligently, and . . . will be content to accept our assent of the objects which appear true to us' .[32] De L'Ortie declared – against the contention of orthodox Huguenots that Bayle's was a 'wicked book' and 'dangerous' to the faith – that the *Philosophical Commentary* was a 'very good book' for showing the errors of all who persecuted those who did nothing against the peace and security of the state.[33]

Charles Le Cène was author of several important works, and a friend of the most famous Huguenot preacher in England in the 1680s, Pierre Allix, who was himself identified as a leading tolerationist who should not be promoted in the orthodox ministers' petition to William and Mary. In the mid-1680s Le Cène and Allix together established the French conformist church in Jewin Street, London. Allix issued several works in defence of the 1688–9 Revolution which defended toleration and redefined heresy.[34] Le Cène's manuscript collection – and his own thinking – is an amalgam of Pajonism, Socinianism, Arminianism and the thought of Ralph Cudworth. It suggests that Le Cène was Christologically Socinian. Le Cène's *Projet* for a new translation of the New Testament was quickly attacked as Socinian, and later condemned as Socinian by the Synod of Brille. As early as 1694 Bishop Burnet recorded that Le Cène lay 'under such suspicions of socinianisme' that unless they were cleared he could not help him.[35] The most important of Le Cène's several tolerationist works was his 1687 *Conversations on Diverse Matters of Religion*, which declared it always better to change one's thoughts in following the light of reason, argued that only persuasion was permitted towards those of other opinions, and contended that if one admitted liberty of conscience one could not condemn heretics unless they erred in matters 'clear and distinct' in the Holy Scripture, focusing on the Apostles' creed. Its second part was a French translation of the leading Socinian John Crell's 1637 *Vindication of Liberty of Religion*.[36] In reviewing the entire work in the *Bibliothèque universelle* in May 1687 Jean Le Clerc declared that Bayle's *Philosohpical Commentary* was on one point merely an 'amplification' of their work. Like Bayle, it attacked the 'injustice' involved in esteeming heretics 'as bad as thieves and robbers, or even worse than them, and to be ranked among those with whom no fellowship or society may be entertained, no promise made and kept' and continued that they 'know not themselves to be heretiques, and would not be such if they knew it; but most strongly believe that they hold opinions concerning matters of Religion, which are true, pious, and altogether agreeable to the word of God, neither do, nor purpose to do wrong to any man'. While thieves invaded other men's rights and 'disturb'[ed], 'the peace and tranquillity of other men', heretics 'lived peacefully with other men, did not know that they sinned, and did not commit anything' against 'the laws of civil society'.[37]

Similar arguments were voiced by Noël Aubert de Versé, who spent parts of 1685 and a year in 1688–9 in England, during which times he was a go-between between Bayle and Robert Boyle, and between Locke and Le Clerc.[38] In the *Historical and Critical Dictionary* Bayle declared Aubert's pseudonymous 1687 *Treatise on Liberty of Conscience* one of four essential recent works on toleration (together with Bayle's own *Philosophical Commentary* and Locke's *Letter Concerning Toleration*). Locke's personal library copy was marked with his 'paraph' mark, often used for works of great significance. The *Treatise* declared that one man's heresy was another man's orthodoxy, and that the erring conscience had the same rights as the orthodox. Aubert's earlier *Le protestant pacifique* – a work both recommended by Locke to his English friend James Tyrrell, and called by the April 1684 synod of Walloon churches in the Netherlands a 'pernicous' book full of 'abominable heresies' – had similarly argued that on the principle of conscience it was necessary for any consistent Protestant to support toleration for Quakers and Socinians and had advocated unity among Christians by the allowance of wide doctrinal diversity.[39]

Similar arguments to those of Aubert de Versé were made by Isaac Papin, who had taken Anglican orders in 1686, sought tutorial employment in England, and spent the mid-to-late 1680s as a correspondent of Jean Le Clerc and Gilbert Burnet. Papin's patron in England was Jacques Cappel, son of the famous Saumur Hebraist Louis Cappel.[40] In *Faith Reduced to its True Principles*, a work which he had written when living before the Revocation in the Bordeaux household of the English merchant William Popple, and which was published from manuscript with a preface by Bayle, Papin argued that statements of faith ought to be confined to 'the proper Terms of the Scripture', and that that which was 'not in the holy Scripture' could not 'be of absolute Necessity to Salvation'. He focused on the Apostles' creed and the proposition that Jesus was the Messiah. He redefined the term 'heretic' to mean 'those who add to the Scripture their own particular Explications' and urged that councils, synods and ecclesiastical assemblies were to be regarded 'neither as Judges, nor as Guides but simply as learned Men'.[41]

In the late 1680s, John Locke attempted to gain a post as tutor for Papin in the household of Edward Clarke. He owned Papin's *Foi réduite*. William Popple, in whose household it had been written, was the English translator of Locke's *Letter Concerning Toleration*. A reader of Le Cène's works from the early 1680s, Locke considered employing Le Cène to work on transcriptions towards Limborch's important tolerationist *History of the Inquisition*, and Le Cène undertook a French translation of his *Letter Concerning Toleration*. In the later 1690s Locke helped to support Le Cène financially in England, having been told that Le Cène faced ruin as the result of orthodox ministers' persecution, that he had been forced to sell his books to feed his family, and that he would otherwise be lost to scholarship.[42] We saw earlier that Souverain was one of the four ministers who visted Maimbourg when he was dying in 1692, and came under the investigation of the orthodox Huguenot ministers. In that year Locke recommended Souverain as tutor to his friend Edward Clarke. He knew of Souverain at that point from Popple. Later correspondence shows that Locke knew Souverain and that he was a tutor for Paul D'Aranda, a Huguenot merchant and second-generation immigrant who was himself alleged to be a Socinian, who was one of Locke's go-betweens to Limborch, and who arranged for the financial support of Le Cène by Locke and Popple. The generally extraordinarily well-informed Claude Rey noted that Souverain was maintained by D'Aranda 'with the help of his friends' as was Le Cène, raising at least the possibility that Locke had finanacially supported Souverain as well as Le Cène. Souverain was the author of an extensive, unpublished, and broadly 'Socinian' (or Artemonite) diatribe against the orthodox doctrine of the Trinity which is, anonymously, recorded among Locke's papers in the hands of Locke's amanuensis and in Locke's own hand.[43] Locke employed Aubert de Versé as a go-between to take books to Jean Le Clerc in 1688–9, recommending his tolerationist thought to Tyrrell, read many of Aubert's works, and noted book recommendations from Aubert.[44] Locke knew Bayle personally from 1686 at the latest, when the correspondence of Sir Walter Yonge suggests that they were already friends, was reading Bayle's 1682 *Letter on the Comets* (the first version of Bayle's famed *Pensées*) in mid-October 1685, very shortly before the most probable dates of composition of his *Letter Concerning Toleration* in November and early December 1685. Locke and Bayle later exchanged books, including their own tolerationist works. Locke knew Jacques Cappel, recording meeting him in London in 1690, and he read his works carefully.[45]

Locke followed very closely the measures undertaken by the orthodox ministers in the Huguenot community in the 1680s and 1690s. Locke's manuscripts include an account, in French, of the declaration of their anti-Socinian orthodox faith by French ministers in 1691, intended for others' subscription, personally endorsed by Locke at the end 'this was prepard but stopd'. Throughout the publication and reception of Limborch's *History of the Inquisition* in the late 1680s and early 1690s, composition of which Locke both encouraged and instigated, both Locke and Limborch saw its tolerationist arguments and its identification of persecution with inquisitorial practices as aimed not just at Catholic practices but equally at contemporary Huguenot practices. Limborch wrote to Locke when composing the work was his 'daily occupation' in September 1690, that 'those whom it least behoved, people who had themselves barely escaped out of the hands of persecutors, have decided to show us an exemplar of the holy office'. In late 1692 Locke replied to another Limborch story that he had a story about the 'French in this country which . . . surpasses it', referring to the report he had just received from William Popple, together with Popple's comments on his *Third Letter Concerning Toleration*. Popple had reported the 'most horrible breach of charity amongst the French refugiez here that ever was heard of', the attempts of orthodox ministers to enquire into the past behaviour of the 'charitable' ministers, including Souverain, who had visited Maimbourg when he was dying to find out 'any by-past conversation of these men that may be an argument of their Heterodoxy'. Popple declared to Locke that 'some of the zealous Orthodox ministers' had animated the 'whole Orthodox Herd' and assembled on the cry of Socinianism 'a perfect Court of Inquisition, to the number of fourscore ministers, and are about making formularies and tests to choak all that have not so wide a swallow as themselves'. In 1694 Locke added in a letter to Limborch that 'the French theologians' zeal for orthodoxy seems to be blazing more fiercely in our colder climate . . . In an assembly convoked for that purpose they accused Cappel, a man, if any among the French, as it seems to me temperate and discreet, as suspect of heresy'. Cappel had refused to answer both when summoned and when visited privately; Locke reported to Limborch that this whole 'storm' was aroused because he had attended the funeral of Maimbourg, a man who was 'not orthodox to a hair's breadth'.[46]

It was, then, in part in the context of reading works by Le Cène, Aubert de Versé and Bayle, among others; in part in the context of many discussions between Locke, Limborch and Popple about the activities by the French ministers against their colleagues suspected of heresy; and in part in the context of Locke's personal knowledge, patronage, and readership of the works of several individuals attacked by orthodox Huguenot ministers for 'heresy', that Locke wrote and published his first three *Letters Concerning Toleration* between 1685 and 1692. All of Locke's *Letters*

Concerning Toleration attack intolerance towards those declared by others to be 'heretics', indicating that 'every church is orthodox to itself and erroneous or heretical to others', and they importantly redefined heresy among those who acknowledged only Holy Scripture as 'their rule of faith' as 'separation' in communion for opinions 'not contained in the express words of . . . Scripture'. For Locke, one was not to 'impose' something as 'a necessary article of faith, unless we should be content also that other doctrines should be imposed upon us in the same manner'. The *Letters* make much of the rest of the case of the other tolerationist works so far described. It was in this context, moreover, that Locke composed the *Reasonableness of Christianity*, with its minimalist Christian credal requirement of faith in Jesus as the Messiah, which was significantly parallel to the arguments of many of these authors.[47]

It was partly in the context of reflecting on the behaviour of the orthodox French ministers that Locke wrote to Limborch of his attempt in the *Reasonableness* to find the truth of Christianity from Scripture itself, the 'opinions and orthodoxies of sects and systems . . . being set aside', and indicated that in Limborch he had found a rarity, 'one theologian' 'for whom I am not a heretic'.[48] This notion of the rarity of Limborch, as thinking Locke's thought not heretical, brings me back to the issue of Huguenot integration in England. Despite the efforts of Rey and 'EE' to define the English as principled full religious tolerationists, the associations that I have sketched of Locke with various individuals among the Huguenots who were extensively tolerationist, and the close parallels of these arguments to Locke's, do not associate them with integration into the mainstream of English society, but indeed the reverse. Locke himself could not publish his theological works with his own name on them in the England of the 1690s and his *Reasonableness* and *Letters* came under a hail of fire as 'Socinian' and even diabolic. Le Cène was supported by Locke, Popple, and D'Aranda because he could not find other employment in England; Papin converted to Catholicism and returned to France, having been unable to find suitable employment in England; and Aubert de Versé reconverted to Catholicism and did the same. Souverain lost his ministerial position in England, left a significant manuscript unpublished at his death, and had his one printed work published anonymously in the Netherlands. Le Cène's, Aubert de Versé's and Papin's works, like Locke's, were published anonymously or pseudonymously. The Trinitarian tolerationist Allix became a dean, but that was due to the largely tolerant Gilbert Burnet's personal appointment, and Burnet himself became increasingly desirous to separate himself in the 1690s from association with a number of tolerationists and alleged 'Socinians' of whom he had been supportive in the 1680s. The tolerationist Huguenots were less integrated in England than in the intellectual community of the 'republic of letters', a republic that was fully tolerationist and central to the 'early enlightenment', but which existed primarily in intellectual space and not in *terra firma*. But that is another story.[49]

NOTES

1   LPL, MS 933, 67; Pierre Jurieu, *Le tableau du Socinianisme* (The Hague, 1690), 559ff.; C. G. Lamothe, *Two Discourses Concerning the Divinty of our Saviour* (1693), 64-8 (mispaginated as 64, 57-60); R. Gwynn, 'Disorder and innovation: the reshaping of the French Church of London after the Glorious Revolution' in O. Grell, J. Israel and N. Tyacke (eds.),

From persecution to toleration: the Glorious Revolution and religion in England (Oxford, 1991), 251–73, esp. 256–8, an extremely important article to which this piece is indebted; *idem, Huguenot heritage: the history and contribution of the Huguenots in England* (London, 1985), esp. 105ff.; B. Cottret, *The Huguenots in England: immigration and settlement, 1550–1700* (Cambridge, 1991), esp. 207ff.

2   LPL, MS 929, 54; LPL, MS 932, 1. These manuscripts trade accusations of distortion, and it is difficult to gain an accurate picture of de L'Ortie's beliefs, and impossible to examine them in the space available. Broadly, it seems that de L'Ortie questioned much of the orthodox Calvinist Huguenot doctrines of the Trinity and satisfaction, questioning the 'eternal generation' of Christ and emphasizing Christ's elevation to glorification, along with many Socinians – to orthodox Huguenots clear evidence of 'Socinianism' – but that he may have diverged from parts of the Socinian understanding of Christ. On the evidence available, de L'Ortie may perhaps best be called a 'Socinianized Arminian' or Amyraldist. Space does not permit discussion here of the significant influence in this period of Socinianism on many Arminians, and vice versa, nor of the significant affinities between Pajonism, Arminianism and Socinianism.

3   LPL, MS 933, 67; LPL, MS 934, 53 (on Daniel du Temps, 'Socinien'); C. Rey, *An Account of the Cruel Persecutions Raised by the French Clergy since their taking Sanctuary here* (1718), 31ff.; S. Mours, 'Les pasteurs à la Révocation de l'Edit de Nantes', *Bulletin de la société de l'histoire du protestantisme français* [hereafter *BSHPF*] (1968), 67–105; John Marshall, 'Locke, Socinianism, "Socinianism" and Unitarianism', in M. A. Stewart (ed.), *English philosophy in the age of Locke* (Oxford, 2000); P. Bayle, *Dictionnaire historique et critique* (Maimbourg L; note E), directed readers to Simon's letters as evidence that Maimbourg had 'openly died an Unitarian, and that he had been so a long time incognito', and Simon's letters discussed Maimbourg's Socinianism as prior to his going to England: R. Simon, *Lettres choisies* (Rotterdam, 1702), *lettre* VII, 77–9.

4   LPL, MS 1029, 65; Rey, *Account*, 31ff.; F. W. Cross, *History of the Walloon and Huguenot Church at Canterbury*, HSQS 15 (1898), 157–8; W. H. Manchée, 'Huguenot clergy list, 1548–1916', *HSP* 11:2 (1916), 263–92 at 291; Cottret, *Huguenots in England*, 181–4; 208–10.

5   LPL, MS 933, 67.

6   On Papin and Le Cène see below. Papin stressed in his *The toleration of Protestants* (1690), 55 (after his conversion to Catholicism) that he had 'always followed the orthodox explications of holy scripture'. I leave aside in this paper for reasons of space the important figure of Jean Le Clerc, who enquired about a position in England or Ireland, was a co-preacher with de L'Ortie in London in 1682–3 and knew many of those considered in this paper. See John Marshall, *Locke and early Enlightenment culture* (forthcoming, 2001).

7   O. Fatio, 'Claude Pajon et les mutations de la théologie reformée à l'époque de la Révocation' in R. Zuber and Laurent Theis (eds.), *La Révocation de l'Edit de Nantes et le protestantisme français en 1685* (Paris, 1986), 209–25; F. Laplanche, *L'écriture, le sacré, et l'histoire: érudits et politques protestants devant la Bible en France au XVII siècle* (Amsterdam, 1986); W. Rex, *Essays on Pierre Bayle and religious controversy* (The Hague, 1965), 142–4; J. Quick, *Synodicon in Gallia reformata* (1692), *passim*.

8   LPL, MS 1029, 65; *BSHPF* (1903), 243; B. Sarazin, 'Les temples et les pasteurs de Mouchamps', *BSHPF* (1909), 547–59 at 558–9; E. and E. Haag, *La France protestante* (10 vols., Paris, 1846–59), vol. 9, 294; A. Paul, 'La deposition d'Aubert de Versé au synode d'Is-sur-Tille (1669)', *BSHPF* (1941), 513–15; P. Morman, *Noël Aubert de Versé* (Lewiston, NY, 1987); E. Kappler, 'La controverse Jurieu-De la Conseillere', *BSHPF* (1937), 146–73; Huguenot Library, London, MS Horsham 22e, vol. 6, 239–60.

9   R. Zuber, 'Papiers de jeunesse d'Isaac Papin', *BSHPF* (1974), 107–43 at 141; I. Papin, *Toleration of Protestants* (1690), 18.

10 LPL, MS 933, 67; C. Frossard, 'Liste de pasteurs des Eglises Réformées de France', *BSHPF* (1858), 426ff.; Cottret, *Huguenots*, 226; Gwynn, 'Reshaping', 259.

11 LPL. MS 933, 67; Cottret, *Huguenots*, 209; Gwynn, 'Reshaping'; E. Wilbur, *History of Unitarianism: Socinianism and its antecedents* (Cambridge, MA, 1945), 532; Frossard, 'Liste de pasteurs', 426–35; S. Mours, 'Pasteurs'; *BSHPF* (1903), 243; Kappler, 'Controverse'.

12 Lamothe, *Two Discourses*, 64–8; Gwynn, 'Reshaping'.

13 Lamothe, *Two Discourses*, 64–8; Gwynn, 'Reshaping', 254–5, 270–1.

14 T. Long, *The Letter for Toleration decipher'd* (1689), 9, 17; L. Levy, *Blasphemy: verbal offense against the sacred, from Moses to Salman Rushdie* (Chapel Hill, NC, 1993), 288–92; J. Force, *William Whiston, honest Newtonian* (Cambridge, 1985).

15 Gwynn, 'Reshaping'; LPL, MS 1029, 65.

16 F. Parrain de Durette, *A Treatise* (1718), 11–12; J. Graverol, *Défense de la religion réformée de ses pasteurs et de ses synodes* (1717); Jean Armand Dubourdieu, *An Appeal to the English Nation* (1718); F. La Pillonière, *Third Defense* (1718), 98–124.

17 A. Snape, *A Letter to the Bishop of Bangor* (1710); *idem*, *A Second Letter to the Bishop of Bangor* (1717); *idem*, *A Vindication of a Passage* (1717); H. Mills, *A Full Answer to Mr Pillonière's Reply to Dr Snape* (1718); Wake in N. Sykes, *William Wake, Archbishop of Canterbury, 1657–1737* (2 vols., Cambridge, 1957), vol. 2, 125–6, cited in Levy, *Blasphemy*, 297.

18 Jean de La Motte, *L'utilité et la necessité des confessions de foi* (1718); *idem*, *Suite de l'écrit intitulé, L'utilité et la necessité des confessions de foi* (1718), 55–6, 59–63.

19 On orthodoxy and intolerance after 1689 see: J. C. D. Clark, *English society, 1688–1832* (Cambridge, 1985); T. Harris, *Party politics under the later Stuarts* (London, 1993); G. de Krey, *A fractured society: the politics of London in the first age of party, 1688–1715* (Oxford, 1985); G. Holmes and W. A. Speck (eds.), *The divided society: parties and politics in England, 1694–1716* (London, 1967); G. Holmes (ed.), *Britain after the Glorious Revolution, 1689–1714* (London, 1969); *idem*, *Politics, religion and society in England, 1679–1742* (London, 1986); *idem*, *The trial of Doctor Sacheverell* (London, 1973); J. Walsh, C. Haydon, S. Taylor (eds.), *The Church of England, c.1689–c.1833: from toleration to Tractarianism* (Cambridge, 1986).

20 B. Hoadly, preface to La Pillonière, *An Answer to Dr Snape's Accusation* (1717).

21 LPL, MS 932, 77.

22 La Pillonière, *Third defense* (1718), 100–4; Cottret, *Huguenots*, 226; Gwynn, 'Reshaping', 259, 270; LPL, MS 929, 67.

23 LPL, MS 933, 67.

24 E. E., *Reflections on two Discourses Concerning the Divinity of our Saviour: written by Monsieur Lamoth in French and done into English* (1692), 1–5, 17–18, 20–2.

25 Rey, *Account*.

26 *Ibid.* On the spectrum of political views after 1689 see J. Kenyon, *Revolution principles: the politics of party, 1689–1720* (Cambridge, 1977); T. Harris, *Party politics*; De Krey, *Fractured society*; Clark, *English society*.

27 [Durette/La Pillonière], *A Treatise Concerning the Abuse of Confessions of Faith* (1718), passim, esp. 6–8.

28 *Ibid.*, 13, 40, 50–3, 79–81.

29 La Pillonière, *Answer to Mr Snape's accusation* (1717), 43–4; *idem*, *Third defense*, 98–124; Rey, *Account*, 16–17, 81; LPL, MS 932, 1. Snape called it a scandal to be associated with Bayle: Snape, *A Vindication of a Passage* (1717), 52–5.

30 P. Bayle, *Philosophical Commentary* (1708), iii–iv, 1–2, 6; *idem*, *Pierre Bayle's Philosophical Commentary*, ed. A. G. Tannenbaum (New York, 1987), title page, 9, 11; *idem*, *De la tolérance: Commentaire Philosophique*, ed. J. M. Gros (1992), title page, 47, 51–2. Bayle's

pseudonym evoked the Quaker George Fox and the Anabaptist David Joris, while his *Supplement* identified Quakers, Anabaptists, Arminians and Socinians as the only full tolerationists in the recent centuries of Christianity: Gros (ed.), *De la tolérance*, 43–4; LPL, MS 933, 67; Marshall, *Locke and early Enlightenment culture*.

31 Marshall, *Locke and early Enlightenment culture*.

32 P. Bayle, *Philosophical Commentary*, 260, 217, 267, 355, 335–7; Tannenbaum (ed.), *Philosophical Commentary*, 145, 122, 148, 189, 178; Gros (ed.), *De la tolérance*, 236, 271–2, 277, 352–3, 337.

33 LPL, MS 932, 1; W. J. Stankiewicz, *Politics and religion in seventeenth-century France: a study of political ideas from the Monarchomachs to Bayle, as reflected in the toleration controversy* (Berkeley, CA, 1960), chap. 6, esp. 218–19.

34 LPL, MS 933, 77; [P. Allix], *Reflections upon the Opinions of Some Modern Divines Concerning the Nature of Government* (1689); [*idem*], *An Examination of the Scruples of those who Refuse to take the Oath of Allegiance* (1689).

35 HL MS R5. Vols 1–10 are Le Cène's manuscripts, very largely his translations of others' works into French. Vols 1–3 include many works of Socinians such as Socinus, Volkel, von Wolzogen and Schlichting translated into French, presumably intended for publication. Vols 6–10 include many works of Arminianism, Pajonism and the thought of Cudworth. On the library collection see E. Briggs, 'Les manuscrits de Charles Le Cène (1647?-1703) dans la Bibliothèque de la "Huguenot Society of London"', *Tijdschrift voor de studie van de verlichting* (1977), 358–78; HSQS 56, 172–3. Jacques Gousset's *Considerations théologiques et critiques sur le project d'une nouvelle version françoise de la Bible* (Amsterdam, 1698) anatomized Le Cène's *Projet* as a compendium of Socinianism, Arminianism and Pajonism: J. Le Clerc, *Epistolario*, ed. M. Sina (Florence, 1989), 225. Le Clerc responded to Burnet's report of Le Cène's Socinianism by distancing himself from Le Cène: *ibid.*, 228.

36 [C. Le Cène], *Conversations sur diverses matières de religion … avec un traité de la liberté de conscience* (Philadelphia [Amsterdam?], 1687), *passim*. The work had formerly been translated into English in 1646 as *A Learned and Exceeding Well Compiled Vindication of Liberty of Religion* (1646) and was later to be translated by Naigeon as *De la tolérance dans la religion*. See J. Vercruysse 'Crellius, Le Cène, Naigeon ou les chemins de la tolérance socinienne', *Tijdschrift voor de studie van de verlichting*, 244; H. Vandenbossche and J. Vercruysse on Le Cène in A. Wissowatius, *Religio rationalis, editio trilinguis*, ed. Z. Ogonowski (Wolfenbüttel, 1982), 63ff.

37 To get as close as possible to contemporary idiomatic translation, I use here the English 1646 translation of Crell's work: *A learned and exceeding well-compiled vindication of liberty of religions*. See Le Cène, *Conversations*, 220–87; *Bibliothèque universelle et historique* (1687), 212–27 (May 1687).

38 Morman, *Aubert de Versé*, chap. 4; Locke MS f 29, 31 (1687).

39 P. Bayle, *Dictionnaire historique et critique*, for Sanctesius (Sainctes), note F; J. Locke, *The Library of John Locke*, ed. P. Laslett and J. Harrison (Oxford, 1965), appendix 2; Aubert de Versé, *Traité de la liberté de conscience* (Cologne [Amsterdam?], 1687), *passim*; *idem*, *Le protestant pacifique* (Amsterdam, 1684), *passim*; Locke, *Correspondence*, ed. E. S. de Beer (8 vols., Oxford, 1976–89), vol. 3, letter 889; E. Briggs, 'A wandering Huguenot scholar', *HSP* 21 (1970), 455–63; Morman, *Aubert de Versé*, 34–5, 40, 58.

40 On Papin and Locke, see S. O'Cathasaigh, 'Bayle and Locke on toleration' in M. Magdelaine *et al.* (eds.), *De l'humanisme aux Lumières: Bayle et le protestantisme* (Paris, 1996), 679–92. On Papin and Bayle, E. Labrousse, *Pierre Bayle* (1964, reprinted 1996), 423–4n; on Papin, R. Zuber, 'Papiers de jeunesse d'Isaac Papin', 107–43; E. Haase, 'Isaac Papin à l'époque de la Révocation', *BSHPF* (1952), 94–122; R. Zuber, 'Spinozisme et tolérance chez le jeune Papin', *Dix-huitième siècle* (1974), 218–27; F. Puaux, *Les précurseurs*

français de la tolérance au XVIIème siècle (Paris, 1881); J. B. Bossuet, *Sixième avertissement*, 673–8

41 [I. Papin], *Foi réduite à ses veritables principes* (Rotterdam, 1687), *passim*; *idem*, *Toleration of Protestants*, 31; Puaux, *Précurseurs*, 115; H. Bots and F. Waquet, *La République des Lettres* (Berlin, 1997), 120–1.

42 Locke, *Correspondence*, letters 2192, 2238; Locke MS f7, 107; Locke MS b2, 101.

43 D'Aranda referred to Le Cène as a noted 'Tolerant, or Arminian, etc.': Locke, *Correspondence*, letters 2192, 2197, 2238; J. Marshall, 'Locke, Socinianism'. D'Aranda was himself declared a 'known Socinian' by the orthodox minister Trouillart: LPL, MS 1029, 65; Rey, *Account*, 38–9; Locke MS e17, 175ff.

44 Morman, *Aubert*, chap. 4. Aubert named Limborch and Le Clerc as witnesses on his behalf in his *Manifeste*, 12–13, 19.

45 Locke MS f8, 239ff.; Locke MS f29, 55; Locke, *Correspondence*, letters 944, 960 1827 (inter alia). See on Locke and Bayle my forthcoming *Locke and early Enlightenment culture* and many papers, including, 'Locke, the Furly circle and toleration'.

46 Locke MS c27, fo. 89r; Locke, *Correspondence*, letters 1567, 1572, 1590, 1608, 1630, 1698, 1692. Jacques Cappel, close friend at Saumur of Jean Le Clerc, had been accused of Arminianism and Socinianism at Saumur in 1682. In 1689 he published a commentary on the Old Testament incuding a treatise on the state of souls after death which did not support the resurrection of the body.

47 [Locke], *Letter Concerning Toleration*, *passim*; *idem*, *Third Letter Concerning Toleration* (1692), *passim*; *idem*, *The Reasonableness of Christianity* (1695). See John Marshall, *Locke and early Enlightenment culture* (forthcoming, 2001).

48 Locke, *Correspondence*, letter 1901.

49 For which, see my *Locke and early Enlightenment culture*. I have also treated of matters discussed at various points in this paper in papers on 'Locke and the Republic of Letters', 'The Inquisition, persecution, toleration and resistance', and 'Orthodoxy and heterodoxy in the Huguenot community' among others, and I am grateful to audiences at the Universities of Denver, Cambridge, London, Durham and Wales, and the North American Conference on British Studies for their comments.

43

The newspaper *The Post Man* and its editor, Jean Lespinasse de Fonvive

Itamar Raban

Jean de Fonvive was a member of the large group of Huguenots who settled in England at the end of the 17th century. Some of them made their living by translating French language works into English, translations that were very successful in the English literary market. His naturalization papers, of 1702, state: 'John Espinass De Fonvive, Son of Henry Espinass by Joanna his wife Born at Fonvive in Perigord in France'.[1] From records in the village of his birth, there remains later evidence, from 1743, of someone with a similar name, whose burial was prevented because of refusal to accept a Catholic ceremony.

In the records of the Huguenot churches in London, no details about the family can be found. In his will of 1737, one spinster daughter appears, Marie Gabriel de Fonvive, as the only heir.[2] Upon her death, in 1761, the next of kin who appear as beneficiaries are in Holland.[3] It is from here that I assume that De Fonvive came to England as a widower, with one daughter. There are several questions regarding the daughter. In her will, the status of 'spinster' appears next to her name, meaning a single woman, or a woman who has never married. Her name appears on the list of spouses of Huguenot soldiers, serving in the English Army who never came to collect the gratuity due them.[4] There is one simple possibility, that she had been engaged to a soldier who fell in the war and remained unmaried to the end of her life. Another possibility which has been suggested is that her appearance on the list was done as a technique to transfer money to her father for his support of the government.

The late date that De Fonvive applied for citizenship, after having already gained a reputation and having lived for many years in London, to which he had fled after the revocation of the Edict of Nantes, suggests that he was part of a large group of refugees who had hoped to see European nations force Louis XIV of France to restore freedom of religion to the Huguenots, and to allow them to return to France. It was actually a new war that broke out, the War of the Spanish Succession, and not the missing sections of the peace treaty of Ryswick, that ended all possibilities of a return to France.

His financial success – as he wrote in a letter of 1705, 'The Post Man bring me above £600 a year'[5]– and his having a coat-of-arms gave him the right to add the title 'esquire' to his name.The use of the French prefix 'de' does not necessarily indicate any association with nobility, but rather his place of origin, which would distinguish him from someone with a similar name. Evidence of his economic success can also be found in a published list of items he had lost, published in 1703: a decorated gold watch, made by a Huguenot craftsman named Decharmes.[6] His daughter, Marie Gabriel, had purchased for him a page from a Bible, illustrating chapter 5 of the Book of Job and dedicated to him. The choice of the Book of Job suggests his ability to recover from his difficult fate as a refugee, but it also shows the strength of religious emotion with which the daughter related to her father.

De Fonvive, upon his arrival in London, immediately settled in a house on Castle Street, near Charing Cross,[7] and continued to live there for the rest of his life, never taking advantage of his economic improvement to move to a different home. We do know from testimonies of the period that this street was in a residential area for many Huguenot refugees. This shows the importance that De Fonvive attached to his being part of the community. He was elected as one of the elders of the Huguenot church in Hungerford Market, and paid the money for the acquisition of a hall for the community when they wanted to convert it into a school.[8]

When he resigned from the editorship of the newspaper in 1720, he became more and more involved with the Huguenot community, and was elected as a director, and hence a trustee of the Hospital for Poor French Protestants that was founded in 1718. He maintained ties with religious figures and young Huguenots, amongst them Pierre des Maizeaux, the enlightened young man who borrowed from De Fonvive a copy of the memoirs of the leader of the Camisard revolt, Jean Cavalier.[9] From the drafts of correspondence, we see the great importance that he attached to preserving the Huguenot tradition and perpetuating his contribution to the era.

His private life style was Huguenot. In his professional life, he took advantage of his origin in order to co-operate with the Delafayes, an immigrant family who had one son who served as the secretary to the English mission which conducted the peace negotiations at Ryswick in 1697–8. In his capacity as secretary, Charles Delafaye was required to report to the Secretary of State, John Ellis, on the developments in the negotiations. Half of the information that appears in his letters was exclusively published by De Fonvive's newspaper, which shows his special connection. When the Delafaye family set up its business in distributing newspapers to subscribers, *The Post Man* was given prominent preference.[10]

De Fonvive had to co-operate with the culture of his English hosts. His most significant connections were with the publishing house of Richard Baldwin, with whom he co-operated all his life. It was this house that published the announcement, of a more personal character, of the death of De Fonvive on 1 February 1737, stating that he 'was a constant and generous benefactor of the poor.' The announcement in *The Gentleman's Magazine* was formal, but did show the importance that he had earned for himself amongst the London community.[11]

Along with the English intellectual John Toland, De Fonvive in 1720 purchased stock in the South Sea Company for the amount of £1000. From Toland's biography, we know that he did this in order to finance charitable activities.[12] Despite the economic crisis that hit England when the South Sea Company collapsed, accompanied by a tremendous number of bankruptcies, it seems that this most difficult blow did not affect De Fonvive's economic strength, either because he had promised to pay the full amount in a number of separate payments, or because his considerable property holdings enabled him to carry the loss. Concerning the charitable goals of his investment, it is significant that they were donated via Lord Molesworth, one of the very few amongst the Tory leaders who became involved with the Huguenot refugees, especially those that settled in Ireland.[13]

De Fonvive gained his status and property through his partnership in two journalism projects. When he first arrived as an immigrant to England, he started making a living as a hired translator, in the service of the publishing house of Richard Baldwin. Thanks to his talents and tremendous knowledge, he was involved in the first attempts of the publishing house to put out a new daily newspaper, and later to produce a newspaper published three times a week.

During this first stage, Baldwin co-operated with another publisher, A. Roper, who was the entrepreneur of the newspaper called *The Post Boy*. After collaborating on a number of joint issues, the partnership broke up. There is no clear reason for the split, but it seems that the different political ideologies – Baldwin was an extreme Whig, while Roper was an enthusiastic supporter of the Tory party – had something to do with it. In those days, support for immigration was one of the notable and known signs of the Whig party, and therefore the announcement of the editor of the pro-Tory newspaper, *The Post Boy* emphasizes the alien character of the newspaper writer: 'For that the author of the said Post Man and Historical Account is Monsiur de Fonvive'.[14]

The partnership between Baldwin and De Fonvive in publishing *The Post Man* began on 24 October 1695, a short time after censorship of the press was lifted, and continued until Baldwin's death in March 1698. When Baldwin was active, the main job of the writer was to translate information that came in from the Continent in the various French language papers, and this worked to De Fonvive's advantage. After Baldwin's death, his widow became the manager, but apparently the newspaper was not her highest priority, and in February 1699 it was printed by the publishing house of F. Leach, 'For the author'. From that moment, the writer was responsible for writing all sections of the paper, except for advertisements, which were the responsibility of the advertisers themselves.

There are many signs pointing to the fact that the connection between De Fonvive and the Baldwin house was maintained. Thus, one can find announcements concerning Anne Baldwin written in italics, a sign of an editorial announcement. The frequent advertisements of books published by Baldwin, which head the columns advertising printed matter, point to the fact that the publishing house of Baldwin continued to accept advertisements for the newspaper. When it was decided in July 1704 to initiate a French-language edition of the newspaper, it was openly announced that the initiative was that of the publishing house of Anne Baldwin, although the printer belonged to another house, apparently because of a shortage of printing presses for carrying out the project.

The ending of De Fonvive's direct partnership with Baldwin was very keenly felt in the editing of the newspaper. In Baldwin's time, one could find stimulating Whig writings, in a simple prose style that dealt with peripheral English issues. The difference between the two periods can be seen when we analyse the content of the papers. At various seasons of the year, storms in the English Channel prevented the arrival of mail from the Continent, mail which brought most of the sources of information, as well as the important French-language newspapers, published mainly in the Low Countries. During days without mail, the newspaper writer had to fill up the paper with more trivial articles, which may have been interesting, but were lacking in any important news from abroad. While in the Baldwin era, these articles dealt with English issues and with news from the court and Westminster, in De Fonvive's time these articles still dealt with European matters, commenting on such issues as the relationships between the rulers and the ruled, the chances of either side succeeding in the continuing Protestant-Catholic struggle, the position of the Huguenots in France and the situation on the various European war fronts.

As long as Baldwin himself took part in the actual writing, he gave expression to his Whig views. After his death, the content of the paper was the exclusive realm of the newspaper writer, De Fonvive, who became a partner, while production, distribution and management was provided by the original publishing house. This new ownership structure did not oblige the newspaper to support any declared political stand, despite the fact that doing so could have benefited the newspaper financially. To emphasize their political identity, party supporters would purchase the newspaper most closely identified with that party. Over the entire run of the newspaper, there were many other rival papers which openly identified with the Whigs. De Fonvive managed to create an image of a paper which maintained a middle-of-the-road approach, despite the fact that his pro-Whig tendency is very much evident: 'If like Fontvive 'tis with a just design to please government or serve the Qween'.[15]

The status of the paper granted it a very special journalistic advantage. Even Marlborough was aware of the advantages of being associated with it. As he wrote to Godolphin, 'If all truth may not be proper in the Gazette, I Desire the favor of you that during this campaign when I send you in your letter, as I do now, a paper of news, You will let it be inserted in the Post Man.'[16]

De Fonvive's journalistic activities were greatly appreciated amongst his professional colleagues, his contemporaries and the political establishment. This becomes clear in the references to him in the memoirs of J. Dunton[17] and in Daniel Defoe's notes in his own newspaper *The Review*.[18] In addition, De Fonvive was offered the editorship of *The London Gazette*.[19] His work was not universally admired, however. When Robert Harley fell from power at the Hanoverian Succession and was imprisoned in the Tower, he felt betrayed by the newspaper men, and expressed his anger against them. Among other things, Harley described De Fonvive as 'a little toothdrawer' who 'has got above £15,000 by news, by cheating the postage and having the common prints come franked'.[20]

Parallel with his editing *The Post Man*, De Fonvive was also busy promoting the news monthly *The Present State of Europe*, which was the translation of a monthly published in French at The Hague called *Mercure Historique et Politique*. This monthly continued to be produced in the years following De Fonvive's retirement from *The Post Man* and apparently relates to Jacques Serces, who wrote, 'A notre ami Mr. de Fonvive qui l'inserta dans la papier de nouvelles quil publie tous les mois'.[21]

Of all the Huguenot writers in England, De Fonvive was the only one with editorial independence. He took the difficult task on his shoulders to be the spokesman for the Huguenot refugees and to explain why the persecution they suffered in France caused them to violate their loyalty to their sovereign.

The political outlook of the Huguenots and the methods by which they desperately tried to make their case known to European leaders and to their own religious fellows, both in France and in the rest of the world, was established outside England and well before the appearance of *The Post Man*. Their standing in the European political and religious world, though, endangered their position in the eyes of the Tory party in England. Similar approaches were seen on the Continent, thus endangering their position with the nations that had absorbed them.

The Post Man was not meant to be a forum for intellectual debate, and De Fonvive's main role as writer was to report events and lead the readers to conclusions in accordance with the Huguenot spirit. His articles commented on the Huguenots' continuing loyalty to the 'legal' king of France, the criteria for citizenship in a society, and the proper relations between ruler and citizen.

There is a clear connection between the time during which the newspaper was written and the force of emotion and frequency of the coverage of the Huguenot issue. Until the end of the war, the great loyalty of the Huguenots is described in their service to the Duke of Savoy, with emphasis placed on the very respectful manner in which they retired from military service when the Duke signed a treaty with Louis XIV, and subsequently switched sides in the war. They swore that they would not take up arms against the Duke of Savoy, as a sign of appreciation of the sanctuary he had granted them. In contrast to this, the treachery of the Irish Catholics was emphasized, since they had defected to the winning side, fighting those who were helping them only the day before. While the war was being fought, the editing was done by Baldwin, and he was not at all hesitant about entering items concerning the Huguenots' contribution to the anti-French alliance, despite the fact that this could cause harm to their image as peaceable civilians. The translated items, which were De Fonvive's responsibility, were composed according to Huguenot political philosophy regarding the proper relation between ruler and citizen, and they added information regarding the great damage done to the French economy caused by the persecutions and the flight of the refugees.

From the conclusion of the war until the end of the 1698s, there is constant repetition of news dealing with the possibility of the repatriation of the refugees to France, based on the relaxation of the restrictions which Louis XIV had placed on them. During those years, the paper published many articles that created a parallel between the exile of the Jews in Babylon and their return to Zion, and the Huguenots' own exile. This was the propaganda developed by the Huguenot exiles in the Low Countries, which was distributed as words of consolation to the entire exile community. Only by December 1698 was it clear to all that the King of France did not intend to ease the situation of the Huguenots in France or to promise any conditions of repatriation to the refugees. From this point, the newspaper focuses on reporting the cruelty of the persecutions in France, the bitter fate of the Huguenot galley slaves, and the need to turn the lands of refuge into permanent homes. The editor makes a historical parallel between the persecutions in France and the Roman persecution of Christianity, which served as comfort and consolation, since everyone knew who ultimately won *that* conflict.

The closing years of the 17th century were especially exciting and it was only at this time, out of all the years of publishing, that there is a mystical explanation of, and belief in, heavenly guidance in the Huguenots' fate. The sobriety that later pervaded the paper made all its reports quite logical, and events were explained in ways that did not conflict with common sense. The intensity of reports of the persecution of the Huguenots was limited by the law that forbade insulting a friendly power. De Fonvive, who had been arrested for an investigation in the past, did not want to take any more chances, so he presented his reports in a way that could not be considered insulting or harmful.

From January 1702 the paper began to report on the rebellion in the Cévennes, but only some two years later did the editor make the connection between the Protestant faith and the rebellion. In the course of the War of the Spanish Succession, there were other uprisings of peoples under legal rule, but the report on the Cévennes revolt was more about human suffering than about the war itself. In 1705 reports about the rebellion cease, and the paper begins to focus on reporting on all the battle fronts, with an emphasis on the Spanish sector. This was because of the fact that the Allied commander was one of the most senior Huguenot refugees, Lord Galway, and many refugees from the Cévennes served under him.

During the war, the paper dealt with analysing methods of government rule in accordance with the criteria that political thinking had created in the past. The allied rulers received good evaluations, as their rule was based on a political contract and accepted the obligations of the state to its citizens, while at the same time the French and Spanish monarchs were described as unfit. In June 1705 it was claimed 'That the King is master of the body, but not of the soul',[22] and two years later the view was expressed 'That the despotick power of the king' negated the due 'submission, reverence and obedience of the subjects'.[23] Many such sentences and phrases were combined with newspaper reports, and they turned Huguenot political thinking into the collective property of the newspaper reading public in coffee-houses, in the street and at home. This public was not concerned with reading books dealing with political and religious thinking.

De Fonvive offered them more acceptable reading material about Europe and foreign events. By this skill he turned the newspaper into a profitable business that provided him with wealth, and even riches, within a short time. The economic prosperity enjoyed by De Fonvive asserts that hatred of the French and the xeno-phobia which characterized the English in those years had not prevented a gifted craftsman from becoming well established and absorbed into English society. Thus is a process which many of his compatriots had undergone, as in those years they had become a part of English commercial prosperity, on the threshhold of the Industrial Revolution.

NOTES

1 HSQS 27, 17.
2 PRO, Pennyman, 1737.
3 PRO, Pennyman, 1761.
4 *Calendar of Treasury books, 1705–06, pt. 3*, 715 (for 24 July 1706).
5 PRO, Portland MSS, vol. 8, 188.
6 *The Post Man*, for 9 December 1703, 11 December 1703.
7 W. H. Manchee, 'Huguenot London: the city of Westminster: Soho', *HSP* 14:2 (1931), 144–90.
8 *Ibid.*
9 A. P. Hands, 'Jean Cavalier: notes on the publication of the "Memoirs"', *HSP* 20:3 (1961), 341–71.

10 M. Harris, 'Newspaper distribution', in R. W. Hunt, I. G. Philip, R. J. Roberts (eds.), *Studies in the book trade: in honour of Graham Pollard* (Oxford, 1975), 139–45.

11 *The Old Whig or the Consistent Protestant* and *The Gentleman's Magazine,* for 3 February 1737.

12 *DNB,* for John Toland.

13 *DNB,* for Molesworth.

14 *The Post Boy,* for 29 October 1695.

15 *The Country Person's Advice,* for 11 August 1706.

16 H. Snyder (ed.), *The Marlborough–Godolphin correspondence* (3 vols., Oxford, 1975), vol. 1, for 6 May 1706.

17 John Dunton, *The life and errors of J.D. late citizen of London* (London, 1705), 249.

18 Daniel Defoe, *Review,* 1 March 1711.

19 PRO, Portland MSS.

20 BL, Portland Deposit, for 17 December 1715. For the idiom, see *Spectator* 358, for 21 April 1712.

21 HSQS 43, 21.

22 *The Post Man,* for 24 June 1705.

23 *The Post Man,* for 6 February 1707.

44

The birth of political consciousness among the Huguenot refugees and their descendants in England (*c.* 1685–1750)

Myriam Yardeni

Huguenot refugees in the era following the Revocation of the Edict of Nantes were assimilated in their different host countries through many channels – economic, social, demographic, religious and cultural.[1] In each country, this assimilation took a different form and followed a different pace.[2] Fastest in England, and slowest in Prussia, this pace was determined by a number of factors, e.g. the interaction between the elite culture of the host countries and that of the new immigrants from France and the capacity of the receiving countries to integrate the successive waves of Huguenots.[3] Important, too, in this process of assimilation was the role played by the secularization of the immigrants.[4]

In Prussia, it was the 'refugee' elites themselves who constituted the main obstacle to total assimilation, while in England these same elites, or at least a part of them, hastened the process. While in Prussia (and formerly in Brandenburg) the refugees enjoyed the status of a 'nation' among other nations, in England they were 'aliens' and not authorized legally to inherit property.[5] However, many of them became denizens or were naturalized in a relatively short space of time.[6]

As the English did not particularly suffer from an inferiority complex toward the refugees, the freshly-arrived French found that they had better learn the language of their new host country as quickly as possible. Some of them did this so well that they were able to achieve notable successes in the fields of culture and communication. The journalists Abel Boyer, Jean de Fonvive and Pierre des Maizeaux come to mind.[7] Outstanding achievements were also reached in the field of historical writing. Rapin Thoyras displayed a deep understanding of the way the British political system functioned and was able to stress the historical significance of the roots of English liberalism, which he discovered in remote Saxon institutions as well as in the love of freedom of the ancient Britons.[8] In this paper, I would like to argue that an important component of the cultural, but also of the social, assimilation of the Huguenots in

Britain was the birth and development among them of a new kind of political consciousness that stemmed from a better theoretical, as well as practical, knowledge of the functioning of British institutions, especially in the ways they were part of a special and illuminating history.

Political consciousness is not necessarily synonymous with politicization. Since its birth, French Protestantism was deeply involved in political issues. An often-cited item in the bibliographies of the French Wars of Religion is Rudolf Nürnberger's book *Die Politiesierung des französischen Protestantismus* (Tübingen, 1948). And it is no accident that the concepts of *politiques* and the *partie politique* are a sequel of the Wars of Religion, nor that Donald R. Kelley was able to establish a link between the beginning of ideology and French Protestantism.[9] In every existential crisis French Protestantism went through, the political aspects of the problems involved are in the forefront of discussion. These crises even constitute an important phase in the development of modern political thought,[10] from the pseudo-liberalism of the Monarchomachs[11] to the heated and enthusiastic defenders of absolutism and divine right.[12] It may not even be an exaggeration to view this phase of the politicization of French Protestantism as a prelude – though never more than that – to Habermas's public sphere.

This politicization was a direct outcome of the existential problems typical of French Protestantism – a movement which, despite the strong aristocratic-military presence within its ranks, and despite its aristocratic leadership during the Wars of Religion, continued to view itself as a minority group.[13] The concern was to discover which political regime would best ensure the movement's survival; this, in turn, may partly help to explain the opportunist switch in French Protestant political thought from 'liberalism' to absolutism and 'divine right' theories.

The birth of political consciousness in French Protestantism is a typical phenomenon of some of the diasporas, especially the one in England and, to a lesser degree, in the Netherlands.[14] It is the outcome of the opportunity the refugees had to compare different options and to make different choices, and the stress here is on the concept of choice, not only in theory, but also 'sur le vif'.

French Protestantism, and especially French Protestantism in the diaspora, approached such a situation for the first time in its history during the Civil War in England, though the problem involved as yet only a tiny elite of pastors, among them 'absolutists' such as Hérault and 'parliamentarians' such as La Marche.[15] But even then, a certain relativism concerning the best possible political system penetrates the heated discussions, as illustrated by the work of one of the most pre-eminent Huguenot controversialists of these years, Moyse Amyraut, who was usually a fervent supporter of royal absolutism: '[it is] just and reasonable that in England monarchy should be limited by the ancient laws of the state, and that the Parliament does well to seek to bring the king back to those limitations if he has really gone too far in encroaching on the rights and liberties of his people'.[16]

Things begin to change radically after the Glorious Revolution, especially during the reign of Queen Anne, when the Huguenots were confronted with the dilemma of how to keep the 'juste milieu' between the Whig convictions and sympathies most of them entertained and the 'duty' of praising a Tory government.

The situation is reminiscent of the tumultuous days of the Civil Wars and the Puritan Revolution. What had changed and created a radically new situation is the presence by this time of approximately 20,000–22,000 Huguenot refugees living in London, divided among some 33 churches, most of them recently founded.[17] Even more important, the French refugees found themselves surrounded by typical forms of British social life that were new to them, such as newspapers and London's coffee-house culture.[18]

For the refugees, this sociability was not yet an offspring of popular or mass culture. Neither is it the sole expression of an elite culture; the elite culture is that of a tiny number of pastors trying through their sermons to direct their flocks through the tortuous hazards of emigration, adaptation and assimilation.[19] Here we can witness the difficult slow birth of a new collective consciousness, promoted by tracts, pamphlets and newspapers in French and in English, in coffee-houses and in the animated discussions typical of the gatherings after the public worship in the Huguenot churches – gatherings feared by pastors who sought to reduce the antagonisms between the extrovert, vociferous Frenchmen and their quiet and more restrained English neighbours.

One of the important questions arising in the tracts, sermons, *journaux* and these fortuitous gatherings is the existence of the British party system and the problems it confronted the refugees with. How were they to behave in such a labyrinth? Should they sympathize with the Whigs, or keep aloof from British problems and stay neutral, or should they, *horribile dictu*, sympathize with the absolutist Tories?

The two best-known French specialists of the British party system, even if they never stayed in England permanently, are Paul de Rapin Thoyras and Emmanuel de Cizé. Thoyras is the well-known author of the *Dissertation sur les Whigs et les Tories*, first published in The Hague in 1717. Emmanuel de Cizé's *Histoire du Whiggisme et du Torisme* was first published at Leipzig in 1717 and then in The Hague in 1718. Both try to penetrate the mysteries of this typically English anomaly that was the party system, an unprecedented phenomenon in history. Perhaps this is the reason they are often unable to distinguish between 'party' and 'faction'. Two modern editors of their texts, Bernard Cottret and Marie Madeleine Martinet, stress correctly that for Rapin Thoyras and Cizé the emergence of the British party system is not a sign of modernity, but an anachronism, deeply rooted in a remote history.[20]

Nevertheless, the very existence of this party system and the possibility of the relatively peaceful co-existence of two 'factions' in the same state, poses problems. In order to answer the questions that arise, Rapin Thoyras and Cizé try to arrive at some generalizations. For both of them it is clear that there is a close relationship between the political conceptions and the religion of the Whigs, on the one hand, and those of the Tories on the other. Of course, they are aware of the fact that there are also exceptions to this rule. Generally speaking, for them the Whigs are Presbyterians and the Tories Episcopalians and even crypto-Catholics. Politically, the distinction between the two parties is equally sharp. Following Cizé, for the Whigs, 'tous les hommes sont nez libres, égaux et indépendants les uns des autres. Rien ne les a engagez à se soumettre au Gouvernement d'un ou de plusieurs de leur espèce, que le désir de vivre en paix et en sureté'.[21]

On the other hand, the principles of the Tories are the embodiment of the absolutism of Louis XIV, evoking strongly the thought that led to the Revocation of the Edict of Nantes: 'Dans le système des Toris, les Rois n'empruntent leur authorité que de Dieu, et par conséquent ils ne sont responsables qu'à lui de leur conduite, et de leur gouvernement . . . Que le Prince envahisse la liberté, qu'il détruise les privilèges, qu'il renverse la Religion de son peuple, il faut le souffrir patiemment'.[22] Rapin Thoyras reached similar conclusions in his work after leaving England in 1702.[23]

Even if it is not too difficult for us to guess where their sympathies lie, Rapin Thoyras and Cizé try to remain objective and unaffected by contemporary events and to frame their arguments in a historical and theoretical discourse. Their preferences and choices are implicit, and are based on moral considerations concentrating more on the individual than on the state. This provides the ideological background to the discussions that pervaded the Refuge in England during the first decades after the Revocation.

For more practical aspects of the birth of political consciousness among Huguenot refugees in England, let us now turn to some of the works of Jacques Abbadie and Jean Armand Dubourdieu.

Jacques Abbadie was one of the most outstanding theologians of his time.[24] Although his refugee itinerary took him through Prussia, the Netherlands, Ireland and England, he knew the English political scene well. His *Défense de la Nation Britannique*, published in 1693, is one of the many responses written against the famous absolutist *Avis important aux Réfugiés* attributed to Pierre Bayle and probably co-authored with his friend Daniel de Larroque.[25]

The *Avis* is scathing about the famous French 'esprit de révolte' and insubordination to legitimate kings, not to say insubordination to the divine right of kings. Abbadie rejects these invectives toward the refugees, who read 'avec plaisir les lardons et les gazettes qui contiennent de nouvelles désavantageuses à la France' and pleads in the name of 'cette liberté de parler' for the refugees to express their views and sentiments.[26]

The political views of Abbadie himself are those of the re-emerging monarchomach theories, strongly influenced by the newly reformulated contract theory: 'nous sommes des sujets et non point des victimes... nous obeissons à des Magistrats et non à des assasins publics'.[27] In every regard, the interests of the society and the collectivity precede those of the individual, even the king. This can be found not only in the theories of contract, but also in the Holy Scriptures: 'Non seulement l'Evangile ne demande point cet abandon des droits de la société, mais il promet principalement ses recompenses à ceus qui s'acquitent fidelement de leurs devoirs envers elle'.[28]

For Abbadie, freedom is one of the foundations of society, not just the 'liberté de conscience', but also the 'liberté d'expression', and even the liberty of free political choice. In this respect, the interests of society and those of the individual are the same, as demonstrated by the choice 'the British Nation' made at the Glorious Revolution.

Minister of the conformist church of the Savoy, Jean Armand Dubourdieu could be considered a second-generation Briton, as his father had also served as pastor in the same church. Dubourdieu states in his sermon *L'orgueil de Nebucadnetzar abbatu de la main de Dieu. Avec quelques Applications particulières aux affairs du temps* (1707), 'There are among us those who subscribe to the thesis of the power of kings; such extreme ideas have undermined our churches. Thanks to God, I did not study my theology concerning the power of kings in the works of Amyraut and Merlat, nor in the *Avis aux Réfugiés*, I have been nurtured since my childhood on the principles of liberty in a free country. I am French by birth, but in this respect I have an English heart'.[29]

Following Dubourdieu, what distinguishes a Frenchman in France from a Frenchman born in England is his attitude towards liberty: 'Qu'irions nous faire en France si la puissance arbitraire demeuroit au même point où elle est? Seroit-ce se servir de sa raison de quitter un pais libre, pour aller chercher des fers . . . j'aime mieux être exilé dans en pays libre, que d'être esclave dans ma patrie'.[30]

Dubourdieu deplores that there are still some 'absolutists among the refugees'. In the preface to his sermon *L'orgueil de Nebucadnetzar abbatu de la main de Dieu*, Dubourdieu, criticized by these fossils, writes that he has decided to reply to his detractors by bringing out the entire sermon for the public to judge.

In several other sermons, Dubourdieu continues to attack Louis XIV and absolutism by comparing the reigns of France and England. In these sermons, one can easily follow the metamorphosis of Dubourdieu into a citizen. What is more, Dubourdieu clearly tries to win over his audience and freedom and 'liberté' become key issues in his preaching. He even praises Archbishop Fénelon because of his love of freedom.[31]

Another important step comes with a pamphlet published in London in 1717, which carries the long title on its cover, *Apologie de nos Confesseurs qui etoient aux galères, au mois de Janvier 1714. Où l'on fait voir que le Sr. R—l a falsifié l'extrait qu'il a publié de leur lettre. Avec des réflexions sur un libelle du même auteur, intitulé, le Coup de Grace pour Mr. R—l.* The table of contents listed on the title page further reveals Dubourdieu's political agenda:

1. Ou l'on fait une Défence Abregée de la Révolution
2. On établit le Droit du Roi GEORGE à la Couronne.
3. On confond la Neutralité recommandée aux Réfugiez, par le Sr. R—l.
4. On justifie la mémoire de GUILLAUME le Libérateur.
5. On défend l'innocence des Protestans Réfugiez,
   Contre les dangereuses Hypotheses, et les
     Calomnies de cet Auteur,
   Avec un Examen du son prétendu Zele pour la Révolution.

I would like to stress one point which seems to me of primary importance, and this is Dubourdieu's attack on neutrality. Dubourdieu argues that the refugees must participate in public discussion and take a clear and unequivocal attitude – in favour of the Whigs, of course. He is scathing towards those who think that, as refugees, they ought always to follow the party of the ruler: 'Si dans l'année 1713 ou 1714 le parti Tory étoit le meilleur, et celui qu'il falloit préférer, parce que c'étoit celui de la Reine, il s'ensuit évidemment que quelques années auparavaut, c'étoit le mauvais parti, et celui qu'il falloit rejetter, parceque le parti opposé etoit celui de la Reine'.[32]

Dubourdieu attacks R—l, probably Pastor Rival,[33] who preaches political neutrality. For Dubourdieu, it is self-evident that the refugees must take a position in favour of the Whigs:

Considerez un peu le cas des Réfugiez: ils sont incorporés dans la Nation par la *Naturalisation*, capables des mêmes emplois, & admis aux mêmes Privileges que les *natifs*, en un mot ils sont compatriotes des *Anglois*, *Anglois* eux mêmes. Dans le tems qu'ils entrent dans le Corps de la Nation, ils la trouvent divisée par deux partis qui ont des principes opposés, & qui se proposent des fins toutes contraires. Un de ces Partis est l'ardent défenseur de la liberté & de la Religion Protestante, l'autre est une faction qui travaille à anéantir la Constitution *civile*, a introduire le pouvoir *Arbitraire*, & par une suite nécessaire, le *Papisme & l'Idolatrie*; s'il faut prendre parti, il n'est pas douteux le quel de ces deux partis là le Protestant François devenu *Anglois* doit choisir. En devenant Anglois ne s'est-il pas engagé à soutenir la Constitution de l'*Angleterre*? entreroit-il dans le Corps de cette nation pour le percer? seroit-ce répondre à l'intention de ces généreux Législateurs qui *passerent* en notre faveur l'Acte de la Naturalisation générale, que de se joindre à leurs ennemis? en un mot le François Protestant, & sur tout le François Protestant naturalisé ne doit-il pas agir de concert, & combattre méme avec les véritables Anglois, & si l'occasion s'en presente *vaincre ou perir avec eux.*[34]

The 'emancipation' of Dubourdieu – and that of the refugees – continues in another pamphlet, *Mephiboseth* (London, 1724). Here he criticizes severely the favourites and the flatterers: 'Après que l'ancienne Rome eut perdu sa liberté, on appeloit les favoris de l'Empereur amis de Caesar, et celui qui tenoit le premier rang dans la faveur, avoit le titre de cher ami, peut on prophaner plus indignement le sacré nom d'ami?'[35] In *Mephiboseth*, the naturalized refugees have not only the right but also the duty to criticize – they are now citizens and, what is more, they are citizens of England.

The way that leads to the birth of political consciousness among the Huguenot refugees in England – and at this stage perhaps mainly in London – includes the widening of both the concept and the sense of freedom. Freedom encompasses not only 'liberté de conscience' or 'liberté de culte'. It signifies the complete panoply of freedoms. Freedom ceases to be a privilege in order to become a civil right and even a human right. Paradoxically, from being a collective need 'freedom' becomes an individual state of mind. This is a slow, but irreversible process, hastening the assimilation and transformation of the refugees in England from strangers to citizens, not only as a collective, but also as individuals.

NOTES

1   M. Greengrass, 'Protestant exiles and their assimilation in early modern England', *Immigrants and Minorities* 4 (1985), 6–81.
2   M. Yardeni, *Le refuge protestant* (Paris, 1985).
3   W. C. Scoville, *The persecution of Huguenots and French economic development, 1680–1720* (Berkeley, 1960); S. Jersch-Wenzel, *Juden und 'Franzosen' in der Wirtschaft des Räumes Berlin-Brandenburg* (Berlin, 1971).
4   M. Yardeni, 'Assimilation et sécularization dans le Refuge', in Yardeni, *Refuge, assimilation et culture* (Paris, in press)
5   B. Cottret, *Terre d'exil: l'Angleterre et ses réfugiés 16e-17e siècle* (Paris, 1985), translated as *The Huguenots in England: immigration and settlement, c. 1550–1700* (Cambridge, 1991); Robin Gwynn, *Huguenot heritage: the history and contribution of the Huguenots in Britain* (London, 1985).
6   Greengrass, 73.
7   G. C. Gibbs, 'Abel Boyer Gallo-Anglus Glossographus et Historicus, 1667–1729: his early life 1667–1689', *HSP* 23 (1978), 87–98, Gibbs, 'Abel Boyer Gallo-Anglus Glossographus et Historicus: from tutor to author', *HSP* 24 (1983), 46–59; Gibbs, 'Huguenot contributions to the intellectual life of England, c.1680–c.1720, with some asides on the process of assimilation', in H. Bots and G. H. M. Posthumus Meyjes (eds.), *The Revocation of the*

Edict of Nantes and the Dutch Republic (Amsterdam, 1986), J. Almagor, *Pierre des Maizeaux (1673–1745), journalist and English correspondent for Franco-Dutch periodicals, 1700–1720* (Amsterdam, 1989); Itamar Raban, 'John Defonvive' (unpublished Ph.D. thesis, University of Haifa, 1991); see also his paper in this volume.

8   N. Girard d'Albissin, *Un précurseur de Montesquieu: Rapin Thoyras, premier historien français des institutions anglaises* (Paris, 1969); M. Yardeni, 'La tolérance rétrospective: la perception de l'histoire des Pays-Bas et de l'Angleterre dans le Refuge huguenot', in C. Berkvens-Stevelinck, J. Israel and G. H. M. Posthumus Meyjes (eds.), *The emergence of tolerance in the Dutch Republic* (Leiden, 1997), 251–67, esp. 259–66.

9   D. R. Kelley, *The beginning of ideology: consciousness and society in the French Reformation* (Cambridge, 1981).

10   Q. Skinner, *The foundations of modern political thought.* vol. 2: *The age of Reformation* (Cambridge, 1978).

11   In her *Le devoir de révolte: la noblesse française et la gestation de l'Etat moderne* (Paris, 1989), Arlette Jouanna places this 'liberalism' in the general context of the 'nobiliaire' ideology.

12   G. H. Dodge, *The political theory of the Huguenots of the Dispersion* (New York, 1947; reprinted 1972); E. Labrousse, 'The political ideas of the Huguenot diaspora', in R. M. Golden (ed.), *Church, state and society under the Bourbon kings* (Lawrence, KS, 1982), 222–83; M. Yardeni, 'French Calvinist political thought, 1534–1715', in M. Prestwich (ed.), *International Calvinism, 1541–1715* (Oxford, 1985), 315–37; J. C. Laursen (ed.), *New essays on the political thought of the Huguenots of the Refuge* (Leiden, 1995).

13   Yardeni, 'French Calvinist political thought'.

14   Yardeni, *Le refuge protestant.*

15   B. Cottret, *Terre d'exil*, 173–97.

16   Moyse Amyraut, *Apologie pour ceux de la Religion sur le sujet d'aversion que plusieurs pensent avoir contre leurs personnes et leur créance* (Saumur, 1647), 90.

17   Gwynn, 91–109.

18   L. Hanson, *The government and the press* (Oxford, 1967); J. A. Downie, *Robert Harley and the press: propaganda and public opinion in the age of Swift and Defoe* (Cambridge, 1979); M. Harris and A. Lee (eds.), *The press in English society from the seventeenth to the nineteenth centuries* (London, 1987); J. Black, *The English press in the eighteenth century* (London, 1987), Black, *Culture and society in Britain, 1660–1800* (Manchester, 1997).

19   M. Yardeni, 'Refuge et encadrement religieux de 1685 à 1715', in Yardeni (ed.), *Idéologie et propagande en France* (Paris, 1987), 117–24.

20   B. Cottret and M. M. Martinet, *Partis et factions dans l'Angleterre du premier XVIIIe siècle* (Paris, 1987), 11, 65.

21   Emmanuel de Cizé, *Histoire du Whiggisme et du Torisme* (The Hague, 1718), 3.

22   *Ibid.*, 13.

23   Girard d'Albissin, 19–20.

24   R. Whelan, 'From Christian apologetics to enlightened Deism: The case of Jacques Abbadie', *Modern Language Review* 87:1 (January 1992), 32–40.

25   Two of the most recent contributions to the controversy concerning the authorship of the *Avis important aux Réfugiés* are E. R. Briggs, 'Bayle ou Larroque? De qui est l'*Avis important aux Réfugiés* de 1690 et de 1692?' in M. Magdelaine, M.-C. Pitassi, Ruth Whelan and Antony McKenna (eds.), *De l'humanisme aux Lumières: Bayle et le protestantisme. Mélanges en l'honneur d'Elisabeth Labrousse* (Oxford, 1996), 509–24; Briggs, 'Daniel de Larroque (1660–1731), author of the *Avis important aux Réfugiés* of 1690 and the beginning of the truly modern Europe', in J. Häseler and A. McKenna (eds.), *La vie intellectuelle aux Refuges protestants* (Paris, 1999), 203–26.

26   Jacques Abbadie, *Défense de la nation britannique, ou les droits de Dieu, de la nature et de*

    la société clairement établis, au sujet de la révolution de l'Angleterre (The Hague, 1693), 81, 3.

27   *Ibid.*, 186.

28   *Ibid.*, 154–5.

29   Jean Armand Dubourdieu, *L'orgueil de Nebucadnetzar abbatu de la main de Dieu. Avec quelques applications particulières aux affaires du temps, ou sermon sur Daniel, ch. IV, vers 29, 30, 31, 32, prononcé dans l'Eglise Françoise de la Savoye, le jour solennel de l'Action de Graces, le 31 décembre, 1706* (London, 1707), préface, a2, r-v.

30   *Ibid.*, a4, r-v.

31   'Je scai que ce *Prélat* étoit un genie Superieur; mais je sais sur tout consister la Superiorité de son esprit, en ce qu'il a senti le poids de ses charmes, quelques honorables qu'on les eût rendües en les couvrant des plus éminentes Dignités, que par ses Réflexions particulières, il a surmonté les préjugez de la Naissance & de l'éducation, qu'il a reconnu que la liberté étoit l'appanage de tous les Hommes, que la Servitude des Peuples étoit une Usurpation des Rois. *Prélat* à jamais digne de nos éloges, digne des éloges de la Posterité en ce qu'il est le seul François de nôtre tems, qui dans le sein du Royaume, ait osé confier au papier ses idées sur le Gouvernement, & à qui cet égard ait donné des Signes de vue & des marques de Liberté'. Jean-Armand Dubourdieu, *La faction de Grande Bretagne* (London, 1716), 14.

32   J.-A. Dubourdieu, *Apologie de nos confesseurs qui étoient aux galères* (London, 1714), 46.

33   On Rival, E. and E. Haag, *La France protestante*, 10 vols. (Paris, 1846–1859; reprinted Geneva, 1967).

34   Dubourdieu, *Apologie*, 145.

35   Dubourdieu, *Mephiboseth: ou Le caractère d'un bon sujet. Sermon sur le II. livre de Sam. Ch. XIX. v. 30* (London, 1724), 24.

45

The Huguenots in Britain, the 'Protestant International' and the defeat of Louis XIV

Robin Gwynn

'A greater opportunity I think was never offered', wrote Henry Compton, Bishop of London on 8 February 1682 to Henry Savile, English Ambassador in Paris at the time of the dragonnades, 'to establish our interest with the Protestants abroad, stren[g]then ourselves and weaken our enemies'.[1] He was referring to the reception of Huguenot refugees in England, and went on: 'But so it is, the poor people have not that encouragement in some parts, as is fit. However I do assure you, there are so many [Englishmen] just to our common interest and the Protestant Religion that they [the refugees] will never want due encouragement'.

This paper springs from an on-going attempt to assess whether Bishop Compton's optimism was justified, and is a progress report on some ways in which the Huguenots contributed to the 'Protestant International', and to Britain's ability to withstand the might of Louis XIV's France over the quarter century from 1689 to 1713. As the opening quotation makes clear, Bishop Compton would have been comfortable with the phrase, the 'Protestant International'. It is a term used by Herbert Lüthy, and recently resumed by the North American historian J. F. Bosher, in considering the significance of a cosmopolitan Protestant diaspora in which merchants were one of the key elements.[2] I will use the term in a somewhat wider sense, because there were other cosmopolitan links – military and diplomatic, for instance – binding together the Huguenot refugees.

How acceptable the term may be to current historians of later Stuart Britain is a moot point. It fits well with Tony Claydon's exploration of the Protestant aspect of William III's propaganda,[3] and a recent thesis by Sugiko Nishikawa argues convincingly that it was not until the early 18th century that the Church of England 'lost the sense that it was a pillar of the Reformed religion in Europe and departed from Protestant internationalism'.[4] On the other hand Steven Pincus, while arguing that Englishmen were not as insular and inward-looking as has often been supposed, perceives a secularizing trend and concludes that 'by the later 17th century most political observers believed the age of religious wars had passed'.[5] In any case, it is only comparatively recently that English historians have developed an appreciation of the importance of Scottish and Irish happenings for events in England, and they may not be ready to take on the full implications of the Protestant International. Their tendency during the 20th century was to ignore the Huguenots.[6] It will be interesting to see whether that changes in the new century.

From the perspective of the Huguenot refugees of the 1680s, England was very much a full member of the European-wide Protestant community that had been engaged in a long battle against Catholicism since the Reformation, a battle that now seemed to be coming to a climax. Thousands of them, indeed, went to war as soldiers. [A new resource on the military aspect of the Protestant International now lodged in the Huguenot Library at University College, London, is a card index prepared by Dr George Hilton Jones. This index identifies over 1,400 individual Huguenot officers in the service of the British crown under William and Anne. Because a very high percentage of these attained reasonable seniority, it is likely that many other officers of lower rank disappeared without trace. Perhaps up to 2,500 Huguenots served as officers under William and Anne in British service. Warren Scoville cites Marshal Vauban's contemporary estimate that France lost 500 or 600 army officers and 10,000 to 12,000 soldiers.[7] For the officers at least, that estimate seems clearly too low.]

The focus of this paper is the French Church of London in Threadneedle Street, the oldest and largest of the 47 Huguenot churches (including 28 in and around the capital) that existed in England by the year 1700. I will argue that its consistory is an overlooked 'missing link', the study of which can shed light on a number of areas of dispute amongst historians that have to do with the Protestant International. The excellent records for this particular church enable identification of all its lay officers in the later 17th century, even if sometimes we know little about them. If only similar records survived for the Savoy church and its annexe l'Eglise des Grecs, the largest and best connected West End Huguenot church! They would make a fascinating comparison: but because key evidence for those congregations had already been lost by 1717,[8] we know far more about the Huguenots of the City and east London than about those in the western suburbs. The conclusions which follow are based on a biographical study of the lay officers at Threadneedle Street investigating family links, work activities, political leanings and where relevant their French background, as well as the work they did for the church.

Reasonably enough, we normally view the Huguenot churches as ecclesiastical organizations, fulfilling their prime aim that God should be worshipped. I want to focus on different, informal functions the consistory fulfilled, in social, economic and political terms. By 'social' terms, I am here thinking of an aspect of the consistory that is normally ignored: its function as a social meeting place and marriage market.

During the half century from 1650 to 1700, 289 laymen served the Threadneedle Street church as elders or deacons. Until March 1688 there were normally 13 elders and 13 deacons at any one time; from then on, 18 of each. The deacons were younger, and having served their term of office, then provided the pool of experienced men from whom the eldership could be selected. Normally both deacons and elders were drawn from significant families in the community. There are hints that around 1670 the quality of the diaconate was briefly in decline,[9] but the social quality of the elders was invariably high.

The Threadneedle Street consistory (using the term here to include both the

Company of Ministers and Elders, and the Company of Deacons) comprised no ordinary group of people. In this 50-year period it included one Physician-General to the Fleet (Paul de Laune); several 'disaffected and suspicious persons' arrested at the time of Monmouth's rebellion; two men (Pierre Barr I, Guillaume Carbonnel) whose remittances and notes of credit delivered Louis XIV's subsidy to Charles II; two (Jean Dubois, Thomas Papillon) who became Members of Parliament; two 'sworn operators to the king's teeth' (George Gosselin, Pierre Blanchers dit de la Roche); one (Joseph Ducasse) who was the sole attendant on Algernon Sidney on the scaffold (and married his daughter); four Upper Bailiffs of the Weavers' Company;[10] two men convicted by Parliament and fined for trading with France during wartime (René Baudouin, Etienne Seignoret); at least a dozen Common Councilmen of London;[11] one foundation Director, one later Governor and 18 initial subscribers to the Bank of England in 1694;[12] and many wealthy merchants and stock dealers.

In the largest consistories in France in the last generation before the Revocation, at Lyon for instance, the elders were increasingly drawn from the best-off families, 'who naturally, often united their children'.[13] So it was in London, where threads of family relationship interwove through the consistory. Pierre Baudry, an elder in the late 1680s, was the son of Jacques Baudry (I), who had served as an elder in the 1640s and the 1660s. He was the younger half brother of Jacques Baudry (II), an elder in the late 1670s. He was the brother-in-law of Nicolas Wicart, another elder in the 1670s, and brother-in-law also of Samuel d'Espagne, who died while in office as elder in 1682. And he married his eldest daughter Lea to Jean, son of Jean Bazin who had served as an elder.

Or consider the substantial merchant[14] and insurance underwriter[15] Claude Hays, son of an *honnorable homme* of Calais,[16] a man whose work was vitally important to the refugees of the early 1680s while he was serving his first term as elder.[17] He married the daughter of David Cognard, an elder in the 1670s. His half-brother Daniel Hays came to England in 1688 and became an elder of the Threadneedle Street church in the 1690s, the same decade as Claude's own son (another Claude) served as a deacon. Claude Hays senior was also the brother-in-law of David Cognard junior, a deacon in the late 1680s. And he married one of his daughters to David Bosanquet and another to Jean de Neu; both became officers of the church in the 1690s.

In the case of the Hays–Cognard–Bosanquet–De Neu connection, the threads of relationship were threads of gold. The consistory had a formidable concentration of wealth and mercantile experience. One indication of wealth is how many of the church officers born abroad either became denizens, or were naturalized – processes that could prove time-consuming, troublesome and expensive, and which there was no point anyone undertaking unless he feared difficulties in passing on money, goods or property. Of the 289 church officers, 189 were certainly born abroad, and 80 per cent of them were definitely endenized or naturalized. Clearly, then, this was a monied group of people. Contrast the Dutch Church of London of the first half of the century, itself far from poor, in which only half the officers had had full or partial English citizenship.[18]

The consistory was in fact very rich indeed. As the period went by, it became increasingly dominated by merchants, who comprised just over half (53 per cent) of church officers with known trades in the 1650s, but nearly four-fifths (79 per cent) by the 1690s. This greater wealth was the direct result of persecution in France. Of those who had become officers of the church before the end of the century, 35 arrived before the Revocation, between 1673 and 1684. (1673 has been taken because that was the year in which the Calais representatives at the Synod of Charenton declared their church was overburdened by the number of refugees already heading for England.)[19] These people stood a better chance of escaping with their capital more or less intact than did later fugitives. Of those 35, 17 came from the major centres of Paris and Rouen. From Paris in this category came François Ammonet, reputed by the French police to be worth 400,000 livres,[20] whose personal goods included 700 oz. of plate,[21] and who became an immediate if short-lived gentleman of the Privy Chamber to Charles II;[22] Louis Berchere, whose son James Louis Berchere became a merchant jeweller or banker in Broad Street estimated to be worth £120,000;[23] and Louis Gervaise, the inspiration behind the foundation of the Royal Lustring Company.[24] The Rouen contingent included Robert le Platrier, who was later joined by his father Jean, merchant, goldsmith, and secretary of the Rouen Consistory. These 35 arrivals also included René Baudouin from Tours, estimated in the 1690s to be worth £315,000;[25] Pierre Lombard from Nîmes, who although described as a tailor was destined to marry a daughter to the younger brother of the Prime Minister, Robert Walpole; and other important merchants with large turnovers like Jacques du Fay from Boulogne, Etienne Noguier from Nîmes and Pierre Renu from Bordeaux.

Another of the 35, Pierre Serrurier, provides an example of a man preparing for his family's exodus. He came in 1682 from St Quentin, where the Le Serruriers were second only to the Crommelins as Protestant merchants. Pierre was the son of Jacques Le Serrurier, a long-standing elder of the St Quentin church, and on 28 September 1685 the local intendant, Chauvelin, reported to Louis XIV:

> Jacques Le Serrurier, marchand de toille, left for London about eight months ago to find a son whom he had set up there. He left his wife [Elizabeth Leger] at St Quentin to gather together all his goods. She left on the 18th or 19th of this month, taking with her all their children and Serrurier's brother, an old bachelor. Their only real estate is the house where they live.[26]

An unscientific 'top ten wealth list' drawn from the church officers across the 50 years might include:

- Pierre BARR from Rouen, whose mercantile activities ranged from the Baltic to the West Indies, and who passed on over £50,000 of Louis XIV's subsidy to Charles II.[27]
- David BOSANQUET from Lunel, a Levant merchant with assets worth £100,000 on his death in 1732.[28]
- Pierre BULTEEL, London born, 'one of the first and best sort of men' in a listing of the principal inhabitants of London in 1640.[29] His son Samuel became a Director of the Bank of England (1697).
- Pierre DELMÉ of Canterbury, whose son Sir Peter was to become Governor of the Bank of England and Lord Mayor of London and to be worth over £300,000 on his death in 1728.[30]
- Daniel HAYS of Calais, Assistant of the Royal African Company, who disposed of £90,000 to members of his family.[31]
- Pierre LE KEUX of Canterbury with his 'very great acquaintance with many

Lords and Commons',[32] who married the daughter of 'rich old Mr [Peter] Marisco', brother of

- Charles MARESCOE of Lille, agent for the Dutch-dominated Swedish tar company, who 'combined East Indian shipping interests with exchange dealings and building speculation'.[33]
- Herman OLMIUS of Lochem, 'a prominent Bank stock proprietor, and one of the commissioners of the Bank subscription of 1709', who purchased Waltham Bury, Essex, from the Earl of Manchester in 1701.[34]
- Thomas PAPILLON, born in Roehampton, who became MP for London and First Commissioner to the Victualling Office under William III.
- Etienne SEIGNORET of Lyon, officially estimated to be worth between £80,000 and £100,000 in the 1690s, who had the largest individual holding in the Million Bank by 1701.[35]

It is a formidable list, and the wide range of places from which these ten people came underlines the way in which the consistory brought together the trading interests of the whole known world. Four of them were born in England. The continuing connection in the church between refugees of a previous generation and newcomers is important. It was not new. Researching the church in the earlier 17th century, Charles Littleton concluded that continued involvement with the French Church of London and growing integration into the English host community were not alternatives, but rather went hand in hand.

> Descendants of immigrants, and frequently long-standing original immigrants themselves, were able to move back and forth between their stranger and English identities quite easily. Rapid and successful integration into English society did not necessarily entail for these immigrants and their children a concomitant abandonment of the French Church and [community]. The elite of the French Church extensively married among themselves, but that does not mean that these intermarrying aliens did not participate in English life or become integrated into the English elite.[36]

What Littleton demonstrates with the De Launes can likewise be demonstrated with successful families like the Delmés, Dubois, Houblons and Papillons. Indeed, the church and its consistory were meeting places where new ideas, money and skills blended with older-established English connections. Wealthy attenders maintained their contacts at the church even while they integrated into English society and ceased to participate as elders and deacons. Thus Thomas Papillon never served as an elder; his one period in office was as deacon, between 1656 and 1659. But he continued to attend services when he could, and in 1699 was allowed special arrangements for receiving communion in his seat on account of his gout. When he died in 1702, he left £100 to the poor of the church and £25 to each of its ministers.[37] Nor can one doubt the reality of his Christian commitment. When in his seventies, and run off his feet as First Commissioner for Victualling the Navy during wartime, he noted

> the whole Old Testament was read over beginning the 17 June 1692, and ending the 26 August 1694, being 2 years, 2 months, 9 days – which makes 795 days. There is in the Old Testament, besides the Psalms, 779 chapters, the 16 days difference comes by reading other Scripture sometimes, on Sacrament days, and on special occasions.[38]

His friend Jean Dubois, born in Canterbury, with whom Papillon had served as a deacon and who like him later became a Member of Parliament, did serve as an elder (1670–2), as did the English-born brothers Jean and Pierre Delmé.

The only member of the Houblon family to hold office in this period was Pierre Houblon junior, a deacon 1651–4, but the Houblons continued to take a very active interest in the affairs of the French church. When Sir John Houblon was chosen as Lord Mayor in 1695, the delighted consistory took the unprecedented step of making a special separation in the ministers' pew to seat him. Over a decade later, he was an important channel of communication with the English authorities on charity distribution and the French 'prophets'.[39] In 1702, Isaac Houblon left £100 to the poor of the Threadneedle Street church and another £200 for Huguenot refugees more generally. His brother Abraham, as executor, entrusted the distribution of both sums to the elders, and it is significant that he knew the poor well enough to make specific recommendations about individuals when handing over the money. Sir James Houblon also left £50 to the poor in 1704.[40] These continuing connections between the descendants of old refugees and new arrivals are important, and show that historians like François Crouzet are unwise in seeking to insist on too sharp a difference between Walloons and Huguenots, or between refugees of the first and subsequent generations.[41]

Such connections also bear on the Huguenot/Walloon role in the foundation of the Bank of England. The tendency for the last generation of historians has been to play it down, and to argue that contemporaries greatly exaggerated it. But after preliminary work on original subscribers to the Bank of England in 1694, I am interested in differences between those of whom I took note and those whom P. G. M. Dickson, author in 1967 of the seminal book *The financial revolution in England*, considered 'Huguenot'. (I know whom he considered in this category because of his generosity in making his working notes available to me 24 years ago.) Surely men attending the French Church of London and serving as its officers in the 1680s and 1690s must have been viewed by their English contemporaries as French, and should be viewed by modern historians as such. David Primerose and Aaron Testas were current ministers of the church when the Bank was launched, and subscribed in 1694; but neither came into Dr Dickson's calculations. Jean Delmé, Jean de Neu and Humfroy Willet had all served as elders in the 1680s, and likewise subscribed in 1694, but they too are excluded. The reason has to do simply with definitions, but it suggests that this subject needs re-evaluation. What is certain is that two ministers and 16 lay officers of this one church (not necessarily in office in 1694 itself) were foundation subscribers to the Bank.

It cannot be argued for London, as Jon Butler has done with regard to New York,[42] that there is no evidence of the 'specific influence of religion in business matters'. It was only natural for a community of inter-related merchants to discuss business, and there is positive evidence that commercial discussion did take place. The Threadneedle Street church was instrumental in the formation and settlement of communities in Ipswich and Rye, for instance; it had to find ways of ensuring that the churches and settlements survived. It organized payments of money to the *galériens* at Marseilles, which required mercantile expertise. A striking example of a commercial development that can only be put down to discussion within the consistory is found in letters patent issued to Francis Ammonett, Claude Hayes and Daniel du Thais in 1682 for the manufacture of draped milled stockings.[43] These three men are not known associated together in any other venture. Ammonet was born in Paris, Hays in Calais, Du Thais in Plymouth. Du Thais had been in England for over 20 years, perhaps all his life, whereas Ammonet was a recent arrival. The only thing these three had in common was that they were all elders at Threadneedle Street in 1682, when the patent was taken out.

Not only were commercial matters discussed, but the consistory of the French Church of London – like its peers in Amsterdam and elsewhere – was an economic powerhouse. Consider the nature of mercantile activity in the later 17th century. A merchant did not need an M.B.A. He needed some liquid assets; these men possessed them. He needed a network of contacts on whom he could rely for advice on cargoes and accurate analysis of markets and individual credit ratings; the Huguenot diaspora provided a network second to none. He needed to be active and motivated; as refugees, these people were both. He needed to be esteemed as trustworthy; who was to be trusted more than those who had run the gauntlet for the sake of their beliefs? The Huguenot refugees had exceptional advantages in all these respects, and in an environment like the London consistory they also had access to the one crucial missing ingredient, local knowledge and support.

The work of D. W. Jones has greatly advanced our understanding of the way in which London trade became 'thoroughly cosmopolitanized' in the 1690s, as Huguenot and other merchant migrants of the 1680s gained a significant share of London's export trade. There was a particularly marked change in exports of old draperies; only 5 per cent of such exports were handled by naturalized or endenized foreigners in the 1680s, 32 per cent or more by 1695.[44] Jones has also shown that the Huguenots were especially important in the Million Bank.[45] The one common factor he perceives in the changes of the 1690s is the importance of wine merchants. However, the present study of an interconnected consistory which was a monolithic Whig bloc suggests that progress can also be made in understanding the implications of political loyalties and genealogical ties.

Naturally, the church officers were profoundly opposed to Louis XIV's activities. They were well informed, and the latest news was eagerly discussed after services; one such discussion landed the church in trouble with the Court, after unguarded exclamations of support for rebellion against the French crown in 1683 were reported to the authorities, just as the Rye House Plot was discovered in England.[46] Apart from news from refugees and from newsletters, many members of the consistory had themselves had unpleasant experiences. Pierre de la Bale had been threatened with arrest in Rouen.[47] Abraham du Gard (I) had been arrested with his wife in France while trying to escape, and suffered severely financially.[48] David Garrick's mother had experienced a particularly unpleasant voyage in making her escape, while his brother died almost immediately after reaching England.[49] Jean Gervaise (I) had been imprisoned, and lost his wife, who abjured. His son, Jean Gervaise (II), probably also suffered imprisonment.[50] Jean de Grave was subjected to the dragonnades – so many soldiers were quartered on him that the charge was 20 crowns a day, then yet more were sent – and forced into hiding before making his escape.[51] Adrien Lernou (I) had been subjected to the dragonnades at Calais, and his son Adrien (II) imprisoned.[52] François Mariette had had houses and vineyards seized to the value of 90,000 livres.[53] Jean le Motteux's father (unless it was he himself) had been forced to abandon five properties around Rouen, and Jean le Platrier had likewise had two houses seized there.[54] Jean Strang had been imprisoned.[55]

Such men needed no persuasion about the reality of the threat posed to the Protestant cause by Louis XIV. Some modern historians have persuaded themselves that Louis was a fundamentally tolerant man who was 'against forced conversions'.[56] The consistory members would have replied that from first hand experience, they knew better. It was not only the French King's designs within France that were of concern. Louis had been guilty of aggression in the 1667 and 1672 wars, and seemed particularly threatening to the whole of Europe between 1678 and 1684. Apart from the Revocation, he was engaged in the 1680s in the destruction of the Palatinate. There was justifiable concern too about the persecution of Protestants that Louis foisted on the Duke of Savoy in Piedmont[57] and events in Orange.[58] In this the church officers simply mirrored the hatred and fear of Louis XIV – 'that savage man', as Lady Rachel Russell called him[59] – prevalent in England. But their constant representations of the refugees' need helped promote an awareness of the Huguenot condition that reverberated in even the most remote areas of England. That was disastrous for James II's policies to assist his Catholic co-religionists because, as the agent Bonrepaus reported to the French Court early in 1686,[60] religion was the pivot round which public affairs revolved in James's reign. It helped prepare fertile ground for the Revolution.

Even more disastrous for James was the flood of refugees that came to England during his reign, all the more since it is now clear that the peak of their arrival was not 1685, as historians have commonly assumed, but mid-1687, just months before the Revolution.[61] Nothing could have been more calculated to undermine James II's relations with his subjects, who equated popery with arbitrary government and feared they might find themselves in the same predicament as the Huguenots. The consistory – while putting nothing down on paper – clearly played a planning role in preparing the ground for refuge. The key connection seems to have been with Paris. François Ammonet was elected elder almost immediately after he arrived in England. But he did not come direct from Paris, where his house became used for (illegal) consistory meetings. He came via Holland, where he helped persuade the Dutch authorities to grant privileges to Huguenot refugees. After he died in 1683, Louis Gervaise (II), a deacon in London in 1684–7, became the contact; French police reported that he regularly revisited Paris to confer with his father and other elders of Charenton on Huguenot matters.[62]

Less obvious than their hatred for Louis XIV, but no less significant, is the political orientation of the church officers within England. It was a subject on which the consistory as a body tried not to expose itself, for at the best of times it was undesirable for the church, a refugee church ultimately dependent on the good will of the authorities of the day, to be drawn into politics. And times were rarely the best. But we have seen how the church leaders as individuals combined their roles in the French church and in English society. The huge majority were English citizens, whether by birth or through their own action. They could not avoid involvement in the English political scene, and some of them did not wish to.

The uniformity on political matters within the ruling elite of the French Church of London is startling. If there is an alternative polarity, one would have to look for it in Westminster, and the unsatisfactory nature of the records for the Savoy makes that impossible. With regard to Threadneedle Street, the situation is as close to being black and white as a historian is ever likely to find in looking at a substantial body of people over a 50-year period. At the time of the English Civil War, the church had been the site of an extraordinary spectacle. Alternating in the pulpit were Louis Hérault from Alençon, a strong royalist who believed in the divine right of kings, and the Channel Islander Jean de la Marche, a violent parliamentarian who was already calling for the execution of Charles I in 1645. While there were many who thought De la Marche went far too far, Hérault had virtually no support whatever; isolated, he had quickly to retreat to the Continent. The consistory was almost entirely composed of parliamentarians, whether moderate or extremist.[63]

Hérault was recalled by royal order at the Restoration, but continued to find little support. 'De la Marche was dead', he reported to the Court, 'but not his spirit'.[64] Isolated again, Hérault was forced to withdraw once more, after a furious spat in which he did his best to blacken the consistory in the eyes of the authorities. Hérault exaggerated, but his perception that at heart the church officers at Threadneedle Street were no friends to the Court was valid enough. In the last quarter of the 17th century there are many who were clearly Whigs, but not one whom the evidence assembled to date suggests to have been a Tory.

Under the conditions of the 1680s, that meant that as well as being wealthy, socially important, and possessed of some local power and consequence, the members of the consistory were also frightened. They were fearful for the London church, fearful for the Protestant cause in England and Europe, in some cases frightened for their personal wellbeing. Fear is one of the greatest motivating forces, and it does not loom large enough in what historians – aware that in the event, the Revolution of 1688–9 passed with negligible bloodshed in England – have written about the 1680s.

Remember, then, that many of the elders if not the deacons had lived through the Civil War in England, that some officers had first-hand recent experience of persecution in France, and that all of them were being reminded week by week as events unfolded across the Channel of what the power of the state could mean for them in Catholic hands. Recall the state's power of imprisonment, torture and execution, the Catholic James II's accession to the throne, and the barbarity of Judge Jeffries's sentences in 1685 at the time of Monmouth's rebellion. Consider the conscious suppression by James II of works describing the plight of Protestants in France, the extraordinary silence of the *London Gazette* in the face of the Revocation, the burning by the public hangman of Jean Claude's *Account of the Persecutions and Oppressions of the Protestants in France* and the arrest of its translator. This is the background against which the members of the consistory had to operate in the 1680s, in the uncomfortable knowledge that the church's past history could be used against them, and that Hérault's outbursts made them a continued object of suspicion. They were, indeed, frightened. Only fear can explain the complete absence of any reference in the consistory minutes[65] to either the Revocation of the Edict of Nantes, or a threatened Quo Warranto against their own church.[66]

Four past or present church officers were arrested and detained at the time of Monmouth's rebellion in 1685, Guillaume Carbonnel, Pierre Houblon, Jacques de Neu and Humfroy Willet, while Isaac (II) de Lillers had his premises searched.[67] The following year a deacon, Pierre Fauconnier, was arrested and his house was searched.[68] The whole church must have uttered a collective sigh of relief at the time of the Revolution. Thomas Papillon could return from Holland, where he had spent much of the 1680s in exile under duress. Joseph Ducasse, who had attended Algernon Sidney on the scaffold, was now able openly to plead his master's case. The censorship which had prevented immediate publication of the situation in France was relaxed. And the consistory could hope that it would no longer be so embarrassed by heavy-handed Court reaction to the English political involvement of its members.

What then can we conclude from this study? On the military side, contemporaries rightly argued that Huguenots would be useful and unswervingly loyal in William's service,[69] and it is known that Huguenot contacts were used as channels of communication between England and Holland in the months before William's invasion.[70] Highly motivated officers who had been trained in the best European army of the day arrived in large numbers, and were crucial in filling the gap left by the many English officers (perhaps two-thirds of the total)[71] who resigned rather than fight against their previous commander-in-chief James II. The victories in Ireland were vital in cementing the Glorious Revolution, and it was Huguenots and Dutch rather than English that bore the brunt of the fighting there.[72]

As for the Threadneedle Street consistory, it is a necessary piece of the jigsaw for any historian trying to piece together what was happening in later Stuart England, and central for anyone seeking to understand the Huguenot influx or assess the significance of the contribution made by the refugees. Those who have written on financial matters have tended to assume that the Huguenot refugees came into a void. Merchants, at least, did not. In the French Church of London they were received into an active, fully functioning, An\glo-European institution of the Protestant International. We have seen that the consistory was a meeting place, where new ideas, skills and resources could blend with older-established English connections, where kin ties could be developed with fellow strangers as well as with Englishmen, where political leanings could be made firm. Kinship and religion and trade and politics were not separate matters, they were closely inter-related, each an integral part of the Protestant International. In recent years historians of the Huguenots have been advancing divergent hypotheses. Since Scoville, there has been a strong minimalist school which wants to downplay the Huguenot impact; Professor Crouzet is its most prominent current exponent.[73] My study of the consistory, and Dr Jones's of Huguenot officers, would suggest that the minimalist school has gone too far, and that its foundations are shakier than its advocates believe.

In recent times, too, historians have tended to downplay the importance of religion. It is good that Professor Bosher has breathed new life into the concept of the Protestant International, a concept supported by the nature and activities of the Threadneedle Street consistory. One thing at least is clear: by their actions, the Huguenot refugees turning up in England (as elsewhere) showed that they had no part in what Emile-G. Léonard once called French 'Protestantism in lethargy'.[74] These, on the contrary, were people for whom Protestant belief had living force. Bolingbroke was not far off the mark when, in a memorial to the Pretender James III in August 1715, he saw 'the whole body of the French refugees' as 'more desperate and better disciplined than any other class of men in England', and the most ready at once to oppose Jacobite invasion.[75]

NOTES

1 LPL, MS 1834, fo. 21r.
2 Herbert Lüthy, *La Banque Protestante en France de la Révocation de l'Édit de Nantes à la*

Révolution (2 vols., Paris, 1959–61), vol. 1, vii; J. F. Bosher, 'Huguenot merchants and the Protestant International in the seventeenth century', *The William and Mary Quarterly*, 3rd ser., 52:1 (1995), 77–100. Ole P. Grell uses a similar term with relation to the 16th-century Protestant diaspora in his essay 'Merchants and ministers: the foundations of international Calvinism' in O. P. Grell, *Calvinist exiles in Tudor and Stuart England* (Aldershot, 1996), 98–119.

3   Tony Claydon, *William III and the Godly Revolution* (Cambridge, 1996), esp. chap. 4.

4   Sugiko Nishikawa, 'English attitudes toward Continental Protestants with particular reference to church briefs, *c.* 1680–1740' (unpublished Ph.D thesis, University of London, 1998), 130.

5   Steven C. A. Pincus, *Protestantism and patriotism: ideologies and the making of English foreign policy, 1650–1668* (Cambridge, 1996), 449.

6   Robin D. Gwynn, 'Patterns in the study of Huguenot refugees in Britain: past, present and future' in Irene Scouloudi (ed.), *Huguenots in Britain and their French background, 1550–1800* (Basingstoke, 1987), 219–36.

7   Warren C. Scoville, *The persecution of Huguenots and French economic development 1680–1720* (Berkeley, CA, 1960), 13. Charles E. Lart believed that 3000 officers were driven out of the French army, but it is not clear on what he based this conclusion: C. E. Lart, 'The Huguenot regiments', *HSP* 9 (1909–11), 491.

8   HSQS 26, 1 (opening entry).

9   Robin D. Gwynn, 'The ecclesiastical organization of French Protestants in England in the later seventeenth century, with special reference to London' (unpublished Ph.D. thesis, University of London, 1976), 71.

10 Paul Doby, Jean Drigué, Daniel Fervaques, Benjamin du Quesne.

11 Pierre Delmé, Paul Doby, Jean Dubois, Daniel Fervaques, Claude Hays (II), Pierre Houblon, Jean Jorion (who was also an alderman), Jacques de Neu, Nathaniel de Neu, Thomas Papillon (also alderman), Benjamin du Quesne, Humfroy Willet. Evidence for Common Councilmen has been drawn principally from J. R. Woodhead, *The rulers of London 1660–1689* (London, 1965).

12 Jacques Auguste Blondel, Isaac Bonouvrier, Jean Delmé, Joseph Ducasse, Jacques du Fay, Louis Gervaise (II?), Daniel Hays, Jean du Maistre, François Mariette, Jacques de Neu (foundation director), Pierre Neveu, Jean le Platrier, Robert le Platrier, David Primerose (minister), Pierre Renu, Etienne Seignoret, Aaron Testas (minister), Humfroy Willet. The future Governor De Lillers Carbonnel did not subscribe in 1694; nor did Pierre des Champs, although he acted as agent for several subscribers.

13 Odile Martin, *La conversion Protestante à Lyon (1659–1687)* (Geneva, 1986), 51.

14 His trading commodities ranged from copper plates to brandy: *Calendar of Treasury Books, 1672–5*, 578; *Calendar of Treasury Books, 1679–80*, 853.

15 Henry Roseveare (ed.), *Markets and merchants of the late seventeenth century: the Marescoe-David letters, 1668–1680* (Oxford, 1987), 583.

16 HSQS 3, 144.

17 FCL, MS 7, 64–6, 80, 84, 89; MS 63, preface, 4; CLRO, ex-Guildhall MS 346, no. 252; *The Currant Intelligence*, no. 42, 13–17 Sept. 1681.

18 Ole Peter Grell, *Dutch Calvinists in early Stuart London* (Leiden, 1989), 269.

19 L. Rossier, *Histoire des Protestants de Picardie* (Paris, 1861), 206.

20 O. Douen (ed.), *La Révocation de l'Édit de Nantes à Paris d'après des documents inédits* (3 vols., Paris, 1894), vol. 2, 24.

21 *Calendar of Treasury Books, 1681–5*, 255.

22 *CSPD, 1682*, 531.

23 Henry Wagner, 'Pedigree of the Huguenot refugee families of Berchere and Baril', *The Genealogist*, NS 23 (1907), 248–51.

24 W. H. Manchée, 'Some Huguenot smugglers: the impeachment of London silk merchants, 1698', *HSP* 15:3 (1936), 410–11.

25 *Ibid.*, 412, 420.

26 Alfred Daullé, *La Réforme à Saint-Quentin et aux environs du XVIe à la fin du XVIIIe siècle* (revised edn., St Quentin, 1905), 193–4, 201, 226.

27 *CSPD, 1651–2*, 575; *1652–3*, 47, 54, 480; *1665–6*, 335; *Calendar of Treasury Books, 1669–72*, 755; *1672–5*, 115, 457; *1676–9*, 1317–21.

28 Grace Lawless Lee, *The story of the Bosanquets* (Canterbury, 1966), 24.

29 *Miscellanea Genealogica et Heraldica*, 2nd ser. 2 (1888), 52.

30 D. W. Jones, 'London overseas-merchant groups at the end of the seventeenth century and the moves against the East India Company' (unpublished D.Phil. thesis, Oxford University, 1970), 186.

31 K. G. Davies, *The Royal African Company* (London, 1957); Huguenot Library, University College, London, Wagner Pedigrees.

32 Joannes H. Hessels (ed.), *Ecclesiae Londino-Batavae Archivum* (3 vols. in 4 parts, Cambridge, 1889–97), vol. 3:ii (Cambridge, 1897), 2740.

33 Roseveare, *Markets and Merchants*. The quotation is from Richard Grassby, 'English merchant capitalism in the late 17th century', *Past and Present* 46 (1970), 92–3.

34 P. G. M. Dickson, *The Financial Revolution in England: a study in the development of public credit 1688–1756* (Basingstoke, 1967), 427; BL, Add. MS 34283, fo. 141.

35 Manchée, 'Huguenot smugglers', 420; D. W. Jones, 'London overseas-merchant groups', 240.

36 Charles Littleton, 'Geneva on Threadneedle Street: the French Church of London and its congregation, 1560–1625' (unpublished Ph.D. thesis, University of Michigan, 1996), 142, 151.

37 FCL, MS 8, fos. 103v, 174r; *Memoirs of Thomas Papillon, of London, Merchant (1623–1702)*, ed. A. F. W. Papillon (Reading, 1887), 382.

38 Papillon, *Memoirs*, 306.

39 FCL, MS 8, fos. 31–2, 245, 251r, 263v.

40 FCL, MS 8, fos. 180–2, 200v.

41 F. M. Crouzet, 'Walloons, Huguenots and the Bank of England', *HSP* 25:2 (1990), 167–78; François Crouzet, 'Some remarks on the *Metiers d'Art*', in Robert Fox and Anthony Turner (eds.), *Luxury trades and consumerism in Ancien Régime Paris: studies in the history of the skilled workforce* (Aldershot, 1998), 268–9.

42 Jon Butler, *The Huguenots in America: a refugee people in New World society* (Cambridge, MA, 1983), 153.

43 Bennett Woodcroft, Subject-Matter Index (made from Titles only) of Patents of Inventions, from March 2, 1617 to October 1, 1852 (2 vols., London, 1854), patent no. 221, where Duthais has been rendered as Guthard.

44 D. W. Jones, *War and economy in th age of William III and Marlborough* (Oxford, 1988), chap. 8. Jones also makes plain that the movement in old drapery exports is not due simply to people switching business.

45 D. W. Jones, 'London overseas-merchant groups', 240.

46 HSQS 58, 104–10.

47 Jean Bianquis and Emile Lesens, *La Révocation de l'Edit de Nantes à Rouen* (Rouen, 1885), 25.

48 *Ibid.*, 28 (Lesens), 73 (Bianquis).

49 David C. A. Agnew, *Protestant exiles from France, chiefly in the reign of Louis XIV* (3rd edn., 2 vols., privately printed, 1886), vol. 2, 447–8.

50 *Miscellanea Genealogica et Heraldica*, 3rd ser., 2 (1898), 59, differs in this from *Bulletin de la Société de l'Histoire du Protestantisme Français* 18 (1869), 551n, and O. Douen (ed.), *La Révocation de l'Édit de Nantes à Paris d'après des documents inédits* (3 vols., Paris, 1894),

vol. 2, 57–9.

51 *HMC*, vol. 75: *Downshire I, pt. 1* (London, 1924), 61–2.

52 Douen, vol. 3, 195.

53 *Ibid.*, vol. 2, 455, 497; vol. 3, 367–8.

54 Bianquis and Lesens, 38, 82–3 (Bianquis), 55–6 (Lesens).

55 *HMC*, vol. 75: *Downshire I part I*, 46, 57, 65, 71; Ruth Clark, *Sir William Trumbull in Paris 1685–1686* (Cambridge, 1938), 51.

56 Ragnhild Hatton, *Louis XIV and his world* (London, 1972), 92–3.

57 *An account of the late persecution of the Protestants in the vallys of Piemont . . . in . . . 1686* (Oxford, 1689), 9, 22.

58 [James Pineton de Chambrun], *The History of the Persecutions . . . in . . . Orange, . . . to . . . 1687* (London, 1689).

59 William Dalrymple (ed.), *Letters of Lady Rachel Russell* (7th edn., London, 1809), 82.

60 Bonrepaus to Seignelay 31 Jan 1686 n.s., 'le principal fondement des affaires de ce pays cy roule sur la Religion': PRO, SP 31/3/163.

61 HSQS 58. Historians may not have realized the timing, but contemporaries did: *HMC*, vol. 29, *Portland III* (London, 1894), 398; Narcissus Luttrell, *A brief historical relation of state affairs* (6 vols., Oxford, 1857), vol. 1, 404.

62 Douen, vol. 2, 23–4, 57–9.

63 Fernand de Schickler, *Les églises du Refuge en Angleterre* (3 vols., Paris, 1892), vol. 2, 86ff., and vol. 3, 197ff.; HSQS 54, 9ff., 25, 35.

64 FCL, MS 6, 609.

65 FCL, MS 7; HSQS 58.

66 Robin D. Gwynn, 'James II in the light of his treatment of Huguenot refugees in England, 1685–1686', *English Historical Review* 92 (1977), 824–5.

67 CLRO, 441/A/2, 37, 42, 61–2.

68 PRO, SP 44/337/125.

69 LPL, MS 941, no. 109 (i).

70 W. A. Speck, 'The Orangist conspiracy against James II', *Historical Journal,* 30:2 (1987), 458.

71 J. Childs, *The Army, James II and the Glorious Revolution* (Manchester, 1980), 206.

72 Childs, *British Army of William III*, 134; Jonathan I. Israel, 'The Dutch Republic and the "Glorious Revolution" of 1688/89 in England', in Charles Wilson and David Proctor (eds.), *1688: the seaborne alliance and diplomatic revolution* (Greenwich, 1989), 40.

73 François Crouzet, 'The Huguenots and the English Financial Revolution', article no. 1 in Crouzet, *Britain, France and international commerce: from Louis XIV to Victoria* (Aldershot, 1996), 224.

74 Emile-G. Léonard, *Histoire générale du protestantisme*, vol. 2: *L'établissement* (Paris, 1961), 331.

75 *HMC.* vol. 56: *Stuart I* (London, 1902), 527. Perhaps the same could still have been said of the next generation of descendants of the refugees in 1745, to judge from the numbers of men offered by Spitalfields silkweavers for service against Bonnie Prince Charlie: Robin Gwynn, *The Huguenots of London* (Brighton and Portland, 1998), 37–8.

Part VIII

Huguenots in Ireland

46

Elites and assimilation: the question of leadership within Dublin's *Corps du Refuge*, 1642–1740

RAYMOND PIERRE HYLTON

Casting the role of the 'elites' into its early modern context – devoid of post-1789 liberalist interpretations – there is an inevitable merger into broad conceptualizations based on leadership, direction, purpose and example. In societies that valued the privilege-principle as its leadership paradigm, the complementary principle was that of responsibility.

When the Huguenot dispersion is considered, this early modern understanding has to be immediately translated into an unprecedented historical situation – one which involved substantial exile communities of refugee Christians. The likelihood of a transplanted elite representing or operating within those communities poses certain questions:

First, to what extent was this elite successfully transferred, and how effectively did it remain intact? Secondly, could it have been transformed by its experiences in exile and how may it have functioned as an agent in the transformation of the greater Huguenot community?

Put another way, how did this elite act as a catalyst for change (i.e. assimilation into the host community), or to what extent did it impede the assimilation process?

In the instance of the Irish *Corps du Refuge*, of which the most significant component was the community in Dublin city, one must raise the qualifications to yet another level. An environment which differed quite radically from that of other French Calvinist refuges in its omnipresent sense of peril, where the certain knowledge of plans for Franco-Jacobite incursions and the awareness of smouldering animosity felt by the majority of Ireland's population cannot have been without effect. It was a situation of sufficient uniqueness as to necessitate the avoidance of the embracing of assumptions which have long characterized the Irish and Dublin refuges as being homogeneous or static or conformable to the general patterns prevailing within the British refuges. These assumptions have all been proven by recent research to be either fraught with error, or subject to modification.[1]

Also, when examining the issues of leadership within a Huguenot-related context, the existence of a threefold elite must be considered. There exists the traditional model provided by the nobility, carrying over from medieval society and far from defunct in the early modern era. The *noblesse d'épée (écuyers)* had been the backbone of the old Huguenot party and, through social convention and historical circumstance, would wield a considerable amount of hegemonic influence within the exile colonies well into the 18th century. The lingering influence of *écuyer* families in Ireland was further buttressed by the disproportionate percentage of noble houses in the French Protestant population of such areas as Dublin, Portarlington, Youghal and Waterford.

Another contributing factor was the scheme to secure a 'Fortress Ireland' to safe-guard the Anglo-Protestant interest against French, Spanish and Jacobite designs by encouraging the plantation of pensioned Huguenot veterans into semi-garrison settle-ments at: Portarlington, Waterford, Cork, Youghal, Carlow, Kilkenny, Birr and Dublin.[2]

The gradual emergence of a mercantile and professional counter-elite to rival noble hegemony was part of the early modern transition, and though there was overlap and amalgamation among individuals within these two elite groupings, an expanding urban environment such as was found in Dublin could only act to encourage the develop-ment of an increasingly influential commercially-based element.

It would be a grave error to discount the pastoral influence: a sort of ecclesiastical elite definitely existed. Leadership was inherent in the role and function of the Huguenot pastorate, whether Conformed or Nonconformist, and whether acting in concert with their consistories or through individual initiative.

A further point to consider is the reality of dealing with what was often a fissured and divided elite. When a community's directing voices are at odds among themselves over the nature and mission of their community one is left with a situation where the rank and file must at times have felt like much of the medieval populace during the years of the Great Schism: where exactly did the true leadership lie? How deeply did a sense of unity and solidarity exist within the *Corps du Refuge*? The controversy over whether to conform or not to the established Church of Ireland, for example, proved `to be of a far more intense than merely denominational considerations. It involved nothing less than the question as to whether or not exile had to be accepted as permanent. To embrace conformity implied a degree of acknowledgement of the possibility that repatriation to France might not be achieved – if ever – for generations to come; which placed Huguenot foreigners into the situation which dictated accom-modation to the Anglophone society and ultimate assimilation into an Anglophone milieu as the indispensible means for self-improvement. However, the expectation of an imminent, triumphal return necessitated the preservation of the unsullied Calvinist forms of worship and, and all that was distinctly Francophone.[3]

Early Ormondite Dublin, 1662–80

The Early Ormondite group, the first Huguenot community in the Irish capital to merit the name, was part-and-parcel of James Butler, 1st Duke of Ormonde's grand schemes for the urbanization, continentalization, and strengthening of royalist Anglicanism within the Ireland over which he presided as Viceroy. Inasmuch as this Huguenot community was Ormonde's creature, the Duke's paternalistic hand was evident at every juncture in its establishment. This was most visibly manifested in the passage of the 1662 Irish Parliament's 'Act for Encouraging Protestant Strangers to Settle and Plant in Ireland', the formation of the conformist French Church which met at the Lady Chapel in St Patrick's Cathedral in Dublin, and in the appointment of Ormonde's own chaplain, Jacques Hierome of Sedan, as the first French Church minister.

Mirroring the Duke's own peculiar vision, this first Huguenot community was to be solidly mercantile; loyalist; and to be carefully nurtured, shepherded and controlled within the confines of Anglican orthodoxy, with episcopal authority clearly set forward, and the use of Jean Durel's translation of the Book of Common Prayer.[4]

Under this framework, it must, however, be stated that the Huguenot worshippers were allowed leeway to the extent that they could preserve certain distinctly Calvinist elements in their services (notably Psalm-singing), and a consistorial form of church governance.

The Early Ormondite community was never substantial enough to have sustained an existence of its own; and, without there being massive, sustained persecution of Protestants in France as would occur in the 1680s, there was little compelling incentive for Huguenots to come to Ireland. After the Duke's fall from power in 1669 the community degenerated rapidly, no independent leadership having emerged. Pastor Hierome, who might have taken the reins of leadership to prevent the colony's eclipse, had much to commend him in terms of scholarship and reputation. However, his dependence on an income based on pluralism of benefices and his predilection for speculative business ventures and political adventurism seems to have diverted him from such goals.[5]

The noble element, as a natural leadership reservoir, was negligible at this juncture, nor did initiative arise from the mercantile families who comprised the bulk of the Early Ormondite community. The long-established Desmynieres family, though well-to-do and active in civic affairs, never evinced overwhelming interest in matters involving their more recently-arrived co-religionists, having been firmly absorbed into the Anglophone establishment. Furthermore, each of the Huguenot mercantile families had previously dwelled in areas of northern France (mainly from around Rouen in Normandy) where the Huguenot element had been urban-based, a very pronounced minority, and – at least from the 1590s on – utterly quiescent in their posture towards constituted authority. Self-assertion was, traditionally, not their strong point.

A potential leader, René de La Mezandière, who was apparently an individual with some leverage at the viceregal court, preoccupied himself in the acquisition of sinecures and ill-starred business ventures.[6]

Late Ormondite Dublin, 1681–91

Whereas the Early Ormondite influx had amounted to little more than a planted colony – and one which did not fare too well at that[7] – the Late Ormondite community was composed of a genuine wave of refugees from persecution who poured into Britain and Ireland in the wake of the *dragonnades* and the increasingly harsh series of government-generated atrocities that culminated in the Edict of Fontainebleau.

That these Late Ormondite settlers were absolutely different from their Early Ormondite co-religionists was perceived by the Duke of Ormonde himself, who was less than enthusiastic in his response. Even though Ormonde was able to re-attain the viceroyalty at Dublin Castle once again (1677–85), his final administration was far less innovative and less fruitful in its accomplishments than his previous tenure of office.[8] Unfavourable comparisons have been drawn to his rather hesitant and subdued response to the *dragonnades* with that of the Crown and administration at Whitehall.[9] Elements of a state of denial over the severity of Louis XIV's policies were followed by grudging acknowledgement and uneasy acceptance of the tidal wave of refugees which swelled the Huguenot population in the Irish capital alone ninefold during the years 1681–4.[10]

One factor lay in the fact that this was not a controlled situation. It was totally unforeseen and difficult to predict in its impact, being potentially volatile. By its very nature, this would have been anathema to the Duke's orderly, structured mind and his hierarchical vision. There was also the factor that these particular refugees were mainly from the southern provinces of France. Most were Poitevins and of professional and artisan backgrounds. Ormonde himself was doubtless fully aware that, though these were Huguenots, they came from a different tradition from the northern merchants of the Early Ormondite years. South of the Loire River, French Calvinists comprised a much larger minority (in many areas even a predominance) within the population and were much more assertive, proactive and independent in their attitudes towards consti-tuted authority. They represented an uncomfortably closer approximation of Ormonde's dreaded Presbyterian menace.[11]

The Duke's worst fears seemed to be confirmed during June–October 1683 when the more ardently Calvinist members among the new refugees began organizing Dissenting conventicles and even collaborating with Anglophone Presbyterian elements active in Dublin. The integrity of the French Conformed Church was con-sidered to be jeopardized and it became all too evident that Pastor Hierome's successor Moses Viridet – himself also one of the Duke's former chaplains – could not cope with the situation. Viridet was not by nature a leader; his actions revealed him as a hesitant and confused individual who was totally out of his depth in such a crisis – and may well have been close to suffering a nervous breakdown.

Forceful action, including use of viceregal troops to disperse the conventicles and some exemplary arrests and detentions, restored the situation – at least on the surface.[12] Viridet was a broken man – he was granted the services of three auxiliary ministers, and allowed to ease into the far less taxing benefice of Arklow, County Wicklow on 16 June 1685.[13]

It was Viridet's successor, Pastor Josuë Roussel who was belatedly to assume a legitimate mantle of leadership and would briefly weld the Late Ormondite Refuge into a presentably coherent community. A Dauphinois by birth, Minister Roussel enjoyed legendary status for his heroic militant resistance to Louis XIV, having been tried *in absentia* at Nîmes and condemned to be broken on the wheel.[14] As such, Roussel commanded a degree of respect amongst his co-religionists which was unique and which permitted him for a time to bridge the gap between the conformist and Calvinist elements. Dublin's Huguenot population might, by late 1686, have approached 650, and the nucleus of a mercantile elite was just beginning to coalesce around the families of David Cossart, Pierre Vatable, Pierre Mariel and Daniel Hays.[15]

No sooner, however, did the Late Ormondite community begin achieving a semblance of identity, than the political climate began to shift abruptly and set into motion the events that would decimate Dublin's Huguenot population. The appointment of Lord Deputy (the Duke of) Tyrconnel in 1687 abruptly stripped away all veneer of administrative protection the refugees had enjoyed; and – as was common with all Protestant Dubliners except Quakers – they fell under suspicion, scrutiny and harassment. In the case of the Huguenots this may have been exacerbated by Roussel's past record as an activist, and by the presence of four Huguenot regiments in the Williamite army which had landed in Ulster. Roussel and other Huguenots suffered imprisonment or detention and as many as 370 individual French Calvinists may have fled to Britain.[16]

In the aftermath of the Battle of the Boyne, the prisoners were released, but the Late Ormondite community could not be patched together again. It had been in a state of flux throughout most of its existence, the experiences of the Jacobite interlude and the War of the Two Kings had shattered it irrevocably. Roussel himself was rapidly losing his vigour, and would die in March 1692; his son and putative successor Charles proving unequal to the task of coping in a transformed Dublin amongst co-religionist newcomers with a far different perspective.[17]

Ruvignac Dublin, 1692–*c*.1740

In 1692, in the wake of the Williamite pacification and Roussel's death, the most substantial wave of Huguenot refugees to enter Ireland, the Ruvignac group, would again alter the equation. It is really only at this stage that the existence of a *Corps du Refuge* can be claimed without question: the numbers, the capital, the skills and expertise of the population in diverse areas are there in evidence. The *écuyers* and the mercantile/professional core were all in place for the first time. Furthermore, there was one individual – one of the Huguenot community's own – who came closer than any to assuming the mantle of leadership. This was Henri Massue, marquis de Ruvigny, Earl of Galway (from 1697), former Deputy-General of the '*Religion Prétendu Réformée*' at the court of Louis XIV, and twice Lord Justice of Ireland.[18]

Even in the case of the Ruvignac years, however, long-held assumptions regarding Galway's leadership, and the very nature of the Irish Refuge itself, must be held up to scrutiny and to some measure of revision. Was the Earl of Galway's leadership ever as enthusiastically endorsed even within his own community as has hitherto been implied? It is a matter of certainty that no one in the 'Huguenot International' had Galway's prestige, that the Earl's position was unique, and that no one else could have been better-placed to function as the guiding hand for the refugee community. While conceding these points, and not in any way disparaging the Huguenot Earl's impact and accomplishments, evidence might lead to reservations regarding the depth and extent of Galway's true leadership role; and both the direction and ultimate effectiveness of such all-embracing policies as he may have advocated.

The greater portion of Dublin's Huguenots (around two-thirds) certainly did not follow the Earl's lead in embracing conformity to the Anglican communion. From the beginning nonconformist congregations were established, flourished and emphatically rebuffed all subsequent overtures the Earl made to them regarding accommodation and compromise. He failed to mend the rift and may even have exacerbated the difficulties among the confessional tendencies. His final plea to the two sides to 'live together as brothers' comes across as a painful, perhaps despairing, admission of frustration.[19] Even at Portarlington, a colony of Galway's own creation, he proved powerless to prevent the quagmire of confessional controversy that was so negatively to affect that community's direction and development.[20]

This defiance of the Earl of Galway's expressed wishes for his community to enter into a conformist arrangement had much to do with the security many must have felt in nostalgia and tradition, but for some who reflected on Galway's pre-exile past, there were other points of contention. There were those who recalled the role played by Galway and his father, the first marquis de Ruvigny as joint Deputies-General at Versailles. There were individuals within the Huguenot community who considered the degree to which the Ruvignys were willing to maintain their loyalty and to accept much of the impositions and legal/illegal disabilities placed upon their co-religionists as being excessive. Some would have even accused Galway of having acted with insufficient vigour during the dragonnade period, and of allowing the controversial Huguenot militant Roux de Marcilly to be sacrificed.[21]

Galway's control over incompetent and insubordinate underlings sometimes appeared to be none too firm; notably in the case of Henri de Mirmand's negative attitude and enigmatic actions during the time of the Earl's ambitious project to colonize Ireland with French families.

To mitigate these critical points, it must also be stated that the Earl of Galway's massive diplomatic, administrative and military responsiblities to the Crown allowed him to spend comparatively little time on Irish affairs. The gout, severe battle wounds and deteriorating health must surely have hampered his effectiveness as an agent for unity and control even within his own bailiwick.[22] It must also be ventured, given the measure of allegiance that he might potentially have commanded among his co-religionists, why – upon the occasion of his death in 1720 – was there not even the remotest suggestion of putting forward a successor to the Earl of Galway as leader of the *Corps du Refuge*? Could it have been that the very notion of a leader had been reduced to an irrelevancy? While it may be argued that there was no one of comparable stature to replace the Earl of Galway, it is equally valid to postulate that the desire to replace what did not exist (i.e. a universally acknowledged head of an International Huguenot movement) was undoubtedly factored into the equation.

We are therefore brought back to the issue: did a *Corps du Refuge* in Ireland ever exist at all? Was it basically no more than legend? Might it not have been merely the hopeful reflection of an ideal more illusory than real? Have historians and scholars been perpetuating yet another myth? Solidarity and unity – how appropriately may these be applied to Dublin's diverse Huguenot population? There certainly had to be a measure of solidarity in the face of a common foe – Roman Catholicism (though it must also be stated that Anglophone Establishmentarians and Dissenters in England, Scotland and Ireland were similarly capable on occasion of sublimating their differences and presenting a united front against perceived threats from the Roman Church). But unity of mission, purpose and even identity was not to be attained.

It is perhaps not to an all-encompassing leadership that one should seek when determining further clues in this direction, but to the 'local worthies', to the entrepreneurs, innkeepers, building contractors; haberdashers; professionals, intellectuals and others who sustained and enriched Dublin's distinctive Huguenot communities well into the latter years of the 18th century. It is on the local level that the occasional semblance of direction may be found. There were always the families and individuals who would emerge, then recede (usually to become anglicized within a short period of time). The Belrieu de Virazels, De Susy Boans, Digues La Touches, Chaigneaus, Maret de La Rives, Boust Laboutries, Jalaberts, Desbrisays, Pomaredes, Blosset de Loches, D'Apremonts, Picards, Mazotins and others certainly achieved prominence, but hardly what would be defined as leadership – and still less of what may be defined as leadership over an identifiable Huguenot Refuge. As the 18th century wore on, the concerns of the Huguenot International (such as it had been) was of less and less concern to each passing generation, whose interests were accordingly more localized; and whose goals became progressively more limited.

It appears that it is not to a deliberate policy orchestrated by the upper echelons of government and society, that the process by which the Huguenot dispersion in Ireland blended in the crucible should be attributed. Rather was it that the very divisiveness and lack of an elite-inspired direction tended to facilitate its ultimate assimilation.

NOTES

1   Samuel Smiles, *Huguenots in England and Ireland* (London, 1889), 294; Albert Carré, *L'Influence des Huguenots Français en Irlande aux XVIIe et XVIIIe siècles* (Paris, 1937), 88; Constantia Maxwell, *Dublin under the Georges* (London, 1936), 67; Raymond P. Hylton, 'The Huguenot communities in Dublin, 1662–1745' (unpublished Ph.D. thesis, University College Dublin, 1985), 148–50 (based upon records in the Dublin Registry of Deeds at King's Inn); Grace Lawless Lee, *The Huguenot settlements in Ireland* (London, 1936), 227; T. P. LeFanu, 'The Huguenot churches in Dublin and their ministers', *HSP* 8:1 (1905), 103, 120–1; HSQS 7, v.

2   *The Statutes at large passed in the Parliaments held in Ireland*, vol. 2: *1634–62*, 498–502 (14–15 Charles II c. xiii); Maurice Craig, *Dublin, 1660–1860* (Dublin, 1980), 3–4; LeFanu 'Huguenot churches', 89–91; HSQS 7, i; Hylton, 66–7.

3   J.-P. Pittion, 'The question of religious conformity and non-conformity in the Irish Refuge' in C. E. J. Caldicott, Hugh Gough and J.-P. Pittion (eds.), *The Huguenots and Ireland: anatomy of an emigration* (Dun Laoghaire, 1987), 285–6, 288, 290–1; G. A. Forrest, 'Religious controversy within the French Protestant community in Dublin, 1692–1716: an historiographical critique' in Kevin Herlihy (ed.), *The Irish dissenting tradition, 1650–1750* (Dublin, 1995), 96–7; T. P. LeFanu, 'Archbishop Marsh and the discipline of St Patrick's, Dublin, 1694' in *HSP* 12:4 (1921), 247.

4   *Irish Statutes*, 498–502 (14–15 Charles II, c. xiii); Craig, 3–4; LeFanu, 'Huguenot churches', 89–99; HSQS 7, 1; National Library of Ireland, MS 2675 (Deeds of St Patrick's Cathedral), 32–3.

5   *CSPD, Addenda 1660–85*, 363 (George Blackall to his cousin, 1672); Hartmut Kretzer, *Calvinismus und Französische Monarchie in 17 Jahrhundert* (Berlin, 1975), 431; National Library of Ireland, Reynal Leslie MS 8007; HMC, *Calendar of the Manuscripts of the Marquess of Ormonde*, NS, vol. 3 (1904), 349 (Lawrence to Matthew); T. P. LeFanu, 'The French Church in the Lady Chapel of St Patrick's Cathedral' in Hugh Lawlor, *The Fasti of St Patrick's* (Dublin, 1931), 285.

6   Thomas Gimlette, *The history of the Huguenot settlers in Ireland and other literary remains* (Waterford, 1888), 192; *CSP Ireland 1669–70 Addenda 1625–70*, 527 (Petition of René de

la Mezandière); Edward MacLysaght, *Irish life in the seventeenth century* (Dublin, 1979), 207, 244–6; HMC, *Calendar of the Manuscripts of the Marquess of Ormonde*, NS, vol. 7 (1912), 81; HSQS 7, 1; HMC, *Tenth Report, Appendix 5: the Manuscripts of the Marquis of Ormonde, the Earl of Fingall, the corporations of Waterford, Galway, etc.* (1885), 61; Philip Benedict, *Rouen during the Wars of Religion* (Cambridge, 1980), 125–51.

7 *CSPD Addenda 1660–85*, 363.

8 James Ernest Aydelotte, 'The Duke of Ormond and the English government of Ireland, 1677–85' (unpublished Ph.D. thesis, University of Iowa, 1975); Carré, 6; National Library of Ireland, Ormond MS 803, 39.

9 Robin D. Gwynn, 'Court policy towards Huguenot immigration and settlement in England and Ireland' in Caldicott, Gough, and Pittion, *Huguenots and Ireland*, 215–17.

10 *Ibid.*; National Library of Ireland, Ormond MS 803, 39; Hylton, 41.

11 J. C. Beckett, *Protestant dissent in Ireland, 1687–1784* (London, 1948), 127, 132–3, 135; Aydelotte, 24; Richard Bagwell, *Ireland under the Stuarts* (London, 1916), 35–8; Thomas Carte, *The Life of James, Duke of Ormond* (London, 1736), 420–21; HMC, *Ormonde Mansucripts*, NS, vol. 7, 12; National Library of Ireland, MS 11971, 77.

12 HMC, *Ormonde Mansucripts*, NS, vol. 7, 65, 81, 89, 93–5, 102, 104, 108–9, 139. 150, 155, 181.

13 British Library, Additional MS 38143 (Government Disbursements 1684–5), 19–20; National Library of Ireland, MS 8007; *CSPD 1684–5*, 261; LeFanu, 'The French Church', 286.

14 National Library of Ireland, MS 8007; LeFanu, 'The French Church', 286.

15 HSQS 7, 2, 116, 144, 146, 207; Royal Irish Academy, Dumont MS 12, n.17; Dublin City Hall, MS DCH (Pipe Water Applications and Miscellaneous Acts of the Dublin Corporation), 28, 34, 406, 469, 474; Irish Registry of Deeds, MSS 7–381–2722; 21–548–12460; 92–198–50375; HSQS 18, 218, 343; HMC, *Report 14, Appendix 5*, 252–4.

16 Trinity College, Dublin, MS 7.4.3 (Irish Protestant emigration to Chester 1689); Carré, 9; *An apology for the Protestants of Ireland* (London, 1689), 5; Hylton, 56.

17 Royal Irish Academy, MS 12, n.17; LeFanu, 'The French Church', 288; National Library of Ireland, MS 8007; LeFanu, 'The Huguenot churches', 110–1.

18 Solange Deyon, *Du loyalisme au refus: les protestants français et leur député-général entre la Fronde et la Revocation* (Lille, 1968), 9, 27–8, 92, 96–7, 159–60; Daniel Ligou, *Le protestantisme en France de 1598 à 1715* (Paris, 1968), 74–5.

19 LeFanu, 'Huguenot churches', 112; *idem*, 'Archbishop Marsh', 253.

20 HMC, *Manuscripts of the House of Lords*, vol. 5: *1702–4*, 49–50; *Formulaire de la consécration et dédicace des églises et chapelles selon l'usage de l'Eglise, d'Irlande* (Dublin, 1702); Lee, 152; D. C. A. Agnew, *Protestant exiles from France in the reign of Louis XIV*, vol. 2 (London, 1871), 107; Raymond P. Hylton, 'The Huguenot settlement at Portarlington, 1692–1771' (unpublished Master's thesis, University College, Dublin, 1982), 37–43, 96–103; Sir Erasmus Borrowes, 'Portarlington' in the *Ulster Journal of Archaeology* 6, 328.

21 Deyon, 9, 27–8, 92, 96–7, 159–60; Ligou, 74–5; J. S. Reid, *A history of the Presbyterian Church in Ireland*, vol. 2 (Belfast, 1867), 458; Maurice Pezet, *L'Epopée des Camisards* (Paris, 1978), 83.

22 Randolph Vigne, 'The good Lord Galway: the English and Irish careers of a Huguenot leader' in *HSP* 24:6 (1988), 543–6.

47

Conditions et préparation de l'intégration: le voyage de Charles de Sailly en Irlande (1693) et le projet d'Edit d'accueil

MICHELLE MAGDELAINE

In the spring of 1692 the canton of Zürich, suffering from a bad harvest, decided to expel the Huguenots who had settled there after the Revocation of the Edict of Nantes. The leaders of the Huguenots in Switzerland, the marquis d'Arzeliers and Henri de Mirmand, in agreement with the Viscount, later Earl of, Galway, developed a plan to settle the refugees in Ireland. Arzeliers composed for William III a 'Project for the Establishment of the Refugees in Ireland', which emphasizes the benefits to the Crown of the Huguenots' settlement in Ireland, as they would be loyal and industrious, in contrast to the 'treacherous' and 'lazy' Irish.

The 'Project' argues that the Huguenots should be allowed to settle in Ireland on very favourable terms: land, tools and supplies should be provided at very reasonable prices, artisans and manufacturers able to set up business easily, privileged by a host of concessions, and the Huguenots able to acquire naturalization immediately upon their arrival. French communities and their churches, each comprising about 50 families (i.e. about 250 to 300 people), should be set up at a day's journey from each other, and would form a network of settlements across Ireland, south-east of the line Dublin-Limerick-Cork. The French churches should be free of ecclesiastical and state interference, able to maintain their own confession of faith and discipline and to convene synods and *colloques* whenever deemed necessary. The 'Project' further requests that in matters of law the settlers be treated as ordinary, Protestant, in-habitants, as long as the privileges given to them specifically are maintained and the existing laws are not contrary to the ecclesiastical discipline.

In March 1693 Charles de Sailly, a former naval officer, visited towns and estates across much of south-eastern Ireland to assess the land for the potential Huguenot settlement. He returned from his travels through Cork, Kilkenny, Tipperary, Waterford, Wexford and Wicklow enthusiastic about the reception he had received from, and the promises made by, those proprieters who had made it known that they would favour Huguenot settlers on their estates. Yet this ambitious plan was never realized, despite all these preparations. Why did the project fail in the end? First, the political conditions were unfavourable. These plans were made during the War of the League of Augsburg, when Germany, through which the refugees would have to travel, was devastated and the English Parliament was chary of supplying additional money indiscriminately.

Finally, the refugees in Switzerland themselves proved unwilling: most of them did not want to move far from the French border. Brandenburg already seemed to them quite far away, and, despite the Edict of Potsdam, they were not drawn to that country. So what would they think of a faraway island? The ultimate failure of this ambitious project shows that integration cannot be forced on to an immigrant population from on high, from the community's leaders. The road to integration is a long one, and the various plans and measures taken here (administrative, political, financial, religious), though essential, were nonetheless not sufficient in themselves to establish the adequate conditions for the Huguenots' integration.

L'exode des huguenots fugitifs se fait de plus en plus important après la révocation de l'Edit de Nantes en octobre 1685 pour atteindre son point culminant en 1686–7. Ils ont afflué vers les Provinces-Unies, l'Angleterre, l'Allemagne, la Suisse, ou plus précisément dans les cantons évangéliques et les états alliés – République de Genève, Principauté de Neuchâtel et Ligues grises. Les fugitifs y arrivent très nombreux et, à la longue, ils sont considérés comme trop nombreux. La Suisse n'est pas un pays riche, elle-même 'exporte' ses hommes dans toutes les armées d'Europe. De plus, une partie de la population craint la concurrence économique que représentent ces réfugiés et trouvent pénible de continuer à payer pour ces gens alors que la vie est difficile pour eux-mêmes à cause des mauvaises récoltes et de la cherté des vivres. Le canton de Zurich avait donc décidé de renvoyer à partir du printemps 1692[1] les huguenots qui arrivaient sans cesse ainsi que ceux qui s'étaient déjà installés. Et l'on craignait que les autres cantons évangéliques ne suivent cet exemple.

Forts de l'expérience qu'ils ont acquise depuis 1685 et conscients de la difficulté de plus en plus grande de trouver des lieux d'accueil, certains personnages, tel comme Arzeliers[2] et Mirmand,[3] se sont déjà révélés comme responsables des réfugiés qui, en Suisse, attendent anxieusement de savoir dans quelle direction diriger leurs pas afin de trouver enfin une nouvelle patrie. Or il y avait déjà un très grand nombre de réfugiés aussi bien aux Provinces-Unies que dans les territoires protestants d'Allemagne et ce dernier pays est ravagé par la guerre de la Ligue d'Augsbourg. Mirmand et les autres chefs du Refuge, en accord avec Galway[4] envisagent alors (1689) de créer des colonies en Irlande.[5] Ils sont certains que leur initiative aura les faveurs de Guillaume III, roi depuis 1688 après le succès de la 'Glorious Revolution', la déconfiture des troupes jacobites à La Boyne et Aughrim et la paix de Limerick (1691) qui consomme la défaite des Irlandais catholiques bientôt soumis aux lois d'exception.[6] D'ailleurs le roi, pour montrer que ce projet lui tient à cœur, nomme quatre commissaires chargés de l'établissement des réfugiés en Irlande, les comtes de Rochester, Ranelagh, Coningsby et Godolphin. Enfin, l'Irlande s'avère le lieu propice à l'accomplissement d'un projet utopique comme celui de la république huguenote à l'île Bourbon, un nouvel 'Eden', symbole de l'innocence première de l'humanité et du paradis terrestre qu'Henri Duquesne[7] avait ainsi voulu fonder en 1689. L'Irlande, qualifiée de 'Canaan'[8] doit apparaître comme une nouvelle Terre Promise où couleraient le lait et le miel. A ces deux projets participe Charles de Sailly,[9] ancien officier de marine qui, après l'échec de l'installation à l'île Bourbon, se met à la disposition des chefs du Refuge.

Ceux-ci désirent à la fois éviter une trop longue errance pour les fugitifs qui sont encore en Suisse mais n'y peuvent demeurer, leur procurer un établissement sûr et se concilier la bienveillance du pouvoir britannique en consolidant l'œuvre de 'protestantisation' de l'île commencée par Elisabeth, continuée par Cromwell, mais toujours à recommencer à cause de la résistance des Irlandais catholiques.

Ils ont appris que les édits d'accueil et de privilèges, si généreux fussent-ils, ne suffisaient pas, qu'il était donc nécessaire de prévoir toutes les conditions matérielles qui rendraient l'installation des huguenots pérenne et de les mettre immédiatement à leur disposition. Quant aux relations avec les autochtones – il en reste! – cela ne pose pas de problème aussi difficile à résoudre qu'en Suisse ou en Allemagne, ce sont des rebelles battus.

Ils ne vont donc pas attendre que Guillaume et Marie[10] organisent l'accueil; ils prennent les devants, et Arzeliers rédige lui-même un 'Projet pour l'établissement des réfugiés en Irlande'[11] inspiré de ceux promulgués par les princes allemands, en particulier l'électeur de Brandebourg en faveur des Suisses en 1684 et le margrave de Bayreuth en faveur des huguenots en 1687. Il soumet son texte à Mirmand et Galway. Ils précisent ce qui leur paraît absolument nécessaire pour que les réfugiés puissent se sentir acceptés mais insistent aussi sur ce que la royauté britannique gagnera en installant en Irlande des communautés huguenotes, tant sur le plan politique (les huguenots, protestants, se montreront évidemment de loyaux sujets), que sur le plan économique (les Irlandais sont, selon eux, 'paresseux', les Français industrieux et inventifs).

Le projet d'édit est divisé en cinq chapitres: 'les moyens de faire l'établissement', la religion, la justice, la police et, finalement, les manufactures et le commerce.

L'exposé des 'moyens de faire l'établissement' est le plus important car, dans l'esprit du rédacteur et des autres responsables du projet, les conditions faites aux réfugiés pour leur transport, leur installation et leurs débuts seront la clef du succès ou de l'échec de ce grand dessein.

A ces malheureux qui ont tout perdu, subi des persécutions, voyagé dans des conditions dangereuses et pénibles, qui, en un mot, se sont littéralement arrachés à leur environnement familier et n'ont pas hésité à se lancer vers l'inconnu pour vivre selon leur conscience, il faut montrer qu'ils sont les bienvenus et leur proposer immédiate-ment la naturalisation, à condition qu'ils demeurent dans l'île au moins sept ans.[12] Il serait bon aussi que leurs enfants conservent ce privilège quand bien même ils quit-teraient l'Irlande pour une terre britannique, jusqu'en Amérique. Ainsi, d'une part les huguenots seront rassurés sur leur sort et, d'autre part, le pouvoir britannique s'attachera, à peu de frais, des sujets reconnaissants et fidèles.

Une question importante se pose avant toute autre considération, celle du trans-port des réfugiés et des frais que cela représente pour les faire venir de Suisse jusqu'en Irlande. Tout un montage financier est proposé: les cantons évangéliques paieraient le voyage jusqu'à la première étape du Würtemberg, ensuite, et jusqu'en Hollande, les souverains britanniques contribueraient aux frais. Enfin les Etats-Généraux des Provinces-Unies subviendraient aux besoins des réfugiés jusqu'à Rotterdam où ils embarqueraient pour l'Irlande. De plus, les choses seraient peut-être plus faciles si les Suisses acceptaient de payer le transport jusqu'à Francfort et si l'on obtenait des vivres à bas prix.

De façon tout aussi urgente, il faut prévoir, en détail et avec le plus d'exactitude possible, où et comment les réfugiés seront installés. D'autant plus que le but n'est pas seulement économique mais surtout politique, l'aspect religieux s'y mêlant, là encore, fort étroitement. Il s'agit évidemment de mettre en valeur les connaissances, le savoir-faire des Français mais peut-être encore davantage de transformer l'Irlande en une île toute huguenote. Ainsi, l'irritant problème de la résistance opiniâtre des catholiques irlandais serait définitivement résolu. Ceux qui ne voudraient pas se convertir seraient relégués dans le Connaught ou exilés. Des églises françaises, comprenant chacune une cinquantaine de familles, c'est-à-dire 250 à 300 personnes, seraient établies à une journée de marche les unes des autres, quadrillant ainsi l'Irlande au sud-est d'une ligne Dublin–Limerick–Cork. Cela renforcerait la présence protestante et donnerait l'exemple de la discipline et du travail.

On distribuera aux immigrants terres, prés, tourbières à prix modique, grains, vin, bière, semences, bétail, outils pour les paysans et les artisans; on les logera jusqu'à ce qu'ils aient construit des maisons. On surseoira pendant quatre ans – voire davantage – à la perception des redevances. Enfin, il faut laisser la liberté d'établissement; si quelqu'un n'est pas satisfait, il pourra s'en aller autre part après avoir rendu ce qui lui avait été accordé, car, observe Arzeliers, le 'cœur humain ... veut moins lorsqu'il lui est le plus permis de vouloir'.[13]

Sur le plan religieux, il paraît indispensable au rédacteur du projet et à ses réviseurs que les églises françaises soient libres, conservent leur confession de foi et leur discipline, convoquent synodes et colloques quand elles le jugeront bon en avertissant simplement le vice-roi d'Irlande. Cela semble exorbitant si l'on songe à la situation qui avait existé en France où aucun colloque ne pouvait se tenir sans la permission du roi et où il n'y avait plus eu de synode national depuis 1659! Mais cela peut signifier que les auteurs du projet se sentent en position de force; grâce aux colonies huguenotes, ils prétendent, l'Irlande va se développer économiquement et connaître enfin la stabilité politique. Cela peut aussi signifier qu'il faut défendre la religion qui maintient la cohésion entre les huguenots et fait partie de leur identité. Dans un but identique, il est proposé d'établir des collèges; ils seraient ouverts aux Anglais et aux Irlandais qui ne pourraient qu'en tirer des avantages d'après les arguments, pour le moins cavaliers, du rédacteur.[14] Il est vrai qu'Arzeliers relève ces points litigieux et craint qu'il y ait une certaine présomption à vouloir imposer dans le pays d'accueil ce qui n'était pas admis en France.

Dans le domaine de la justice et de l'administration, on veut, paradoxalement, que les colons soient traités comme les habitants mais que les privilèges accordés soient maintenus et que les lois existantes ne soient pas contraires à la discipline ecclésiastique.

Quant au dernier chapitre, 'des manufactures et du commerce', il demande au roi 'd'accorder aux manufacturiers et aux marchands les privilèges les plus avantageux que faire se pourra', de faire faire des avances diverses aux entrepreneurs. Mais la prudence est recommandée et il est rappelé que si les princes allemands ont accordé des privilèges aux réfugiés, ceux-ci ont été jugés exorbitants par leurs sujets et suscité parfois des réactions violentes.

Afin de ne rien laisser au hasard, Charles de Sailly est chargé d'évaluer les possibilités offertes aux Français. Le récit de son voyage est conservé.[15] Il part de Dublin le 2 mars 1693 au 4 avril 1693 et parcourt la majeure partie de l'île, se rendant chez les seigneurs, protestants évidemment, qui se sont déjà fait connaître comme favorables à l'établissement de huguenots sur leurs terres et chez d'autres encore qu'on lui recommande. Il n'oublie pas les propres terres du roi. Sa première étape est pour Kilkenny, puis Clonmel située dans une région qui est le 'jardin de l'Irlande'. Il y aurait place pour au moins 600 familles, on pourrait y établir des industries, cultiver le chanvre et le lin, fonder un collège. Malheureusement, il y a plus de papistes que de protestants! A Cashel où il arrive le 9 mars, tout est ruiné mais les seigneurs ne sont pas favorables à l'installation d'immigrants qui ne paieraient pas de taxes. Il voyage ensuite dans les comtés de Tipperary, Kilkenny, dans ceux de Waterford, Wexford et Wicklow (14 et 15 mars), où pourraient vivre, selon lui, plus de 2000 familles et cela serait nécessaire car 'si l'on ne prend pas des mesures pour abaisser les papistes qui sont plus de deux hommes pour un et fortifier les protestants, on craint qu'ils ne se soulèvent avant qu'il soit sept ans!'[16] Puis il s'arrête sur la Blackwater à proximité de Youghal. Le 18 mars il arrive à Cork et observe que 'tout le pays, de Rathcormack à Cork, n'est qu'un vrai désert propre à faire des ermitages'.[17] De là, il se rend à Macroom, le 'Montpellier de l'Irlande'[18] mais là encore, ce ne sont que ruines. A Blarney, terre du roi dans les environs de Cork, on pourrait installer les 600 premières familles qui doivent arriver dans le courant de l'année. Son périple l'emmène ensuite à Bandon, Kinsale, de nouveau à Cork le 28 mars. Il s'arrête à Waterford où tout lui semble remarquable: le pays propice à la culture du chanvre et du lin, à l'élevage, le port en eau profonde, la ville enfin où pourraient travailler toutes sortes d'artisans mais aussi des chirurgiens et des médecins, où l'on pourrait établir un collège important. Enfin, par Thomastown et Castledermot, il revient à Dublin le 3 avril.

Il est plein d'enthousiasme devant l'accueil qu'il a en général reçu et les promesses qui lui ont été faites mais cependant conscient des difficultés qui peuvent se présenter si l'on ne recueille pas assez d'argent ou si la protection du roi et du Parlement fait défaut.

Mirmand, à qui tous rendent compte, se réjouit certes de l'avancement du projet et de sa préparation minutieuse mais reste cependant très prudent comme il l'était depuis le début de l'entreprise car il était 'toujours dans la prévention que cette affaire échouerait faute d'argent'. [19] Et c'est en effet à un échec qu'aboutit cette entreprise si bien préparée, malgré les quelques centaines de réfugiés qui arrivèrent en Irlande et se fixèrent soit dans des villes où existait déjà une communauté huguenote, soit en fondant de nouvelles communautés, comme Portarlington établie par Galway.

Pourquoi cet échec, alors que, semblait-il, rien n'avait été laissé au hasard? En effet, tenant compte des expériences vécues dans d'autres pays du Refuge, les organisateurs du peuplement huguenot de l'Irlande avaient prévu dans les moindres détails ce qui était indispensable à leur établissement et à leur intégration dans les meilleures conditions. Mais les événements, tout d'abord, ont joué contre eux: quand Zurich décide de renvoyer les réfugiés au printemps 1693, la guerre ravage l'Allemagne, les Français ont pratiqué dans le Palatinat la politique de la terre brûlée dès 1688–9 rendant la route du Rhin impraticable. Les fugitifs sont obligés d'emprunter la route de terre, par Nuremberg et Cassel.[20] Guillaume III mène une campagne difficile et n'a pas d'argent pour les réfugiés, le Parlement trouve que la guerre coûte cher et presse la reine Marie de renoncer au projet.

De plus, dans leur désir d'établir des huguenots en Irlande, les auteurs du projet n'ont-ils pas été trop optimistes, voire présomptueux? Sailly, en particulier, qui estime qu'en quelques années, on pourra installer plus de 6500 familles! Alors que l'Irlande est affaiblie et que les seigneurs espèrent accueillir des gens qui pourront investir de l'argent et non des misérables qu'il faut commencer par aider.

Enfin, les responsables du Refuge, dans leur désir de mettre leurs coreligionnaires à l'abri du besoin et donc de toute tentation de revenir dans le royaume au risque de renier leur foi, n'ont-ils pas oublié qu'ils avaient affaire à des êtres humains qui pouvaient manifester leur volonté propre? La majorité d'entre eux, petits artisans, paysans, espéraient encore que le roi changerait d'avis et qu'ils pourraient rentrer en France. Ils ne voulaient pas trop s'éloigner des frontières; déjà le Brandebourg leur paraissait bien lointain et ne les attirait pas spontanément malgré l'Edit de Potsdam. Alors, que dire d'une île lointaine? . . .

Il ne suffisait donc pas d'organiser le mieux possible, avec la meilleure volonté du monde, l'établissement de ces huguenots pour permettre une rapide intégration, il aurait aussi fallu préparer davantage les populations, ménager des susceptibilités bien compréhensibles et, surtout, ne pas oublier que les réfugiés pouvaient désirer autre chose que ce que l'on voulait leur imposer. Le chemin de l'intégration est un long chemin et les mesures administratives, politiques, financières et religieuses, si elles sont absolument nécessaires, ne sont pas suffisantes.

NOTES

1 Lettre de Paul Reboulet, pasteur de l'Eglise française de Zurich, à Henri de Mirmand, de 25 décembre 1691: Bibliothèque publique et universitaire (BPU), Genève, MSS Court, no. 17, vol. M.

2 Gaspard Perrinet, marquis d'Arzeliers (1645–1710), d'une famille dauphinoise et dont le père avait été député général des Eglises de France de 1644 à 1653, s'était réfugié tout d'abord à La Haye puis à Berne; il fit partie du Comité secret de la Suisse et fut représentant du roi d'Angleterre à Genève déjà avant 1703.

3 Henri de Mirmand (1650–1721), d'une famille du bas Languedoc, fut président de chambre au présidial de Nîmes et ancien de l'Eglise. Réfugié tout d'abord en Suisse, à Zurich, il se mit au service de l'électeur de Brandebourg et joua un rôle très important pour l'établissement des réfugiés. Marie de Chambrier, *Henri de Mirmand et les réfugiés de la révocation de l'Edit de Nantes (1650–1721)* (Neuchâtel, 1910).

4 Henri de Massue, marquis de Ruvigny (1648–1720), vicomte (1691) puis comte (1696) de Galway a été choisi par Louis XIV pour succéder à son père en tant que député général des Eglises protestantes et fut le dernier détenteur de cette charge. Il se réfugia en Angleterre et passa au service de Guillaume III. En 1693, nommé lieutenant des forces en Irlande, il projeta de repeupler l'île avec des huguenots: Chambrier, 69–71, appendice.

5 *Ibid.*, 201 (citation des 'Mémoires de Mirmand').

6 Maureen Wall, 'The age of penal laws (1691–1778)', dans T. W. Moody and F. X. Martin (eds.), *The course of Irish history* (Cork, 1978), 217–31.

7 Henri Duquesne était le fils aîné de l'amiral Abraham Duquesne, à l'origine d'un projet de

république à l'île d'Eden (l'île Bourbon) en 1689.

8 Chambrier, appendice no. 1 ('Mémoires de Mirmand', 18).

9 Charles de Sailly, gentilhomme bourguignon, s'était fixé en Irlande où il reçut des terres en 1692: Chambrier, 214.

10 Souverains conjointement; la reine Marie était la fille de Jacques II chassé par la 'Glorious Revolution' en 1688.

11 BPU, Genève, MSS Court, no. 17, vol. M. fos. 70–73. Le texte remplit trois folios recto-verso et le recto d'un quatrième. Chacun est divisé en deux colonnes: à gauche les articles, à droite les 'raisons et observations', c'est-à-dire les arguments à employer pour convaincre les souverains. De plus, Arzeliers, reprenant la copie après réflexion, a parfois ajouté des observations supplémentaires.

12 Charles avait continué la politique d'Elisabeth et de Cromwell. Le Parlement d'Irlande avait promulgué en 1662 une loi, confirmée en 1672, pour encourager l'immigration de réformés français. Enfin, en 1674, les Français reçurent le droit de naturalisation et l'entrée gratuite dans les corporations pendant sept ans, moyennant le serment de 'Supremacy'.

13 'Projet d'établissement', chap. 1, article XX.

14 *Ibid.*, chap. 2, article X, 'raisons et observations' (voir note 10).

15 BPU, Genève, MSS Court, no.17, vol. M, fos. 93–110; ce texte a été publié dans le *Bulletin de l'histoire du protestantisme français* 17 (1868), 591 ff.

16 *Ibid.*

17 *Ibid.*

18 *Ibid.*

19 Chambrier, appendice no. 1 ('Mémoires de Mirmand', 20).

20 Lettre de Mirmand à Galway de 27 mai/6 juin 1693: BPU, Genève, MSS Court, no. 17, vol. M.

48

The integration of the Huguenots into the Irish Church: the case of Peter Drelincourt

Jane McKee

Most of the Huguenots who worked as clergymen in England and Ireland after the Revocation of the Edict of Nantes tended to remain with their own people, serving a French church and a French community which remained, to a large extent, separate from the surrounding society. In spite of the efforts of the authorities in Ireland[1] and also, occasionally, in England[2] to ensure conformity to the Anglican rite, many Huguenots refused to use Jean Durel's French version of the Anglican prayer book. Even where the congregation was conforming the order of service was not entirely Anglican.[3] Full integration into the English and Irish Churches, with its implication of the loss or dilution of Huguenot or even of French identity does not seem to have been an important aim for many Huguenots or for many of the Huguenot clergy. It was usually in later generations that real integration took place, and that clergy of French origin succeeded in reaching the highest offices in the English or Irish Church. The best example of this gradual integration in Ireland is perhaps the Chenevix family, where it was Richard Chenevix, a grandson of the original immigrant Philippe Chenevix, who became Bishop of Killaloe in 1745, before moving to the see of Waterford and Lismore in 1746.[4]

Yet there were Huguenot clergymen of the first generation who were granted substantial preferment in the Anglican Churches of Ireland and England. This study will examine the factors which appear to have favoured their integration and advancement, before going on to analyse the career of one of the most successful of these men, Peter Drelincourt who became Dean of Armagh in 1691.

Factors which favoured assimilation

In spite of the doctrinal and liturgical differences which separated the French 'Eglise Réformée' and the Church of England, the idea that a member of the French Reformed Church could take orders in the English Church was not without distinguished precedents by the second half of the 17th century. Anthony Wood noted that nine French Protestants were incorporated into Oxford University between 1625 and 1657.[5] Of these, most were medical, but at least two were clergymen who were entering the service of the Church of England, one of them being Pierre or Peter Dumoulin the younger, son of the famous Pierre Dumoulin who had been one of the pastors of Charenton before being exiled to Sedan and who was one of the great polemicists of the Eglise Réformée in the early- and mid-17th century. Doctrinal differences between the Church of England and the Eglise Réformée had tended to be underplayed in France and there was a much greater rapport between the Eglise Réformée and the English Church than between the Reformed community in France and Dissenters in either England or Ireland, although the Dissenters had attracted some Frenchmen during the Civil War, most prominently Louis Dumoulin, brother of Peter.[6] Ordination into the Anglican churches could therefore be seen as an acceptable path to follow, although it was not one which was followed by many of those who fled in the 1680s.

Most of the members of the Huguenot clergy who came to England and Ireland towards the end of the century stayed with the French churches and therefore with the French community. Even some of those who eventually made careers in the Anglican churches began their ecclesiastical careers in England in the French churches before moving into service in the Church of England or Church of Ireland. Jacques Abbadie, who served in the Savoy church in London, before acquiring his deanery of Killaloe in Ireland in 1699 when his health became a problem, provides one example of such a career pattern.[7] Louis Saurin was also minister at the Savoy church before he too moved to Ireland and received preferment in the Irish church, becoming Dean of Ardagh in 1726.[8] A third similar case was that of Peter Allix who obtained permission from James II to set up a French church in London before being granted preferment in 1699 in the Church of England.[9]

Of the immigrant Frenchmen who became Anglican, five became deans in Ireland. They were, in order of appointment, Peter Drelincourt who was appointed Dean of Armagh in 1691; John Icard who succeeded to the deanery of Achonry in 1695; Jacques Abbadie who became Dean of Killaloe in 1699; Peter Maturin who was made Dean of Killala in 1724, and Louis Saurin who became Dean of Ardagh in 1726.[10] Drelincourt, Icard and Abbadie were appointed more than twenty years earlier than either Maturin or Saurin and, although all the deaneries were remote from Dublin, Drelincourt, in Armagh, was dean of the primatial see. In England, Peter Allix became Treasurer of Salisbury Cathedral; Samuel de l'Angle, a Prebendary of Westminster, while Jacques Pineton de Chambrun and Jean Mesnard were made Prebendaries of Windsor, and a number of other Huguenots became rectors of parishes.[11]

Some of these Frenchmen who received benefices in the English and Irish Churches were already well known as theologians and writers, or as victims of persecution. Peter Allix had been a minister attached to the Paris church at Charenton and was well established as a scholar and polemicist before reaching England.[12] Jacques Abbadie had served in the French church in Berlin before the death of his protector the Elector of Brandenburg brought him to England.[13] He was also the author of a number of religious works, most famously his treatise on the truth of the Christian religion.[14] Jacques Pineton de Chambrun had become famous as a victim of extreme ill treatment during the *dragonnade* in Orange in 1685 and for his subsequent escape to Geneva of which he published an account, *Les larmes de J. Pineton-de-Chambrun, qui contiennent les persécutions arrivées aux églises de la principauté d'Orange depuis l'an 1660; la chute et le relèvement de lauteur avec le Rétablissement de S.-Pierre en son apostolat ou sermon sur Jean XXI*, of which an English translation was published in 1687.[15]

Others were closely related to famous personalities. Maturin's father, Gabriel, was imprisoned in the Bastille for 26 years and was another celebrated victim of persecution.[16] Peter Dumoulin, as we have already seen, was a son of the famous Pierre Dumoulin of Charenton and Sedan; Peter Drelincourt was the youngest surviving son of Charles Drelincourt, minister of Charenton for almost fifty years and the author of many religious works; Louis Saurin was of noble family and a brother of the famous Huguenot preacher of the refuge, Jacques Saurin, while the de l'Angle brothers were nephews of Samuel Bochart and one of them, also Samuel, had been one of the ministers at Charenton for eleven years before moving to England in 1682.[17]

Several of them came to England or Ireland under the wing of a powerful patron. In Germany, Abbadie had enjoyed the favour of the Elector of Brandenburg, and he came to England with Marshal Schomberg. It was also at the behest of King William that he received preferment in Ireland. We know relatively little of the life of Jean Icard who is much less well-documented than the other Irish deans, but he served as a military chaplain for a number of years, in Ireland, in England and in Flanders, and this may well have gained him patronage to help him to this deanery.[18] Chambrun and Jean Mesnard came to England as chaplains of William of Orange.[19] We do not know the circumstances of Peter Drelincourt's arrival in England, but he arrived in Ireland in the household of the Duke of Ormond and became his domestic chaplain there in 1681.[20]

In some cases also, the benefices received by French clergymen seem to have followed the publication of books or pamphlets favourable to the authorities. Abbadie, for example, wrote a *Défense de la nation Britannique, où les Droits de Dieu, de la nature et de la société sont clairement établis au sujet de la révolution d'Angleterre contre l'auteur de l'Avis important aux Réfugiés* (1692), in which he defended the Williamite settlement and provided a funeral oration in praise of Queen Mary and, by the King's command, a narrative account of the Assassination Plot. Subsequently, his health in London became a problem, and it was at the King's request that he was given preferment in the Irish Church. Peter Drelincourt too, as we shall see, published a pamphlet or pamphlets which pleased his protectors. For others, however, political involvement brought problems. Peter Dumoulin was a royalist in England during the Civil War, at considerable cost to his career, while Peter Allix, who wrote a defence of the Christian religion in 1688 which was dedicated to King James, further lost favour upon the advent of King William after publishing his *Examination of the Scruples of those who refuse to take the Oaths* in 1689.[21]

Linguistic competence seems to have had some influence upon preferment. Peter Allix learnt English very well and quickly and published many works in that language. Drelincourt was also fluent and, as Maturin arrived as a child, he can also be presumed to have become fluent. We know nothing about the linguistic competence of the others, but there was one famous case, that of Jacques Abbadie, where lack of linguistic competence was an obstacle. King William wished him to become Dean of St Patrick's Cathedral in Dublin, but because of his poor English he was not appointed there but to the post of Dean of Killaloe in the west of Ireland, which post was less comfortable, more remote and financially inadequate to meet his needs.[22] Archbishop Boulter stated in his letter of recommendation to Lord Carteret, the Lord Lieutenant, in September 1726 that Abbadie's deanery and preferments were only worth about half of what Dublin would have brought him.[23]

Finally, all the deaneries to which Frenchmen were appointed were in Ireland. The Irish Church was often used at the end of the 17th and in the 18th century to provide preferment for Englishmen where none was available in England and it is therefore not surprising that the most senior Huguenot members of the Anglican clergy of the period should have been appointed to benefices in Ireland.[24]

In general, therefore, while few members of the clergy of the Eglise Réformée left the service of the French community when they came to the British Isles, those who did and who were successful in their ecclesiastical careers were usually men who were already famous or well-connected, or who had been close to powerful protectors, often in the role of chaplain, or who had provided some kind of significant service to their benefactor. Their command of the English language and their political allegiances also had a significant influence upon their ecclesiastical careers. Abbadie's advancement was adversely affected by his poor command of the English language, while Allix, whose English was excellent, seems to have seen his ecclesiastical career stagnate as a result of having displeased King William.

Peter Drelincourt

Of all these men, Peter Drelincourt seems to have been the most successful in terms of ecclesiastical preferment. His appointment as Dean of Armagh in 1691 made him the earliest of the French deans, and the deanery of Armagh was more prestigious and, with the parish of Armagh, more financially rewarding than that of Killaloe, which was the next French appointment in 1699. Primate Boulter writes of an income of £120 per annum for Abbadie in Killaloe in the 1720s, while Drelincourt's deanery and parish were valued at roughly the same time at approximately £880.[25] In social terms too, he became integrated into British society more successfully than many of the other Huguenots, his daughter Ann becoming a member of the aristocracy under the title Lady Primrose, after her marriage to Hugh, Viscount Primrose in 1739.[26]

His career follows some of the patterns outlined above. He came from a very prominent family. His father, who served as one of the pastors of Charenton for nearly fifty years (1620–69), was celebrated as a writer of sermons and polemical works, but was especially famous for his pastoral works. Both his *Catéchisme ou instruction familière* and his *Consolations de l'âme fidèle contre les frayeurs de la mort* ran to many editions during the 17th century and later. In addition two of Peter's brothers were also well-known figures. Laurent, the eldest, was a minister of the Eglise Réformée and a celebrated Huguenot poet. His *Sonnets chrétiens*, published in 1677, had already had six editions by 1680 and went through many more editions during the 18th century. They were even used in some parts of the Refuge as a textbook for schoolchildren.[27] Another brother, Charles, was Professor of Anatomy at Leyden and had been the private physician of William and Mary before they came to England.[28] He published many medical works, but was also a man of great general erudition and was said by

Pierre Bayle to have an exceptional understanding of Theology and of the French language.[29] Peter was therefore very well connected, and at least one historian attributes his deanery to the influence of his brother in Holland with William and Mary.[30]

He also had other powerful patronage. The Duke of Ormond, who may have had some contact with Peter's father during the exile of the Stuarts under the Commonwealth,[31] employed him to supervise the studies of his grandson at Oxford from 1678 to 1681. Drelincourt's years with the young James Butler in Oxford were not entirely successful, as he was criticized for his inability to impose discipline upon his charge, for his financial management and for his wisdom, particularly when he intervened in a schoolboy row. However, Ormond seems to have regarded him favourably, for he subsequently took him into his own household, with the post of 'domestick chaplain'. It was while Ormond was Lord Lieutenant of Ireland and with his support that Drelincourt entered the Irish Church in 1681 and received his first preferments as Precentor of Christ Church Cathedral in 1681 and Archdeacon of Leighlin in 1683, before being appointed Dean of Armagh in 1691, three years after the death of his protector in 1688, but at a time when his former pupil, now the second Duke of Ormond, was in high favour with King William.[32] There he stayed for over 30 years, rising no further in the Church, despite efforts in 1705 to engage the support of the second Duke of Ormond, now near the end of a very unsuccessful period as Lord Lieutenant of Ireland, for further preferment. Ormond did have another short period as Lord Lieutenant (1710–11), but his career was never again as brilliant or his influence as great as it had been earlier, and his support for the Jacobite cause was soon to lead to his exile from the British Isles. Drelincourt's fortunes seem therefore to have remained linked to those of the Ormond family, but his failure to progress to a see may also have been influenced by the fact that he was an outsider. Although the Irish Church was often used for advancing the careers of Englishmen who could not obtain preferment in England and although, as we have seen, all five Huguenots to rise to the level of Dean did so in Ireland, there were those among the Irish who objected strongly to the advancement of outsiders and there was considerable debate, from 1707 onward, concerning the desirability of making the Irish Church more Irish.[33]

Drelincourt's career may also have been helped by early exposure to English society. He seems to have arrived in England earlier than many of his contemporaries and to have had, at an early stage of his career, an excellent command of the English language. He may have been in England as early as 1661, for a letter from Jean Durel to Charles Drelincourt in that year states that one of Drelincourt's sons is staying in London.[34] Certainly, when he arrived in Oxford with the young Lord James Butler in 1678, it was not for the first time, for he wrote in a letter to the Duke of Ormond that he had already spent a considerable amount of time at the University.

> J'estime et j'honore extrémement cette belle université où pour mon avancement parti-
> culier j'ai passé plus d'une fois un temps assez considérable.[35]

He was therefore familiar with English society and its ways. He also had a very good command of the English language by the time he accompanied Lord James to Oxford for, although he wrote to Ormond himself in French, his correspondence with Lord James's father, Lord Ossory, with Sir Robert Southwell, who supervised the

Oxford operation, and with others was in a very correct and idiomatic English. Indeed, by 1692, English is creeping into his French in his correspondence with John Ellis, as if it were in the process of becoming his first language.[36] That this command of the language was significant for his career is confirmed by a letter from Lord Arran, who wrote to his father the Duke of Ormond in 1683 to try to secure advancement for Drelincourt and Ormond's other domestic chaplain, a Mr Wilson, while retaining their services as preachers for Christ Church Cathedral, which, as he writes, 'I think will be no small satisfaction to your Grace, when you come over, for good preaching is very rare with us here.'[37]

Drelincourt also differed from most of the other Huguenot immigrants in marrying a British woman. Correspondence with John Ellis in around 1681 shows Drelincourt making serious efforts to find a wife. Mention is made of his financial circumstances and of someone in France, but he says that he is much more interested in Ellis's sister, showing a clear desire for assimilation into his new society.[38] This sister is unlikely to be the Mary he eventually married, but his wife brought with her an estate in Wales which bordered on that of a Mr Ellis, so there may have been some link. There is some uncertainty about the background of Drelincourt's wife, but it is likely that she was a daughter of Peter Morris who was for a short time Dean of Derry and who had a daughter named Mary.[39] Mrs Drelincourt was one of the executors of the will of his son Theodore in 1731, and Theodore's daughter Mary Margaret received a bequest from Dean Drelincourt and is described in his will as his goddaughter.[40] Peter Morris is also recorded in his will as the Revd Peter Morris of Killenshir in the Co. of Denbigh going to Ireland[41] and we know that Mrs Drelincourt had estates near Wrexham in Denbighshire.[42] It is also likely that she was a sister of Edward Maurice who was Bishop of Ossory 1754–5. He was co-executor of her brother's will in 1731 and his bequest of books to what is now St Canice's Library in Kilkenny in 1756 contained a number of books which had belonged to Peter Drelincourt.[43] Mrs Drelincourt survived her husband by many years, dying in 1755, and their daughter Ann was married in 1739 to a man who had been born in 1716, so it is probable that this was a very late marriage for the Dean. It certainly cemented his position in society, for his daughter married a viscount, but if the marriage took place late, as seems likely, it cannot have had any great influence on his ecclesiastical career. It is, however, indicative of his active pursuit of assimilation into his new society.

Finally, like some of the other immigrant entrants to the Anglican churches, Drelincourt produced one or perhaps two pieces of writing which were politically significant. Both were pieces of propaganda designed to entice the Huguenots to settle in Ireland. The first, in French, is anonymous, but it dates from 1681 when Drelincourt, as we saw earlier, was already in Ireland and a chaplain in Ormond's household. It could be described in modern terms as a publicity leaflet for Ireland, written in French and targeting the Huguenot market. Ireland is presented as a land of milk and honey, offering many opportunities in farming, manufacturing and commerce. It is a country where the Protestant church is powerful:

> La Religion Protestante y a la Justice, le Pouvoir, et toute l'Authorité en main; soutenue d'une bonne Armée de dix mille hommes, répanduë dans tout le Pays en diverses Garnisons, et composée de Soldats Protestans: Leurs Officiers, Ceux de Justice, et de Police, les Magistrats, et les Gouverneurs le sont aussi.[44]

He goes on to claim that taxes are low, the right to property is respected; the Huguenots have been very well received and are treated like native-born (Protestant) Irishmen; they have a French church; money has been collected for them; good will surrounds them; and naturalization will be easily and cheaply obtained.

Such a piece of writing must have found favour with Ormond who had lived in France and knew the French language well, but it was destined primarily to be read by a French audience and to attract Huguenots to Ireland where Ormond was anxious to welcome them for the skills and economic benefits they could bring. The second pamphlet was published in Dublin in 1682, this time under Drelincourt's name and destined to be read by English speakers, since it was written in English. This pamphlet, *A speech made to His Grace the Duke of Ormond, Lord Lieutenant of Ireland, and to the lords of His majesties most honourable Privy Council, to return the humble thanks of the French Protestants lately arriv'd in the kingdom and graciously reliev'd by them,* is mentioned in a letter dated 16 November [probably 1681] where Drelincourt asks Ellis to ensure its publication in London and states that he wrote it out of gratitude for the welcome given to the refugees to Ireland:

> Vous aurez sans doute appris la manière obligeante et charitable avec laquelle on a reçeu icy les protestans françois qui y sont arrivez despuis peu, J'ay peur que personne ne songe a publier la generosité de ces Messrs du conseil du Roy et de cette ville. C'est pourquoy je vous prie de ne pas manquer de faire donner ce memoire qui est de l'autre coté, je viens de le faire moy-même, faites-le mettre, je vous prie dans la première gazette qui s'imprimera a Londres . . . [45]

He also states later in the letter that he has already shown it to the members of the Privy Council who approved it and want it to be published in London. Its fulsome thanks on behalf of the second wave of Huguenot refugees to Ireland were written, it would appear, without any consultation with the refugees, and the pamphlet seems to be designed primarily to enhance the writer's reputation with those who mattered, at a time when he was casting about for a new career, after leaving that of tutor.

In conclusion, then, Drelincourt was less celebrated than many of the other entrants to Anglican holy orders, but he had influential family connections, especially through his brother Charles who knew William and Mary, and he found, in the Duke of Ormond, a very influential protector to further his career. He arrived well before the Revocation of the Edict of Nantes in 1685 and may have benefited from being one of a smaller number of immigrants. He seems also to have arrived at quite a young age and to have been more prepared than many of the other Huguenot immigrants to leave the tight circle of French society and become fully integrated into English life and customs, gaining a command of English which must have been of considerable assistance in helping him make a good impression on those who could assist him to make his way in the world. However the decisive factor, if, as seems likely, he was the author of *De l'état présent d'Irlande*, must surely have been his activity as a pamphleteer. His role in helping to attract Huguenots to Ireland to swell the ranks of the minority Protestant population and bring new skills to its economic development would have been of considerable value to the Duke of Ormond and, together with his other services to the Duke and his family, would have accounted for the rapid preferment which formed the basis of his future prosperity.

NOTES

1 Ruth Whelan, 'Liberté de culte, liberté de conscience? Les huguenots en Irlande 1662–1702', in Jens Häseler and Antony McKenna (eds.), *La vie intellectuelle aux Refuges protestants* (Paris, 1999), 69–83.

2 Charles Weiss, *Histoire des réfugiés protestants de France depuis la révocation de l'Edit de Nantes* (Paris, 1853), 263–76.

3 R. Whelan, 'Sanctified by the Word: the Huguenots and Anglican liturgy', in Kevin Herlihy (ed.), *Propagating the Word of Irish Dissent, 1650–1800* (Dublin, 1998), 75–94.

4 D. C. A. Agnew, *Protestant exiles from France* (London, 1871), vol. 2, 271–3.

5 *Ibid.*, vol. 1, 19–21. Their foreign qualifications were recognized by Oxford and they were given an Oxford degree.

6 Charles Drelincourt in Paris exemplified this desire to find common ground with English Anglicans, but his *Lettres sur l'episcopat d'Angleterre* (Paris, 1660) also reflect the difficulty of attempting any real *rapprochement*. The letters begin with a real desire to accept the English episcopacy, but they also demand tolerance for the system of the Eglise Réformée and grow increasingly impatient with the lordliness of the English hierarchy.

7 Agnew, *Protestant exiles*, vol. 2, 96–102.

8 *Ibid.*, 273; Emile and Eugène Haag, *La France protestante* (Paris, 1846–59; reprinted Geneva, 1966), vol. 9, 184.

9 Agnew, vol. 2, 208–13.

10 H. Cotton, *Fasti Ecclesiae Hibernicae: the succession of the prelates and members of the cathedral bodies in Ireland* (Dublin, 1848), vol. 1, 413, 478; vol. 2, 33, 53; vol. 3, 188, 338; vol. 4, 80, 84, 93, 105.

11 Agnew, vol. 2, 96–118, 208–26, 271–5.

12 Haag and Haag, vol. 1, 61–6.

13 *Ibid.*, vol. 1, 7–11.

14 Jacques Abbadie, *La vérité de la religion chrétienne* (Rotterdam, 1684).

15 Haag and Haag, vol. 8, 245–8.

16 Agnew, vol. 2, 274–5.

17 *Ibid.*, 220–1.

18 *Memoirs of the Reverend Jaques Fontaine, 1658–1728*, ed. Dianne Ressinger, Huguenot Society New Series 2 (London, 1992), 147, 213

19 Agnew, vol. 2, 111, 116.

20 Drelincourt to John Ellis, 29 April 1681: BL, Add. MS 28875, fos. 216–17.

21 Haag and Haag, vol. 4, 430–1; Agnew, vol. 2, 208–13.

22 Toby Barnard notes the reluctance of 17th-century clergymen to reside in the country because of the discomforts and dangers involved. See T. Barnard, 'Improving clergymen', in A. Ford, J. McGuire and K. Milne (eds.), *As by law established* (Dublin, 1995), 142.

23 Agnew, vol. 2, 101

24 Barnard, 'Improving clergymen', 141.

25 'The case of the Quare Impedit brought by the Crown against the Archbishop of Armagh & Nathanael Whaley Clerk the Present Rector of Armagh for the rectory of Armagh', no date: Public Record Office, Northern Ireland, T545(1). The P.R.O.N.I. dates the manuscript to between 1722 and 1730.

26 Sir James Balfour Paul (ed.), *The Scots peerage* (Edinburgh, 1910), vol. 7, 111.

27 'Avertissement du libraire', in L. Drelincourt, *Sonnets chrétiens* (Amsterdam, 1746).

28 Haag and Haag, vol. 4, 314–17.

29 Pierre Bayle, *Dictionnaire historique et critique* (3rd edition, Rotterdam, 1720), 1019.

30 G. L. Lee, *The Huguenot settlements in Ireland* (London, 1936), 200.

31 J. McKee, 'Pierre Drelincourt et sa contribution à la vie intellectuelle en Angleterre et en Irlande', in Jens Häseler and Antony McKenna (eds.), *La vie intellectuelle aux Refuges protestants* (Paris, 1999), 272.

32 Cotton, vol. 2, 33, 53.

33 Barnard, 'Improving clergymen', 141.

34 B. Armstrong and E. Labrousse, 'Une lettre de Jean Durel à Charles Drelincourt', *Bulletin de la Société de l'histoire du protestantisme français* (April–June 1967), 263–97.

35 Drelincourt to Ormond, 17 July 1679: *Historical Manuscripts Commission, Calendar of the manuscripts of the Marquess of Ormond, K. P. preserved at Kilkenny Castle*, new series, vol. 5 (Hereford, 1908), 156.

36 Drelincourt to John Ellis, 20 October 1692: BL, Add. MS 28877, fo. 413; Drelincourt to Ellis, 11 April 1693: BL, Add. MS 28878, fo. 78. John Ellis, like Peter Drelincourt, was a protégé of the Ormond family, employed as secretary first to Thomas, Earl of Ossory and, after his death in 1680, to the Duke of Ormond. He came to Ireland as secretary to the Commissioners of the Revenue, but left again in 1689 to become secretary to the second Duke of Ormond before gaining favour with William III and later with George I. He occupied a series of public offices and amassed a considerable fortune.

37 Arran to Ormond: HMC, *Calendar of the Manuscripts of the Marquess of Ormond*, New Series, vol. 7 (London, 1912), 25.

38 Drelincourt to Ellis, 23 August (2 letters) [1681], 17 September [1681]: BL, Add. MS 28894, fos. 77–82

39 J. B. Leslie, *Derry clergy and parishes* (Enniskillen, 1937), 35.

40 J. B. Leslie, *Armagh clergy and parishes* (Dundalk, 1911), 218–19.

41 Leslie, *Derry clergy*, 35.

42 BL, Add. MS 12563–A (Map, dated 1747).

43 The present curator of St Canice's Library, Mr Hugh Campbell, has identified some of these books.

44 [P. Drelincourt], *De l'état présent d'Irlande, et des avantages qu'y peuvent trouver les protestans françois: en une lettre d'un des chapelains de monseigneur le duc d'Ormond, viceroi d'Irlande, a un de ses amis en Angleterre* (Dublin, 1681), 5.

45 Drelincourt to Ellis, 16 November [1681]: BL, Add. MS 28894, fos. 83–4.

49

Good faith: the military and the ministry in exile, or the memoirs of Isaac Dumont de Bostaquet and Jaques Fontaine

DIANNE W. RESSINGER

The wave of Huguenots who settled in England and Ireland after 1685 produced two rare full-length autobiographies which are written from, in turn, the military and the ecclesiastical viewpoint. Both are powerful and revealing documents on many levels, describing in detail the lives of two Protestant families in France before 1685 as well as in exile in England and Ireland. Isaac Dumont de Bostaquet, a nobleman from Normandy, and Jaques Fontaine, a minister from Saintonge, wrote vastly different accounts of hardship, defeat and the ultimate triumph of faith in a difficult time. Beyond their importance as Huguenot documents, their memoirs are important first-person accounts of international events in the late 17th century, particularly Dumont's description of William III's Irish campaigns and Fontaine's account of conditions in England and Ireland. Dumont de Bostaquet's memoirs have never been available in English, and these comments are based on a translation in progress, with much material yet to interpret. His manuscript was an important source for Thomas Babington Macaulay, who brought it to the attention of French editors Charles Read and Francis Waddington who published it in 1864. Their edition of Dumont's memoirs has often been used to illustrate aspects of the diaspora to Ireland.

The two Huguenots reflect different extremes of integration into life in England and Ireland. Each made observations about his host society, from which Dumont remained generally aloof while Fontaine participated fully, though contentiously. Both memoirs were meant for private family use, and neither was published until more than 100 years after the death of the man who wrote it.[1]

Captain Isaac Dumont de Bostaquet's recollections give many personal details, but are far more objective than the Reverend Jaques Fontaine's. Nearly half of Dumont's manuscript concerns his years as a cavalry officer, describing his role as eyewitness to the Glorious Revolution and William III's Irish campaigns of 1689–92. The Reverend Jaques Fontaine casts himself as beleaguered hero of his recollections, offering an intimate self-portrait. A judgemental and analytical man, in looking back he found fault with himself as well as with others. Each of the two men was certain of the importance of his life story and felt a deep need to relate his part in events he considered significant in a turbulent lifetime.

The two Huguenots had little in common except that both were men of action and both were Protestant. Dumont de Bostaquet was a pragmatic realist and a soldier, accepting hardship as a fact of his life in exile. Jaques Fontaine was an idealist who set high standards for himself and others; hoping for the best, he expected the worst. Frequently convinced that he would be treated badly, this often became a self-fulfilling prophecy, and disappointment made him critical and self-righteous. The results of their different viewpoints are two widely different eyewitness accounts of the refugee experience in England and Ireland.

The life stories of these two men will be familiar to historians of the Huguenot movement. Since there are no comparable full-length autobiographies, Dumont is often used to represent the military and nobility in exile while Fontaine speaks for the ministry. The pitfall in seeing them as representative is that looking back is always subjective, coloured by personality and perception and distorted by choice as well as by accident and opportunity.

Twenty-six years – a generation – separate the births of Isaac Dumont de Bostaquet and Jaques Fontaine, both from notable families in France. Captain Dumont was born in 1632, the Reverend Fontaine in 1658, the same year as the first of Dumont's children. Dumont was cheerfully aware of his privileged status – his aristocratic connections[2] nearly drown us in a sea of Norman nobility. Fontaine was eager to convince his descendants of his family's noble origins,[3] although he claims to disdain nobility as meaningless in the face of life's realities. Both men were deeply mindful of family members who sacrificed conviction in order to preserve their comfortable lives in France, and both suffered exile, failed expectations, and relative impoverishment for the sake of faith.

Though he left a number of grown children in France, the children who shared Dumont's exile were under 10 years of age when he wrote his story, finishing it when he was 61 years old. Fontaine's story was also told in old age – he was 64 – and all but one of his children had gone, most of them to Virginia. He was determined to maintain family solidarity, while Dumont knew that this was an impossibility. He had seen his family torn apart by the diaspora – his children who remained in France included a daughter born after his escape whom in fact he would never see.

The major trait the two men shared was belief in the benevolence of the 'Providence' which had directed their lives. Each had extraordinary faith in God's plan which he trusted in spite of the disruptions and discomforts of life in exile.

France

Dumont's privileged early life and education in France took place amongst his elite family connections, and he paints a colourful picture of the daily life of a *seigneur* in the mid-17th century. Military and government service were a family tradition just as service to the Church was Fontaine's heritage. Dumont was an only son and benefited from the best education available to a young Huguenot nobleman. At 13 he attended the Protestant academy at Saumur[4] for two years, followed by exclusive riding and military academies in Rouen and Paris. In 1652 he briefly entered military service, but soon returned to Normandy where he married and for many years lived the life of a country gentleman.

Fontaine's early life in France was less colourful and refined than the aristocratic Dumont's, but like Dumont he was raised by a widowed but assertive mother. His education, extensive by standards of the time, was somewhat haphazard. A series of indifferent teachers preceded his attendance at the College of Guyenne, where he earned his Master of Arts degree in 1683. His education was arranged 'by those who preferred thrift to my advancement' as the family suffered increasing persecution in the early 1680s.[5]

Dumont de Bostaquet was to marry three times. In 1657 he married the first of three 'shadow' wives about whom we know everything and nothing. We know everything about the maze of his litigious in-laws, but we know almost nothing about the three women as individuals. He rarely calls them by name, and they seem almost interchangeable – portrayed as passive and uninvolved. His first two weddings show Protestant *noblesse* at play under the protection of the Edict of Nantes – they are anything but solemn with horses, dogs, lackeys in elegant livery, music and *masques*. He married a third time in 1679 to the woman with whom he shared persecution and exile. Marie de Brossard is described as no longer young, but with a spirit 'solid and intelligent, sustained by wisdom and piety'.[6] In exile she was forced to be selfsufficient, and must have been a woman of resource, for she managed family affairs during Dumont's long absences in Ireland.

Dumont seems not to have known his children intimately, for he rarely mentions them as individuals. He had a total of 19 children, several of whom died as infants or young children. It was clearly a man's world, and the only child he describes in any depth was his son and namesake, Isaac. The birth of his children by three wives spanned the 31 years between 1658 and 1689.[7]

Family life for Fontaine by comparison seems extremely intimate. In his memoirs he created a deeply felt portrait of his wife Anne Elisabeth, whom he married soon after escaping with her to England; it was a true and lifelong partnership. She must have been impressive in every sense; serene, intelligent, spirited yet devout, with firm opinions which she was not afraid to express. She was certainly a match for her volatile husband, who had great regard for her. Their eight children were all born in exile, between 1686 and 1701.[8]

Both Dumont's and Fontaine's stories of persecution and escape are detailed and exciting, well-known and often quoted. In 1685 Dumont, 53 years old, faced with the prospect of dragoons in a home filled with women and young girls, felt he had no choice but abjuration, though it shamed him deeply.[9] He finally left France in 1687, forced by circumstance to abandon a pregnant wife, 11 children, an 80-year old mother, and extensive property holdings. He escaped to Holland, where the family was reunited in The Hague the following year. There Dumont enrolled as a captain of cavalry in Louvigny's regiment of Red Dragoons and joined William, Prince of Orange, on his expedition to England in 1688.[10]

Fontaine, remembering his escape in his memoirs, portrays himself as a brave but indignant single man of 27 with few responsibilities, embarked on an exciting adventure. He dashed about the countryside urging resistance, disguised as a country gentleman to keep out of the clutches of dragoons who had taken over his home. His bold escape in an open boat near La Rochelle, however, looks like child's play compared to the agony of Dumont's arrival in Holland, wounded, alone, and devastated at leaving his family behind.

Exile: England

Dumont's initial impression of England, landing with William's forces at Torbay in November 1688, is one of military splendour described in extravagant language, and his account then turns to the logistics of landing, lodgings, and marching in unfamiliar terrain. His comments on his early days in England lack descriptions of personal contact with the English. He says simply, 'We enjoyed observing the islanders' way of life',[11] and nothing is said of interaction beyond an occasional remark on the habits of local citizens with whom he lodged. His attention is on military matters as part of a liberating force rather than as an individual in contact with local populations.

His first substantive comment about life in England has to do with seeing an Anglican church service, and is probably the passage most often quoted from his memoirs. He writes, in part:

> At Exeter I saw the Anglican church service for the first time, and I was surprised that all of the outward appearance of papism had been retained . . . But because all this was so unlike the simplicity of our Reformed service, I was not edified by it.[12]

Fontaine's assessment of the Anglican church is remarkably close to Dumont's. Ordained by the Presbyterian Synod at Taunton in 1688, he remained staunchly nonconformist. He writes:

> Th[e] splendour [of the English church] did not impress me. I preferred the simplicity of worship that I had professed from childhood to all the grandeur, pomp, magnificence and riches of the Episcopalians. I decided then to labour with my own hands and preach the Gospel in its purity of doctrine and simplicity of ceremony.[13]

Dumont brought only his pregnant wife and two small children from The Hague to live in Greenwich in the summer of 1689; his older children remained in France. In Greenwich they found a complete support system; the presence of the senior Marquis de Ruvigny and his family at the Queen's House there brought many prominent refugees to live in or visit the town.[14]

The following description, with its striking lack of any mention of Englishmen, was written in the summer of 1689:

> We have found good company here, especially the family of the Marquis de Ruvigny. His generosity and mercy toward the unhappy refugees provides a sanctuary to those in need . . . My wife received the help she needed in giving birth to our child; . . . [a]nd the Marquis de Ruvigny and Madame Chardin did me the honour of presenting him for baptism . . . at the Queen's House.[15]

Though his financial security was limited, there was no question about how Dumont would earn a living and provide for his family; he was a cavalry officer, supported by the military. Combining his highborn and his military connections, Dumont was able to make a pleasant transition to life in England. During his long absences in Ireland in the service of King William III, his family functioned wholly within the Huguenot community in Greenwich. Because his needs were met by his aristocratic, military, and family contacts, he had little need to participate in English society, a pattern which would continue in Ireland. He had the additional comfort and security of leaving Marie and their three children in the safe Huguenot haven at Greenwich.

Jaques Fontaine also wrote an idyllic description of his arrival in England in November 1685 after 11 days at sea in a small boat,[16] but the idyll soon turned to poverty, bitterness, and frustration. In contrast to Dumont's Greenwich experience, there was no ready-made support system in elegant surroundings to ease the transition into life in the west of England. His was a daily struggle in a small house in a back street, dealing with a system he neither understood nor accepted. Within two years of his arrival in England, he married and had his first child, engaged in the grain trade with relatives remaining in France, started a school for teaching French, and began a profitable cloth manufactory. Fontaine described all of this in great detail, and all of it required extensive interaction with the English economy and social structure. From the day of his arrival in England he was forced into competition and conflict with local citizens. His constant assertions of being cheated by local businessmen as well as by relatives with whom he attempted to do business in France show his developing suspicion and scepticism.[17] That it seems often to have been true is unfortunate and says much about the reality of life in exile.

Fontaine's alienation can clearly be seen as an expression of his feelings of isolation from the English and later Irish towns in which he lived. His failure or inability to embrace local customs and practices resulted in contempt for the very people with whom he was forced to associate in his need to support his family. He lived in several communities but remained detached, not accepted in them, facing his difficulties with an arrogant and uncompromising attitude. Fontaine spent nearly 10 years in England, and when he left he never looked back.

In comparing the language skills of the two men, Dumont's description of his furlough from Ireland to rejoin his family at Greenwich in November of 1690 is telling:

> [W]e landed and went in search of lodgings, [and] slept comfortably at the home of a peasant, and the next morning we hired horses to travel . . . [to] Chester. A young Englishman who had crossed with us joined us, bargained for everything we needed, and was useful to us during the whole trip.[18]

Although he does not specifically discuss speaking English, it seems safe to say that his command of the language was rudimentary. He had spent two years in England and Ireland when he wrote this, and he still needed help with transactions in English. Protected within the French regimental fellowship, he had little need to speak English because his contact with the populace was limited.

Fontaine, on the other hand, was thrown instantly into the local economy. He comments about his first purchase of bread in the new country: 'the man we were with spoke poor French. I asked him to repeat it several times, thinking I had misunderstood him, but he repeated that each biscuit cost only a halfpenny'. Quickly realizing that one could make money buying English grain and shipping it to France, he decided to go to the grain market, 'choosing an interpreter who was not very bright' so as not to give away his plans. Obviously his English was limited, but necessity forced him into business immediately. After six weeks he received a proposal of marriage from his English host's sister, who had 'a servant repeat this to me in the worst possible English [which] I understood as well as she did, but pretended not to follow'.[19] He had made remarkable progress with his English. He must have found necessity a good teacher but he really had no choice.

Exile: Ireland

Dumont and Fontaine took their families to Ireland to live at about the same time, Dumont in 1692 and Fontaine in 1694. Their experiences in Ireland continued and even magnified what had happened to them in England.

Dumont's move to Ireland came because of the pension he had been granted on the Irish Establishment for his service in William's Irish campaigns.[20] He tells us, surprisingly, that his wife was willing to leave Greenwich and 'definitely wished to go to Ireland and insisted that I stop thinking of anything but our journey'.[21]

In Dublin Dumont was once again surrounded and supported by old friends and military companions, his attitudes determined by his loyalty to his regiment and to Ruvigny, now Lord Galway. Dumont's name appears as *ancien* in the registers of the French Church of St Patrick between 1692 and 1697, when he removed to Portarlington, appearing in the registers there in November of 1698.[22] Little is known of his life in Dublin, but in Portarlington Dumont was among the retired military men who shared the same fate. Recent research shows that Portarlington was not the golden Valhalla for retired officers which has often been described, but was a significant colony of exiled Huguenot families of shared experiences and ideals. Disagreement and controversy occurred there as elsewhere.[23]

When he decided to bring his family to Ireland, Dumont had already spent considerable time there as a captain of cavalry in Lord Galway's regiment (formerly the Duke of Schomberg's, who had been killed at the Battle of the Boyne). Dumont fought in and described several major engagements in the campaign, including the Boyne, and was closely and personally allied to Lord Galway. Unfortunately his memoirs end just six months after he had brought his family to Dublin. We have no commentary on Huguenot society there, and even more regrettably, we do not have his first-hand account of the colony of pensioned military officers at Portarlington. His comments on Dublin are limited to a few vague phrases and the final paragraph of his long manuscript:

> Six months and more have passed since my arrival in Ireland. Here we have known the happiness of being among our friends and the even greater joy of having . . . with us our pastors from Greenwich . . . And so after six years of pilgrimage, I am at Dublin. The arrival of Milord Galway has given us real joy and touched us with sweet pleasure in this strange country. Yet here I think constantly of my family in France, and I pray to God to bless them along with my family here which is happier serving God as we do in full liberty. They join their voices to mine, praying for the deliverance of our family in France and for our reunion . . . [24]

Though there is no account of the last 16 years of his life, his memoirs make another extremely important contribution, as they are the only substantial eyewitness account of an officer in one of the three Huguenot regiments which played a significant role in William III's victory in Ireland. In addition to identifying many of the officers in the Huguenot regiments, his first-hand narrative was used by Macaulay as a major resource in his *History of England from the accession of James II*, which influenced generations of historians. Macaulay, in describing the reign of William and Mary, the Battle of the Boyne, and the sieges of Limerick and Londonderry made extensive use of Dumont de Bostaquet's manuscript.[25]

In common with many Huguenots, including Fontaine, Dumont had almost nothing to say about either Ireland or the Irish – they might almost have been invisible.[26] His comments are limited to observations of the poverty and desolation caused by the military campaign in which he had participated. In Ireland he had no more need to integrate himself or his family into the local economic or social structure than there had been in England. He stayed within the safe confines of Dublin's and Portarlington's Huguenot communities.

Fontaine took his family to Ireland in 1694 in order to practise as a Calvinist minister. He found his place in Cork among 'a few French people eager to have a minister but [who] did not have the means to pay one'.[27] Though he ended his life in the security and comfort of the large Huguenot community at Dublin, Fontaine's first 15 years in Ireland were filled with isolation, failure, betrayal, and attack, hating and hated by the native Irish. There is much historical drama in his recollections of his early years in Ireland, but overall it was a grim if colourful period in his life.[28]

In 1699 Fontaine moved his family to the remote Bere Peninsula in order to establish a farm and fishery there, taking with him 13 French soldiers who had retired after serving in William's Irish campaigns. The fishery failed, the soldiers left, and by 1702 he was deeply in debt, for which he characteristically blamed others. His family was twice attacked at their remote home by French privateers who finally destroyed most of his property, wounding and taking him prisoner for a time. The result of this ruin was compensation by the Irish government, and he received a pension which provided security for the rest of his life and an education for his children. The family's final move was to St Stephen's Green, Dublin, in 1709. A measure of his feelings when at last he arrived in Dublin is that in the final pages of his memoirs there is an end to the vituperative comments about Ireland which had dominated his previous descriptions. After the long years of strife and disruption he at last found peace among Dublin's Huguenots.

Children

If an immigrant family can be said to have successfully integrated into the host society when its children have become a part of that society and contributed something to it, then both the Dumont and the Fontaine families failed to integrate in Ireland. Of Dumont's children no son survived to leave the protection of the Huguenot community at Portarlington and take his place in the Irish establishment, and his daughters never left the colony there. By contrast, all of Fontaine's children left Ireland and integrated most successfully into life in the British colony of Virginia. Correspondence between those in England and those who went to Colonial Virginia provides a marvellous study of assimilation in progress through two generations.[29]

In Portarlington only Dumont's daughter Judith-Julie remained with him until his death in 1709; his two youngest sons entered military service in Holland, where the eldest died at age 23 in 1706, and the fate of his youngest son is unknown after that date. After Dumont's death Marie Magdelaine, the daughter whom he had never seen, came from France to Ireland. She married in Portarlington, but nothing is known of her two daughters who survived. Judith-Julie had six children by two marriages, and of Dumont's children only she left known descendants in Ireland. Judith-Julie's second marriage, after her father's death, was to Antoine Ligonier de Bonneval, conformist minister of the French Church at Portarlington. Their descendants were the Vignoles family, through whom Dumont's memoirs were preserved and made known to Macaulay.[30]

Dumont and Fontaine were both separated at the end of their lives from all of their children except, in each case, one daughter. It is easy to imagine how precious Judith-Julie was to her father Isaac Dumont de Bostaquet, a man who lost by death or distance 18 of the 19 children he fathered. Fontaine was lonely but consoled by the success and close contact his children maintained in spite of the distances which separated them.

Attitude to France

Regardless of all other comparisons that can be made, Dumont and Fontaine were in exactly the same position before leaving France. Leave or remain, each of them was a ruined man unless he were willing to abjure. Both had much to lose, but the ways in which they remembered and regarded their home country were very different.

Dumont took great pride in the endless family connections which shaped his identity. In exile he looked back with longing and nostalgia to his extended family, his estates in Normandy, and to the children left behind. He learned later of the bitter aftermath of his escape – his condemnation *in absentia* as a criminal, persecution of family members, the death of his mother and some of his children. The last sentence of his memoirs is a prayer for the deliverance of his family still in France and for their reunion. Dumont's deep sadness and yearning for his lost and lovely life there is one of the most touching aspects of his memoirs.

By contrast, Fontaine's attitude to France was one of hatred and blame, and he felt contempt rather than sorrow for family members who elected to stay behind. In England and Ireland he was more than once cheated by relatives still in France, and he was relentless in his hatred of the French privateers who attacked him twice at his home on the Bere Peninsula. Even his attitude to his fellow refugees is often far from generous. In refuge Fontaine expresses scorn for France, viewing her difficulties from afar with triumph in his belief that the kingdom had been destroyed by casting out the Huguenots. His extreme point of view was expressed in his memoirs: 'Never think that France will enjoy prosperity while she oppresses God's elect'.[31]

Good Faith

In the opening 50 pages of their respective memoirs Dumont refers to God 13 times, Fontaine more than 60, reflecting the more central role of religion in the Fontaine family. Differences in their interpretations of God throughout their lives reveal their self-identities as well as their personalities, professions, and perspectives.

Dumont typically 'praises, blesses, thanks, and loves' God who 'saves, protects, preserves, and sustains' him. In adversity Dumont did not express anger at God, but resignation. His convictions remain constant through his memoirs. He saw God as benevolent, believing that those who love Him will find eternal happiness, and when disaster struck he saw it as God's punishment. For example, after a string of mis-fortunes in 1673 which included the death of his second wife and the complete destruction by fire of his *château* at Fontelaye, he wrote 'I regarded these repeated blows as the effect of God's anger toward me. I reflected on them as much as my human weakness was capable of, and throwing myself into the arms of His divine providence, I tried to endure all my unhappiness with constancy'.[32]

As a minister, Fontaine's preoccupation with religious ideas and practices was more complex and all-consuming. Describing events in his early life he used such expressions as God 'commanded, deprived, thwarted, directed, judged'. He saw mercy and promise on occasion, but generally saw himself as a young warrior and the religious crisis in France as war. In 1685 he was unmarried and without dependents, while Dumont was a man of 53 with a large household and a great deal of property to safeguard. However reluctantly, Dumont abjured before he finally left the country in 1687.

While Fontaine's religious principles and commitment cannot be doubted, there is no question that he revelled in the adventure of the upheaval of persecution, and with youth's intense emotion, he saw God as vengeful and demanding. But he experienced an awakening, and from the moment of his arrival in England his descriptions of God – written 37 years after the fact – change. Surely he would not himself have been aware of what his own writing revealed about the effect of freedom of worship on his view of God. He began to use such phrases as 'infinite mercy, grace, pity, deliverance', and that God 'helped, provided, comforted, strengthened, rescued' him and gave him solace in a life otherwise marred by bitterness and resentment.

It is ironic that the violence in France brought out a corresponding fury in Fontaine, a minister and thus supposedly a peaceable man, which Dumont, a professional soldier but apparently a gentler nature, never expressed. Fontaine was often hostile, and on occasion he showed a shocking streak of violence. He writes appallingly of an incident at Bearhaven:

> one of [the] robbers lived in a cave in a rock among some of my Irish tenants . . . [I] climbed down towards him, pistol in hand, and called to him to surrender, or I would fire at him. He threw himself on the ground and surrendered peacefully. I seized him by the hair, my pistol in my hand, in case he made the slightest resistance . . . I sent him to Cork where he was hanged and quartered. I received a reward of £40 and many thanks from the government and men of importance . . . loved doing strict justice to the Irish in my position as Justice of the Peace . . . I sent eight or 10 to prison at Cork every assizes . . . I was the one to be feared in the county . . . [33]

Dumont, being older, experienced rather more peaceful conditions as a young man in France, which shaped a soldier who seldom expressed bitterness or hostility. A captain of cavalry for four years in England and Ireland, he never mentions killing anyone.

Conclusion

In order for an author to consider his reminiscences important enough to write down, they must contain elements of surprise and excitement in his own mind. His objective is to capture the interest as well as the admiration or sympathy of those for whom they are created. When Dumont, almost at the end of his travels, and Fontaine, definitely at the end of his, reached Dublin, the upheavals had been endured and surmounted and each of the two men had found peace. There was really nothing left to tell.

It had been fairly easy to accept a new environment on good faith as Dumont did, for he was not forced to struggle to support himself and his family within it. Others directed his actions, and he seems to have lived happily enough on the outside looking in. Fontaine, on the inside with both feet, remained uneasy about his place in a social structure he did not always fully grasp. Though he would have denied it, throughout his years in England and Ireland his writing shows his hunger for the importance which contacts with such men as Lord Galway could give him. Important men were – and had always been – Dumont's world, and he moved easily within the upper reaches of Huguenot society in exile.

However different their backgrounds, ages, personalities, professions, families, and the experiences they recounted, Dumont and Fontaine ended in almost exactly the same circumstances. Each lived fairly comfortably in retirement, supported and consoled – in the company of other exiles – for the loss of financial security and home-land, in which he had lost faith. In the shelter of a Huguenot community, each man had a pension of 5 shillings per day provided by the Irish government. Each had lost the comfort of continuity and stability, and each had suffered disruption after dis-ruption in an effort to find a practical way to live in exile. But whatever they had lost, in the end each man retained his faith that God's plan for him had been essentially good no matter how incomprehensible.

Dumont had faith in military order and the wisdom of leaders, and in the good intentions and generosity of others. Fontaine had an equally strong faith that others will usually act badly and for selfish gain, and that authority is usually corrupt. But both men believed in themselves and the rightness of the sacrifice they had made to preserve religious freedom. In lives filled with disruption, faith provided the only real continuity.

Was it worth it? Dumont looks back to France with longing to the family he left there, while Fontaine looks ahead to America. The reality of their last years in Ireland was far more humble than what their expectations in France would have provided, but they were able to share their lives with others who had made the same sacrifices of economic security, homeland, and continuity. Their faith had become their identity.

NOTES

1 The complete history of the two holographic manuscripts written by Jaques Fontaine in Dublin in 1722 is given in the introduction (pp. 13–21) to *Memoirs of the Reverend Jaques Fontaine*, ed. Dianne W. Ressinger, Huguenot Society of Great Britain and Ireland New Series No. 2 (London, 1992), the first complete English version of this text [hereafter Fontaine, *Memoirs*]. Quotes from Fontaine used in this paper come from this edition. Quotes from the memoirs of Dumont de Bostaquet follow the pagination of Charles Read's and Francis Waddington's edition of the manuscript: *Mémoires inédits de Dumont de Bostaquet, gentilhomme normand, sur les temps qui ont précédé et suivi la révocation de l'Edit de Nantes, sur le refuge et les expéditions de Guillaume III en Angleterre et en Irlande*, eds. C. Read and F. Waddington (Paris, 1864) [hereafter Dumont de Bostaquet, *Mémoires*]. The author of this paper is currently preparing a full-length English translation of Isaac Dumont de Bostaquet's memoirs.

2 Dumont wrote a lengthy genealogy of his family which gives details of related noble families in France as early as 1370, but unfortunately gives few dates. Dates of birth for his parents' generation are not given. Isaac was born in 1632, his parents Samuel Dumont and Anne de La Haye *c.*1600. It seems reasonable to date the family's adherence to the Protestant faith from some time around the date of the marriage of Isaac's grandfather Geffroy Dumont, Lord and Patron of La Fontelaye, Bostaquet, Viboeuf, and Bellemare. He married Elisabeth Rémond as his second wife, and they gave their sons typical Huguenot Old Testament names (Samuel, Abraham, Isaac, Jacob) during the last quarter of the 16th century. Dumont de Bostaquet, *Mémoires*, 327–36.

3 Fontaine, *Memoirs*, 25–7.

4 Fontaine's father and uncle also attended the famous Protestant academy, known for its high academic standards, at about this time. *Ibid.*, 50.

5 This comment precedes a description of educational methods used to teach philosophy at the College of Guyenne, 1682–3. *Ibid.*, 78.

6 A description of the three weddings can be found in Dumont de Bostaquet, *Mémoires*, 29, 47, 80.

7 A complete list of Dumont's children, including a history of the Vignoles family as well as a correction of mistakes made by Read and Waddington in their 1864 Introduction, is given in T. P. Le Fanu, 'Dumont de Bostaquet at Portarlington', *HSP* 14 (1929–33), 226–7.

8 For a complete list of his children and grandchildren see Fontaine, *Memoirs*, 223 (Appendix 1)

9 Dumont de Bostaquet, *Mémoires*, 107.

10 *Ibid.*, 218.

11 *Ibid.*, 217.

12 *Ibid.*, 223.

13 Fontaine, *Memoirs*, 133.

14 A detailed history of the Huguenot community at Greenwich, using baptismal and burial records as well as diaries of contemporaries Samuel Pepys and John Evelyn, is given in Randolph Vigne, 'In the Purlieus of St Alfege's', *HSP* 27:2 (1999), 257–73. Not only are prominent Huguenot families identified and their contributions described, but many less famous Huguenot names are given from parish registers. Dumont de Bostaquet is discussed at some length, and the baptismal record of Henri, Dumont's son, in July 1689 is noted as part of the St Alfege register.

15 Dumont de Bostaquet, *Mémoires*, 246.

16 Fontaine, *Memoirs*, 124.

17 *Ibid.*, 123–9.

18 Dumont de Bostaquet, *Mémoires*, 296.

19 Fontaine, *Memoirs*, 123–6.

20 Le Fanu, 'Dumont de Bostaquet', 212.

21 Dumont de Bostaquet, *Mémoires*, 318.

22 Dumont is recorded in the registers for the French Conformed Church of St Patrick's in Dublin in 1694 until May 1697 as *ancien*: HSQS 7, 93, 146, 147, 150, 152. Thereafter he is frequently entered as *ancien* in the French Church at Portarlington: HSQS 19, which also contains the record of his death and burial in 1709. See also Le Fanu, 'Dumont de Bostaquet', 216.

23 For recent articles concerning the interpretation of the Huguenot communities in both Dublin and Portarlington, see John S. Powell, 'Rethinking Portarlington', *HSP* 27:2 (1999), 246–56; Ruth Whelan, 'Points of view: Benjamin de Daillon, William Moreton and the Portarlington affair', *HSP* 26:4 (1996), 463–89; Raymond P. Hylton, 'Dublin's Huguenot communities: trials, development and triumph, 1662–1702', *HSP* 24:3 (1985), 221–31.

24 Dumont de Bostaquet, *Mémoires*, 324.

25 The Dumont memoirs are Royal Irish Academy, Dublin, MS 12 N17. Information on the manuscript's location was kindly provided by Prof. Ruth Whelan during the Huguenot Round Table Conference at the National University of Ireland, Maynooth, May 1999. In a footnote in chap. 14 of vol. 3 of *The history of England from the accession of James II* (London, 1855), Lord Macaulay writes, 'There is some interesting information about Ruvigny and about the Huguenot regiments written by a French refugee of the name of Dumont. This narrative, which is in manuscript, and which I shall occasionally quote as the Dumont MS, was kindly lent to me by Dr Vignoles, Dean of Ossory'.

26 Ruth Whelan, in 'Persecution and toleration: the changing identities of Ireland's Huguenot Refugees', *HSP* 27:1 (1998), 20–35, states that the 'French refugees became colonizers in Ireland, where they were concerned at least as much with domination as with the preservation of their own liberty'. This certainly applies to Fontaine's and Dumont's attitudes to the Irish. In addition, the Fontaine children, as colonizers in Virginia, owned many slaves. It is difficult to understand how, as children of persecution, they were able to embrace slavery, but not only did they tolerate it, indeed most southern branches of the extended family owned slaves through the generations until the American Civil War of 1861–5. See also note 29.

27 Fontaine, *Memoirs*, 146.

28 *Ibid.*, 160 ff.

29 Surviving correspondence between Peter Fontaine and Maryann Fontaine Maury, representing the Virginia branch of the family, and John and Moses Fontaine and their sister Elizabeth Fontaine Torin in Wales are in Colonial Williamsburg Foundation's Manuscript Collection, MS 68.3 (Fontaine/Maury Papers, Part I); MS 90.5 (Fontaine/Maury Papers, Part II). A study of Fontaine's children and their contributions to colonial America is given in my unpublished paper 'This side the water: a Huguenot family in Virginia', prepared for the conference 'Out of new Babylon: the Huguenots and their diaspora', College of Charleston, Charleston, South Carolina, 1997.

30 Le Fanu, 'Dumont de Bostaquet', 226–7.

31 Fontaine, *Memoirs*, 116.

32 Dumont de Bostaquet, *Mémoires*, 79.

33 Fontaine, *Memoirs*, 160.

50

Writing the self: Huguenot autobiography and the process of assimilation

RUTH WHELAN

The title of the conference, and the volume of essays resulting from it – 'From Strangers to Citizens' – embodies an assumption that used to be quite current, and often still is, in studies on immigration. Consciously or unconsciously, the title expresses the experience of early modern immigrants in these islands as a 'story line', that is, as a linear narrative, expressing a linear process that moves from being foreign to being assimilated to the receiving society.[1] That is what the term assimilation means. Strangers become similar to the citizens of the society of destination, and, in the process, they engage in 'a complete sequence of experiences whereby the individual moves from one social identity to another', to quote a recent study.[2] And, of course, if we tell the story from the end, rather than the beginning, then this assumption is correct. In Ireland, and I think also in England, the only remnant of their original social identity that descendants of Huguenots retain today is their genealogies and their foreign names, and in many cases, even their names have been assimilated to the naming processes of the receiving society.[3] It is my purpose in this paper, however, to address the story of integration and assimilation from the beginning. Telling it from the beginning will show, I believe, that the processes of migration and integration were less linear and more uneven than the title of the conference suggested. But how do we tell the story from the beginning?

In the same study of migration quoted above, R. C. Ostergren observed that 'the key to understanding the migrational process lies in being able to isolate the psychological situation of the individual in the context of his changing milieu'.[4] Other specialists agree with this approach, pointing to the important 'glimpses' that the life stories of immigrants provide 'into the lived interior of migration processes'. Life stories, according to these specialists, give us some sense of the way migrants 'continually construct and reconstruct understandings of themselves and their larger social circumstances'.[5] Unfortunately, such life stories by immigrant Huguenots are in short supply compared, for example, to English Puritans or Quakers of the same period.[6] Some have survived, however, whether in the form of memoirs, or short escape narratives, and they do provide unique insights into the migrational process. In a very insightful article, Carolyn Lougee Chappell used extant escape narratives to trace the ways that Huguenot immigrants negotiated their identity in the changed and changing circumstances of exile.[7] In this paper, I want to continue that process of exploration by focussing on one of the longer Huguenot autobiographical narratives, the regrettably incomplete life story of Isaac Dumont de Bostaquet.[8] But I shall concentrate at least as much on the form as on the content of his story.

If we accept the findings of the study by Emmanuèle Lesne, which attempts to define the poetics of early modern French memoirs, Dumont de Bostaquet's life story offers a unique challenge to interpreters. In her view, Dumont's Memoirs are resistant to classification because of what she calls their polymorphism, meaning that they take successively different forms, and that, therefore, they can be situated within a number of different generic categories. 'How can we classify Dumont de Bostaquet's Memoirs', she asks, 'since they are at one and the same time, military, religious and political?'[9] – 'personal' should also be added to her list of categories, as I shall show. But it is precisely because of their polymorphic form that Dumont's Memoirs offer important glimpses into the lived interior of the migrational process, as he experienced it. The form arises, in part, out of the successive phases of his migration, and points to the disparate nature of that particular experience of migration. It therefore calls into question the 'story line' I referred to above, since there is no linear movement from stranger to citizen in this account. In fact, while one major shift occurs in Dumont's social identity, other aspects of that identity remain more stable, in what might be called a kaleidoscopic process of adaptation to the receiving societies through which he passed before settling in Ireland. Furthermore, his Memoirs are not just a record of that process, they also actively participate in the reconstruction of a social identity for the self and others in an implicit or explicit dialogue between the narrator and the stated or implied reader/s, as we shall see.[10]

The polymorphism of Dumont's Memoirs is partly explained by the sequential composition of the different parts of the life story, eight in all. However, while the manuscript is divided into eight separate parts, it was probably written over a period of six years, possibly started sometime in 1687, and definitely completed in April 1693, and may be organized into six sequences.[11] Each of these sequences coincides either with his arrival in a new country or place of refuge, or with a new set of experiences. The first and longest sequence, which treats his early life and escape from France, was completed probably in the first half of 1687. The second records the safe arrival of the child of his third marriage, Judith-Julie, and later his third wife in Holland, and was probably written at The Hague in April 1688. A third sequence – covering parts three and four – was composed in Greenwich in December 1689, and records his role in the descent on England with William of Orange's army. The fourth, and quite short sequence, was completed in Lurgan on 9 May 1690, and gives an account of his experiences during the early stages of the Irish campaign.[12] A fifth sequence contains his own eyewitness account of the Battle of the Boyne and the Siege of Limerick, and may have been written at Greenwich towards the end of 1691.[13] A sixth and final sequence, ranging over parts seven and eight was completed in Dublin on 3 April 1693 just after Dumont had moved to Ireland,[14] where he remained for the rest of his life. These Memoirs were written in at least four different places, and they record a wide variety of experiences. If we focus our attention less on the experiences themselves –

the traditional way of reading memoirs – and more on the way they are told, then a connection emerges between narrative form, or forms, and Dumont's shifting concept of self, as he constructs it retrospectively.[15]

A problem arises immediately from this assertion, quite simply because the form of Dumont's life story seems both accidental and, as Lesne has argued, unclassifiable. Accidental it is, up to a point. Dumont seems to write his life impulsively, as a response, even a reaction, to his changing circumstances, and with a sense of urgency to record his own unique testimony of the events he witnessed, or the testimony of others, which he has garnered.[16] It is also unclassifiable, to a certain extent, but not in the terms that Lesne has employed. The 'serial narrative form' adopted by Dumont places his life story somewhere between the diary, 'written to the moment', and the memoir, composed 'from a retrospective time and stance', to use the categories articulated by Felicity Nussbaum.[17] The resulting indeterminacy of form, with its resistance of narrative closure, makes Dumont's Memoirs particularly valuable as a story of the configuration and *re*configuration of social identity. Because his indeterminable narrative enacts his changing motivations and purposes in writing, allows contradictions to exist, and does not seek to harmonize dissonance.[18] It thereby produces an inconclusive textual self that expresses the often painful business of renegotiating identity as *process* rather than conclusion, as complexity rather than coherence.

It is important, however, not to overlook the significance of the retrospective viewpoint of Dumont's story, even if this is sequential and sometimes more immediate than is usual in the composition of memoirs.[19] Autobiographical retrospect is a heuristic stance, a remembering of experience and an investigation of self that is seeking to make sense of the past.[20] All the more so when the writer is a refugee, whose frames of reference have been suddenly and brutally changed. The *dragonnades*, the Revocation and its aftermath provoked a crisis of teleology in French Protestantism from which Dumont is by no means exempt. His serial retrospective may be understood as a reply to that crisis, as a quest for a moral order capable of providing the structures to enable him to understand his life, and redeem it from incoherence. Without attempting to reduce the polymorphism of the Memoirs to narrative unity, I follow Frank Kermode in arguing that there is 'a moment of interpretation' in Dumont's life 'that gives sense and structure to the whole'.[21] That moment, I believe, is his coerced conversion to Roman Catholicism. From this privileged viewpoint, the apparently unrelated sequences of Dumont's Memoirs coalesce into a kaleidoscopic narrative reconstruction of lost identity and a narrative rehabilitation of a lost self. Three aspects of that process are of interest: the loss of cultural identity, the loss of religious identity, and the loss of political identity. For reasons of narrative clarity I shall address them in turn, but with the understanding that in reality they form a psychic whole in the lived interior of Dumont's migration process.

While the experience of moving between deeply rooted local cultures may greatly enrich the lives of immigrants, the initial sensation is one of displacement, dispossession and cultural dislocation. This was certainly the case for Dumont de Bostaquet. When news of the imminent arrival of the soldiers from Rouen was bruited abroad, the local Protestant nobility gathered at Dumont's home to make plans. He was for immediate flight, but was persuaded not to leave his family unprotected.[22] He then proposed to follow certain members of his family into exile once he had managed to turn his property into a capital sum that would enable him to provide for them abroad.[23] But when they were surprised trying to escape with his help and protection, he was identified and had to flee ahead without making such provision, in order to avoid arrest. When he arrived in what he describes as the sanctuary of Holland[24] he was, therefore, alone. We know from what he wrote about this period in his life that he acted swiftly to re-establish contact with friends, kin, and, most importantly for him, his pastor. All of these efforts could not repair the loss of the family he had been forced to leave behind in France, however. And, in my opinion, his initial motivation in writing what he describes as a faithful account ('récit fidèle') of his life to that date (that is, 1687) was to reconstruct in narrative form the family and kinship network that was now lost to him in exile. Because telling stories about the past is one of the ways people generate and reproduce a culture, thereby shaping cultural identity.[25]

Both the content and the form of the first of the six sequences support this understanding of the Memoirs. In this the longest part of his narrative, Dumont nostalgically recreates his story as a member of the rural French nobility, and a paterfamilias who went to great pains to build up his patrimony and preserve it for his multitudinous offspring. The title he ascribed to this sequence suggests that this was a self-conscious use of narrative to reconfigure in exile a narrative identity centred on place and kin. He calls this part a 'récit fidèle [. . .] pour servir de mémoire à ma postérité' ('a faithful narrative designed to serve as a memorandum for my posterity'). I follow the 17th-century lexicographer, Furetière, in translating this use of 'mémoire' in the singular as 'memorandum'. Furetière's definition of 'mémoire' is important here. He observes that '[un mémoire] est un escrit sommaire qu'on donne à quelqu'un pour le faire souvenir de quelque chose' ('a memorandum is a summary account given to someone to make her or him remember something').[26] In other words, Dumont configures his Memoirs from the outset not simply as an act of memory for personal use (which is another possible meaning of the word 'mémoire', used in the singular, albeit in the feminine form), but as an act of communication with the stated reader/s, namely his posterity. And, as we learn at the end of this first sequence of the Memoirs, this part of his life story is also an imagined dialogue with his immediate descendants, that is, his children, whom he addresses directly in closing as 'mes chers enfants' ('my dear children').[27]

There are a number of things worth noting about the relationship of form to content, as Dumont configures it here. Like all autobiographical narratives, Dumont's life story is clearly designed to save the self, and the cultural identity of that self, from oblivion by handing on an account of his own past to future generations ('ma postérité'). But there was a particular urgency in his case, since the very existence of French Protestants as a religious and social grouping was being wiped out by a brutal drive to conformity in 'the all Catholic France' of Louis XIV, to use an expression of Dumont's contemporary, Pierre Bayle.[28] Although full-length Huguenot memoirs, like Dumont's, are rare, the impulse to collect and create documentary evidence of a way of life – and the destruction of that way of life – is not. For example, the extant papers of Abraham Tessereau, one of the King's secretaries in the 1650s, contain many eye-witness accounts, titled 'mémoire', or 'mémoires', collected in the 1680s to provide a reliable story for posterity of the dismantling of French Calvinism, to quote Elie Benoît, who later incorporated them into his monumental history.[29] This wider social framework reactivates the essentially legal context in which the word 'mémoire' was used. By writing his life, Dumont puts the official historiography of French Calvinism on trial, and leaves a trace, a memorandum, to guide posterity to a truer account of their past, which is his present.[30]

But there is another related and, perhaps, less obvious aspect of the writing of memoirs in order to preserve and transmit the past to future generations. The impersonal 'postérité' to whom Dumont addresses his Memoirs becomes the deeply personal 'mes chers enfants' by the end of the first narrative sequence. When, contrary to his plan, Dumont arrived alone in Holland, he founded what might be termed a patrilocal emigration[31] for which he had, however, been unable to provide financially. His recreation of his life in France as an imagined dialogue with his children may be interpreted as a configuration of the life story as a patrilocal text, that is, a kind of patrimony in narrative which is all the dispossessed exile can now pass down to his children. Implicitly, Dumont's discursive presentation of the past is a narrative space designed both to preserve the social identity embedded in the past,[32] and to make his immediate descendants remember it and embody it as a living memory. Thus, the life story, as Dumont and others practice it, is an exercise in cultural conservation. The Memoir as memorandum is constructed as a means of transposing the past into a collective identity in the present.[33]

Transmitting the factuality of the past is not the only concern, however. Like many authors of aristocratic memoirs in this period,[34] Dumont is also driven by a desire to pass on the exemplarity of the past, that is, to draw out the lessons to be learned from his own story, and convey them through the narrative to his descendants.[35] There is a problem with this, however, since the lessons to be drawn from his life are not always exemplary. Like so many other French Calvinists at the time of the Revocation, Dumont signed a formulary of abjuration in order to protect himself, his family, and his property from the destruction wrought by the billeting of soldiers on those who refused to convert to Roman Catholicism. The words he uses to describe this act communicate a loss of self and a sense of lost bearings. He speaks of abjuration as a temptation and a tragedy; a crime, a sin and a failure; a weakness and a fall.[36] The sense of guilt that these words express is complicated by the fact that Dumont's social standing started what he calls a conflagration.[37] Others in the local community, including members of his own family, followed his bad example, as he terms it, which only serves to increase his self-reproach.[38] It is significant that once Dumont reached Holland, he lost no time in making a public act of repentance for his abjuration (in The Hague, 27 June 1687), and recording this liturgical act, known as *reconnaissance*, in his Memoirs.[39] Carolyn Lougee Chappell has written about the ways that the liturgy of *reconnaissance*, and its open admission of what was seen as the wrongdoing of abjuration, shaped Huguenot escape narratives, and, more generally, autobiographical narrative. If her insights are applied to Dumont's Memoirs, they point to another possible level of meaning, which it is fruitful to explore.

The longer personal memoir (as opposed to the short escape narrative) written by Huguenots is more often than not set in a moral and theological narrative frame that can help the writer make sense of dislocating experiences. Dumont is no exception. In fact, he shares a tendency with his co-religionists to allegorize his life story in biblical terms, although so allusively, at times, that this is easy to overlook. It is invidious to select one of these allusions in preference to any of the others, and yet one allegorization in particular seems to weave together the implications of so many of the discrete reminiscences and explicit references to the Bible in his life story. This is how Dumont sums up the days leading up to the arrival of the *dragons* in Normandy, when he was kept busy with the family wedding in Paris, the pleasure trip to Versailles, and the settling of various properties and debts:

> Mais, hélas! l'homme propose et Dieu dispose; nous ne songions qu'à affermer notre habitation lorsque nous devions prendre des mesures plus prudentes; et semblables aux premiers habitants de la terre, on bâtissoit et l'on se marioit sans voir les nues prêtes à crever pour inonder la terre que nous habitions: toutes les provinces du royaume étoient la plupart exposées à la persécution des dragons.[40]

There is a twofold biblical reference here, both to the Flood, and to Jesus's use of it as an analogy for the end of time.[41] Both of these references are used allegorically by Dumont to make some sense out of experiences that defy understanding: the *dragonnades* are presented as a cataclysmic event bringing a whole world to an end. Symbolic narrative of this kind opens a window into the horror felt by French Protestants in those crucial years before the Revocation, but I am more interested in the way its teleological implications shape Dumont's entire life story.

There is a tragic wryness in the moral frame used by Dumont to interpret his prudence as a paterfamilias, which he has sketched so fondly, as less than prudent in the circumstances that overtook him.[42] The moral reference is also present in his use of the allegory of the Flood, which was visited on the world, we are told, because of the great wickedness of humankind.[43] Again and again, in the sermons preached at the time of the Revocation, ministers reacted to the bewilderment of their flocks, who were wondering why such things were happening to them, by pointing to their sinfulness and lack of faith. Dumont implicitly accepts this explanation when he allegorizes his own experience in terms of the Flood, and uses a lexis associated with sin and guilt to interpret his own behaviour, particularly, his abjuration.[44] Such acceptance of personal moral responsibility could be crushing were it not for the explicitly providential context in which it occurs, 'man proposes but God disposes'. Dumont displays an unquestioning trust in the inscrutable providence of God,[45] and frequently makes reference to this unseen but deeply felt presence in his life. What this means, of course, is that there is a 'shadow dialogue', to use Lougee Chappell's term,[46] with the ultimate interlocutor, namely God, going on in Dumont's Memoirs. This most important dialogue of all has been overlooked by critics, which is a pity, since it links Dumont's memoirs to the tradition of spiritual autobiography, that deeply personal form of narrative practised in early modern France.[47] But, in this case, it is spiritual auto-biography with a Calvinist tone.

The tone is set from the opening lines of Dumont's Memoirs, where he presents his narrative as an exercise in introspection that will lead him to amend his life.

> Ce n'est point un sentiment de vaine gloire qui me fait mettre sur le papier le récit de ma vie, mais un pur effet du loisir que nous donne la Providence dans ces heureuses provinces où pouvant en toute liberté réfléchir sur le temps qui s'est écoulé depuis ma naissance sans un véritable progrès pour le ciel, je voudrois faire un meilleur usage de ce qui me reste de jours que je n'ai fait par le passé.[48]

This opening caveat is, in a sense, simply a variation on a defining commonplace of autobiographical narrative, present in such writers as far apart as Julius Caesar and

Jacques-Auguste de Thou, who promise to avoid false modesty and false pride.[49] But the religious note struck here, and again in the closing sentence of the first part, where Dumont offers his life story to his children as a model to help them to avoid the evil and follow the good he has done,[50] points to another possible sense. There is a tradition of introspection and confession within French Calvinism that stresses the importance of self-examination in the presence of the unseen but ever present God. Believers are urged to examine their lives for signs of grace and election, which are demonstrated not only by repentance for sin, but also by the acts of goodness that have been accomplished by divine grace.[51] The mixture of self-confidence and self-reproach, the configuration of the paterfamilias as both provider and betrayer in Dumont's Memoirs, are inspired, I think, by this Protestant religious practice of the examined life. This means, of course, that his life story is, in the deepest sense of the term, a confession. It is a confession made first and foremost before God, and simultaneously, but almost at one remove, before the wider community in what might be termed a narrative version of the ceremony of *reconnaissance*. In this way, Dumont re-establishes continuity with a more authentic self – the one preceding abjuration – and rehabilitates it.[52] He also recaptures exemplarity, since the recognition of wrong frees him to transmit to the next generation the values he all but lost, and the lessons he learned from his own unhappy experience. The life story is the site, then, where an eroded religious identity is restored through a quasi-liturgical act of memory.

So far a picture is emerging of Dumont's Memoirs as a story of conservation and restoration of the social and religious past within the present. But there is in fact a sequence of this autobiographical narrative, namely the military sequence, that is oriented not toward the past, but rather toward the future. The social and personal identity of the Huguenots of France was a site of conflict between the way they defined their fidelity to God, and the drive of Louis XIV's political regime towards religious and social conformity.[53] Huguenots like Dumont resolved this conflict by creating a hierarchy of loyalties, wherein their fealty to King and country was subordinated to their primary loyalty to the Reformed faith, which they believed was of divine origin.[54] This hierarchy of loyalties was expressed in their flight from France, although this was forbidden by royal ordinance, and in their transfer of fealty to the respective monarchs of the receiving societies. Dumont inscribes this dual action in the life story by referring to the France he has fled as 'mon ingrate patrie',[55] and by framing the second sequence of his Memoirs as an exemplary narrative of his own transfer of fealty to the Protestant William of Orange.[56]

The language he uses to describe this shift in identity is significant. He speaks of his newly found 'attachement fidèle et passionné pour un Etat et pour un prince à qui je dois le secours de ma misère et le repos de ma conscience'.[57] Yves Durand has identified this kind of language as typical of early modern clientelism and fealty,[58] and Dumont uses it here to express a political choice in favour of one of France's historic enemies. Although some Huguenots denounced their co-religionists as traitors for making choices of this kind,[59] Dumont apparently effects the transfer of fealty without qualms. Why? Because King and country have betrayed him ('*ingrate* patrie'), setting him free to resolve the conflict he felt in France by a transfer of fealty to a Protestant sovereign and state, where his primary loyalty to God and the Reformed faith can be reconciled with his political commitment. This sequence of the Memoirs is, therefore, a performative narrative in as much as it not only represents a significant shift in identity, but also makes that new political identity real by the simple act of recording it in the binding language of fealty. In this way, the Memoirs become a set of identity papers, or passport between the culture of origin and the culture of destination, a place of negotiation between past and future.[60]

However, the undeniable shift in Dumont's political identity should not be taken to mean that he has assimilated to the society of destination, or become a citizen rather than a stranger, on the contrary. In exact counterpoint to the title of the conference, Dumont still describes France as his 'patrie', and thinks of the receiving society as 'étrange',[61] which indicates that he continues to see himself as French, and to think of France as home, like so many other first generation Huguenot refugees.[62] What has changed is his political solidarity, but this is based on a shared Protestantism rather than on assimilation to the social identity of the receiving society. This becomes quite obvious in both the language and content of the final sequences of the Memoirs, where Dumont sketches his part in William of Orange's military campaigns. As soon as the refugees got wind of William's projected descent on England, according to Dumont, 'tout le monde s'empressa à lui donner des marques de son zèle et de son attachement à son service'.[63] The language of fealty and clientelism recurs quite appropriately here, but it is also accompanied by a providential discourse.

William is referred to as both 'notre héros' and the 'libérateur' designated by God to save England from the popish tyranny of James II; while the Huguenot military are described as signing up for a 'guerre sainte'.[64] At significant moments in the narrative, Dumont sees Providence at work to save William from potential disaster, or facilitating his 'liberation' of England and Ireland.[65] And, in one very illuminating moment in the Memoirs, he expresses the hope that God will inspire William III to liberate Dumont's own homeland, France, from oppression.[66] For Dumont, then, God, Protestantism, William and William's battles are all of a piece, and his allegiance to all of these has brought him to a place of ambivalence towards France. France is home and yet, he believes, it should be invaded by one of its historic enemies, with whom he himself identifies. In other words, he has moved into a kind of cosmopolitan sense of identity that ignores national boundaries in favour of a commitment to the Protestant International, as it has been called.[67] This is a form of adaptation, based on the recognition of a shared religious and political ideology, and it necessarily involves a shift in identity, which makes it possible for him to move easily between Holland, England and Ireland. Yet, in each of these countries it is the Protestant interest that forms the focus of Dumont's concerns and reaps the benefits of his activities as a Huguenot cavalry officer, rather than the local cultures, particularly when these are Roman Catholic.[68] So, although he identifies with a religious tradition and a political cause, he still remains a stranger in very significant ways. The latter sequences of the Memoirs portray, then, a cosmopolitan Protestant officer who seems at variance with the paterfamilias, deeply rooted in the social network of the local nobility – whether Protestant or Catholic – of Normandy, who writes the opening sequence of the Memoirs. Or is he? This brings me to my final observation.

Although Dumont enlisted in one of the Huguenot regiments who were to participate in William's campaigns, he was almost excluded from the descent on England as the result of an accidental injury to his arm sustained during the time the troops were waiting to embark. His friends advised him to withdraw, but Dumont refused to accept their advice. The reason he gives in his Memoirs sheds an important light on his motivation.

> Leurs conseils charitables n'étoient pas de mon goût: je voulois avoir part à la gloire de ce grand dessein et suivre ce troisième Guillaume en Angleterre, comme mes pères y avoient suivi le premier qui étoit notre duc de Normandie.[69]

'Gloire' is a loaded word in 17th-century France, and is almost untranslatable, since it carries with it the whole weight of a civilization. It is a term associated with heroism, merit, and an aristocratic culture of self-aggrandizement and self-fulfilment, which brings with it public recognition of the worthiness of certain actions or attitudes.[70] By using it to describe the descent on England, Dumont not only reveals his admiration for the enterprise, but also his desire to share in the reflected glory that would be his as a result. Furthermore, as the reference to his forefathers suggests, participation in William's campaign meant for Dumont that he could reconnect with a family tradition of heroism and cosmopolitanism, and translate a glorious past into his present, which, as we have seen, he thought of as less than glorious in some respects.[71] The military experiences portrayed in the life story bring together Dumont's social, religious and political identity and renegotiate it to produce a new and positive sense of self, which is simultaneously rooted in the past and oriented towards the future. In other words, the latter sequences of the Memoirs are a site of rehabilitation and reconstruction of lost identity, brought about by story telling. In this way, the self diminished by abjuration and exile can transmit to his posterity a glorious tale of commitment to the Protestant cause, of triumph over adversity, and of providential protection. It is story as memorandum, lest they forget. And, perhaps, it is story as invitation, beckoning them to follow what is, once again, an exemplary life.

This study of Dumont de Bostaquet's Memoirs leads to two kinds of conclusions, firstly, concerning both the genre itself, and, secondly, the processes of assimilation. The problems of categorization encountered by Emanuèle Lesne when confronted with Dumont, to which I alluded at the beginning, stem, in my opinion, from the way she and others define the genre. In his groundbreaking essay, written in 1971, Marc Fumaroli introduced a distinction, later followed by Lesne, between two kinds of memoir writing: the confessional memoir of personal moral reflection, on the one hand, and the aristocratic or 'worldly' ('mondain') memoir of self-aggrandizement and self-justification, on the other.[72] As I hope I have shown, this distinction breaks down in the case of Dumont de Bostaquet, whose writing of the self belongs to both of these categories simultaneously. Consequently, rather than using the distinction to exclude Dumont from a poetics of the genre, as Lesne has, it would seem more appropriate to call the definition itself into question, since it is incapable of accounting for all of the extant examples of memoir writing in 17th-century France.[73] French Protestantism may have been the object of exclusionist politics in the reign of Louis XIV, and may therefore be less familiar, but this only means that we still have things to learn about the *mentalités* of the time.

Dumont's Memoirs reveal that in 17th-century France the 'moi' (or self) is not always 'haïssable' (or hateful) as Pascal expressed it.[74] As we have seen, it is possible to write personal and confessional narratives in this period where the self and the world are perceived negatively and where self-examination does not lead to self-abnegation,[75] but to a more measured sense of both personal weaknesses and strengths. This may in part be the result of certain liturgical and religious practices particular to French Calvinism, as I have suggested, namely, the habit of seeking signs of grace and election in a moral attitude to the everyday world with its rights and wrongs, rather than in a rejection of it. The sensibility that expresses itself in this way is not, however, exclusively Calvinist.[76] It is the result of a peculiar social and narrative alchemy that brings together aristocratic, political and religious attitudes, which enable Dumont to recapture a certain heroic sense of self and redeem his life from incoherence. But the impetus behind the narrative (and actual) quest for meaning does arise out of the experience of being a Calvinist in 17th-century France, and the loss of self-identity that entailed, particularly as a result of abjuration. For all its incomplete and indeterminable qualities, Dumont's life story functions, then, to renegotiate and prove his faithfulness to the self, family and God whom he feels he has betrayed. By dedicating himself to the service of the Protestant king, he weaves these different strands of his life together, and turns loss into the hope of the political redemption of the country he still thinks of as his own.[77] His Memoirs are a narrative of lost identity recovered, a narrative that reflects the processes by which that identity was renegotiated, and a narrative intended to perpetuate that identity in the future.

Finally, it must be conceded that we cannot draw any general conclusions about the processes of integration and assimilation from one set of Huguenot memoirs. However, there are striking similarities between Dumont's life story and what we know about these processes from other sources, and these similarities are worth dwelling on for a moment. Firstly, the emphasis on the conservation and transmission of the culture of origin in Dumont's Memoirs calls into question, to quote W. Petersen, 'the usual notion that persons universally migrate to change their way of life'.[78] In fact, the Huguenot migration was quite clearly conservative in as much as the refugees were only seeking a place where they could resume their old way of life.[79] So much is obvious in Dumont's narrative expression of conservative impulses, but these also appear in real life. For example, the characteristic clustering of Huguenots in settlements often according to provincial origins, their group coherence, and language retention, at least in the first generation, all bear witness to their desire to retain their original social identity. Secondly, the restoration of an eroded religious identity is of central importance in Dumont's life story. It also finds expression in the historical reality of the immigrants through the central importance of the ethnic church, that is, the widespread practice of religious nonconformity on the part of the Huguenots who settled in these islands.[80] In fact, leaving aside examples of individual integration and assimilation, it is possible to argue that, like Dumont de Bostaquet, Huguenot immigrants lived simultaneously in two worlds. On the one hand, they lived in a social world where cultural traditions and familiar religious rites were perpetuated, and, on the other, they inhabited an economic and political world where adaptation to the society of destination was necessary to survival.[81] Caught between these competing impulses to conserve and to adapt, they did not move smoothly from one social identity to another. The strangers, whose Protestantism made them less wholly strange, were still slow to become citizens, at least in the first generation.

NOTES

The author would like to dedicate this essay in memory of Elisabeth Labrousse (1914–2000), scholar, teacher, and friend.

1   See J. H. Miller, *Ariadne's thread: story lines* (New Haven and London, 1992), 18.
2   The quotation is from R. C. Ostergren, 'Swedish migration to North America in trans-atlantic perspective', in I. A. Glazier and L. de Rosa (eds.), *Migration across time and nations: population mobility in historical contexts* (New York and London, 1986), 127. Ostergren does not accept the linear view of assimilation, however. I am influenced here by R. Benmayor and A. Skotness 'Some reflections on migration and identity', in R. Benmayor and A. Skotness (eds.), *Migration and identity* (Oxford, 1994), 1–18. See the essays by E. Barrett, and B. van Ruymbeke in the present volume, which also question the common notion of assimilation. For some reflections on different kinds and stages of adaptation by Huguenots to the receiving society, in this case Ireland, see R. Whelan, 'Sanctified by the Word: the Huguenots and Anglican liturgy', in K. Herlihy (ed.), *Propagating the Word of Irish Dissent, 1650–1800* (Dublin, 1998), 93–4.
3   See the essay in this volume by C. Lougee Chappell, 'What's in a name?'.
4   Ostergren, 'Swedish migration', 134. The gender-specificity is, obviously, in the original.
5   Benmayor and Skotness, 'Some reflections', 14.
6   See G. Gusdorf, 'De l'autobiographie initiatique à l'autobiographie genre littéraire', *Revue d'histoire littéraire de la France* 75 (1975), 957–94.
7   C. Lougee Chappell, '"The pains I took to save my/his family"': escape accounts by a Huguenot mother and daughter after the Revocation of the Edict of Nantes', *French historical studies* 22 (1999), 1–64.
8   I. Dumont de Bostaquet, *Mémoires sur les temps qui ont précédé et suivi la Révocation de l'Edit de Nantes*, ed. M. Richard (Paris, 1968). All references are to this edition.
9   E. Lesne, *La poétique des mémoires (1650–1685)* (Paris, 1996), 36.
10 Benmayor and Skotnes, 'Some reflections', 15, see the life story as 'participating in a process of negotiating new identities'. A similar position is advanced by Lougee Chappell, '"The pains I took"', 36–7.
11 The manuscript is held at the Royal Irish Academy, Dublin, Ms 12 N 17. The following inscription in a contemporary hand is barely legible on the cover: 'Registre faict en Holande à La Haye le mois d'apvril mil six cent quatre vingt huict. Continué en 1689 en Angleterre à Greenwich en decembre. Finy le mois d'apvril 1693 à Dublin en Irlande', which, of course, seems to call into question my own dating above. But it is most likely that April 1688 marks the date of completion of parts one and two, and that part one was started and finished at the earlier date. There is also a marked change in tone in part two, where Dumont's fondness for his children changes for a time to bitterness (see *Mémoires* (from n. 8), 150, 155), which may be taken to indicate that part two represents a new stage in Dumont's reminiscences. Furthermore, throughout the manuscript there are many changes in the quality of the ink and, indeed, the handwriting, suggesting that the manuscript was written in more than six stages. A more detailed analysis of the manuscript might result in greater precision.
12 Dumont, *Mémoires*, 232.
13 *Ibid.*, 262.
14 *Ibid.*, 279.
15 I am guided here by P. J. Eakin, 'Narrative and chronology as structures of reference and the new model autobiographer', in J. Olney (ed.), *Studies in autobiography* (New York and Oxford, 1988), 32–41.
16 Dumont explicitly excludes material from his Memoirs that has not been witnessed (by

himself or a third party), or which is not unique to him, for example, events that are reported in the gazettes; see Dumont, 164, 232.

17 F. A. Nussbaum, 'Toward conceptualizing diary', in Olney (ed.), *Studies in autobiography*, 128.

18 I am guided here by Nussbaum's conceptualization of diary, *ibid.*, 128–40.

19 For example the fourth sequence, completed in Lurgan on 9 May 1690.

20 See J. P. Miraux, *L'autobiographie, écriture de soi et sincérité* (Paris, 1996).

21 F. Kermode, *The genesis of secrecy: on the interpretation of narrative* (Cambridge, MA, 1979), 16, 136. Kermode is in turn influenced by Dilthey and Starobinski.

22 Dumont, 96, 98.

23 *Ibid.*, 106.

24 *Ibid.*, 147.

25 E. Tonkin, *Narrating our pasts: the social construction of oral history* (Cambridge, 1992), 97, 112.

26 See A. Furetière, *Dictionnaire universel* (The Hague, 1690); also M. Fumaroli, 'Les mémoires du XVIIe siècle, au carrefour des genres en prose', *XVIIe siècle* 94–95 (1971), 10.

27 See Dumont, 146. The conceptualization of memoir writing as a dialogue with one's children is a commonplace of the genre of personal or family memoirs.

28 See P. Bayle's indignant denunciation of the politics of conformity as it affected the Protestants of France, *Ce que c'est que la France toute catholique sous le règne de Louis le Grand*, ed. E. Labrousse, R. Zuber, H. Himelfarb (Paris, 1973). The treatise was originally published in 1686.

29 Abraham Tessereau, 'Memoires et pieces pour servir à l'histoire generale de la persecution faitte en France contre ceux de la religion reformée depuis l'année 1656, jusqu'à la Revocation de l'Edit de Nantes', held in Archbishop Marsh's Library, Dublin. See E. Benoît, *Histoire de l'Edit de Nantes* (Delft, 1693–5), vol. 1, unpaginated 'Preface generale'. On Tessereau, see T. P. LeFanu, 'Mémoires inédits d'Abraham Tessereau', *Proceedings of the Huguenot Society* (hereafter *HSP*) 15:4 (1937), 1–20.

30 Furetière gives mostly legal examples to illustrate the meaning of the word 'mémoire'; see Fumaroli, 'Les mémoires du XVIIe siècle', 10, 12–13. According to Fumaroli and Lesne (*La poétique des mémoires*, 35–51), the writing of memoirs over against official historiography is common during the Fronde; however, neither critic mentions that protest-memoirs were also written by French Protestants at the time of the Revocation.

31 I borrow this expression from H. C. and J. M. Buechler (eds.), *Migrants in Europe: the role of family, labor and politics* (New York, 1987), 294.

32 See Tonkin, *Narrating our pasts*, 46.

33 *Ibid.*, 97, 111, 135.

34 See Fumaroli, 'Les mémoires', 23–4.

35 I am drawing here on P. Ricoeur, 'Memory and forgetting', in R. Kearney and M. Dooley (eds.), *Questioning ethics: contemporary debates in philosophy* (London, 1999), 9.

36 For example, Dumont, 97, 98, 102, 103, 134, 135. E. Labrousse, 'Le Refuge huguenot', *Le genre humain* 19 (1989), 149, notes the crippling remorse that oppressed so many of the French Protestants who abjured.

37 Dumont, 104.

38 *Ibid.*, 106; indeed, according to Dumont, the authorities were counting on his social standing to draw others into the Roman Catholic fold (99, 102).

39 *Ibid.*, 153, see also 135.

40 *Ibid.*, 94: 'But alas! man proposes and God disposes; we gave thought only to leasing out our property, when we should have been taking more prudent measures; and, just like the early dwellers on the earth, we were building, marrying and giving in marriage, not noticing that the clouds were ready to burst and flood the earth where we dwelt. All the provinces

in the kingdom were, on the whole, subject to persecution from the soldiers.'

41 See Gen. 7 and following, and Matt. 24:36–9; these verses occur in what is known as the 'little apocalypse', which both Matthew and Mark use to close the Jerusalem ministry of Jesus.

42 This dovetails with another biblical allusion used by Dumont to set his abjuration in a moral light, namely, 1 Cor. 3:19; see Dumont, 135 where he dismisses as folly (before God) the so-called wisdom he displayed in trying to save his property by abjuring.

43 Gen. 6:5.

44 See also, Dumont, 150: 'J'ai joui de beaucoup de bien, mais n'en ayant pas fait un aussi bon usage que je devois, Dieu m'en a privé' ('I had the privilege of owning a great deal of property, but since I did not make as good a use of it as I should have, God took it away from me').

45 See, for example, Dumont, 135, where he quotes the classic biblical text on inscrutable but adorable divine providence, Rom. 11:33.

46 Lougee Chappell, '"The pains I took"', 10.

47 Fumaroli, 'Les mémoires', 28–30 and Lesne, La poétique des mémoires, 92–113.

48 Dumont, 23: 'It is not feelings of vainglory that make me write down the story of my life, but simply the leisure bestowed on us by Providence in these happy provinces where, being able to reflect in freedom on the time that has passed since my birth without any real progress towards heaven, I want to put the rest of my days to better use than I have in the past.'

49 Y. Coirault, Revue d'histoire littéraire de la France 75 (1975), 937. Fumaroli, 29.

50 Dumont, 147.

51 See, for example, J. Claude, Examen de soymesme pour bien se preparer à la communion (Charenton, 1682). In the second rule for self-examination, Claude urges his readers to examine the motivations for their actions, and points out that if they find that the idea of God inspires their virtuous acts then they may take this as a sign of the truth of their faith. In the fourth rule, Claude reflects at length on the doubts and inner torment that afflict believers who change their religion under duress, and offers reassurance by insisting that repentance is a sure sign that they are not cut off from the hope of salvation. He returns to this theme in the fifth rule, pointing out that resistance to the very tempting advantages of abjuration is a sure sign of regeneration. I do not wish to imply that Dumont has read Claude's treatise, although this is certainly possible. The treatise does, however, express a tradition of self-examination in the presence of God, which seeks to affirm the good, and not simply emphasize the wrong in a believer's life. The relevance of such a treatise to the times is borne out by the developed reflections on the spiritual problems that arise out of abjuration. The date of publication of the first edition, 1681, which coincides with the dragonnades, is surely not an accident. However, while the likelihood of Dumont's being influenced by embedded religious and/or liturgical practices is very strong, it must also be admitted that, after 1650, writers of memoirs were generally influenced by Augustine's Confessions (see Fumaroli, 27–32; Lesne, 102–113).

52 See Lesne, 109–110 for a reflection on the narrative implications of confession for autobiography; and Lougee Chappell, 10–14, for the shadow dialogue with the wider community.

53 For a reflection on this conflict of identity, see O. Millet, 'Intolerance, friendship and urbanity: Balzac and his Huguenot correspondents', in R. Whelan and C. Baxter (eds.), Toleration and religious identity: the Edict of Nantes and its implications in France, Britain and Ireland (Dublin, 2000).

54 See M. Yardeni, 'Problèmes de fidélité chez les protestants français à l'époque de la Révocation', in Y. Durand (ed.), Clientèles et fidélités en Europe à l'époque moderne. Hommage à Roland Mousnier (Paris, 1981), 297–314.

55 Dumont, 191: 'my ungrateful homeland'.

56 *Ibid.*, 150.

57 *Ibid.*, 150: 'enthusiastic and loyal commitment to a State and a prince to whom I owe financial succour and a peaceful conscience'. See also 171, where Dumont speaks of the freedom of conscience he enjoys under William of Orange.

58 Y. Durand, 'Clientèles et fidélités dans le temps et dans l'espace', in Durand (ed.), *Clientèles et fidélités*, 9.

59 See P. Bayle, *Avis important aux Refugiez sur leur prochain retour en France* (Amsterdam, 1690), 269, and Yardeni, 'Problèmes de fidélité', 303.

60 I owe this insight to discussions with Carolyn Lougee Chappell during the London colloquium. Professor Lougee Chappell has developed this approach to Dumont's Memoirs, and to Huguenot Memoirs more generally, in some as yet unpublished papers on the subject.

61 Dumont, 279.

62 Myriam Yardeni has studied the wider implications of this phenomenon amongst the refugees in her essay, 'Problèmes de fidélité'.

63 Dumont, 174: 'everyone hastened to show him signs of zeal and devotion to his service'.

64 *Ibid.*, 173–74: 'our hero' and 'liberator', a 'holy war'; see also, 188, 191, 199, 202, 233.

65 *Ibid.*, 197, 202, 234, 260.

66 *Ibid.*, 191. This hope was widely nourished among the refugees, see Yardeni, 'Problèmes de fidélité', 309.

67 M. Prestwich (ed.), *International Calvinism, 1541–1715* (Oxford, 1985); also, Yardeni, 307.

68 Dumont also had problems with the rites of the Church of England, when he encountered them for the first time in Exeter; see Whelan, 'Sanctified by the word', 74–94. For the wider implications, particularly for Ireland, of Dumont's identification with the Protestant interest, see R. Whelan, 'Persecution and toleration: the changing identities of Ireland's Huguenot refugees', *HSP* 27:1 (1998), 20–35, and the ensuing comment and rejoinder: C. E. J. Caldicott, 'On short-term and long-term memory', and R. Whelan, 'Remembering with integrity', *HSP* 27:2 (1999), 279–83.

69 Dumont, 176: 'Their charitable advice was not to my taste: I wanted to participate in the glory of that great enterprise and follow the third William to England, as my forefathers had followed the first one who was our Duke of Normandy'.

70 According to Furetière, 'gloire se dit . . . de l'honneur mondain, de la loüange qu'on donne au merite, au sçavoir et à la vertu des hommes'. See M. Prigent, *Le héros et l'état dans la tragédie de Pierre Corneille* (Paris, 1986), for an interesting reflection on the concept of *gloire*.

71 I owe this insight to the discussions that followed my paper at the London colloquium, and wish to record my thanks here to Caroline Lougee Chappell and Michelle Magdelaine for their perceptive comments.

72 See Lesne, 421, where this distinction is drawn very sharply as she concludes.

73 I am drawing here on the paper I gave to the Faculty of Arts Research Seminar, at the National University of Ireland, Galway, on 16 February 2000, 'Defining a genre: Huguenot autobiography'. I am grateful to the Dean of the Faculty, and to Dr Jane Conroy of the Department of French for the invitation.

74 B. Pascal, Pensée 597, *Pensées*, ed. L. Lafuma (Paris, 1963).

75 See Fumaroli, 32, for the notion that confessional memoirs in this period lead to the 'extinction of the self'.

76 On the question as to whether Calvinism can be spoken of as a distinct culture, and of its interaction with other cultural traditions, see P. Benedict, 'Calvinism as a culture? Preliminary remarks on Calvinism and the visual arts', in P. C. Finney (ed.), *Seeing beyond the word: visual arts and the Calvinist tradition* (Grand Rapids, MI, 1999), 25–7.

77 Dumont, 191.

78 W. Petersen, 'A general typology of migration', in C. J. Jansen (ed.), *Readings in the sociology of migration* (Oxford, 1970), 65.

79 See *ibid.*, 55 for this definition of conservative migration.

80 Ostergren, 'Swedish migration', 136–138 outlines these conservative characteristics in immigrant settlements. On the question as to whether the concept of ethnicity may be applied retrospectively to the Huguenots, see the essay by B. van Ruymbeke in the present volume. R. D. Gwynn, 'The distribution of the Huguenot refugees in England', *HSP* 21 (1965–70), 404–36, and 'The distribution of Huguenot refugees in England: London and its environs', *HSP* 22 (1970–76), 509–68, notes the predominance of nonconformity in England; for Ireland, see Whelan, 'Points of view: Benjamin de Daillon, William Moreton and the Portarlington affair', *HSP* 26:4 (1996), 463–89, 'The Huguenots, the crown and the clergy: Ireland 1704', *HSP* 26:5 (1997), 601–10; and 'Sanctified by the Word', 74–94. This last article reflects (among other things) on Dumont's eventual acceptance of Anglican rites, and tries to identify different kinds of adaptation to the receiving society on the part of Huguenot immigrants.

81 I am influenced here by Ostergren, 138–9.

Part IX

German and Huguenot immigrants in Britain and Ireland in the 18th century

Part D

51

The English reception of the Huguenots, Palatines and Salzburgers, 1680–1734: a comparative analysis

ALISON OLSON

In 1687, again in 1709, and yet again in 1732, substantial groups of Continental refugees fled their homelands seeking asylum in England. The first were Huguenots fleeing France after Louis XIV's Revocation of the Edict of Nantes; the second, Germans, labelled Palatines, fleeing from a variety of villages in the southern Rhenish area for a number of different reasons; and the third, Protestant Salzburgers, threatened with renewed persecution by the local bishop. They were three of what the English called 'swarmings', all rather similar in some respects, such as numbers (10– 15,000 on each occasion) and local support (welcomed by 'the Quality', but despised by the lower ranks). But there was a world of difference in English reactions to the three groups: the Huguenots were generally welcomed with compassion and encouraged to stay in England; the Palatines met so much hostility and raised such fundamental questions that many of them had to be sent off to the American colonies; lastly the Salzburgers, like virtually all arrivals after the Palatines, quickly, quietly, and by pre-arrangement were shunted off to the American colonies in order to keep those volatile issues from disrupting national politics again.

Why did such a reversal take place in so short a time? We must begin by trying to understand why the Palatines encountered such a hostile response when the Huguenots had generally received a sympathetic greeting two decades before. Six town governments, for example, had offered money or shelter to the Huguenots. None helped the Palatines, and when the national government attempted to distribute small groups of them to provincial towns, the towns sent them back to London. The initial charity drive for the Palatines in 1709 raised one third of the amount the Huguenot collections had brought in 1686. After this the 1709 Palatine charities dried up whereas Huguenot fundraising had continued from 1686 until 1709. Huguenot settlement in England had been encouraged for almost a decade; after the first shiploads of Palatines arrived ministers instructed the British representative at The Hague to discourage any more from coming and took steps to repeal the Naturalization Act which had created a procedure by which immigrants could apply for citizenship.[1]

Two superficial explanations for the change come to mind: the Palatines were of a lower social rank than the Huguenots, and unlike the Huguenots, the Palatines became pawns in a virulent partisan rivalry. But beyond these lay a more telling difficulty. The deteriorating ability of foreign communities already in England to help fellow immigrants from their homeland put pressure on government to take up the responsibilities that the stranger communities could no longer meet. The increasingly effective government offices were indeed becoming able to handle these responsibilities, but now Englishmen had to ask themselves whether they really wanted the government to do so. The rancorous public debate that ensued raised issues so divisive that Queen Anne's harried government dispatched as many Palatines to the colonies as it could and future governments, worried about the recurrence of the disruption, rushed to send all potential Continental immigrants to the colonies before they could raise the volatile issues again.

In the quarter century between the Huguenot and the Palatine 'swarmings' the ability of established foreign communities to care for new arrivals eroded. There had been only seven French churches in London when the Huguenots arrived, but these churches had been willing, able and organized to help their refugee compatriots. The only French church of any size was the Threadneedle Street congregation, whose members had tended to be somewhat aloof from the rest of the London Huguenots, but they were very well organized. The churches had for several decades elected representatives to a French Committee of London which handled the payment of ministers' salaries and the distribution of charity to needy French. The French had their own bankers, merchants of considerable wealth such as Thomas Papillon.[2]

In the 1680s the French churches, working with the nominal support of the Archbishop of Canterbury and the remnant of an inefficient committee set up by James II, had been able, largely on their own, to rent land and unoccupied buildings around Spitalfields where the Huguenot refugees had first gathered to distribute supplies, and to move some of the refugees out of London and resettle them in the English provinces.[3]

In 1709 the six Lutheran churches in London, too, contained men of wealth and standing, even some bankers, but they lacked both the will and the organization to help the Palatines. We do not have the full records of the Lutheran churches that we would like, but it does appear that the Lutherans had no committee, and only two Lutheran ministers – one at the German Church at the Savoy and the other at court – working to help the new arrivals, and serving on Queen Anne's commission set up for the purpose.[4] They simply did not have the resources to rent lands or buildings or to give out supplies; many of the Palatines had to be put out in the parks, where they tried to raise money by selling trinkets. The Lutheran communities could chip in for insurance for refugees resettled outside London, but they depended on the government to move them.

The Lutheran predicament reflected a general decline in the ability of most stranger communities – Huguenots briefly excepted – to serve as buffers between new immigrants and English society. Churches suffered when some of their members prospered, married into English families and moved their homes and their shops away from their original neighbourhoods. The reduced groups, made up on the whole of the less successful members, were left behind to cope with later arrivals whose vocational skills were generally weak, whose wealth was limited, and whose ranks did not include many home-trained ministers to replenish the initial supply. When sudden waves of immigrants appeared, the resources of the established groups were strained beyond capacity, as the struggling German chapels were with the Palatines in 1710.[5] Since the groups were unable to handle basic needs like housing, employment, or keeping order, as their Tudor predecessors had done, there was nothing to keep the issues from becoming sore points between the foreigners and the natives.

The problems of the foreign churches were further compounded by the Toleration Act of 1689, which allowed Nonconformist Protestant denominations in England to have their own preachers, teachers, churches, and services without legal impediment, but formally excluded them from the Church of England. The Archbishops would have liked to keep the foreign Protestant churches under the Church of England in order to ease their assimilation, and encourage Anglican influence over Protestant churches on the Continent.[6] Parliament's excluding refugee churches from the Archbishop's authority undermined the Primate's authority and divided the stranger communities between those who had the wherewithal to support a church on their own and those who conformed to the Church of England because they were too poor to do without its help.[7]

As the fragmenting ethnic communities struggled, the British government moved into more and more of their functions. Charity drives fell under government direction; so did employment and even the upkeep of some of the immigrants' church buildings. The government's contribution to the maintenance of the remaining French refugees began to increase and by 1709 the government found it necessary to take up the question of whether it should aid the foreign refugees as it had not before, for now it was far more capable of doing so. Just how much the government was generally strengthened by the Glorious Revolution is under considerable debate. What is not really debatable is the government's increased ability to transfer groups of foreign refugees to the colonies, thanks to the creation of the Board of Trade. The Board was established in the wake of the Glorious Revolution, created by an Act of Parliament in 1696, with members to be picked by the King. The government had given almost no assistance to Huguenots wishing to relocate in the colonies in the 1680s, but almost immediately took up the possibility of sending Palatines there in 1709, and one of the major reasons it was able to do so was the availability of the Board of Trade to help.

In May 1709 the Board of Trade began taking up the Palatine question at nearly every meeting, corresponding with the Lord Treasurer, the Attorney General and the Ordinance Board, and from May through July it was regularly attended by the two overworked and exhausted German ministers. In May the Secretary of State, Lord Sunderland, wrote the board directing them 'to consider of a method for settling the said Germans in some part of this kingdom' and expressing his own preference – though not, he admitted, that of the Queen's – for resettlement in the colonies.[8] Six weeks later when the Palatines were still coming over, the British envoy in Rotterdam assumed they were headed for the colonies: 'The expenses may be great but are necessary if you are in want of these people for the Plantations, as my Lord Townshend seems to be of opinion you are'.

One of the jobs of the Board of Trade was to assist foreign refugees to move to the American colonies and the Board early undertook responsibilities that earlier government committees had declined. In 1699, for example, a group of Huguenots petitioned for help in getting to Virginia and the Board agreed to get them land on which to settle.[9] In 1706 the Board agreed not only to arrange for the purchase of land, but also to pay for transportation of refugees to Pennsylvania.

With government strong enough to take responsibility either for helping refugees get to America or for assisting them at home, English people had to ask whether, in fact, they really wanted the government to do either. Two general questions were at the heart of the extensive pamphlet and Parliamentary debates on this decision. First, either as the would be patrons of European Protestantism or simply as a people whose distinguishing feature was humaneness, should the English feel obliged to aid fellow Protestants – or any people – in need? Second, whatever the moral argument, was it in the English economic interest to encourage immigration because more bodies led to more wealth? The question concerning English Protestantism had been around since the Reformation and the assumptions behind it had faced increasing attack since the mid-17th century wars with the Netherlands, another Protestant power; the other issue was new. But both now prompted new debates over English character, English interests and the appropriate English role in a Protestant world.

First should the English welcome the Palatines as fellow Protestants since the Anglican Church was still seeking to be at least the moral leader of all European Protestant churches? The Archbishop of Canterbury made this the theme of one of his appeals for support of a charity brief.[10] The author of *The Reception of the Palatines Vindicated* argued for refugee aid on grounds of 'supporting the Protestants abroad and relieving and protecting them at home'.[11] But opponents insisted that the Palatines had not come to escape religious persecution at all, but had left their worn-out lands simply in expectations that the streets in England and America were paved with gold. In the 1680s Louis XIV's increasing discouragement of Protestants, culminating in his Revocation of the Edict of Nantes, had been well known in England, but in 1709 there was no comparable evidence that the Palatines had been persecuted, so it was hard for them to play on English sympathy or desire for the island to serve as a refuge for perse-cuted Protestants. The best their supporters could do was claim that they had been 'forced to leave by the oppressive exactions of the French',[12] meaning the French armies that had fought over their lands.

The British government did its best to weed out Catholics and sent at least 1000 of them back home, but the very fact that Catholics were ever even in the group argued against religious motivation for the initial flight. The government knew this: they had on hand a 1705 declaration of the Catholic elector John William promising liberty of conscience, a 1707 statement from a 'disinterested person' testifying to the sincere execution of the Elector's promise,[13] and even a statement from the Lutheran con-sistory denying that persecution existed.[14] Prince George's chaplain and a Palatine supporter, the Reverend Anton Boehm, admitted that few of the Palatines had prayer books and fewer still had Bibles. That might be explained either by their poverty or by confiscation of some goods along the way, but it is certainly significant that though the group for whom occupational records remain included eight school masters, it included no ministers. It may be significant, too, that shortly after their arrival 'large numbers' of them, who could have had no previous familiarity with the Anglican church, were taking Anglican Communion in preparation for initiating the naturalization procedure. Even the editor of the *Daily Courant*, a Palatine supporter, had to acknowledge that 'there was no reason to think that Palatines had less freedom in their homeland than they would have anywhere else'.[15]

But if the Palatines had been driven out of their homelands not by religious oppression but by an undefined 'arbitrary oppression' of Louis XIV, was that enough to require the English to welcome them? No, argued those who defined Englishness as Protestantism and the English mission as aid to the enemies of Antichrist. Yes, argued those who defined the essential quality of Englishness not as Protestantism, but as humaneness, a quality that set the English off from other people and obliged them to open their doors to any kind of refugee who had fallen on hard times. Since the Palatines were suffering from oppression or want, the argument ran, they were proper objects of charity; turning them away would show want of humanity to strangers: 'God willed the children of Israel to love the Strangers because they were Strangers in the Land of Egypt'.[16] Again and again papers reminded readers that the Palatines were 'the objects of French barbarity'[17] whose distress had been compounded by a harsh winter and a subsequent shortage of bread. 'Never call yourselves charitable, kind to strangers and the like, while your Parochial Constitutions will not suffer them to sleep under a Roof in the Nation'.[18] 'The kindness shew'd to these poor people will help to wipe out the Blots that be on our characters as Englishmen abroad . . . it will be an unanswered return upon those that shall hereafter reproach us . . . with . . . want of Humanity to Strangers'.[19]

Here again there were doubters. Did the Palatines really need help, or were they simply coming to England in search of the easy life? Even the Board of Trade had doubts. They had heard on good authority that the Palatines were lured to London by a book whose title page was in gold and whose appeal was that English streets were paved with gold.[20] If they had any reasonable willingness to work, argued one highly placed opponent, they would have been perfectly comfortable if they remained at home'.[21] The only reason for their distress, the critics generally urged, was congenital laziness, and if they came to England to avoid work, that was no reason to give them charity.[22]

Moreover, the summer of 1709 followed a bad winter in England as well as in Germany and the poor harvest that followed nearly doubled bread prices on the island. For the English poor 'it was . . . natural . . . to complain that the Multitude of Foreigners made the markets continually rising, and would soon devour the land'.[23] Charity should begin at home, should it not, where 'our own native Poor were starving without any manner of Provision made for them'.[24] So the argument that kindness to strangers was part of the humanitarianism that defined English character simply prompted more controversy over the Palatines.

The Palatine supporters then took up quite a different argument: refugees were a potential economic resource. Far from devouring the land, extra population would enrich it. The 1709 Naturalization Act, for example, had opened with 'Whereas the Increase of People is a Means of Advancing the Wealth and Strength of a Nation . . .'[25]

The question whether population added to national wealth had been discussed since early in the 17th century, at least since the time of Sir Francis Bacon; the intensity of the discussion had picked up during the Restoration and even more so after the publication of Sir William Petty's *Political Arithmetic* in 1690. Petty calculated the value to the country of each man, woman and child at £80 over twenty years.[26] Palatine supporters cited Petty's general remarks on the subject: 'Princes are not only Powerful, but Rich, according to the number of their people'.[27] 'Labour is the Father and Active

Principle of Wealth, as Lands are the Mother'.[28] Lord Sunderland, Secretary of State, advised the Board of Trade that the Queen preferred keeping the Palatines in England, since the 'Addition to the number of her Subjects would in all probability produce a proportionable increase in their Trade and Manufactures'.[29]

The Palatine supporters developed the argument, sometimes citing the government statements verbatim: 'numbers of people are known to strengthen a nation'[30]; 'The Multitude of People is the Interest of the Nation'[31]; '. . . the increase of People is a means of advancing the wealth and the strength of a Nation'[32]; 'It is a Fundamental maxim in Sound Politicks, that the Greatness, Wealth, and Strength of a Country consist in the number of its Inhabitants'[33]; 'Number of People are a Means of Advancing the Wealth and Strength of a Nation'.[34] The Bishop of London used the same words in his letter instructing Anglican ministers to collect charitable contributions for the Palatines.[35]

But the argument that increasing a nation's population necessarily enhanced its wealth was already being questioned by the time of the Palatines' arrival. Was it enough for the newcomers simply to increase population, without bringing any particular skills? Petty would have said 'yes': husbandmen were one of the main 'Pillars of any Commonwealth'.[36] But the Board of Trade worried that the Palatines were 'more fit for the almshouse than the workhouse' and their concern actually reflected Defoe's own argument in 'Giving Alms no Charity' (1704) that giving jobs to the destitute poor would take work away from the industrious poor.[37] Defoe himself thought the Palatines industrious, but he did not credit them with any skills except farming and referred only to settling them on the land or using them as farm labour.[38] A government census of 1232 of the refugees showed 100 tailors or weavers, 110 carpenters and masons, and 35 smiths. But the vast majority – 800 – were simply husbandmen.[39]

Could they be trained? They may possibly have picked up some skills in the camps; one report commented on their settlements in the parks 'almost all sorts of trades are carrying on'.[40] Thomas Firmin, Sir Matthew Hales, and Josiah Child had all argued that religious and vocational training could make the poor, be they English or foreign, useful to society and Defoe echoed that Palatines could pick up any skills a community needed.[41] But a number of critics disagreed: the Germans were too 'stupid' and 'slavish' for vocational training. Significantly, while Huguenot financier philanthropists like Papillon set up vocational schools to retrain the Huguenots, no one stepped forward to help the Palatines.[42] Their indolence was supposed to be so great that if the English encouraged them to settle they would 'be confirmed in that laziness they are already too prone to'.[43]

But more serious than that, the opponents argued, suppose one did train them: would not they be in a position to take jobs away from English labourers? As with earlier immigrants, 'the common People had a Prejudice and, as it were, a natural Aversion to them, and the merchants had some jealousie of their Manufacturers and Trades'.[44] The government tried to resettle groups in towns outside London, but the local populace sent them back.

Most doubtful, even if the Palatines did add to the useful work force, could they actually fit into English society? Were they capable of becoming citizens? Again, Defoe, as their strongest defender, certainly thought so. The key was simply to distribute them in small groups of 30 or 40 Palatines throughout the country and they would pick up English language and custom. In making this point, Defoe followed his argument in the *True Born Englishman*, a poem he had written in response to John Tutchin's *The Foreigner* in 1700. *The Foreigner* had attacked William III's Dutch advisers as 'Vermin', a 'boorish, cheese eating race born in bogs'. Giving titles and lands and offices to them was awarding them to outsiders, a group fundamentally different from (and inferior to) the English, and taking their proper inheritance away from true-born Englishmen. Defoe, in opposition, had argued that foreign groups were not so different from the English; they could and did assimilate easily, and the so-called *True Born Englishman* was actually a composite of all the foreign groups that had settled on the island at various times and blended with the existing inhabitants.[45]

The *True Born Englishman*, in turn, derived from Defoe's reading of Locke. In *The Essay Concerning Human Understanding*, which had first appeared in 1690, Locke had interpreted character as outlook, as approach to life and society, a mental structure of beliefs created over an individual's lifetime from the interaction of the mind and the senses of the body. According to Locke, the mind created ideas and representations of things from materials provided by the senses, and the totality of the creation amounted to one's character. Since impressions could come from the most broadly defined cultural environment, one's mental outlook, essentially one's character, was the result of experiences with family, state and community, neighbourhood, school and work-place. Far from being a 'stranger' to every place in the earth's environment, as the soul was, one's character was rooted in the experiences of one's early upbringing and also one's later life. One's personal identity depended on one's consciousness of this; so did one's national identity.[46]

But what experiences were most decisive in this shaping? Many writers went along with Defoe in considering climate and physical environment the fundamental character shapers: 'The climate may this modern breed ha' mended'; 'Borrowing new blood and manners from the clime'.[47] This argued well for the Palatines. The critics, of course, did not concur. Those who like Locke himself thought education the principal shaper of character, reverted to the argument that the 'stupid Germans' were too dull and lazy to be educable. This assumption supported the idea of sending refugees to the colonies where all they needed was land to make a living by farming, which most them already knew.[48] In the colonies, moreover, foreign settlers could produce raw materials which would in turn provide jobs for Englishmen at home. Two thousand men in the colonies, wrote Thomas Archdale expansively, equated 100,000 at home.[49] An estimate made by one of the Georgia Trustees somewhat later was more conservative (one colonist equalled four Englishmen) but to the same mercantilist point.[50]

Other writers like the Earl of Shaftesbury thought that the most important factor shaping national character was the political constitution of the state, which itself determined the citizen's response to and participation in his own government. This argument had worked in favour of the Huguenots, who had fled ecclesiastical despotism to enjoy the comparative toleration of England, and whose co-religionists in London, descendants of the refugees who had come a century earlier, were now running their own candidates for Parliament.[51]

It did not do particularly well for the Palatines, who were assumed to come from despotic principalities where the inhabitants seem to have accepted the government unquestioningly and to have left primarily for jobs, not freedom. Some of their supporters argued that the Palatines really did come to escape despotism. More often they were labelled 'slavish', fighters for their tyrants and oppressors 'more fit to be slaves or vassals'. They were of no use to England; in the colonies, at least, they would not do much damage.

So the argument went on, though the Palatines were ultimately skilled, some in England, some back in the Rhineland, and some in America. Decade after decade the same two questions festered, each time groups of Continental migrants sought an English home. In 1732 when the Bishop of Salzburg's renewed persecution produced an exodus of Protestants from his domain, the questions threatened to unsettle the government once again. Gone for good was any serious reliance on London's German community which was even weaker in the 1730s than it had been before. So the relief of the Salzburger refugees fell to two Anglican institutions, the Society for the Propagation of the Gospel and the Society for Promoting Christian Knowledge, both working with Parliament. Together they organized charity drives, strove to regulate the number of immigrants who gathered to leave Salzburg, managed the brief appearances of the refugees so they would not directly confront any Englishmen, arranged with ship captains to transport them directly to farmland in the colonies, and ultimately pressed colonial governments to grant them citizenship which was recognizable in other colonies, but not in Britain. Were they appropriate objects of this public charity? Were they more economically useful in the colonies than in England? Would colonial society assimilate them, vocationally unskilled, politically unskilled, ecclesiastically untested, but clearly not Anglican?[52] The beauty of the forced relocation of immigrants in the colonies was that the government never had to answer these questions.

From the settlement of Georgia to the fighting of the American Revolution, Continental refugees appealing to England for sanctuary were consistently sent to the American colonies, making those 40 years among the most free from ethnic violence in English history. The English had passed on to the colonies their uncertainties about 'what it takes to be English'. But on the other side of the ocean, this created a new question: were there looser, even lower standards for Americanness than for Englishness? Forty or so years after Georgia was founded, the Americans decided they did not really want to know.

NOTES

1 *London Gazette*, 4–6 Aug. 1709; *The State of the Palatines for fifty years past to this present time* (London, 1710), 11; Gilbert Burnet, *History of his own time* (London, 1857); Narcissus Luttrell, *A brief historical relation of state affairs from September 1678 to April 1714*, vol. 6 (Oxford, 1857), 446; *A view of the Queen's and Kingdom's enemies in the case of the poor Palatines* (London, 1709), 7. For London's consistent opposition to the naturalization of foreigners, see William Maitland, *History of London* (London, 1960), 507, 511, 650–1, 658, 693, 704–5; *The Present State of the British Island* (1725). The debates for 4 and 12 Feb. 1708 and 3 Jan. 1711 are in *The Parliamentary history of England from the Norman Conquest in 1066 to the year 1803*, vol. 6 (London, 1810), 780–3. Included is a 13-point paper circulated during the debate opposing naturalization. Two reasons were that aliens would endanger the constitution because they would be loyal to their own princes and that aliens would send their 'treasures' to their homeland. For the Naturalization Act see Caroline Robbins, 'A note on General Naturalization under the later Stuarts', *Journal of Modern History* 34 (1962), 176; A. H. Carpenter, 'Naturalization in England and the

American colonies', *American Historical Review* 9 (1904), 293; *Daily Courant*, 6 Aug. 1709; HSQS 18, xi; Dickinson, 'Poor Palatines', *English Historical Review* (1967), 484; Jonathan Swift, 'Thoughts on Various Subjects', in *The prose works of Jonathan Swift*, ed. Herbert Davis, vol. 1 (Oxford, 1965), 242; Philip Otterness, 'The 1709 Palatine migration and formation of German immigrant identity in London and New York', paper given at the Washington Seminar in Early American History, 4 Dec. 1997, 21.

2 Reginald Lane Poole, *A history of the Huguenots of the dispersion at the recall of the Edict of Nantes* (London, 1880), 79; HSQS 50, 8, 19; Robin D. Gwynn, 'The distribution of refugees in England, II: London and its environs,' *HSP* 22:6 (1976), 523; D. N. Griffiths, 'Huguenot links with St George's Chapel, Windsor', *HSP* 22:6 (1976), 496–508.

3 Roy A. Sundstrom, 'Aid and assimilation: a study of the economic support given French Protestants in England, 1680–1727' (unpublished Ph.D. thesis, Kent State University, 1972), 230–1; Malcolm Thorp, 'The English government and Huguenot settlement, 1680–1702' (unpublished Ph.D. thesis, University of Wisconsin, 1972), *passim*; HSQS 51, 1–3, 17, 22–3, 27, 32, 37; 'The English government and the relief of Protestant refugees', *English Historical Review* 9 (1894), 663–72; HSQS 49.

4 The German visitor von Uffenbach, visiting London in 1710, spent a month among well-connected Germans in London and never heard the Palatines mentioned: *London in 1710, from the travels of Zacharias Conrad von Uffenbach*, ed. W. H. Quarrell and Margaret Moore (London, n.d.), 27–62.

5 Bernard Cottret, *Huguenots in England: immigration and settlement, 1550–1700* (Cambridge, 1985), chaps 4 and 5; *London in 1710*, 12, 15, 17–27.

6 William Wake, later Archbishop of Canterbury, argued essentially for a comprehensive Anglican Church in May 1689: *An Exhortation to Mutual Charity and Union among Protestants in a Sermon preached before the King and Queen at Hampton Court, May 21 1689* (London, 1689), 15, 18 (BL, Pamphlet 694 e7).

7 'The Case of the Dutch and French Protestant Churches in England since King Edward the Sixth', GL, MS 7424, 52. This is not dated, but probably written in connection with the Coetus's effort at getting foreign churches exempted from the Occasional Conformity Bill, 11 Feb. 1711/12: GL, MS 7412/2, 127. See also *A Proposal of Union amongst Protestants: from the Last Will of the Most Reverend Doctor Sandys* (London, 1679), 2, 4. The Wake MSS at Christ Church, Oxford contain several letters from churches on the Continent asking Wake to take them under his protection. In appealing for help for Bohemians driven into Poland and Prussia in 1716, Wake came close to suggesting that he was actually looking for Continental churches that could fit under the Anglican umbrella: *Good Brother*, London, 1 July 1716 (BL, Pamphlet 1782–2). In 1717 Wake was actually talking about an 'Anglo-Gallican Church' and also the possibility of the King's serving as a mediator among different Protestant churches in Germany. See William Beauvoir to Wake, 1 Feb. 1717/8 and 14 May 1718 and James Caesar to Wake, 23 April 1717: Christ Church, Oxford, Wake MS 28, 105, 115, 123. Bishop Gibson either reviewed or drew up himself an 'Abridgement of Considerations under which the King of Great Britain should work to the Reestablishment of the Reformed Church of France': Lambeth Palace Library, Gibson MS 932/79.

8 See, for example, minutes of 4, 6, 12, 18, 23 and 30 May 1709: *Journal of the Commissioner for Trade and Plantations from February 1708/9 to March 1714/5* (London, 1925; reprinted Lichtenstein, 1969), 26, 28, 32, 33–4, 37, 39.

9 *Acts of the Privy Council, Colonial*, vol. 2, no. 783 (7 March 1700). Records of the Privy Council's deliberations are in the PRO, Colonial Office 5/1311, fos. 11, 13.

10 Lambeth Palace Library, Lambeth MS 953, 94 (not dated).

11 *The Reception of the Palatines vincidated in a fifth letter to a Tory Member* (London, 1711), 31. But in 1709 this argument was open to the complaint that since the Act of Toleration

took foreign churches out of the supervision of the Archbishop of Canterbury, the Church of England could no longer appropriately claim to be the patron of all European Protestantism.

12 *The Post Boy,.* 4–7 June 1709.

13 Walter Allen Knittle, *The early eighteenth century Palatine emigration* (Philadelphia, 1936), 9.

14 *Daily Courant,* 6 Aug. 1709.

15 *Daily Courant,* 8 Aug. 1709.

16 *Reception of the Palatines,* 15.

17 Daniel Defoe, *A brief history of the poor Palatine refugees, 1709,* ed. John Robert Moore, Augustan Reprint Society Publication 106 (Los Angeles, 1964), 30.

18 *Defoe's Review,* 2 July 1709, 154.

19 *Ibid.,* 16 Aug. 1709, 229.

20 Knittle, 14.

21 *View of the Queen's and Kingdom's enemies,* 6.

22 Clarendon to Dartmouth, 8 March 1710: *New York colonial documents,* ed. Edmund B. O'Callaghan, vol. 5, 195–7.

23 *Reception of the Palatines,* 16

24 *View of the Queen's and Kingdom's enemies,* 7.

25 Sundstrom, 'Aid and assimilation', 200.

26 William Petty, 'Political Arithmetick or a Discourse concerning the Extent and Value of Lands' (London, 1690), in *The economic writings of Sir William Petty,* ed. Charles Henry Hull, vol. 2 (Cambridge, 1899), 267.

27 William Petty or Capt John Graunt, 'Natural and Political Observations mentioned in a following index and made upon the Bills of Mortality' (5th edn., London, 1676), in *Economic writings,* ed. Hull, vol. 2, 377.

28 William Petty, 'A Treatise of taxes and contributions' (London, 1662) in *Economic Writings,* ed. Hull, vol. 1, 68. See also articles on 'Nicholas Barbon, projector' and 'Sir William Petty; political arithmetic', in William Letwin, *The origins of scientific economics* (London, 1963), 48–75, 114–46.

29 PRO, 388/76, fo. 54 (3 May 1709).

30 Burnet, *History of his own time,* 863.

31 *Reception of the Palatines,* 37.

32 *London Gazette,* 31 March–4 April 1709.

33 *Reception of the Palatines,* 4.

34 *Daily Courant,* 6 Aug. 1709.

35 Lambeth Palace Library, Lambeth MS 953, fos. 93–4 (6 July 1709).

36 Petty, 'Political Arithmetick' in *Economic writings,* vol. 2, 259.

37 Karl de Schweintz, *England's road to social security, 1349–1947* (Philadelphia, 1947), 55.

38 *Defoe's Review,* 6 Aug. 1709, 215–16; *The Palatines' Catechism or a true description of their camps at Blackheath and Camberwell* (London, 1709), 4.

39 *State of the Palatines,* 7.

40 *The Boston Newsletter,* 13 March 1710, reporting news from London, 16 Aug. 1709.

41 *Defoe's Review,* 15 July 1709, 157.

42 David Owen, *English Philanthropy, 1660–1690* (Cambridge, 1964), 17–19.

43 Clarendon to Dartmouth, 8 March 1710: *New York colonial documents,* vol. 5, 195–7.

44 *Reception of the Palatines,* 7.

45 John Tutchin, 'The Foreigners, a poem' (London, 1700) in John Tutchin, *Selected Poems, 1685–1700,* ed. Spiro Peterson, Augustan Reprint Society Publication 110 (Los Angeles, 1964); Daniel Defoe, 'True Born Englishman' in *The works of Daniel Defoe,* vol. 2 (New York, 1908), 242.

46   John Locke, *An Essay concerning human understanding*, bk. II, sect. 1 (London, 1967), 89–98; James Gibson, *Locke's theory of knowledge and its historical relations* (Cambridge, 1960; originally published 1917), 114–9; Neal Wood, *The politics of Locke's philosophy* (Berkeley, CA, 1983), 61.

47   Defoe, 'True Born Englishman', 242.

48   *Palatines' Catechism*, 4.

49   Library of Congress, Washington, Archdale MS, 1694–1706, quoted in Knittle, *Palatines*, 151. Daniel Defoe argued against this, pointing out that in the colonies they would produce more of certain products than the trade would allow: *Defoe's Review*, 19 July 1709, 181–3.

50   *Reasons for establishing the Colony of Georgia with regard to the trade of Great Britain* (London, 1733), quoted in Leonard W. Cowie, *Henry Newman: an American in London, 1708–43* (London, 1956), 230.

51   HSQS 50, 8, 19.

52   Alison Olson, 'The Palatines and the Salzburgers: two eighteenth-century groups of refugees and their reception in England,' paper given at the American Historical Association conference, December 1992; Olson, 'The Palatine reception in England and America: changing ideas of ethnicity at the beginning of the eighteenth century', paper given at the Massachusetts Historical Society, November 1993.

52

The Naturalization Act of 1709 and the settlement of Germans in Britain, Ireland and the colonies

William O'Reilly

Between the Glorious Revolution and the outbreak of the Seven Years War in 1756, large numbers of German Protestant immigrants of various regional and religious backgrounds travelled to Britain, Ireland and the British American colonies. Building on networks of religious, political and economic interest established in the 17th century, these migrants found in Britain protection and refuge from the many confessional struggles taking place in Continental Europe. Yet these 18th-century German migrants required a new series of justifications to gain continued most favoured support from the British Crown, granting them freedom to settle in Britain or later in Ireland and British America.[1] These efforts made greatest use of the pre-existing Protestant diaspora in London in particular, of a number of philanthropic associations and also of groups within the Anglican Church who favoured the sponsorship and settlement of Continental Protestants in the British lands. In 1709 the confluence of these efforts, together with the passage through Parliament of a new General Naturalization Act, led thousands of Germans from the lands on both sides of the Rhine to arrive in London; an immigration which English economic writers had sought for decades and yet which was to prove an unmitigated disaster.[2] The so-called 'Palatine Migration' became a test case of English governmental support for the continued recruitment and settlement of foreign Protestants in Britain, a case which was to see Tory versus Whig policies, mercantilist economic reasoning and ideas of population all challenge the German Protestant hope of finding a 'new Canaan'.[3]

Protestant refugees from the Continent played several valued roles in English society. As skilled and unskilled labour and as reformed brothers in Christ, where the continued support of such groups did not challenge domestic or international policies, public and governmental support translated to hospitality for these Protestants. When mercantile and political interests dictated caution, however, and German Protestants were seen as some form of threat to national well being, hospitality turned to hostility.[4] Yet supporters for the continued settlement of Protestants in Britain were found throughout most sectors of society. The Anglican 'Society for Promoting Christian

Knowledge' (SPCK), founded in 1698/9, maintained strong relations with Pietist Lutheran ministers in the German lands, most especially at the most important contemporary seminary for the training of German Lutheran missionaries, Halle.[5] The Revd Thomas Bray, founder of the SPCK, also founded, in 1701, the Society for Propagating the Gospel in Foreign Parts (SPG), the first missionary arm of the Anglican Church in the Americas. Two of the most significant individuals to connect the German Halle Pietists and the SPCK and the SPG were Heinrich Wilhelm Ludolf (1655–1712), living in London since the 1670s, secretary to the Danish embassy at the Court of St James and later emissary of Prince George of Denmark, consort of Queen Anne and co-founder of the SPCK; and Anton Wilhelm Böhme, Lutheran chaplain in London during the reign of George I.[6] Ludolf was appointed commissioner for the Palatine refugees in London in 1709 and retained an important role in mediating between the varied interests of the refugees, the Crown and Protestant interests in the SPCK and Halle.

Equally important in this debate were a number of contemporary English economic writers, whose writings reflected and fed the revolution in trade taking place since the later 17th century.[7] Writing on trade reached an all time high in the first decade of the 18th century in Britain, reflecting the emerging debate on the significance of the economic role of the colonies and the concerns about what effects colonial trade growth would have on British society.[8] Charles Davenant, Josiah Child, William Petty, John Carey, John Pollexfen and Matthew Hales were all interested in the emergence of a new social and economic society in Britain and wrote on the subject of British improvement.[9] A fellow contemporary of these writers was Daniel Defoe, whose voluminous output has attracted much attention from social historians,[10] literary scholars,[11] biographers,[12] and scholars of colonial theory.[13] Yet in his day Defoe was best known as the author of *The True Born Englishman: a satyr* (1701), a defence of King William and his Dutch and Huguenot allies against those who opposed the growing influence of foreigners in English political and social life. Defoe attacked the nationalist jealousies of his fellow English and satirized their trenchant refusals to accept foreigners and their skills.[14] Only one of many apologies for foreign immigrants in England written by Defoe, he was perhaps the greatest public advocate of Protestant immigration to England and while his prolific output as a writer is well known, his consistent support for the settlement of Protestant refugees in Britain and her colonies and his demands for a cheap and expeditious means of incorporating these immigrants into British society as quickly as possible (through acts of naturalization or otherwise) is less well known. This paper will outline the relationship between contemporary 18th-century economic ideas, economic and political circumstances and government policy in England in the late mercantilist period through the examination of the role of Daniel Defoe in the arrival and subsequent treatment of German Protestant refugees in London in 1709 as part of the 'Palatine Migration' of that year.

Public discussion of the suitability of accepting German Protestants in Britain as full subjects of the Crown centred on the range of legal options and forms of redress open to Government. The debate usually expressed itself in terms of whether foreigners should be offered naturalization, that is, whether a cheap and convenient way should be offered to immigrants to allow them to acquire the legal rights of native-born subjects. Both its proponents and its detractors believed, probably wrongly, that such an offer, by means of a general naturalization act, would inspire a large number of foreign Protestants to travel to Britain. The questions were considered in Parliament on more than a dozen occasions from the Restoration in 1660 until such an act was finally passed in 1709. At the same time, the new profusion of economic tracts, pamphlets, and broadsides that issued from the presses after the Restoration gave the naturalization issue an important place in their pages. Daniel Defoe entered this established debate with vigour.[15]

A general naturalization act was sought to replace the existing means by which an alien could change his status. There was denization by a grant of the Crown, and naturalization by a private act of Parliament. Both were time-consuming and expensive and few immigrants bothered to obtain naturalization or denization under these customary procedures in either the 17th or 18th centuries. In fact the chief disabilities of being an immigrant, namely the inability to own property and the obligation to pay alien duties and taxes, probably caused little hardship to most immigrants.[16] The act of 1709 embodied the proposals that had long been debated. It stated that any person born out of allegiance of the Queen who received communion in some Protestant church in Great Britain, who took the oath of allegiance and supremacy, and who made certain decreed declarations in open court, would, after the payment of a fee of one shilling, be deemed a natural-born subject of Great Britain. In the event, the 1709 act became the focus of a heated partisan dispute between Whigs and Tories and it was repealed only three years after its passage through Parliament. Immigration was, then as now, a controversial issue. But despite the fury it provoked, it remains very doubtful that such a naturalization act was really the right measure for the end that was sought, which was to entice large numbers of immigrants, especially German Protestant immigrants, to come and settle in Britain and her colonies and thus expand the nation's population.

And population was the central concern. Around the time of the Restoration, fears began that England's population was too small. Economic writers proclaimed the pressing need for more people and a general naturalization was hailed as the common solution. The observation that England was 'not half peopled' became a commonplace, and proposals for a naturalization to increase population appeared in the works of Josiah Child, Carew Reynell, John Houghton, Charles Davenant and many other economic writers. An anonymous tract. 'The Grand Concern of England' (1673) declared 'a general naturalization of all foreign Protestants' is 'absolutely necessary at this time' since there was 'nothing so much wanting in England as people'.[17]

One of the few consistent principles of mercantilist theory was the insistence that a nation had to be populous to be economically powerful. In 1697 Defoe published 'Some Seasonable Queries on . . . a General Naturalization'. The pamphlet urged the passage of the naturalization bill then pending in Parliament. In 1698, in 'Lex Talionis', Defoe wrote that 'no number of foreigners can be prejudicial to England'; a million immigrants 'of whatever nation' could employ and people by their consumption of the nation's provisions.[18] These views were further elaborated upon in 'Giving Alms no Charity' (1704) where Defoe maintained that even two million foreign subjects 'could do us no harm' since 'multitudes of people make trade, [and] trade makes wealth.'[19] Defoe never doubted that immigrants would quickly be assimilated by English society; he insisted that the 'true-born Englishman' had been a foreigner only a few generations ago. His fictional writing also bears out this belief: Robinson Crusoe's father was an immigrant from the Hanseatic city of Bremen. The heroine of

'Roxana' had come from France with her refugee parents when she was ten years old. 'Those nations which are most mixed are the best', Defoe wrote in the preface to the 1703 edition of 'The True Born Englishman', and 'have the least of barbarism and brutality among them.' This was also the man who, at the age of 43 years, changed his name from Foe to the rather more foreign and exotic sounding 'Defoe', acquiring an air of Continental cosmopolitanism.

Defoe had, then, encouraged the attraction and settlement of foreign Protestants in Britain from the start of his career. After the election of 1708 in England, a new Whig coalition government pressed through Parliament a number of acts which had long waited on the books. One of these was the Naturalization Act, which Tories had long opposed and Whigs had long canvassed, and which received royal assent on 23 March 1709.[20] Within a few weeks of the act being passed, German Protestants began to arrive in London.

Initially, at least, individuals were recruited – tempted – to uproot from their native territories in Germany, with the clear intention of attaining an economically and socially more comfortable living standard in their adopted home. Migration was most often dissuaded, if not outright banned, by German rulers. The Elector of the Palatinate made several attempts, between 1651 and 1663, to compensate for de-population within his area by inviting foreign subjects to settle, with the promises of immunity from taxes and protection in return for their farming the land left fallow by the departed Palatines. In this case, the offer was accepted mainly by migrants from Switzerland, the Tyrol and the Spanish Netherlands.[21] Numerous reasons other than religious persecution may have prompted more than 13,000 Palatine people to leave their homes in the period 1709–1711 and travel initially to England, but it was the immediate threat of religious persecution which caused them to seek protection from the onslaught of the French Catholic army.[22]

As had been the case in Zurich, where emigrants to Brandenburg and to North America had been organized by Pastors, it was a Pastor from the Rhineland-Palatinate who stirred interest among his fellow landsmen, a people who were 'ruined and utterly spoiled' by the French invasion of 1707, to migrate initially to England, with a view to receiving the Crown's permission to travel to the English colonies in North America.[23] In 1708, a war which took on all the guise of a Protestant–Catholic conflict was raging in Europe between Louis XIV of France and a European confederation which included England and many of the German states. During military sorties on the English army, the French had many times invaded the Rhineland-Palatinate area, and it was as result of one of these attacks that in April 1708 a Lutheran minister named Joshua de Kocherthal led a group of nine families (41 people in all, of whom 15 were Lutherans and 26 Calvinists) from the area to seek refuge in England. Their pleas to Queen Anne for protection and financial aid were sympathetically heard, as she ordered that they be paid an allowance of one shilling per head, per day, and that de Kocherthal was to be paid the money for distribution among the others. Furthermore, they were to be made 'free denizens of Britain without charge', which gave them permission to settle on British soil either in England or in any other of the new colonies.[24] De Kocherthal quickly decided to set forth with the group for America, and in October they set out on board the *Kingsale* for New York, arriving on 18 December 1708 in Buzzard's Bay, New England, after a considerable delay due to bad weather.

It was news of de Kocherthal's success in attaining Crown support in England, together with his pamphlet which promoted migration, 'Aussfuhrlich- und umstandlicher Bericht von der beruhmten Landschaft Carolina', which brought the first wave of the Palatines from their homes in the areas of Assenheim, Heidelberg, Mannheim, Speyer and Worms to the port of Rotterdam.[25] It has been suggested that the English ambassador in Frankfurt-am-Main actively engaged in promoting migration, and that it was he who was responsible for the distribution of de Kocherthal's pamphlet.[26] This may very well have been true, for the speed with which the migrants were shipped from Rotterdam to London, and the very positive reception with which they were greeted, all point towards the execution of a well-planned state-sponsored venture. Before the main groups of Palatines ever reached England, a Whig sponsored bill in the House of Commons granted the right of naturalization to all foreign Protestants who settled in Britain. Many Members of Parliament argued – citing the successful integration of the Huguenots as an example – that foreign Protestants settling on English soil would, if granted the right of naturalization, increase the wealth and power of Britain. The bill was passed with little debate and great speed, being read in the House of Lords on 11 March 1709, and receiving Royal assent on the 23rd of the same month.[27] In reality the act could not have been known of before most Germans left their German homelands to travel to England: the act was passed at the end of March and the first Palatines arrived in London in May after several months travel. The Act of 1709 did not provoke Palatine migration, although the disastrous results of poor Palatines arriving in London certainly did assist the repeal of the Act in 1712.[28]

Between April and October of that year, approximately 13,500 people travelled from Rotterdam to London, from the areas already mentioned, but also from along the Rhine tributaries, the Neckar and the Moselle and from the region between Speyer and Mainz. Problems were encountered relatively early on by the authorities on the English side, when overcome with these 'herds' of Palatines.[29]

This issue of the 'authenticity' of the Palatines claims of religious persecution, remembering that this was initially the predominant, if not sole, reason, for their speedy transfer to Protestant English soil, soon came to the fore. British authorities had believed that the migration was that of a group of conscientious Protestants fleeing the wrath of Catholic France, until they discovered that approximately one quarter of the fugitives were Catholics.[30] As many Protestants and Catholics were married to each other, the women amongst them were offered the option of converting to the Protestant faith, or returning to Germany, while the men could additionally choose to enlist and fight for Queen Anne in Portugal. Perhaps as many as 3000 chose to return, and they were all given free passage to Rotterdam and a grant of five Guilders to cover the cost of their trip from Rotterdam.[31] The remaining number – perhaps as many as 9000 – were all housed in the London area around the Tower ditch. They lived in terrible conditions, with often as many as 100 to a house, and on 9 May 1709, John Tribbeko and George Ruperti, two clerics from the Palatine group itself, reported that some of their number were very sick, and others had died of hunger and overcrowding. Health soon improved when the Palatines were moved to barns, rent being paid by private individuals and philanthropists. By late May, 6500 were accommodated in tents on Blackheath, Greenwich, and Camberwell commons. In a warehouse owned by a Sir Charles Cox lodged 1400 immigrants, and the surplus number were lodged in Her Majesty's 'Ropeyard' at Deptford.

Resentment, at the expense incurred in housing the Palatines in a time of rising prices and unemployment, caused many English people to question the sense and value of the governmental action. Defoe countered challenges that German immigrants would take English jobs. There was no lack of work in England, he wrote, and the additional labour of naturalized foreigners would raise wages and more than proportionately increase the demand for labour. But the Palatines were poor and a common objection to the Naturalization Act had been that all beggars of Europe would be attracted to England. Defoe had earlier complained that England was 'burdened with a crowd of clamouring, unemployed, unprovided-for poor people'.[32] A settlement of the Palatines on the land was the best solution; but this must be a planned settlement. Projectors who wished to employ them would be unwilling to provide the necessary security to the parish where they were to be settled. It was proposed to form colonies of Palatines in the New Forest and these would ultimately form self-sufficient communities, while remaining small enough to necessitate the intermingling of German immigrant families with native English ones. The scheme would achieve the twin objectives of settling the Palatines and of improving the land that lay in waste and economically barren.

Meanwhile, a continuous stream of Palatines continued to arrive in England during the summer months of 1709. Attempts were made to teach the refugees English and a short grammar and bilingual phrase-book was printed, entitled 'A Short and Easy Way for the Palatines to Learn English, oder Eine Kurze Ausleitung zur Englischen Sprach zum Hutz zur armer Pfalzer/nebst angehangsten Englischen and Deutschen ABC' (London, 1710).[33] Approximately one thousand bibles, testaments and prayer books were also distributed, and religious services were offered, twice weekly, by three German ministers and other local clerics. Nonetheless, realization that local hostility was building up, and pressure on the Government to ascertain the truth in the rumours that the Palatines were simply seeking free transportation to the British colonies, resulted in a Crown commission being established. One of its members, Roger Kenyon, who visited the Blackheath camp in August 1709, wrote: 'What freak brought these poor creatures hither is not easy to guess, but it seems there has been some books sent hither among them . . . with flattering descriptions of Cariline [sic] and they are mad to go thither.'[34]

Indeed, the Committee went on to proclaim those responsible for bringing the Palatines to England 'enemies to the nation' and declared: 'The inviting and bringing over the poor Palatines of all religions at the public expense was an extravagant and unreasonable charge to the Kingdom and a scandalous misapplication of public money.'[35]

Thus the Government, ever wary of growing public disquiet at the Palatines' presence in the capital, instigated various actions in order to dispose of the Palatines as quickly as possible. Six hundred and fifty Palatines were finally sent to North Carolina, when the Honourable Christopher de Graffenried acquired a grant of 10,000 acres of land at the exceptionally favourable rent of five shillings per 1000 acres, for the Palatines. A number were settled in Chester, the Corporation of Liverpool accepted 130. The colonists in Jamaica agreed to accept a number, as did those of Antigua, St Christopher, Nevis, and possibly even the Canary Islands.[36] Of course, the Queen's guarantee of a grant of £5 per Palatine to an individual or parish was an incentive to English landlords and corporations to accept the Palatine settlers, and this also suited Queen Anne, who had always favoured their settlement within Britain. Apart from those mentioned above, a further 650 were settled in Britain, 322 entered military service, 141 children were 'purchased by the English', suggesting they became indentured servants or apprentices, and 56 became domestic servants. A further 2814 embarked at the end of December 1709 for New York.[37]

Of those who remained, 3073 persons were sent to Ireland.[38] As early as 1694, it had been proposed by the Baron de Luttichaw to the English Government to settle one thousand Protestants from Silesia in Ireland, in an attempt to bolster Protestant numbers and bring industry to the country.[39] Thus the proposal of the Lord Lieutenant, the Marquis of Wharton, and the Privy Council in Dublin, that the Queen should settle a number of Palatine families in Ireland was not a new one. The refugees were discussed in the Irish House of Commons on 20 and 24 August 1709, and it was agreed: 'That it is the opinion of this House that her Majesty by sending over a proportion of Protestant Palatines into this Kingdom has very much consulted the strengthening and securing the Protestant interest in Ireland . . . That it will very much contribute to the security of this Kingdom that the said Protestant Palatines be encouraged and settled therein.'[40]

A subsidy of £25,000 was granted for the initially proposed number of 500 families, but this number was exceeded early on, as between 4 and 7 September 1709, 794 families (2971 persons, 1135 of whom were under the age of 14 years) arrived in Dublin. On 14 October a further 100 persons (25 families) arrived and on 24 January 1710, two children arrived alone.[41] These 3073 persons constituted the original Palatine settlement in Ireland. Not since the arrival of the Huguenots in the preceding century had such a significant number of foreigners settled in Ireland. Initial Government and native Irish reaction to the Palatines seems to have been quite similar on both occasions, in fact.[42]

Five hundred and thirty eight families (2098 persons) were immediately dispatched into the country to a number of estates, and the remaining 258 families (970 persons) stayed in Dublin. Confusion seems to have existed among these families, for by January 1710 many of those who had been sent into the country returned to Dublin, having believed that Queen Anne was to give them rent-free lands in Ireland. Certainly it appears that some agents or individuals were continuing to incite the Palatines with propagandist texts, for they referred to broadsheets and pamphlets which they claimed had been circulated in the Palatinate promising them rent-free land in Carolina and Pennsylvania, if they agreed to migrate there.[43] As the possibility of reaching the American colonies from Ireland was slim, many of the families returned to England (232 did so between April and November 1710). Although many were encouraged to go directly to Hamburg from Dublin, most refused and insisted on travelling to England, where several hundred were reported to have ended up begging on the streets.[44] Even the Commissioners in Dublin accepted that 'some turbulent and mutinous persons' were encouraging the Palatines in their belief that they would fare better were they to return to England. The difficulty with which the Irish Governmental Commission was faced – that of trying to dispel local fears and hostilities, and at the same time trying to find employment or a useful purpose for the Palatines, resulted in the Irish House of Lords complaining to the Queen about the large numbers of indigent and useless Palatines, a group who had been cast over on to the backs of the Irish at a time of extreme dearth and poverty.[45]

Palatine dissatisfaction with the settlement offered them in Ireland remained, a more than favourable settlement which offered an initial immediate grant of eight acres of land per head, more often than not in areas of prime agricultural land, a further monetary grant of 40 shillings per family, per annum, for seven years, to cover the cost of farm stock and utensils, and their land was to be granted in leases of three lives, a lease type unimaginable for the native Irish. Significant groups continued to leave the country. The report of one Mr Crockett, who attempted to do just that, testifies to their determination, and the continuing resentment with which they were viewed by those who were trying to help them: 'They made no further return for his kindness: on the contrary some of them threatened to throw him into the sea when he went on shipboard to persuade them not to proceed on their journey.'[46]

By 21 November 1711, two years after the Palatines first arrived in Ireland, only 40 per cent of the original number remained, that was 312 families (1218 persons), and 50 per cent of these were in Dublin, although the original plan had been to disperse them in rural areas amidst the Gaelic Irish. In the early months of 1712, the numbers dropped further when more of the Germans fled the country, and little more than 1000 remained.[47] The Treasury in London, still subsidizing the venture, saw that of the original grant of £24,000 given for the Irish Palatines, only £4878 7s 6d remained, and that this would only support the remaining number for a further 15 months. Whether it was realization of their financial predicament, final contentment with, and acceptance of, some type of a future in Ireland, or simply that they had enough travelling and had lost their *Wanderlust*, the drift homewards ended by August 1712. At this time, the Palatines were settled in a few small and scattered colonies around the country, in Limerick, Kerry, Wexford, Tipperary and Carlow, where a small area still bears the name 'Palatinetown'.[48] The Limerick settlements were by far the most important, as it was Sir Thomas Southwell, a member of the Irish parliament who had already accepted ten Palatine families, who agreed to take the greatest number of those remaining in Dublin, in September 1712. Those families not on the Southwell estate remained elsewhere in negligible numbers, and constituted a minority of the total Palatine community in Ireland. This September settlement on Southwell's property, at the villages of Courtmatrix, Killeheen and Ballingrane, was to found the basis for future Palatine expansion, eventually having small colonies at Adare, Pallaskenry, Ballyriggin, Ballyorgan and Glenosheen in Co. Limerick, Kilnaughtin, Bally-macelligott and Castleisland in Co. Kerry and Kilcooly in Co. Tipperary.[49] From the detailed enumeration which was carried out at St Catherine's in London in 1709, the families that settled at Courtmatrix (30 Palatine families), Killeheen (25 families) and Ballingrane (50 families) – the major settlements which circled the town of Rathkeale – can be traced in the records, and it appears that 48 of the families resident on the Southwell estate in 1720 were among this early group of migrants.[50]

Despite the best attempts by Daniel Defoe and others to advance the settlement of German Protestants in Britain and Ireland from 1709 onwards, the favoured outcome was not attained. Within a few years of their arrival only a handful of Palatines remained in England and many families established in Ireland had left the country or would do so in the proceeding decades, preferring to re-establish themselves in the American colonies. Defoe's cherished plans for settling Germans on the land and turning them to the improvement of England's trade had come to nothing. Nevertheless he did not relinquish projects to encourage German settlements. Indeed, he set forth recommendations similar to the one that he had endorsed for the Palatines in his *Tour* and in a number of his later works (*Atlas Maritimus* (1728) and *A Plan of the English Commerce* (1730)).[51] The issue, however, had been decided in 1709, at the time of the General Naturalization Act and the Palatine migration. The plan of increasing England's population by receiving immigrants had been discredited, and Defoe's hopes thereafter of seeing a settlement of immigrants on the waste lands of England, in Ireland and in the Colonies were futile. His schemes had failed. Yet Defoe's writings on the subject have a continuing importance to historians. They provide a detailed picture of the ideas about immigration, land, and population of England's most productive early economic writer, and his engagement in the Palatine affair reveals the connection in the early 18th century between economic ideas, commercial and administrative circumstances, and legislative procedure.

Without Defoe's constant efforts on behalf of European Protestants and his continued support for their establishment in Britain, the settlement of 1709 might have been terminated before it ever came to pass.

NOTES

1   I am grateful to the Millennium Research Fund of NUI, Galway for support in carrying out the research in this paper. Renate Wilson, 'Continental Protestant refugees and their protectors in Germany and London: commercial and charitable networks', *Pietismus und Neuzeit: ein Jahrbuch zur Geschichte des Neueren Protestantismus* (Göttingen, 1994), vol. 20, 107–24, here 107–8.

2   Daniel Statt, *Foreigners and Englishmen: the controversy over immigration and population, 1660–1760* (Newark, 1995), 121–41; Walter A. Knittle, *The early eighteenth-century Palatine emigration: a British government redemptioner project to manufacture naval stores* (Philadelphia, 1936).

3   H. T. Dickinson, 'The "Poor Palatines" and the parties', *English Historical Review* 82 (1967), 464–85.

4   For a general discussion of the changing views of European Protestantism in Britain, see: Ernest Gordon Rupp, *Religion in England, 1688–1791* (Oxford, 1986); William Reginald Ward, *The Protestant evangelical awakening* (Cambridge, 1992).

5   Recent studies of the role of Halle and German Lutheran mission work are: Daniel L. Brunner, *Halle Pietists in England: Anton William Böhm and the Society for Promoting Christian Knowledge* (Göttingen, 1993); Arno Sames, *Anton Wilhelm Böhme, 1673–1722: Studien zum ökumenischen Denken und Handeln eines halleschen Pietisten* (Göttingen, 1989); Edmund McClure (ed.), *A chapter in English church history: the minutes of the Society for Promoting Christian Knowledge for the years 1698–1704* (London, 1888).

6   For Ludolf's missionary activities, see: S. G. Simmons, 'H.W. Ludolf and the printing of his *Grammatica Russica* at Oxford in 1696', *Slavonic Papers* 1 (1950), 104–29; Joachim Tetzner, *H.W. Ludolf und Rußland* (Berlin, 1955).

7   D. C. Coleman, *The Economy of England, 1450–1750* (Oxford, 1977).

8   Jacob M. Price, 'The Imperial economy, 1700–1776', in P. J. Marshall (ed.), *The Oxford history of the British Empire*, vol. 2: *The Eighteenth Century* (Oxford, 1998), 98; Statt, *Foreigners and Englishmen*, 22.

9   On the debate concerning England's 'waste lands', see Keith Thomas, *Man and the natural world: changing attitudes in England 1500–1800* (Harmondsworth, 1987), 15.

10   For example, Roy Porter, *English society in the eighteenth century* (London, 1991).

11 Including Bram Dijkstra, *Defoe and economics: the fortunes of Roxana in the history of interpretation* (New York, 1987).

12 Laura Anne Curtis, *The elusive Daniel Defoe* (New Jersey, 1984) and Peter Earle, *The world of Defoe* (London, 1976).

13 Fakrul Alam, 'Daniel Defoe as a colonial propagandist' (unpublished Ph.D. thesis, University of British Columbia, Canada, 1984).

14 Daniel Defoe, *The True Born Englishman* (London, 1700), 618–23; Jack P. Greene, 'Empire and identity from the Glorious Revolution to the American Revolution', *Oxford history of the British Empire*, vol. 2, 212.

15 Defoe was, after 1712, to become an apologist for the slave trade. See Daniel Defoe, *Review* no. 44 (10 January 1713), 89: 'No African Trade, no Negroes; no Negroes, no Sugars . . . that is to say, farewell all your American Trade, your West-India Trade'. He also became financially involved in the 'South Sea Bubble' in 1720: Daniel Defoe, *The trade to India critically and calmly considered* (London, 1720); Glyndwr Williams, 'The Pacific: exploration and exploitation', *Oxford history of the British Empire*, vol. 2, 554.

16 Daniel Statt, 'The Birthright of an Englishman: the practice of naturalization and denization of immigrants under the later Stuarts and early Hanoverians', *HSP* 25 (1989), 61–74; HSQS 17; Statt, *Foreigners and Englishmen*, 128: 'But the Tory argument that the naturalization act was responsible for bringing the Palatines to England is untenable. Immigrants as poor as the Palatines could have gained little or nothing by becoming naturalized subjects, and almost none of them took advantage of the act. Of the 933 persons known to have been naturalized under the act in the year 1709 almost all bore French names.'

17 *The Harleian Miscellany* (12 vols., London, 1808–11), vol. 8, 13–61, 23–5: Statt, 'Defoe and immigration', 297.

18 Daniel Defoe, *Lex Talionis: or, an enquiry into the most proper ways to prevent the persecution of the Protestants of France* (London, 1698).

19 Daniel Defoe, *Giving Alms no charity* (London, 1704), 5–8, 23; P. N. Furbank and W. R. Owens (eds.), *Daniel Defoe: 'The True Born Englishman' and other writings* (London, 1997), 231, 234.

20 Statt, *Foreigners and Englishmen*, 127.

21 Hans Ulrich Pfister, *Die Auswanderung aus dem Knonauer Amt, 1648–1750. Ihr Ausmass, ihre Strukturen und ihre Bedingungen* (Zürich, 1987), 206.

22 Ludwig Hausser, *Geschichte der Rheinischen Pfalz nach ihren politischen, kirchlichen und literarischen Verhaltnissen* (Heidelberg, 1924), vol. 2, 840. See also: Herbert Zielinski, 'Klimatische Aspekte Bevölkerungsgeschichtlicher Entwicklung', in Arthur E. Imhof (ed.), *Historische Demographie als Sozialgeschichte: Gießen und Umgebung vom 17. zum 19. Jahrhundert* (Darmstadt, 1975), vol. 2, 944–9; Joachim Heinz, *'Bleibe im Lande, und nähre dich redlich!': Zur Geschichte der pfälzischen Auswanderung vom ende des 17. bis zum Ausgang des 19. Jahrhunderts* (Kaiserslautern, 1989), 43; Wilhelm Abel, *Agricultural fluctuations in Europe* (New York, 1980), 184.

23 Vivien Hick, 'The Palatine settlement in Ireland: the early years', *Eighteenth-Century Ireland* 4 (1989), 113.

24 *Ibid.*, 113–14.

25 Joshua Harrsch de Kocherthal, *Aussfuhrlich- und umständlicher Bericht von der Berühmten Landschaft Carolina in dem Engelländischen America* (4th edn., Frankfurt am Main, 1709).

26 Julius Goebel, 'Neu Dokumente zur Geschichte der Masseneinwanderung im Jahre 1709', *Jahrbuch der deutsch-amerikanischen historischen Gesellschaft von Illinois* (Chicago, 1913), 181.

27 Hick, 114–15.

28 Statt, *Foreigners and Englishmen*, 128.

29   Hausser, *Geschichte*, 840.

30   Richard Hayes, 'The German colony in County Limerick', *North Munster Antiquarian Journal* 1:2 (1937), 43, writes 'Two thousand of them turned out to be "Papists"'.

31   Hick, 116.

32   Furbank and Owens, *Daniel Defoe*, 252.

33   Hick, 117.

34   HMC 35, *Kenyon MSS*, 442–3, no. 1, 116 (2 August 1709).

35   Hick, 43.

36   *Ibid.*, 118.

37   BL, Harleian MS,7021, fo. 280.

38   Rüdiger Renzing, *Pfälzer in Irland: Studien zur Geschichte deutscher Auswanderer-kolonien des frühen 18. Jahrhunderts* (Kaiserlautern, 1989), 22.

39   *Calendar of Treasury Papers*, 346, for 20 February 1694.

40   *Irish House of Commons Journal*, vol. 3, 1709.

41   Hick, 119–20.

42   J. L. Mc Cracken, 'The social structure and social life, 1714–60', in F. W. Moody and W. E. Vaughan (eds.), *A new history of Ireland (1691–1800)* (Oxford, 1986), vol. 4.

43   For example 'Propositions of the Lords and Proprietors of Carolina to encourage the transporting of Palatines to the Province of Carolina', in PRO, State Papers, Queen Anne, 84/232, 415 (5 July 1709).

44   Hick, 122.

45   J. G. Simms, 'The Protestant Ascendancy, 1691–1710', in *New history of Ireland*, vol. 4, 26.

46   Hayes, *German colony*, 47.

47   Helmut Blume, 'Some geographic aspects of the Palatine settlement in Ireland', *Irish Geography* 2 (1952), 172–9.

48   McCracken, 'Social structure', 41.

49   Hayes, 'German colony', 48.

50   P. J. O'Connor, 'Palatine families on the Southwell Estate 1709–12 to 1720', *Irish Palatine Association Newsletter* 2 (1991).

51   Daniel Defoe, *Atlas maritimus et commercialis* (London, 1728); *idem, A tour through the whole island of Great Britain*, ed. G. D. H. Cole (2 vols., London, 1928); *idem, A plan of the English commerce* (4th edn., Dublin, 1728).

53

German immigrants and the London book trade, 1700–70

GRAHAM JEFCOATE

When Anton Wilhelm Böhm, a Pietist from Halle, arrived in London shortly after the turn of the 18th century he found lodgings with a German family in Bedfordbury near Charing Cross and temporary employment as a teacher of local German children. The Strand area and the liberty of the Savoy had long been favoured by German-speaking residents of London as it had by Huguenots and other expatriate communities. St Mary's in the Savoy, a Lutheran chapel usually known as the Marienkirche, had been founded to meet their spiritual needs in 1694 but it also provided a focus for a rapidly growing community, providing services such as a parish school. It was not the only Lutheran congregation in London at the turn of the 18th century. Chapels had been founded to serve communities that flourished in the City (Hamburg Lutheran Church in Trinity Lane, 1669) and around the court at St James's (Deutsche Hofkapelle, 1700). During the 18th century, a further Lutheran chapel was opened in Alie Street, Goodman's Fields, east of the City, to serve the growing community of German sugar refiners in the area (Georgenkirche, 1762). In addition to these Lutheran chapels, German-speaking Calvinists, Catholics and Jews had their own meeting places in London throughout the period.[1]

These places of worship are evidence for a growing and sustained resident community of German speakers. Significant German immigration to London had begun in the second half of the 17th century and increased rapidly throughout the 18th. The great majority of this immigration was from northern Germany and had economic causes, although refugees from Catholic repression in southern Germany (such as the well-known case of the Palatines who arrived in London in 1708) also swelled the numbers. The accession of a German dynasty to the British throne in 1714 played only a relatively indirect role in terms of German immigration. Germans were attracted to London as Europe's most vibrant commercial centre, providing opportunities for enterprise and entrepreneurship, and as a hub of a growing Atlantic trade. Links with the port cities of Hamburg and Bremen were especially strong. Some trades (such as sugar refining or bookbinding) became near-monopolies for German immigrants in the course of the century. One credible estimate suggests there were about

16,000–20,000 Germans in London by the end of the 18th century, the equivalent of a medium-size contemporary German town.

German bookselling in London is recorded from the first decade of the 18th century and its origins are closely associated with Pietism, the Lutheran reform movement. Anton Wilhelm Böhm (1673–1722) was himself a close collaborator of August Hermann Francke, Pietism's leading personality in the period. Francke's *Waisenhaus* or Orphanage founded in 1698 at Halle an der Saale developed rapidly into a network of charitable and missionary institutions; in the first three decades of the century it was to achieve an extraordinary impact in a wide range of fields and across three continents.[2] The Pietist sense of mission was crucial both in the opening of a German bookshop on the Strand ca. 1710 and even in the much later foundation of a German printing press in Gerrard Street in 1749.

Johann Christian Jacobi

Johann Christian Jacobi, the first German bookseller in 18th-century London, was another disciple of Francke, sent specifically to open a bookshop through which Pietist literature could be distributed. He set up shop 'near Somerset House' in the Strand about 1709. In 1712, his address is given as Southampton Court, Southampton Street, Covent Garden, but by 1717 he had premises in the Exeter Change on the Strand, which provided cheap retail space, with 'lock up' facilities, for a number of foreign booksellers in this period (including Huguenots) and was close to the German chapel in the Savoy. Jacobi's activities need to be regarded as part of the Pietist enterprise in England during the first decades of the century; an enterprise based on close links between Francke at Halle and the Society for Promoting Christian Knowledge in London. The strength of these links was largely due to Böhm. Since his arrival in London in 1701, Böhm had established himself within the SPCK and had developed a close working relationship with Joseph Downing, the SPCK's printer and bookseller. It was Downing who issued the great majority of Pietist works prepared for the press by Böhm, including translations and the first German-language editions printed in London during the period.[3]

In practice, Jacobi appears to have developed a modest book shop aimed at the growing German market based largely on SPCK items and others imported from the Pietist book shop at Halle, especially German Bibles, Psalters and prayer-books. He clearly provided Downing with a retail outlet for his products serving a small but potentially valuable market. His name occurs some 14 times in imprints between 1710 and 1717, sometimes described simply as 'the German bookseller' and often in partnership with Downing. The titles published by Jacobi himself are almost exclusively Pietist-related texts in English or German, but include a periodical (only one copy of which has been preserved) and an edition of a London guidebook in French. Our knowledge of his bookselling activities, slender as it is, allows us to draw some preliminary conclusions about the German element in the London book trade in this period:

1. It was located in the proximity of the Strand, one of the traditional centres of German settlement, and outside the direct control of the Stationers' Company which regulated book trade activity in the City itself.

2.   Its stock balanced local publications (both Downing's and Jacobi's own) with imported titles focusing almost entirely on the message of Lutheran Pietism. Nevertheless, some early diversification is discernible (for example, some titles in English and a French-language guide to London).
3.   It was relatively short-lived; suggesting the model may not have been sustainable.

Johann Christoph Haberkorn

After Jacobi's apparent withdrawal from the retail trade around 1717, and Böhm's death five years later, there is no evidence of any serious German bookselling (and only occasional examples of German printing) until the late 1740s. Between March and June 1749, Johann Christoph Haberkorn (d. 1776), (who had been present in London from at least 1746) acquired a property on the north side of Gerrard Street and, with his partner Johann Nicodemus Gussen, set up the first German press in London using imported *fraktur* types (i.e. German black letter). They state the purpose of the press very clearly in the preface to one of their first major publications, a German *New Testament* printed by them and also sold by Andreas Linde, a German bookseller recently established in Catherine Street, Covent Garden:

> And it happened, that according to God's will, in this place too (that is to say, in the city of London), a German printing shop was set up a little time hence, entirely in order to print good, improving works that would promote true Christianity . . .[4]

Significantly, they mention the potential markets for their publications in their preface: not only the German-speaking population of London but also the rapidly growing communities of Germans in the North American colonies. In December 1750, the same month the publication of the New Testament was announced, the pair was briefly arrested, rather oddly for printing a Catholic devotional book for the bookseller James Marmaduke. Incidentally, this was the first in a series of often somewhat bizarre misfortunes that were to characterize Haberkorn's personal life and career.

Despite this uncertain start, Haberkorn (whose partner Gussen is no longer mentioned after 1753) appears to have built a substantial and successful printing business, with a little associated bookselling, enabling him to move into larger premises in fashionable Grafton Street about 1761 and to take at least one apprentice (in 1763).

Haberkorn remained quite closely associated with German community life throughout his years in London and chose eventually to return to Germany itself. Printing for the German-language market, and especially for the growing Lutheran parishes, remained a cornerstone of his business. As the proprietor of London's only printing press with the capacity to print in German using *fraktur* types, we must assume all genuine German-language imprints from London in this period are associated with his press. Much ephemeral, unattributed or surreptitious work remains to be uncovered, however, although Haberkorn's distinctive ornaments often make his work readily identifiable. They confirm, for example, that he printed in London for

Nicolaus, Count Zinzendorf, the founder of the Moravian community. He was certainly never a stranger to controversy.

Nevertheless, Haberkorn recognized from the beginning that no sustainable printing or bookselling business could be built on these foundations alone. Diversification and expansion were essential to survive as a foreigner in an overcrowded and notoriously risky trade. His very first known imprint had been a poem in honour of the wedding of a Lutheran pastor, printed significantly in English rather than in German.

Apart from printing in the local vernacular, Haberkorn appears to have specialized increasingly in foreign-language books (especially French and Italian), culminating in an extraordinary edition of Boccaccio's *Decamerone* (1762), a work as far removed from Halle Pietism as one can imagine.[5] Many of his titles were printed at the expense of the author and required a capacity to combine letterpress with engraved material. He was responsible for a number of the key architectural and design books of the period, including Thomas Chippendale's *The gentleman and cabinet-maker's director* (1754 and 1755). Above all, he was closely associated with the King's favoured architect, Sir William Chambers, most of whose major publications he printed, including the well-known accounts of Chinese style and of the gardens and buildings at Kew. The quality of these titles, both in terms of presswork, the integration of text and print and page layout, suggests a printer prepared to experiment and to innovate.

Andreas Linde and Christlieb Gottreich Seyffert

Andreas Linde set up shop in Catherine Street, a somewhat insalubrious street linking the Strand with Covent Garden, shortly after Haberkorn and Gussen in Soho. He had been in London since at least 1743. Like Haberkorn, Linde sought to diversify his business, in his case by combining bookselling with bookbinding and selling stationery. He also claimed royal patronage (however doubtfully), as for example in the title to an important catalogue issued in 1753, where he describes himself as 'stationer to His Majesty and to His Royal Highness the Prince of Wales, and bookseller to Her Royal Highness the Princess of Wales'.

Nevertheless, a majority of the titles printed for Linde (or sold by him) have a German connection. Of particular interest are the original works translated by the German author Christlob Mylius, a London resident in the early 1750s, including an important German edition of Hogarth's *Analysis of beauty* printed by Haberkorn using *fraktur* types and published jointly with Schmidt of Hanover in 1754, a very rare and early example of Anglo-German co-operation in the publishing field.[6] Apart from German-language translations and devotional works, there is a high proportion of theological controversy in English centring on the perceived menace of the Moravians. If Haberkorn (disguised) was printing Zinzendorf's works, then Linde was openly selling attacks on them.

Linde largely gave up bookselling in the late 1750s, selling his stock by auction in November 1758. His successor as the principle purveyor of German books in London, Christlieb Gottreich Seyffert from Leipzig, is perhaps the least known of the German members of the London trade since the only recorded copies of two major catalogues issued by him in 1757 were destroyed in Berlin in the Second World War. Their titles show he was a major importer of books from Germany but most of Seyffert's surviving imprints are in English or French, with a bias towards the satirical. He was also the London agent, in succession to Linde, for such major international scholarly enterprises as the annual series of commentaries on natural science and medicine printed in Leipzig. From 1757 to 1760, Seyffert's shop was 'opposite St Anne's Church' in Dean Street, Soho, after which he moved to Pall Mall. He appears to have given up his bookselling business about 1764 and disappears from view.

Carl Heydinger

With Haberkorn's return to Germany about 1767, and Linde and Seyffert's withdrawal from the field, a market niche was created which was to be filled by Carl (or Charles) Heydinger. By 1768 Heydinger was referring to himself in imprints as 'imprimeur et libraire' or 'Buchdrucker und Buchhändler'; from that same year we have his first surviving advertisements on leaves forming part of the final gathering of books printed and sold by him. One of these lists works in German, French and Latin, mostly imported; another includes a number of German and English items, some printed by Heydinger's German predecessors in the London trade, including Haberkorn and Linde, offered at prices between 4d and 10s 6d. Although Heydinger was to achieve much during his two decades of printing and bookselling in London, he too was perceived by contemporaries as having ultimately failed to establish a sustainable business.

Conclusions

Success in 18th-century publishing depended on a number of factors, including access to distribution networks, effective advertising and, above all, shares in the copyright or outright ownership of successful titles. But 18th-century German members of the London book trade also had to seek a fine balance between specialization and diversification.

Demand for German-language books remained low. German-speaking Londoners do not appear to have been conspicuous consumers of German books at any time during the 18th century, and only the churches and schools represented a steady, if small, market.

Despite a temporary fashion for all things German later in the century, English-speaking Londoners showed no sustained interest in the German language or its literature. In contrast with other language areas, and particularly northern, central and eastern Europe, the English-speaking world remained almost completely immune to the pleasures of the German language or its literature throughout the period. There were frequent complaints later in the century that London Germans themselves, mostly active in trade and commerce, often sought to shed their German roots or were at least unenthusiastic readers. German literature enjoyed little prestige in England, after all, and German books were widely regarded as poorly produced and expensive. Pressures of assimilation also meant, for example, that second-generation Germans might themselves not be fluent German speakers.

If the 'market conditions' were unfavourable to those hoping to establish a distinctly German branch to the trade, then other, more practical problems added to their difficulties. Although Latin and foreign-language books were not subject to import duties, the overheads in bringing them from Leipzig, or from other centres of the German book trade, must have been considerable. Adverse winds and, in the latter part of the century, naval action in the North Sea could delay deliveries by many weeks.

Printing and selling German books in 18th-century London was probably not in itself a viable business. In order to make a living, each of the German immigrants in the London book trade invariably saw expansion and diversification as the answer. Diversification could mean printing or selling books in foreign languages other than German or at least establishing a specialist niche of some kind. It could mean selling stationery or undertaking orders for binding. It might also mean (for Heydinger) importing and marketing patent medicines from the apothecary at Halle. The stock of a German bookseller often included current and antiquarian titles, both imported and inherited from London precursors. The need to diversify also meant that Heydinger, for example, remained both a printer and a bookseller at a time when much of the London trade specialized in one branch or the other.

The failure of Germans to establish a sustainable business within the London book trade in this period might well be explained in this need to balance specialization and diversification. This way of doing business must have been associated with considerable overheads, for example costs associated with importing books, maintaining a back list and producing promotional material (for example, full-scale catalogues) while retaining the capacity to print in a number of languages with both *fraktur* and *antiqua* types.

If Haberkorn, Linde, Seyffert and Heydinger can be described as establishing a distinctly German branch to the London book trade in the period between 1750 and 1770, then the major factors affecting its development might be summarized thus:

1. The market for German-language books, among Germans resident in London and perhaps (at least until an indigenous trade developed) among Germans resident in British colonial possessions in North America, remained the cornerstone of the business.
2. This market remained relatively small and largely confined to those of German origin.
3. Commercial judgements needed to be made between printing German books in London and importing them, often expensively, from Germany itself.
4. To survive and prosper, German members of the London book trade needed to expand or specialize and certainly to diversify their businesses. Printing in German and English could be expanded into other languages. Specialist areas of publishing such as plate books, 'fancy' printing, religious controversy or satire might be explored. Bookselling might be supplemented by other services and products.
5. Businesses continued to be mainly located in the area of the Strand or Covent Garden, with a tendency to move to more fashionable streets to the west as they developed.
6. Despite considerable successes over a number of years, most German booktrade initiatives were perceived by contemporaries as failing in the long run.

The line between success and failure in the 18th-century London book trade was a narrow one and it seems clear that most German initiatives in this area were indeed relatively short-lived. Although I do not think we should necessarily take contemporary perceptions of failure at face value, no sustainable model of a successful book trade outlet with distinctly German characteristics appears to have emerged before the 19th century. I feel, however, that we need to understand much more about contemporary retailing beyond the book trade before we can evaluate properly the evidence we have.

That evidence suggests at least a succession of enterprising individuals prepared to innovate and diversify in order to succeed. In the process, they produced lasting work of great interest and high quality. Their products, and the context in which they were made, tells us much about the opportunities and constraints of building sustainable models for a non-indigenous book trade. I believe they also provide us with important evidence for the way in which language-cultures interrelated in the period.

A Provisional Checklist of German Members of the London Book Trade, 1710–70

JOHANN CHRISTIAN JACOBI

'Near Somerset House, Strand'; Southampton Court, Southampton Street, Covent Garden; Exeter Change, The Strand, ca. 1709–17.

JOHANN CHRISTOPH HABERKORN

North Side, Gerrard Street, Soho, ca. 1749–60 (with Johann Nicodemus Gussen to ca. 1753); Grafton Street, Soho, ca. 1761–67.

ANDREAS LINDE

Catherine Street, Strand, ca. 1751–60 [widow still there in 1766 and at Bridges Street, near Covent Garden, ca. 1767–74].
Bibliotheca curiosa, being a catalogue of the libraries of Messrs. Jager and Brande, apothecaries to His Majesty, both deceased; and of a reverend and learned clergyman, [1753]; A catalogue of curious and usefull books in all languages and sciences, the most of them lately imported. . . . Which will be sold very cheap, . . . on Thursday, December 5, 1754; A catalogue of the quire-stock and copies of a bookseller, going into another way of business; to be sold at the Queen's Arms Tavern, in St Paul's Church-Yard, on Tuesday November 28, 1758.

CHRISTLIEB GOTTREICH SEYFFERT

'On the corner of King's Street, Soho', 1757; 'opposite St Anne's Church', Dean Street, Soho, 1757–60; Pall Mall, ca. 1760–4.
Catalogue of new books lately imported in [the] French, Latin, and German languages, and in [al]most all faculties, 1757; Catalogus neuer teutscher Bücher, aus allen Wissenschaften, 1757 (both destroyed).

CARL HEYDINGER

'At the sign of the Moor's Head, Moor Street near Compton Street, Soho', ca. 1766–7; Grafton Street, ca. 1768–70; No. 274, 'opposite Essex Street', Strand, ca. 1771–5; No. 6, Bridges Street, Strand, 'opposite the Theatre Royal, Drury Lane', ca. 1776–80; Queen's Court, Great Queen Street, Lincoln's Inn Fields, 1780–4.
Catalogus librorum latinorum, graecorum, hebraicorum, &c. . . . Qui venales prostant Londini apud C. Heydinger, bibliopol. in platea vulgo dicta the Strand. Londini, 1773.

NOTES

1 See Susanne Steinmetz, 'The German churches in London, 1669–1914' in P. Panayi (ed.), *Germans in Britain since 1500* (London, 1996), 49–71.

2 Francke's foundation (formally, the *Franckesche Stiftungen zu Halle*) was dissolved by the Communist authorities of East Germany but revived after German reunification in 1990.

3 See Graham Jefcoate, 'Joseph Downing and the publication of Pietist literature in England, 1705–1734' in J. L. Flood and W. A. Kelly (eds.), *The German book, 1450–1750: studies presented to David L. Paisey* (London, 1995), 319–32.

4 *Das neue Testament unsers Herrn und Heilandes Jesu Christi, verteutscht von D. Martin Luthern: mit jedes Capitels kurtzen Sum[m]arien, und nöthigsten Parallelen. London: gedruckt und verlegt bey Joh. C. Haberkorn, und Joh. N. Gussen; wie auch bey Andreas Linde, Papierhändler, und Buchbinder zu Ihro Königl. Hoheit Printz George, in Katherine-street, in den [sic] Strand, 1751.* Quoted and translated from the 'Vorbericht an den Leser', dated '22 Dec. 1750'. The New Testament was sold for 1s 6d.

5 *Decamerone di Giovanni Boccaccio cognominato principe Galeotto[.] Londra: presso Giovanni Nourse libraio di S M Britannica, 1762.* Haberkorn is revealed as the printer in the colophon, 'Nella stamperia di Giovanni Haberkorn, l'anno 1762'. The title-page is set in a consciously 'archaic' style deemed appropriate for the subject (compare Haberkorn's work on the edition of the first volume of *The antiquities of Athens, measured and delineated*, printed in the same year).

6 *Zergliederung der Schönheit, die schwankenden Begriffe von dem Geschmack festzusetzen, geschrieben von Wilhelm Hogarth. London: bey Andreas Linde, J. H. K. der verwitteten Prinzessin von Wallis, Buchhändler, und in Hannover bey J. W. Schmidt, 1754.*

54

Naturalization and economic integration: the German merchant community in 18th-century London

Margrit Schulte Beerbühl

Integration and assimilation are complex processes which depend on a variety of economic, social, political and last but not at least on individual factors. In this paper I will focus only on the economic integration of a small group of German immigrants, the merchants. German merchants had played an prominent role as members of the Hanse in late medieval and early modern England. In the 19th century the big international houses of German origin like the Barings, the Schroders or Rothschilds also made an important contribution to the British commerce, as Stanley D. Chapman has shown in several articles.[1] The 17th and 18th centuries, however, remain the dark ages in the history of the German merchants' community in Britain.

The closure of the London Steelyard in 1598 did not lead to a complete breakdown of the economic relations between both countries. The German market remained of importance to England and vice versa. The British trade with Germany had started to grow again from the late 17th century, although it did not show the rates of growth of some other British overseas markets.[2]

German merchants also became increasingly interested in gaining access to the British markets. In Germany mercantile activities were restricted by the political fragmentation of the country. The German states did not have any colonies, and therefore had no direct access to colonial products. Between 1688 and 1755 the British Empire did not only grow very rapidly, but also very visibly. The export and re-export markets were the most expansive sectors of the British economy. London became the seat of the empire and the world's foremost trading and financial centre. The visible expansion of British commerce offered economic opportunities to German merchants, which they could not find at home.

After the loss of their corporate privileges the German merchants had to reshape their economic relations with Britain The access to the commercial empire became the acquisition of British nationality. In part one of my paper I will therefore focus on the economic function of British nationality and the size of the German merchant community in the 18th century as far as it may be derived from the naturalization records.

Economic integration did not stop with the acquisition of British nationality. It was generally followed by a variety of other activities, such as membership of trading companies insurance companies, and other important economic institutions as well as partnerships with English merchants. In part two of my paper I will look into some of these aspects.

I

Until the middle of the 19th century British nationality could be acquired either through denization or naturalization. Denization was a partial nationality, while naturalization conferred the full rights of a natural-born subject. Denizens were excluded from some important economic rights, therefore foreign overseas merchants sought naturalization. Naturalization was acquired through a private act of Parliament and was a costly affair. In the middle of the 18th century its fees amounted to about £65. Only a minority of foreigners ever acquired British nationality.

Not all foreigners were affected in the same way by the alien laws. The majority of immigrants seemed to have lived without many disadvantages. Only a small wealthy group of foreigners was affected by them, for they could neither acquire real property nor inherit or bequeath property. Foreign merchants, especially, had to face a number of economic disadvantages which weighed heavily upon them and impeded their competitiveness. They had to pay double taxes, and could neither own a British ship nor become members of the big trading companies. As some big London companies such as the Russia or Levant Companies retained their trading monopolies in the 18th century, foreigners were more or less excluded from trading to these countries.

Daniel Statt thought the alien duties to be one of the most important disabilities suffered by aliens, but the navigation acts were at least as important.[3] Henry Peterson, a Danish subject, had traded for more than 16 years between Denmark and London. He applied for British nationality in 1660, because the 'late Act of Navigation had made him incapable of his trade'.[4] The few German merchants, who continued to live in London in the 17th century, only started to acquire British nationality after the passing of the first navigation act. The Hanseatic merchants had traditionally been overseas traders with far reaching trade links to the Baltic and other European regions. Many of them also possessed their own ships. As the navigation acts excluded foreigners from the profitable colonial markets unless they were British subjects or subjects of the producing countries, they were a crucial impediment to foreigners. Therefore the number of Germans who applied for British nationality began to rise after 1660.

As there were no immigration controls in Britain until the outbreak of the French Revolution we do not know much about the number of immigrants nor about the number of German merchants among them. According to the estimates of Gregory King there were no more than about 10,000 merchants and traders in London in 1688. Only 2000 belonged to the wealthy elite of overseas merchants. Gary De Krey estimates that about 30 per cent of them were of foreign birth.[5] More details about the nationalities may be derived from D. W. Jones's and Perry Gauci's data. Among the list of 68 considerable import and export merchants of foreign birth which Jones compiled from the London port books of the 1690s 21 were Germans. Perry Gauci has counted 18 German from the 1692 poll tax assessments for the city of London.[6] As 10 names appear in both lists, the total number is not more than 30.

More information can be obtained with the help of the naturalization records. They have been completely preserved.[7] Unfortunately they do not mention the profession of the naturalized persons. Therefore it is necessary to consult further sources. With Jones's and Gauci's data as well as some German sources it is possible to identify 41 naturalized foreigners of German birth as merchants for the period 1660 to 1700. It is likely that many more belonged to this group. Of a total of 174 Germans who were naturalized, 73 came from the Hanseatic towns of Hamburg, Bremen, Danzig and Lübeck. Many names of these Hanseatic immigrants originated from well-known merchant families.

The impression that merchants, especially, sought British nationality can be confirmed for the period 1715–1800. There are some sources available from the 18th century, which make it possible to work out a professional profile of the naturalized subjects. The German 'Geschlechterbücher' or family books and especially the London directories, which start in the 1730s, become valuable sources for identifying the professions of the Germans. Because of London's leading role in the commercial world at that time, it is likely that a great part of the foreign merchants lived in London and therefore should be recorded in the directories.[8]

The total number of naturalizations was low between 1715 and 1800. Only 446 male Germans were naturalized, although the Germans were the largest group of naturalized British subjects after 1715. With the help of the above mentioned sources as well as some other sources I have been able to identify the professions of 316 Germans.

Table 54.1   Professions of naturalized foreigners of German birth, 1715–1800[9]

Profession	numbers
merchants	263
brokers	13
furriers/skinners	3
Esquires	3
children	2
sugar refiners / sugar bakers	14
nobility	2
trades (tailor, mason, dyer, watchmaker)	5
professions (doctors of divinity,of physick, apothecary)	5
captains	2
musician/musical intrument maker	2
freemen (City of London)	2
unidentified	130

The breakdown of the professions conveys a homogeneous picture. Of the 316 identified Germans 263 were merchants. The four groups of brokers, furriers, esquires and the two children may be added to the 263 merchants, so that the total number amounts to 284. Retired merchants were often termed esquires in the 18th century. Except for the three esquires listed in the table the others have been identified as merchants. Therefore it is likely that they also belonged to this group. The two children were naturalized with a view of succeeding to the merchant houses of their father and uncle and therefore should be also added to this group. Unfortunately nothing is known about the business of the two Germans who were freemen of the City of London. It cannot be ruled out that they were also traders.

Among the 130 which have not yet been identified, many more were probably merchants. They were not recorded in the directories, because they either did not stay in London or were not thought important enough to be mentioned. So the final numbers are likely to be even higher.

The viewpoint that naturalization was crucial for entrance into the commercial world of the British Empire can be further supported by the time at which naturalization was acquired by the merchants. The British law of nationality did not have any residential requirements until the reform of law in 1870. According to Daniel Statt a residence of 10 or 20 years was common before naturalization in the 17th century.[10] The average time of residence before naturalization seems to have been shorter in the 18th century. There are cases in which German and Russian merchants did not stay in England prior to their naturalization, but these cases are rare. They had usually stayed for some years in London before deciding to apply for naturalization. From the biographical sources of some German merchants we get the impression that the years of residence were not of prime importance, but rather the decision to open a merchant house. Herman Jacob Garrels and Anthony Hinrichs, for example, had worked as employees in London for at least seven years. They applied for British nationality the moment they decided to set up their own merchant house.[11] Others who came to Britain with the intention of opening a merchant house, like John Frederick Schroder, applied for naturalization shortly after their arrival. In a few cases the London directories mention the names of German merchant houses before the naturalization of their owners. Their difficulties were evidently serious, for in all cases they got British nationality within the next few years after their first mention in the directories.[12]

From the number of merchants among the naturalized subjects, as well as from the time of acquisition, we may conclude that naturalization was the key to economic integration. It removed the disabilites of aliens and opened the door towards further economic as well as social integration. Naturalization was generally followed by a variety of further activities.

II

As the majority of the naturalized merchants did not intend to trade on a local level, but rather on a bilateral, if not on an international one, their names can be found in several influential companies of the 17th and 18th centuries. They became members in the Eastland Company, the Russia, or Levant Companies. Theodore Jacobsen, for example, the agent for the Hanseatic towns and Steelyard master, was the first German to enter the Eastland Company after its reform in 1673. He also belonged to the group of tobacco merchants, who started the attack on the old Russia Company at the end of the century.[13] After the reform of the Russia Company in 1698, which opened membership to all British subjects on payment of an entrance fee of £5, several German merchants entered the Company. Some also became members of the Court of Assistants. From the 1730s onwards until the decline of the company in the early 19th century at least one German belonged to the Court of Assistants.[14] German merchants are also found among the governing members of the South Sea Company[15] and the insurance companies.[16]

Besides membership in trading or insurance companies, partnerships with English merchants must be regarded as an important sign of integration into the British merchant community. The establishment of partnerships with Englishmen required a more intimate co-operation with each other than with mere trading partners. As joint partners, merchants had to place a lot of confidence in the reliability, skill, integrity and honesty of each other. Partnerships also involved relations which went beyond simple commercial ones. Therefore they are crucial indicators of integration and assimilation.

In the 18th century the big London merchant houses were generally composed of several partners. The London directories convey an excellent impression of such partnerships, their changes and their extension. Some of them can also be pursued for several generations. The directories, however, do not mention all partners. In general they only name major partners, minor ones are often hidden behind the 'Co', but even major partners cannot always be found in the name of the house.[17] Despite these reservations the directories are a valuable source for tracing partnerships. They reveal a multi-faceted picture.

Partnerships with Englishmen can be found among the first generation of immigrants. Andrew Grote from Bremen was at first partner of Paul Kruger, a naturalized merchant from Hamburg. Later on, in 1766 he opened a banking house under the name of Grote & Prescott. His partnership with the Englishman George Prescott did not only last for the rest of their lives but even through the following generations. Other German merchants seem to have preferred partnerships with their fellow countrymen at least in the first generation. Since the beginning of the 18th century a numerous group of merchants from Hamburg had settled in London. They all belonged to the mercantile elite of Hamburg and were more or less all related to each other. Several of them can be traced for at least two generations in the London directories. Among them were members of the Amsinck, the Mello, and the Dorrien families. The first generation of this group exclusively established partnerships with their relatives. Only the second generation took Englishmen as partners.[18]

The decision to work with certain partners depended much upon the personal experience of the individual merchant. In a period when communication and transport was slow and overseas trade involved considerable risks, members of the family appeared to be the most trustworthy partners.[19] The success of the big merchant and banking houses of the Schroders, the Rothschilds and other well-known families of the 19th century resulted from their strong family ties. The preference of family members or other near relatives cannot necessarily be regarded as a lack of integration but rather as part of a mercantile strategy to reduce partnership risks.

Stuart Jenks and Andrew Pettegree have drawn our attention to wills as a valuable group of sources in evaluating the process of integration and assimilation into the host community.[20] They referred to the nomination of English executors or testators and to the provision for gifts to Englishmen as indications of the move beyond the immigrant community. No research has so far been undertaken into the wills of the 18th century. The few wills I have looked into also reveal close relations with English merchants. Henry Peter Kuhff, a merchant from Frankfurt, for example, named as his executors Sir John Lubbock and Alderman John William Anderson, two well-known English merchants.[21]

Other sources reveal that German merchants had established friendly relations with English merchants. Samuel Holden, for example, the governor of the Russia Company and director of the Bank of England, started his career in Russia with Matthew Shiffner as partner. This was not only the beginning of a lifelong mercantile partnership, but also of a personal friendship. Holden became the guardian of the Shiffners' sons John and Henry, whom he had sent to England to be educated.[22]

Others became respected and well-known members of British society. Nicholas Magens did not only gain a reputation as a successful merchant, but also as a well-known writer of economic tracts. Theodore Jacobsen, who started as a merchant in the Steelyard, later became a well-known architect. He was also member of the Royal Society of Arts and a Fellow of the Society of Antiquaries.[23] Since the Act of Settlement in 1701 naturalized British subjects were debarred from becoming members of Parliament. The wealth and respectability of their fathers and grandfathers, however, laid the foundations of the political careers of Henry Shiffner, Alexander Baring, John Duntze and Magens Dorrien.

Not all of the German merchants were successful, but on the whole the German merchant community of the 18th century conveys the impression of a prosperous and well-integrated group. Their position as directors of insurance companies or members of the Court of Assistants as well as their personal and economic relations with well-known English merchants reveal their social and economic advancement and their integration into English society.[24] The key to integration and success was the acquisition of British nationality. The advantages which the Germans derived from British nationality however, were not one-sided. They came from German merchant families, which possessed their own mercantile networks. In other words they brought with them new customers for British and colonial products. They thereby helped to expand the British Empire and commerce and contributed to making it work.

NOTES

1   For the Hanse, see Terence H. Lloyd, *England and the German Hanse, 1157–1611: a study of their trade and commercial diplomacy* (Cambridge, 1991); for the 19th century see Stanley D. Chapman, 'The international houses: the Continental contribution to British commerce, 1800–1860', *Journal of European Economic History* 6 (1977), 5–48; S. D. Chapman, *Merchant enterprise in Britain: from the Industrial Revolution to World War I* (Cambridge, 1992), esp. part II, 3.

2   According to Elizabeth Karin Newman, Germany accounted for 25.2 per cent of England's re-exports to Europe and 18.5 per cent of Europe's exports to England in the middle of the 18th century. Elizabeth Karin Newman, 'Anglo-Hamburg trade in the late 17th and early 18th centuries' (University of London Ph.D. thesis, 1979), 292ff.

3   Daniel Statt, 'The birthright of an Englishman: the practice of naturalization and denization of immigrants under the later Stuarts and early Hanoverians', *HSP* 20 (1989), 61–73, 64.

4   He became a denizen on 17 October 1660. It is not quite clear from the records if he was the same person who took the oaths for his naturalization in 1660. HSQS 17, 79, 80, 81.

5   Gary Stuart de Krey, *A fractured society: the politics of London in the first Age of Party, 1688–1715* (Oxford, 1985).

6   D. W. Jones, *War and economy in the age of William III and Marlborough* (Oxford, 1988), Tables 8.3 and 8.4; see also Peregrine Gauci, *Strange politicians: the overseas trader in state and society 1660–1720* (forthcoming).

7   The records for the 17th and 18th centuries were compiled and edited by W. A. Shaw in HSQS 17 and HSQS 27.

8   The author is working on a project on 'British nationality and commerce: the contribution of German and Russian-German merchants to the making of the British Empire.

9   Compiled from the London *Directories*, the bankruptcy records, Deutsche Geschlechterbücher, Sun Fire Registers, Royal Exchange fire policies, and the Common Council Journals of the City of London.

10 Statt, 67.

11 Margrit Schulte Beerbühl, 'Das Tor zum Welthandel. Ostfriesische Kaufleute werden britische Staatsangehörige', in *Quellen und Forschungen zur ostfriesischen Familien- und Wappenkunde* 4 (1998), 98–109.

12 The house of Peter Henry Kuhff appeared in Kent's *Directory* in 1759 for the first time. He was naturalized in February 1762.

13 See R. W. K. Hinton, *The Eastland trade and the common weal in the seventeenth century* (Cambridge 1959), 161ff; Jacob M. Price, 'The Tobacco adventure to Russia: enterprise, politics, and diplomacy in the quest for a northern market for English colonial tobacco, 1676–1722', *Transactions of the American Philosophical Society*, new series, vol. 51 (Philadelphia, 1961), 108

14 Among them were Abraham Korten from Elberfeld, Matthew Shiffner, a Russian-German, John Anthony Rucker and his nephews from Hamburg.

15 Theodore Jacobsen became one of the directors of the South Sea Company.

16 Arnold Mello, a merchant from Hamburg, was one of the directors of the London Assurance from 1766. Henry Peter Kuhff from Frankfurt, was a director of the Royal Exchange Assurance from 1777 and the government of the Phoenix Fire Office was almost entirely composed of German sugar refiners in the early 1790s (W. Lowndes, *A London Directory* (1795); *Kent's Directory for 1777* (1777)).

17 The house of Peter Henry Kuhff, for example, appeared under the name of 'Kuhff & Comp' from 1759. From 1774 its name was changed to 'Kuhff, Grellet, & Co'. Only his will mentions that his house had three partners after 1773 if not earlier, each having equal shares. The third partner was his brother Frederick Charles. As the latter was never naturalized, nothing more is known about him.

18 John Dorrien, a descendant, opened a banking house with the Englishman Carlton in 1772. The house subsequently came to be known as Dorrien, Mello, Martin and Harrison.

19 Hermann Jacob Garrels from Leer, for example, took his brother as a partner after he had failed with Anthony Hinrichs. George William Soltau continued alone after he went bankrupt with Paul Amsinck.

20 Andrew Pettegree, 'Thirty years on: progess towards integration amongs the immigrant community of Elizabethan London' in John Chartres and David Hay (eds.), *English rural society 1500–1800. Essays in honour of Joan Thirsk* (Cambridge, 1990), 297–312; Stuart Jenks, 'Hansische Vermächtnisse in London ca. 1363–1483', *Hansische Geschichtsblätter* 104 (1986), 35–111; Stuart Jenks, 'Leben im Stalhof', in Jörgen Bracker, Volker Henn and Rainer Postel (eds.), *Die Hanse. Lebenswirklichkeit und Mythos* (2nd edn., Lübeck, 1989), 210–15.

21 See will of Paul Amsinck. He left all his money to family members in Hamburg, London and Oporto. He also made a special provision of gifts to some English friends. Among them were Thomas Eames, merchant, and father-in-law of Paul Amsinck the younger. (PRO Prob 11).

22 The most important trading partner of Walter Shairp, Russia merchant and consul in

Petersburg, was the London House of Amyand, Uhthoff & Rucker. He also entertained a close friendship with Henry Uhthoff of this house. Uhthoff was born in Bremen.

23   Philip Norman, 'Notes on the later history of the Steelyard in London', *Archaeologia or miscellaneous tracts relating to antiquity* 61 (1909), 409.

24   Nicholas Magens did not only gain a reputation as a most successful merchant, but also as a well-known writer of economic tracts. Theodore Jacobsen, who started as a merchant in the Steelyard, later on became a well-known architect. He was also member of the Royal Society of Arts and a Fellow of the Society of Antiquaries. Norman, 409.

55

'A dearer country': the Frenchness of the Rev. Jean de la Fléchère of Madeley, a Methodist Church of England vicar

Peter Forsaith

'Ubi Christiani, ibi patria'[1] wrote Jean de la Fléchère to Charles Wesley in 1759, explaining why he had resisted his mother's imploring requests to return to his native Switzerland. Having been in England some nine years he was considering his future: he was too deeply rooted in English life, and too heavily involved with the Methodists, to return to Europe. Twenty years later his sentiments were the same 'as I was "born again" in England, that is, of course, the country which is dearer to me'.[2] Like many others he found England strange at first, but congenial and secure.

John Fletcher of Madeley (as he became known) is a name to conjure with in Methodist historiography, and indeed hagiography. Although the notion of his being Wesley's 'designated successor' is now debunked, his claims to fame remain as the prime Arminian polemical champion and as the outstanding saint of early Methodism whose apostolic ministry in the Ironbridge Gorge area of Shropshire coincided with the most significant period of industrial developments there. While the prospect of Fletcher leading the Methodists after John Wesley's death is speculation, this free spirit is nonetheless generally recognized to be, with John and Charles Wesley, the third person of the triumvirate which headed Methodism in the latter part of the 18th century.

What is less generally recognized is that Fletcher himself – vicar of an English parish – was in fact a French-speaking Swiss, Jean Guillaume de la Fléchère, born in Nyon, Switzerland in 1729, the youngest child of a well-to-do family. He studied at Geneva University, rejected the prospect of becoming a minister in the Swiss church, tried a military career and then travelled to England in 1750 becoming tutor to the family of Thomas Hill, M.P. for Shrewsbury. He experienced an evangelical conversion which both confirmed a strong latent childhood spirituality and gave new substance to his misgivings about Calvinism. His religious enthusiasm became something of an embarrassment to his employer but in 1757 he was ordained into the Church of England, and in 1760 became Vicar of Madeley in Shropshire.

Giving himself sacrificially to parish work, he overcame strong initial opposition to exercise a remarkable ministry among the colliers and ironworkers. In the 1770s he was embroiled in the acrimonious Calvinist controversy, becoming prominent by his able defence of Wesley's Arminianism. His 'Plan of Reconciliation' argued that Arminianism and Calvinism counterbalanced each other, and were both necessary for a holistic gospel – that the truth lies in the paradox. Exhausted by his parish work his writing and his asceticism, and seriously ill with tuberculosis he recuperated in Switzerland in 1778–81 where he briefly exercised a cautious and unofficial ministry.

On his return to England he proposed to Methodism's leading woman preacher, Mary Bosanquet, daughter of a prominent London Huguenot family. Married in 1781, they ministered together in Madeley until his death in 1785 after which she continued his work for a further 30 years, until her own death in 1815.

In his letters to Charles Wesley between 1757 and 1760 there is a striking incidence of French names. Closer analysis reveals that Fletcher was involved in the French churches in London, and was exercising a ministry in a Methodist setting among French Protestants. Further; the names given suggest that it was mostly among Huguenots that Fletcher was moving in his early years in England. Interaction between Methodists and French émigrés was possibly greater than is generally recognized, and Fletcher himself owed perhaps as much spiritually and theologically to the French churches as to the Methodists.

It is to the examination of those links, and what they signify, that this paper is directed. In it I shall concentrate upon Fletcher's letters to Charles Wesley, many of which are in French, in the years 1758–60 in order to give instances of links with French and Swiss origin communities in London, and to explore his ministry among French-speaking congregations (including those churches which Wesley acquired). I shall also touch on his marriage to a member of a leading Huguenot family, and suggest some areas for further enquiry about the overlap between Huguenots and early Methodists.

Writing in 1781 Fletcher himself stated that after his arrival in England 'one Mr Des Champs, a French Minister, to whom I had been recommended, procured me the place of tutor to the son[s] of Mr. Hill ... [where] I applied myself to the study of divinity'.[3] This brief remark raises a curtain upon the world into which Fletcher entered in his early years in England.

'Mr Des Champs' is surely Jean des Champs who was in Geneva in 1723–7 and became a minister of La Petite Savoie chapel from 1749. He would be in a key position to introduce Fletcher to French networks in London, and perhaps to influence him theologically also. Des Champs records how he received 'innumerable visits of all foreigners of a certain order, for whom I have been a kind of bureau d'addresse'.[4]

Knowledge of Fletcher's early years in England is scant but in a long letter to his father in 1752 to he wrote of:

> Les dames Thomasset chez qui je vais quelques fois, s'établissent assez bien ... j'y trouvé une Assemblée de Suisses plus nombreuse que vous n'en pouvez avoir à Nyon.[5]

Again, there is a ready identification as the Misses Thomasset gave a Bible at the inauguration of the Swiss Church at Moor Street in 1762: whether the 'Assemblée' was religious or social (or both) is impossible to discern[6] It may well indicate the existence of a Swiss congregation in London by then. That Fletcher was within a religious environment at this time is clear from a letter five years later to Charles Wesley:

By this time I was a strict Legalist. I spent part of the day in reading the Scriptures and in prayer, thinking that my repenting added to those duties, would skreen me from the wrath to Come . . . thought myself both meek and patient but the frequent proofs which my calling oblig'd me to make of those Christian virtues shew'd me soon what little share I had of them, . . . How many prayers growns fastings tears sighs watchnights Did I go thro' and all I vain, . . . However I exhorted and reprov'd as I had an opportunity.[7]

In what community of faith would he learn the 'duties' of reading the Scriptures and private prayer, the obligation of his calling; go through fastings and watchnights, and exhort and reprove? Such features could well be associated with French-speaking churches which were numerous and active in the west end of London where he lived with the Hill family at St James during Parliamentary sessions. Moreover, his employer's francophile inclinations would doubtless encourage him. Some of his pupils' exercise books in French survive.[8]

His own evangelical experience was precipitated by his attempting to exhort while in St Albans – he made the mistake of preaching to a Methodist, who turned the tables on him. So in London he 'inquir'd after the Methodists a[nd] came to west street and Hog Lane'.[9] Wesley's West Street chapel had once been a French Church,[10] but Hog Lane 'Les Grecs',[11] was one still. And here the letter changes from the impersonal to the personal: 'I soon Could trace all my experience in *your* preachings only one thing I could not account for *you* preach'd forgiveness of Sin, and power over [it] as being given at the Same time' [my emphases].[12] Does this indicate, as it seems to, that Charles Wesley was preaching in a most fashionable French church pulpit as well as the Methodist chapel? That is the inference.

It was to West Street that Fletcher went directly from his priestly ordination at the Chapel Royal, St James[13] to assist John Wesley administer the sacrament. His diaconal ordination, a week before by Bishop Beauclerk of Hereford, is recorded as at Spring Gardens Chapel.[14] At this time Jean des Champs, coincidentally or otherwise, was a minister of both Spring Gardens and the Chapel Royal.

Fletcher was preaching at West Street three mornings a week in 1758, though to numbers of just 20 or 30; he was concerned to ensure that in his summer absence a M. Bernon 'would take upon him preaching to the *French in my place*' (at both West Street and Spitalfields).[15] He also entreated Charles Wesley to preach for both of them,[16] implying that Charles too was preaching in French.

The Wesleys had also acquired a Huguenot chapel at Spitalfields, and in February 1758 Fletcher wrote: 'I still preach *at Spittlfield in French and the* Lord brings some hundreds to hear.'[17] While Spitalfields, with its population of working people close to his base at the Foundery, was very useful for John Wesley's work,[18] it was West Street, leased in 1743, which occupied a particular place in his affection.[19] As a consecrated building it enabled the Wesleys to celebrate the sacrament (with the elegant 'Fenowillet' communion service) as a mark of conformity. Known in its Huguenot times as 'La Tremblade' or 'La Pyramide', Wesley termed West Street 'The Chapel', as did Fletcher.

In 1759 Fletcher was preaching, in French, at the Sunday service at West Street 'avec les dispositions de Jonas' and later 'Je prêche pour tenir la Chapelle ouverte jusqu'à ce que Dieu envoie un ouvrier selon son cœur'.[20] That Easter Charles Wesley had hurried westwards to be with his wife for the birth of a child, so Fletcher celebrated the sacrament also: 'J'ai prèché et administré le sacrement à West street quelques fois pendant ces Fêtes.'[21]

Among congregations which had been formally Methodist for 15 years, yet seem to have retained a significant French presence, Fletcher was assuming a quite specific ministry. When in early 1760 the Countess of Huntingdon offered Fletcher the opportunity to minister daily to those who gathered in her London home, he stipulated that it should not interfere with his preaching in French. This was a priority activity for him. He translated at least one of Wesley's sermons into French.[22]

He found his own lodging in the winter of 1759/60, basing himself in St James's, close by Mme Carteret[23] who lent him a frank to write to Charles Wesley: 'Votre frere parut fache quand je lui dis que j'avois pris un chambre pres de St James's, il dit qu'il aimeroit mieux en paier la rente pour rien, plutot que de me voir perdu *parmi les riches*'.[24]

Although Fletcher was moving among the well-to-do, his ministry was focused upon the poor, a pattern to become characteristic of him: 'I do not make haste to get acquainted with those that are on high; methinks it suits me better to converse with the poor and illiterate I have more freedom to say before them *have mercy on me a miserable sinner*'.[25]

Relationships with women were not always his strong point, and one widow clearly misunderstood his intentions. To extricate himself he sent an open letter via M. Bernon [see 16 Aug 1758] but a year later the affair still pursued him: 'Mon aventure *avec la Veuve* a fait chemin jusqu'à Shrewsbury'.[26] The lady's identity is uncertain. On his return to London in late 1758 he discovered malicious gossip had gone the rounds, and he was all but heckled out of the pulpit.[27] Then followed difficulties with one Mlle Amirauld:[28]

> je suis obligé de me rennoitre le plus grand fou de Londres pour m'en être laissée imposer si longtems par cette femme, elle est grand Actrice et a contrefait le Role de Didon de façon a tromper pour quelques heures au moins un homme moins simple & moins crédule que moi: Mais d'être sa dupe pendant des années entières c'est ce que l'on poura à peine croire sans me croire digne *des petites Maisons* [Bedlam].[29]

One is reminded of controversies years before with the 'French prophets'.[30]

In 1759 Charles Wesley offered Fletcher a salaried ministry seemingly to work among French-speaking elements of London Methodism.

> Quelle idée monstrueux . . . Quoi! les travaux de mon ministère sous vous (si ulli sint) mériteroient *un salaire, moi* qui n'ai fait que déshonorer Dieu jusqu'ici, et qui ne suis pas en état de faire autre chose pour l'avenir.[31]

It becomes inadvisable then, on the basis of these letters, to insist upon strict demarcation between French Protestants and Methodists in London, certainly at West Street. Among these people Fletcher, with Charles Wesley (for whom he had sought a French Bible[32] and to whom he wrote in French), was working. The letters, incidentally, make no mention of the collapse and rebuilding of part of West Street in late 1759. By December 1759, Fletcher was also preaching (according to Tyerman at Lady Huntingdon's instigation) to French prisoners at Tunbridge.

Following his removal to Madeley, Fletcher's immediate links to the French community inevitably declined although he maintained some contacts. He mentions several times that a M. Buhet is acting as his banker.[33] He also asked Charles Wesley to buy books by French authors: Voltaire, Quesnel and others, and was surprised by the excellence of a Catholic work by a Père Guilloré. He mentions his bookseller: Verden, another Huguenot name.[34] He continued to share his Frenchness with Charles Wesley so in 1765: 'Je suis bien aise que vous ayez lu du Cerceau sur la poësie Françoise c'est un bon ouvrage, aussi bien que Fénelon sur l'Eloquence'.[35] In 1776 Fletcher asks Charles Wesley to remember him to Mrs Carteret[36] and in his last known letter requests him to peruse some writings, and suggests 'you could direct me both as a *Poet* and a *French* man'.[37]

Fletcher never lost his Swiss roots or his empathy with French Protestants. When in 1765 he ventured to preach out of doors he noted 'l'expression françoise parmi nos freres protestants de Languedoc, est *precher au desert*'.[38] which expression conveys strong Huguenot metaphor.[39] Returning in 1770 to continental Europe his visit to the Protestants of the Cévennes mountains was for Fletcher a high and holy moment.[40] The Cévennes was also the ancestral home of David Bosanquet, driven out in 1685, who became a successful London merchant and whose grand-daughter Mary was to become Mrs Fletcher.

John Fletcher met Mary Bosanquet in London around 1757.[41] She (perhaps with a streak of her grandfather in her) left the family home rather than compromise her new-found religious faith. She first exercised a ministry among the Methodists in Leytonstone, then moved to Yorkshire, all the while treasuring secretly her fondness for John Fletcher. He too acknowledged to Charles Wesley in 1763 that: 'la personne qui se presenta alors à mon imagination étoit Miss Bosanquet, Son idée me poursuivit pendant quelques heure le dernier jour & cela si chaudement que j'aurois peut-être perdu mon repos.'[42] It was not until 1781 that he opened his heart and she accepted his proposal of marriage. At their wedding was John Valton, one of Wesley's preachers with a French ancestry. Husband and wife together visited Dublin in 1783, where Fletcher preached (in French) to a French congregation taking as his text 'Call to remembrance the former days, in which, after ye were illuminated, ye endured a great fight of afflictions'.[43]

We pass now from the pieces of the jigsaw to draw some tentative observations from the emerging picture. The irregular relationship between the established church and the Methodists, or more particularly 'Mr Wesley's people' (to borrow Lady Huntingdon's phrase) was a recurring issue throughout John Wesley's life. Increasingly strained relations led to Fletcher proposing to Wesley in 1776 a plan for the formation of a 'Methodist Church of England': its content is revealing, and begs the question: from where did Fletcher draw the model for such a body?

Fletcher sketches a 'daughter church', under the 'protection of the Church of England' in which Wesley is allowed to be *episcopus* in all but name. Appeal is made to 'the liberty of English men, and Protestants, to serve God.'[44] Similarities can be detected with the features of the Savoy Chapel model of the French church in London: notably independence within an episcopal superintendency and ordination, anti-dissent and Moderators (post-Wesley). Worship would be evangelical in nature, while also sacramental. Such a scheme, characterized by a desire for reform of the established Church, may arguably have owed its ecclesiology to Fletcher's early experience in London.

There may be deeper symbiosis here. Methodist historians have for nearly a century reflected upon Halévy's suggestion that John Wesley saved England from a French Revolution.[45] Social conditions in England were sufficiently different from those in France that such a thesis is hardly a realistic proposition; Rack summarizes the flaws in the thesis;[46] and a response has been that, if anything, Methodism precipitated a deeper revolution in terms of the social implications of the Methodist κερψγμα. ('proclamation'). Social conditions in the two countries were very different in part because of the disappearance of the entrepreneurial (Protestant) middle ranks of society from France. But the Halévy thesis might then be reworked to ask whether the 'Wesleyan reformation' was made possible by the religious legacy of the Huguenots? Further, for our purposes, how deeply was Fletcher of Madeley, with his personality, his churchmanship and his doctrinal stance instrumental in that transaction?

I am not a theologian, but I have hinted at areas where Fletcher's doctrine may owe much to continental Protestant thinking. Professor Patrick Streiff, whose biography of Fletcher should shortly be available in English, has traced something of Fletcher's doctrinal roots through the currents of the Reformed traditions of mid-Europe in the 17th and early 18th century. Fletcher's approach could hardly have come from someone rigidly schooled in either the Church of England establishment or in the academies of English Dissent. Yet his doctrinal influence upon the emerging Methodist movement, especially in America, was colossal; an influence which anonymously makes itself felt still in the continuing spread of Methodism, and in the significance of holiness themes in Pentecostalism.

In the final analysis Fletcher's Arminianism does not reject entirely the Calvinism he learned in Geneva but modifies it to achieve a creative encounter between two presumed exclusives. If Methodism had severed its umbilical cord to Continental pietism when Wesley fell out with the Moravians, it is arguable that through Fletcher a reconnection was made to the themes of European Reformed thought, and that for this his London years were highly formative.

Methodist and Huguenot historical studies run close at some points, but too rarely intersect. Milburn's 1985 article 'Early Methodism and the Huguenots', dealt with Wesley's links with French individuals in the 1740s and notes French/Swiss origin names linked to early Methodism – Delamotte, Perronet, Rouquet, Valton, Gilbert (with whom Fletcher might have travelled to the West Indies) and not disregarding Molly Vazeille who so disastrously wed John Wesley.[47] Within Fletcher's letters is further evidence of later interaction and we must consider that there was a stronger, and more intricate, relationship than may have been generally acknowledged. Geoffrey Milburn asked:

> Is it possible that the most fundamental debt which Wesley owed to the Huguenots in England is that he glimpsed in them a model as to the kind of community into which Methodism might evolve, and the position it might occupy in the English religious spectrum?[48]

The answer looks more and more like 'yes'; and further, that the man to whom Wesley looked as scholar and saint, if not successor, was key to that relationship.

NOTES

Fletcher's letters to Charles Wesley are indicated in the text by date alone; those to other recipients are indicated by recipient and date. Fletcher's use of underlining to emphasize words and phrases has been retained in the quotations used here, set as italics. All the letters cited are within the Methodist Archives deposited at the John Rylands University Library, Deansgate, Manchester [hereafter JRULM], unless indicated otherwise, and are located within either the Fletcher folio volume or Folder Fl.36.1.

A full list with references is to be found in Patrick Streiff, *Jean Guillaume de la Fléchère/John William Fletcher, 1729–1785: ein Beitrag zur Geschichte des Methodismus* (Frankfurt, 1984), 493ff.

1   September 1759. 'Where there are Christians, there is my country'.
2   To T. York, 18 July 1779.
3   To C. Bosanquet, 22 September 1781. In Luke Tyerman, *Wesley's designated successor: the life, letters and literary labours of the Revd John William Fletcher* (London, 1882), 488–9, Joseph Benson, *The life of the Revd John W. de la Fléchère* (2nd edn., London, 1805), 22.
4   Uta Janssens-Knorsch, *The life and 'Mémoires secrets' of Jean des Champs (1707–1767)*, Huguenot Society New Series 1 (London, 1990), 41–2.
5   To M. de la Fléchère, 7 March 1752.
6   W. H. Manchée, 'The Swiss church of Moor Street', *HSP* 17:1 (1942), 53–63.
7   10 May 1757.
8   Shropshire Records and Research Centre, Attingham Papers 112/13/5–8.
9   10 May 1757.
10 Frank Baker, 'The early experiences of Fletcher of Madeley', *Proceedings of the Wesley Historical Society* [hereafter *PWHS*] 33 (June 1961), 29n. See also G. E. Milburn, 'Early Methodism and the Huguenots', *PWHS* 45:3 (December 1985), 77.
11 Satirized in Hogarth's 'Noon'. See Robin Gwynn, *Huguenot heritage: the history and contribution of the Huguenots in Britain* (London, 1985), plate 18.
12 10 May 1757.
13 13 March 1757.
14 Fletcher's ordinations are in William R. Davies, 'John Fletcher's Georgian ordinations and Madeley curacy', *PWHS* 36 (June 1968), 139. The actual certificate is in JRULM.
15 18 February 1758. A Huguenot Bernon family is recorded in New England: G. Andrews Moriarty, 'Notes on Huguenots in Boston, Massachusetts', *HSP* 19:4 (1956), 190.
16 16 August 1758.
17 18 February 1758, A congregation of 4000 was estimated in 1769: 'John Wesley and Professor Liden, 1769', *PWHS* 17:1 (1930), 2.
18 John C. Bowmer, 'John Wesley's Huguenot chapels', *PWHS* 27 (1949–50), 25–6.
19 Milburn, 'Early Methodism', 77.
20 22 March 1759; (April) 1759.
21 (Late April) 1759.
22 'Salvation by faith'. Also possibly 'Awake thou that sleepest'.
23 William Minet and Susan Minet (eds.), *Le Livre des Témoignages de l'Eglise de Threadneedle Street*, HSQS 21 (1909), 45 (François Carteret, 16 ans, 2 December 1747).
24 15/22 January 1760.
25 18 February 1758.
26 29 September 1759.
27 12 December 1758. See Melville Horne, *Posthumous pieces of the Revd John W. de la Fléchère* (Madeley, 1791). The letter is not found in the Fletcher MSS.
28 Moïse Amyrault was a noted Protestant radical of the 17th century. Some of the Amyrault

family came to England: C. E. Lart, 'The Protestant churches of Angers and Saumur', *HSP* 15:1 (1934), 42.

29 22 March 1759.

30 Kenneth G. C. Newport, 'Early Methodism and the French Prophets: some new evidence', *PWHS* 50:4 (February 1996), 127–40; Hillel Schwartz, *The French Prophets: the history of a millenarian group in eighteenth-century England* (Berkeley, CA, 1980).

31 4 September 1759.

32 (April) 1759.

33 Peter Buhet was a goldsmith in St James's. Goldsmiths were often also bankers: *PWHS* 26, 21; HSQS 26, 21 (Suzanne Buhet baptized 5 November 1709); HSQS 11, 109 (Boüet).

34 26 December 1763. W. H. Manchée, 'Marylebone and its Huguenot associations', *HSP* 11:1 (1915), 111.

35 10 May 1765.

36 11 May 1776.

37 19 December 1782.

38 10 May 1765.

39 Schwartz, *French Prophets*, 114–15.

40 Benson, *Life*, 138–40.

41 To C. Bosanquet, 22 September 1781.

42 9 September 1763.

43 Hebrews x: 32.

44 *The Journal of the Revd John Wesley,* ed. Nehemiah Curnock (8 vols., London, 1909–16), vol. 8, 331–2.

45 Elie Halévy, *A history of the English people in 1815* (reprinted, London, 1987); Bernard Semmel, *The Methodist revolution* (London, 1973).

46 Henry D. Rack, *Reasonable enthusiast: John Wesley and the rise of Methodism* (Epworth, 1989), 171ff.

47 Milburn, 'Early Methodism'.

48 *Ibid.*

56

Archibishop Thomas Secker (1693–1768), Anglican identity and relations with foreign Protestants in the mid-18th century

Robert Ingram

In the last year of his life, Thomas Secker, Archbishop of Canterbury continued to devote his time and energy and to use his political capital to promote the relief of persecuted Continental Protestants.[1] By the late 1760s, the Waldensians, a Reformed group living in Piedmont and known in England also as the Vaudois, had been suffering at the hands of the Dukes of Savoy and their armies for many centuries. The English press had regularly chronicled their persecution, the English state had offered refuge to them since the late 17th century, and the English people had contributed to subscriptions for them since Cromwell's day. While little had been done on their behalf during the Seven Years War, not long afterwards Secker took up their cause.

> The Vaudois had been for some Years soliciting for a Brief, having formerly had several. I thought it not convenient immediately after the War, nor after the Brief for the American Colleges. But now [1767] I proposed it, first to the Lord Chancellor & the Lord President, then to the King: who all approved it. And it was ordered in Council.[2]

Secker's efforts on behalf of the Vaudois should strike the reader as novel, for English relations with and aid to foreign Protestants in the mid-18th century has been almost wholly neglected by historians of the Church of England,[3] of the English state,[4] and of Secker himself.[5] Yet perhaps nothing illustrates more clearly the Georgian Church's self-image than its relations with foreign Protestants. Likewise, those inter-confessional relations highlight important dilemmas and challenges facing defenders of Anglican orthodoxy such as Thomas Secker.

During Secker's career, Protestants in France, Poland, Hungary, Moldavia, Turkey, Piedmont, Switzerland and Germany wrote or sent emissaries to England to report on Roman Catholic persecution, to request financial aid to rebuild churches, or to seek supplemental income for their ministers. Some sought English assistance to help them flee Catholic Europe and settle in North America. Others, like the Huguenots of the late 17th and early 18th centuries, sought refuge in England and left English authorities with large numbers of permanently resident francophone Protestants, many of whom desired government bounties without ever intending to conform to the established Church. In dealing with these expatriated Protestants and their numerous requests for aid, the Church had to address several difficult questions, the answers to which highlight Anglican identity in the mid-18th century. What should the Church do at home regarding the evangelical revival and Protestant nonconformity? How best might religious refugees be assimilated into English society?[6] Was the Church of England a catholic Protestant one or a national Anglican one?[7] What were the nature and limits of England's self-proclaimed role as 'protectress of European Protestantism?'[8] How did the English religious and political leadership reconcile that international role with their defence at home of an Anglican 'Constitution in Church and State?'[9] For orthodox Anglicans like Secker, relations with foreign Protestants raised a further series of ecclesiological and theological questions. Should the Church of England treat as equals non-episcopal foreign congregations? And what threat did supporting those foreign nonconformist congregations pose to Anglican orthodoxy within England?

In the mid-18th century, Thomas Secker helped to shape the answers to these questions. He assumed the primacy in April 1758 not only as one of the most respected and competent Anglican churchmen of his day, but also as a noted friend of the Protestant cause. When considering Secker's involvement while archbishop in English charitable efforts for foreign Protestants, a few salient points come to light. First, the English granted considerable aid to foreign Protestants in the mid-18th century. This involved the leadership at the highest levels of church and state, and aid generally came in three forms – guaranteed refuge in English territories, direct financial grants, and diplomacy. Parliament sometimes granted money to specific foreign Protestant groups, but most often financial aid came from the Civil List, from royally-sponsored church briefs, from individual donors, or from land grants in North America. Second, while assistance was usually forthcoming, church and state often offered aid for markedly different reasons, and a tangled knot of motivations underlay the decisions of both church and state in their dealings with Continental Protestants. On the whole, the episcopacy's response could best be characterized as altruistic, yet with a palpable sense of underlying unease. While people regarded it as a duty to persecuted brethren in Catholic Europe, fears of thereby encouraging heterodoxy in England always lurked, especially for an orthodox churchman like Secker. The state, on the other hand, seemed to have cared primarily about the larger geopolitical implications of English aid.

This essay does not examine the reasons why the English offered relief to Continental religious refugees. Rather, it considers the ways the Church of England's leadership – and Thomas Secker in particular – dealt with the perceived threat to Anglican identity posed by pressing for aid to the religious refugees during the mid-18th century. For while orthodox Anglicans thought it incumbent upon them to support Continental Protestants, they also were often uneasy about the potential consequences of doing so.

Questions of ecclesiology, liturgy, and theology – concerns central to Anglican identity – most worried orthodox churchmen like Secker when dealing with emigré congregations in England. Most of the foreign congregations were nonconformist and did not follow the Anglican liturgy. While Anglican ecclesiology privileged episcopacy, orthodox Anglicans had, since the Reformation, argued that hostile political circumstances prevented most Continental Protestant churches from maintaining episcopacy.[10] This allowed them to avoid unchurching those Protestants living in Catholic states bent upon establishing confessional uniformity. By the mid-18th century, however, this rationalization no longer worked, as it became evident that many Continental churches had chosen long since never again to adopt episcopacy. Secker and other orthodox Anglicans worried what message native English nonconformists might take from Anglican countenance, even support, of foreign Protestant congregations in England. Might English nonconformists demand full civil liberties since the Church of England supported and helped provide relief for those who worshipped in non-episcopal churches? As a result, Secker used all available means to persuade foreign congregations to adopt the Anglican liturgy and come into the fold of the established Church.

Secker had occasion near the end of his life to reflect at length about the relationship between foreign Protestant churches in England and the established Church.[11] In early 1767, the Artillery Church, a French nonconformist chapel in Bishopsgate, London, asked John Moore, lecturer of St Sepulchre's, to preach an anniversary sermon commemorating the Revocation of the Edict of Nantes. Before accepting the offer, Moore had his father, himself rector of St Bartholomew the Great, approach Secker about the matter. Though advising against accepting the invitation, Secker referred Moore to Richard Terrick, who as Bishop of London had direct episcopal jurisdiction over foreign congregations in London. Terrick, however, saw no prohibition to accepting the invitation, and there the matter rested until the Artillery Church's minister Jacob Bourdillon wrote Secker arguing that ordained Anglican ministers should be able to conduct services in French nonconformist churches. Clearly Moore had told Bourdillon of the archbishop's initial qualms about his preaching the anniversary sermon, and Secker's response to Bourdillon points to the ambiguities faced by orthodox Anglicans when dealing with foreign Protestants in England.

Upon more considered reflection, Secker accepted Bourdillon's argument that ordained Anglican ministers faced no canonical barrier to *preaching* in nonconformist churches. He agreed that neither the relevant Edwardian and Caroline statutes nor the seventy-first canon that Bourdillon had cited prohibited Anglican clergy from preaching in nonconformist churches. Neither did he see any prohibition in Canon 71 forbidding them from leading religious services in private houses.[12] 'I see no other Law, that hath any Appearance of putting a Negative on Mr Moore', he concluded.

Yet this was as much as Secker was willing to concede, and he rejected wholly Bourdillon's argument that ordained Anglican clergy might conduct religious services in nonconformist chapels. For Secker reminded Terrick that every ordained Anglican clergyman had 'subscribed a Promise at their Ordination, that they would use the Form in the Common Prayer Book prescribed, in the publick Prayer & Administration of the Sacraments, & none other'. And here Secker explicitly drew the connection between French nonconformist churches and native English Dissenting ones.

But if a man uses, perhaps alternately, our form in one Congregation, and a different Form or none in another, & explains his Subscription to mean only, that he would use the established Liturgy as often as he officiated in the established Church: surely this is taking a considerable Step further. Were he to divide himself thus between the established Church and an English dissenting congregation, it would be universally condemned. So far indeed the Cases differ that the Dissenters were of our Church, & Separated themselves from it; & the French, not. But the Interpretation of the Subscription Promise might be extended equally to both Cases.

Later, he would insist that 'there is no more Reason, why a Foreigner, not episcopally ordained, shd be allowed to administer the Sacrament in the Church of England, than why an Englishman, not episcopally ordain'd should'. Secker ended the letter with a rambling rumination on the nature and origin of ecclesiastical authority, considering especially the problem of ordaining Scottish Episcopal priests and American bishops.

Secker's reflections highlight the problems of identity and authority posed by foreign Protestants in England to defenders of Anglican orthodoxy,[13] for churchmen like him held 'a strong attachment to the Catholicity and Apostolicity of the English Church as a branch of the Universal Church Catholic, within which he does not include willfully non-episcopal churches'.[14] And his ambivalent response to foreign Protestant churches in England shows the tensions they created among Anglican churchmen – on the one hand, the foreign Protestants were refugees from Catholic Europe who looked to England as a haven from religious persecution while on the other hand, their non-episcopal origins made unlikely their whole-hearted acceptance by orthodox Anglicans. The ambivalent reception given resident foreign Protestants is illustrated most clearly in the operation of the Royal Bounty to aid Huguenot refugees resident in England.

Soon after assuming the see of Canterbury, Secker began receiving letters from French Protestants and their agents in England. Within a few months appears in his log correspondence from John James Majendie, who over the next decade emerged as one of Secker's most frequent and intimate correspondents and who served as the chief liaison between French Protestants and the English church-state. The eldest son of a late 17th-century refugee Huguenot minister, John James took Anglican orders and rose to prominence as tutor to Queen Charlotte and her two oldest sons, as the preacher at the French chapel in the Savoy, and as a prebendary of Windsor.[15] Among other prominent resident supporters of the French Protestant community in London were Louis Dutens, Benjamin du Plan, Jacques Serces, Jean des Champs, and César de Missy.[16] One of the most frequently discussed issues between these French agents and Secker was the operation of the Royal Bounty, established in the late 17th century to aid destitute French Protestants refugees in England. What their work on the Bounty demonstrates are the ways the Anglican leadership battled against religious heterodoxy, even among those taking refuge in England from religious persecution elsewhere.

Following the flight of the Huguenots after the Revocation of the Edict of Nantes, the English provided relief for them through a variety of *ad hoc* charitable means.[17] This brought only limited relief to the destitute refugees, though, and in November 1695, William III reminded the House of Commons of the 'miserable circumstances of the French Protestants who suffer for their religion' and urged the body 'to provide a supply suitable to these occasions'.[18] In April 1696, the House responded by adding to the Civil List an annual bounty of £15,000, with £12,000 designated for the laity and £3000 for French ministers. The money for distressed clergy was either granted directly to individual clergymen or, more commonly, to individual congregations to help them supplement their minister's salary. In 1726, George I reduced the grant to £8591, with £6872 6s for the laity and £1718 4s for eligible clergy. The Royal Bounty would remain funded at this level until the turn of the 19th century.[19]

The administration of the Bounty fell to three groups. The Lords Commissioners – composed normally of the Archbishop of Canterbury, the Bishop of London, the Lord Mayor of London and others appointed by the Crown – oversaw the administrative process. The members of the French Committee were either recent refugees or descendants of earlier immigrants chosen by the Lords Commissioners, who actually distributed monies from the Bounty. Finally, the work of the French Committee was audited by the English Committee, a supervisory board composed of prominent Englishmen and members of the 'French' community.[20]

The job of distributing the £15,000 annual grant fell originally to the French Committee. In November 1739, however, the Lords Commissioners established a separate Ecclesiastical Committee, composed of four French ministers and a lay treasurer, whose sole function was to administer the funds to the ministers.[21] While some historians have examined the French Committee's work distributing the Bounty to laymen, none have examined closely the work of the Ecclesiastical Committee. Yet the Church of England, by way of its representation on the Lords Commissioners, tried to use the Ecclesiastical Committee to promote conformity to Anglican liturgical forms among the Huguenot churches. And it is on the Church's contact with the Ecclesiastical Committee that this essay will focus.

In a letter thanking Secker for helping secure tax-exempt status for the Bounty, Majendie raised a point that was to cut to the heart of the Ecclesiastical Committee's work and purpose.

> And now, My Lord, I must beg Leave to inform your Grace that a Meeting of the Ecclesiastical Committee, lately held to draw up the new List for your Grace's signing . . . at which meeting neither the Revd. Mr. Serces nor myself could be present, on account of Illness, it had been resolved, contrary to the established Rules & Practise observed hitherto, to introduce into the said List a nonconforming congregation with a Pension of £20 pr annum.[22]

The Revd James Barnouin was the initiative's ringleader, and what ensued from Majendie's complaint to Secker was a debate that showed clearly the ambivalence the Anglican leadership felt regarding the established Church's relations with the refugee Huguenots, for while Secker wanted to aid them, he did not at the same time wish to promote Protestant nonconformity in England. Secker was most concerned to encourage Huguenot conformity to Anglican forms of worship, and in this, he represented the extreme example of a broader stream of Anglican opinion regarding them.[23] His aims and methods can be seen most clearly in the dispute with Barnouin regarding eligibility for Bounty support.

Within a year after Secker became Primate, Barnouin, longtime minister of the nonconformist French Church at Southampton,[24] queried whether 'there is any

Clause, wherein some particular priviledges have been granted of their Churches that should conform to the Church of England, whereby those that should not conform should be excluded from all benefits arising from thence?'[25] Under the terms of the Act establishing the Bounty, conformist congregations had received payments to help them pay their clergy. While individual nonconformist clergy could receive Bounty funds, nonconformist congregations were barred from receiving grants to help them hire clergy. But the origins of the policy were murky, so that there were no clear legal barriers to opening the Bounty's coffers to nonconformist congregations.[26]

The argument between Barnouin and Secker began in May 1759, when Barnouin challenged the legality of denying monies from the Bounty to nonconformist French congregations.[27] Barnouin pointed out that there was no written or, to his knowledge, implicit prohibition against funding the nonconformists. 'After this Nation had [since Edward VI's reign] received . . . with so much humanity the French Protestants', it would be hard to believe that William III and Parliament 'would have excluded these same Protestant Churches from the Benefices of the bounty Granted for the support of the French clergy in General'.[28] Appealing to a history of amicable inter-confessional relations, he noted furthermore, that 'the Divines of the Church of England have always, ever since the time of the Reformation held a friendly Correspondence with the Churches of France; have always looked upon their Ministers as Brothers & have always put a great difference between them, and those they call schismaticks'.[29] Why also, he wondered, would the government have established pensions for non-conformist French churches in Ireland but not intended relief to be granted to those attending nonconformist French churches in England. Meeting with Secker in person a week later, Barnouin went even further, contending 'that most of the French Protestants who come over, are averse from the Church of England, & many of them think it almost as bad as the Church of Rome'.[30]

Barnouin's appeal to Secker was timed to coincide with his petition to the Ecclesiastical Committee to grant Bounty monies to the French nonconformist congregation in Southampton that he led. Interestingly enough, the application was forwarded to the Committee by Benjamin Hoadly, Bishop of Winchester and the *bête noir* of 18th-century orthodox Anglicans. Not surprisingly, Hoadly recommended funding Barnouin's congregation. For, he wrote Majendie, 'I have enquired thoroughly into it; & am fully convinced that the granting it would be for the public good, the Interest of Religion'.[31] Equally unsurprising was Secker's opposition to Barnouin's scheme.

Secker rejected Barnouin's arguments primarily on the grounds that they would unnecessarily encourage religious heterodoxy in England. To begin with, he worried about the scope of the Bounty's activities, presumably concerned that it offered support even to nonconformist ministers.[32] He thought it was 'less advisable to give to nonconformist congregations, than to others, because it tends to discourage a needless separation'. Indeed, since most French Protestants in England were not recent refugees, Secker believed the laity had had ample time and opportunity to conform. 'And few of the Fr. Laity', he argued, 'have Objections of Conscience against the Service of the Established Church to which they have now had sufficient time to reconcile themselves'.[33] Barnouin would resign from the Ecclesiastical Committee over Secker's refusal to expand benefaction,[34] but Secker remained firm that the Bounty should be used not only to aid those legally qualified but also to promote conformity to Anglican ecclesiological and liturgical forms among resident French Protestants. When replacing Barnouin on the Ecclesiastical Committee, care was taken to appoint someone who would promote these aims, and it is not surprising that all three French ministers nominated to fill the position served conforming French churches in London.[35]

The guidelines for administering the Bounty to French Protestants, then, provided one means by which Secker could encourage conformity among the French refugee congregations in England. And it appears that the Committee followed those guidelines to the letter,[36] and this determination to adhere strictly to the guidelines extended even to requests from eminent persons. In 1759, for instance, the Duke of Grafton asked Secker to grant Bounty funds to an impoverished cleric named Viel, 'a Frenchman by Birth & a minister here'.[37] Poor, married with three children, and in Anglican orders, here was a French refugee cleric who seemed to fit ideally the Bounty's purpose. Secker soon passed Grafton's request along to Majendie, asking him whether Viel qualified under the Bounty's terms.[38] After looking into the matter, Majendie reported that prior to taking Anglican orders, Viel had been a Roman Catholic priest in France and was thus prohibited from receiving Bounty aid under George II's strictures given in 1729.[39] In turn, Secker denied Grafton's request, though he granted Viel money out of his own pocket 'as I have done for sev'l years past, & shall do with more pleasure in time to come, on account of your Graces good opinion of him'.[40] Despite the fact that Grafton was a powerful man, Secker denied his request that would have, in effect, bent the rules of Bounty administration. As a man of rank Grafton might have expected preferential treatment; that Secker refused to grant such treatment suggests that he and the rest of the Ecclesiastical Committee sought to follow the established rules of administration regardless of the petitioner's eminence.

By way of conclusion, the case of Jean Louis Gibert and his followers from France suggests the kinds of situations when questions of ecclesiology, liturgy, and theology among foreign Protestants were secondary for orthodoxy Anglicans like Secker. In April 1761, the Huguenot clergyman Gibert went to London to ask the authorities to help the Protestants in France 'from the Hardships, which they now suffer'd on account of their Religion'.[41] In any peace negotiations concluding the current war with France, he asked the English to press the French government to grant a general toleration for Protestants. If that proved impossible, he asked whether 'the King wd furnish them with money to come over into England'.[42] After consulting leading government ministers, Secker counselled Gibert that requesting a toleration would slow down peace negotiations and might incite the French government to impose even harsher penalties on the Protestants. Instead,

His Majesty directed me to say in His Name, that both Humanity & Religion disposed him to pity & relieve them, but that he thought nothing could be attempted by him without Danger of hurting them, whilst they continued in France; but that as soon as they had quitted it, they should have every Mark of his Protection & Favour & Bounty . . . [43]

The plan proposed was for the group to come to England, reassemble, and then depart for North America where it would establish a colony. After a meeting with

Secker on 23 April 1761, Gibert returned to France not to be heard from again until early January 1763 when there arrived a letter from a 'M. Gautier' announcing the imminent arrival in England of Gibert and his refugee Protestants.[44]

Gibert's arrival coincided with the last stages of the negotiations of the Treaty of Paris. Sensing the time was ripe, he and his followers, buoyed by George III's assurances two years earlier, had escaped into Switzerland en route to England.[45] Upon receipt of this news from Majendie, Secker immediately alerted Charles Wyndham, 2nd Earl of Egremont and one of the secretaries of state, adding that the refugees were 'well worth having'.[46] Egremont advised taking up the matter with the Treasury, which Secker did by contacting Bute, bringing him fully up-to-date on the situation and encouraging expediency, since Gibert had now arrived in London to help settle arrangements for his followers in Switzerland.[47] But, when Bute was forced from office and replaced by George Grenville, the character of the negotiations became bitter, and it is here that Secker's skill as a politician, the measure of his political weight, and his commitment to aid persecuted Continental Protestants shone through.[48]

Grenville initially held only a tenuous grip on his office as the King's first minister and this coincided with several serious domestic and financial issues facing his government, a situation Secker would exploit when pressing Gibert's cause. From the outset, Grenville expressed his reluctance to offer financial aid to Gibert's Huguenots, but he promised to work with George III to resolve the situation.[49] In the end, he sought to resolve the matter behind the backs of both the Archbishop and the King by contacting Gibert directly and ordering him 'to stop the disembarking of the French Protestants for wm he is concerned, till the means of their subsistence shall be regulated; but not intimating how or when such Regulation is to be made'. After hearing this news from Gibert, Secker demanded a private joint-audience with the King to discuss the matter with him and Grenville, explaining that '[t]his appears to me [so] unsuitable to the assurances wch I have in the Kings name by his Order two years ago, that I shall think my self guilty of neglecting my Duty to his Majesty, unless I remind him of them'.[50]

Though Grenville worried about the cost of supporting the refugees,[51] Secker won the day. George III welcomed Gibert and the French refugees 'to stay in England, till a proper Destination abroad can be found for them. And these may in the mean time be maintained out of the public money allotted for the Relief of Prisoners'.[52] He also granted to the refugees £1000 from his personal resources.[53] The King did, however, caution those Huguenots still in France to remain there until notice had been sent regarding proper provision for them in England, though '[b]y this he doth not mean to discourage them from the Intention of becoming his Subjects, which he is very desirous that they should'.[54] After months of wrangling during which Secker continually hounded Grenville and his subordinates at the Treasury regarding late payments and unkept promises,[55] Gibert and his followers set sail from Plymouth on 2 January 1764, and arrived in South Carolina four months later where they established the successful colony at New Bordeaux.[56]

Aside from his evident conviction that these refugee Protestants deserved the church-state's help, what strikes one here is that Secker made no mention of the theological belief of Gibert and his followers. While conformity to Anglicanism was expected of those refugees who remained in England, nonconformity among those just escaping Catholic France seemed fine, so long as they practised their nonconformity far away, in North America. Grenville's utter lack of enthusiasm for the project also indicates more than the fact that the English government was in financial straits after the Seven Years War. For encouraging the flight of French Protestants *after* the war with France rather than *during* the war must have seemed an investment with little hope of immediate gain.

This essay forms part of a larger project on Thomas Secker and Anglican identity in the mid-18th century.[57] My central argument there runs thus: the Church of England faced myriad social, political, cultural, and intellectual challenges to its hegemony and threats to its identity between the Hanoverian Succession and the American Revolution. The Church's leaders were fully aware of these challenges, and Thomas Secker spearheaded efforts to reform, revitalize, and protect the Church and its identity in response to the challenges – to *reform* not by radically transforming the institution's structure or theology but instead by making the institution operate efficiently and by staffing it with more professional clergy; to *revitalize* by seeking an aggressive role for the Church both at home and abroad; and to *protect* by defending Anglican ecclesiology, Trinitarian orthodoxy, and the institution's ancient rights and privileges.

Neglected by nearly all historians of the mid-18th-century Church of England, however, have been Anglican relations with foreign Protestants. This is unfortunate because the central themes regarding Anglican identity that one finds when addressing issues of pastoral care, Church-State relations, and theological debate also come to light when examining the Anglican relations with refugee Protestants in Hanoverian England. Persecuted Continental Protestants may have been, in Secker's words, 'well worth having' in England. But they came at a price, and that price, he feared, might just be the undermining of everything he had spent his entire career to defend.

NOTES

William Gibson first suggested that I study Secker and has been a source of encouragement, advice, and help ever since. I would also like to thank Nigel Aston, Richard Drayton, Jeremy Gregory, Martin Havran, Peter Nockles, Lois Schwoerer, and Stephen Taylor for their comments on an earlier draft of this paper. Melanie Barber of Lambeth Palace Library also provided much help.

Abbreviations used in the notes:
Autobiography: John S. Macauley and R. W. Greaves, eds., *The autobiography of Thomas Secker, Archbishop of Canterbury* (Lawrence, KS, 1988)
Works: Beilby Porteus, ed., *The Works of Thomas Secker, L.L.D., late Lord Archbishop of Canterbury: to which is prefixed a review of his life and character* (London, 1825).

1   The best introductions to Secker's life are Leslie W. Barnard, *Thomas Secker: an 18th-century Primate* (Sussex, 1998); Aldred W. Rowden, *The Primates of the four Georges* (London, 1916), 248–309; and *DNB*.
2   *Autobiography*, 59, 68. The next summer Secker again helped to organize the Vaudois relief efforts.
3   Chief among those who have considered the Anglican dimension of English relations with Continental Protestants have been Norman Sykes and John Pinnington. See Norman Sykes, *Daniel Ernst Jablonski and the Church of England: a study of an essay towards*

Protestant union (London, 1950); Sykes, *William Wake, Archbishop of Canterbury, 1657–1737*, vol. 2 (Cambridge, 1957), ch. 6; Sykes, *From Sheldon to Secker: aspects of English Church history, 1660–1768* (Cambridge, 1959), ch. 4; Sykes, 'The 17th and 18th Centuries' in C. R. Dodwell, ed., *The English Church and the Continent* (London, 1959), 73–94; John Pinnington, 'Anglican openness to foreign Protestant churches in the 18th century', *Anglican Theological Review* 51:2 (1969), 133–49. A recent valuable contribution on this subject has been made by Sugiko Nishikawa in her unpublished dissertation, 'English attitudes toward Continental Protestants, with particular reference to Church Briefs, c.1680–1740' (Ph.D., University of London, 1998).

4   See, for example, Robin Gwynn, *Huguenot Heritage: the history and contribution of the Huguenots in Britain* (London, 1985) and Irene Scouloudi (ed.), *Huguenots in Britain and their French background, 1550–1800* (London, 1987), neither of which consider the Huguenot assimilation after the 1720s.

5   Barnard, 211.

6   For a discussion of the problems 18th-century European states faced in assimilating religious minorities, see W. R. Ward, 'Anglicanism and assimilation; or mysticism and mayhem in the 18th century' in W. M. Jacob and Nigel Yates (eds.), *Crown and mitre: religion and society in northern Europe since the Reformation* (Bury St Edmunds, 1993), 81–91. For the initial assimilation of the Huguenots into English society, see Gwynn, *Huguenot Heritage*, ch. 10.

7   C. J. Podmore, 'The bishops and the brethren: Anglican attitudes to the Moravians in the mid-18th century', *Journal of Ecclesiastical History* 42:4 (1990), 622–3.

8   Colin Haydon, *Anti-Catholicism in 18th-century England, c. 1714–80: a political and social study* (Manchester, 1993), 23.

9   Boswell reports that Johnson took umbrage at Secker's toast to 'Constitution in Church and State' rather than to the more traditional 'Church and King'. George Birkbeck Hill (ed.), *Boswell's Life of Johnson*, vol. 4 (Oxford, 1934), 29.

10 Norman Sykes, *Old priest and new presbyter* (Cambridge, 1957), 69, 81–2. See also Peter Benedict Nockles, *The Oxford Movement in context: Anglican High Churchmanship, 1760–1857* (Cambridge, 1994), 146.

11 Secker to Richard Terrick, 23 September 1767: LPL, Secker v. 7, fos. 227–30. Unless otherwise noted, the Secker quotations in the following four paragraphs refer to this letter.

12 Gerald Bray (ed.), *Anglican canons, 1529–1947* (Bury St Edmunds, 1998), 363.

13 This point is explored in relation to the Moravian Church in Podmore, 'The Bishops and the Brethren' and Podmore, *The Moravian Church in England, 1728–1760* (Oxford, 1998), ch. 7.

14 P. B. Nockles, 'Change and continuity in Anglican High Churchmanship, 1792–1850' (unpublished University of Oxford D.Phil. thesis, 1982), li.

15 'Henry Lewis Majendie' in *DNB*.

16 For more on Huguenot agents in mid-18th century England, HSQS 43, 44.

17 Between 1681 and 1694, charitable donations totalling £90,174 were collected for the Huguenots in Anglican churches on the order of the English monarchs. Roy A. Sundstrom, 'French Huguenots and the Civil List, 1696–1727: a study of alien assimilation in England', *Albion* 8:3 (1976), 221.

18 Quoted in Roy A. Sundstrom, 'Aid and assimilation: a study of the economic support given French Protestants in England, 1680–1727' (unpublished Ph.D. dissertation, Kent State University, 1972), 54.

19 HSQS 51, 37.

20 Sundstrom, 'Aid and Assimilation', 56–60.

21 The original members of the Ecclesiastical Committee were the Revs. Paul Convenent, Stephen Abel Laval, James Barnouin, John Peter Stehelin, with Peter Tirel serving as

treasurer. John James Majendie served on the Ecclesiastical Committee from 1749 to 1784. HSQS 51, 38 and 40, n3.

22 John James Majendie to Secker, 29 January 1759: LPL, MS 1122/II, fo. 115:.

23 Jon Butler, *The Huguenots in America. A refugee people in New World society* (Cambridge, MA, 1983), ch. 1.

24 Barnouin served as minister of the French Church at Southampton from 1736 until 1797. Edwin Welch (ed.), *The minute book of the French church at Southampton, 1702–1939* (Southampton, 1979), 8–9.

25 Isaac Jean Barnouin and Thomas du Bisson to Secker, 1 May 1759: LPL, MS 1122/II, fo. 119.

26 Pinnington, 143–4.

27 The appeal probably resulted from a dispute earlier in the year among French committee members regarding the issue. John James Majendie to Secker, 29 January 1759: LPL, MS 1122/II, fos. 115–6. Secker's notes on the subject furthermore suggest that Barnouin had raised a similar issue with Archbishop Thomas Herring in 1750 only to have it rejected. Thomas Secker's observations on French nonconformist churches' claim to share Queen Anne's Bounty, 8 May 1759: LPL, MS 1122/II, fos. 123–5.

28 Indeed, Barnouin argued that 'it appears that King William who procured this money for the French Protestants was so far from intending, that the French Churches, that had or would conform to the Church of England, should have any exclusive advantage in the distribution of this money, that he open'd in his own Palace a French Chapel according to the Confession of Faith, the Liturgy, and Discipline formerly in use amongst the French Protestants in France . . . ', Isaac Jean Barnouin and Thomas du Bisson to Secker, 1 May 1759: LPL, MS 1122/II, fo. 119.

29 *Ibid.*

30 Secker's notes on a conversation with M. Barnouin, 9 May 1759: LPL, MS 1122/II, fo. 127.

31 Benjamin Hoadly to John James Majendie, 17 April 1759: LPL, MS 1122/II, fo. 121.

32 Secker wrote, 'The substance of what I said to M. Barnouin was only, that I should have been fearful of extending it [the Royal Bounty] so far, had the proposal been made in my time; and therefore should be more unwilling to extend it further, and take in the nonconformist Congregations also'. Secker to John James Majendie, 19 May 1759: LPL, MS 1122/II, fo. 130.

33 Secker's observations on French nonconformist churches' claim to share Queen Anne's Bounty, 8 May 1759: LPL, MS 1122/II, fo. 125:.

34 Isaac Jean Barnouin to Secker, 21 January 1760: LPL, MS 1122/II, fo. 167

35 John James Majendie to Secker, 24 January 1760: LPL, MS 1122/II, fo. 169–70. The Revds Henri de Rocheblave, Jean des Champs, and Samuel Mauzy served, respectively, the French Royal Chapel, the Savoy Church, and St Martin Orgars.

36 For example, see the petitions from Anne Gonsalve (LPL, MS 1122/II, fos. 74, 76, 78); M. de Flandrin (LPL, MS 1122/II, fo. 133), and M. Montbrun (LPL, MS 1122/II, fos. 187, 189).

37 Augustus Henry Fitzroy, 3rd Duke of Grafton to Secker, 28 January 1759: LPL, MS 1122/II, fo. 96.

38 Secker to John James Majendie, 8 February 1759: LPL, MS 1122/II, fo. 97.

39 John James Majendie to Secker, 11 February 1759: LPL, MS 1122/II, fos. 98–9.

40 Secker to Augustus Henry Fitzroy, 3rd Duke of Grafton, 15 February 1759: LPL, MS 1122/II, fo. 100.

41 Secker's notes on a meeting with Gibert, 24 April 1761: LPL, MS 1122/III, fo. 170.

42 *Autobiography*, 47.

43 Secker's notes on a meeting with Gibert, 24 April 1761: LPL, MS 1122/III, fo. 170.

44 M. Gautier to John James Majendie, December 1762: LPL, MS 1122/III, fo. 174.

45 'On this, as soon as Peace was made, M. Gibert came over with some hundreds, and more

were coming', Secker wrote: *Autobiography*, 47.

46   Secker to Charles Wyndham, 2nd Earl of Egremont, 6 January 1763: LPL, MS 1122/III, fo. 176.

47   Secker to John Stuart, 3rd Earl of Bute, 31 March 1763: LPL, MS 1122/III, fo. 184.

48   Bute wrote Secker on 8 April announcing his 'retirement' and notifying him that the matter regarding Gibert had been referred to Grenville. John Stuart, 3rd Earl of Bute to Secker, 8 April 1763: LPL, MS 1122/III, fo. 186. Three days later, Grenville contacted Secker, writing that he was aware of the Gibert matter but that he awaited a review of the relevant papers to discuss his thoughts. George Grenville to Secker, 11 April 1763: LPL, MS 1122/III, fos. 189–90.

49   Secker to John James Majendie, 17 April 1763: LPL, MS 1122/III, fo. 193.

50   Secker to George Grenville, 25 April 1763: LPL, MS 1122/III, fo. 197.

51   Secker later recalled Grenville's concerns. 'But, as they were all poor; not being allowed in France to sell any part of their real or even personal Estate, Mr. Grenville was afraid of the Expence, for which there was no fund': *Autobiography*, 47.

52   Secker's notes to J. L. Gibert regarding French Protestants, 29 April 1763: LPL, MS 1122/III, fo. 198.

53   Secker gave them £52 10s.: *Autobiography*, 47.

54   Secker's notes to J. L. Gibert regarding French Protestants, 29 April 1763: LPL, MS 1122/III, fo. 198.

55   The arrangement settled upon was for Gibert and his followers to be settled in Plymouth until transport to America could be secured for them. John James Majendie also was to secure the financial assistance of the local French community there who would advance the refugees money against credit from the Treasury. From the correspondence, a pattern of avoidance on the Treasury's part appears. On 19 May, Secker sent letters to Grenville announcing that a Plymouth merchant had volunteered to administer the disbursement of funds to Gibert and his followers (BL, Stowe MS 119, fo. 159). Not receiving a response, Secker sent Caesar de Missy back to the Treasury with another letter, instructing him not to return until he had received a written response from Grenville or one of his aides. (BL, Stowe MS 119, fo. 156). Charles Jenkinson responded that he was handling the matter while Grenville was away, but that he could not locate the relevant papers (LPL, MS 1122/III, fos. 208–9). The matter regarding the Plymouth merchant would not be resolved until Grenville returned to town in late June and ordered the immediate payment of the funds to Gibert and his followers (LPL, MS 1122/III, fo. 210). As late as January 1765, though, the Treasury was still delaying payment to the refugees (BL, Add. MS 38204, fo. 43).

56   Arthur Henry Hirsch, *The Huguenots of colonial South Carolina* (Durham, NC, 1928), 38–43.

57   My doctoral project at the University of Virginia is entitled 'Anglican hegemony in a polite and commercial age: Thomas Secker, the Church of England, and the Atlantic world, 1715–1770'.

57

What's in a name?: self-identification of Huguenot *réfugiées* in 18th-century England

CAROLYN LOUGEE CHAPPELL

This paper began in autobiography – that is, in autobiographical narratives – and moved on to autobiographical notations of a quite different sort. The larger project from which it derives, tentatively entitled 'Writing the diaspora: escape memoirs and Huguenot identity', endeavours to collect and study all extant first-hand memoirs of escape from France in the era of the Revocation, both those that recount only the emigration and those that do so as part of a larger telling of a life story.[1] Such escape memoirs are scarce, which is, as Robin Gwynn has remarked, somewhat surprising: 'One wishes there were more original memoirs to set alongside those by Jaques Fontaine, Dumont de Bostaquet and others that have survived. Some have disappeared from view even over the past century; where are all the sources known and used by [Samuel] Smiles?'[2] To date, I have identified 51 such narratives. They yield many insights into Huguenot lives in exile, including the experience of integration and assimilation, as Ruth Whelan's and Dianne Ressinger's papers in this volume show. The memoirs' limitations, too, are important, however. A minute swath of the social hierarchy finds voice through them: almost exclusively ministers and nobles, from time to time a rare artisan. And female voices are nearly absent: of the 51 memoirs I have found, only eight were written by women. This narrowness led me to ask whether there might be some other first-hand source that might be broadly construed as 'auto-biographical' or self-reflexive in a way that would afford entrée particularly to the experiences of women and of a broader segment of the social hierarchy than the highly literate alone.

Many studies of integration have focused on areas of adjustment and measures of assimilation that are less likely to involve women than men. So, for example, measures of structural assimilation in the 18th century that rest upon such secondary-group formalities as workforce participation, civic activity, residential locations, admissions to educational institutions, or association memberships over-represent men. Similarly, analyses of receptional assimilation that rest upon written or pictorial opinion are much more likely to find men's expressions of prejudice or stereotyping than women's, simply because men wrote and illustrated more than women did. Primary-group affiliations (friendships, informal patronage relations) in which women might be more prominent are more difficult for the historian to penetrate.[3] So are many indicators of cultural assimilation in private life: rituals, codes of behaviour, linguistic usages, dress, speech, food, bodily care.[4]

The literary critic of autobiography John Paul Eakin once wrote that autobiography 'attempts, as it were, to pronounce the name of the self'.[5] Naming and autobiography alike – both through language – give identity and continuity to the self. Just as autobiography is naming, so naming, which is consubstantial with self-awareness, is an autobiographical act.[6] Now as it happens, this rapprochement of naming and autobiography – as obscure as it sounds – may provide the entrée we seek into women's experience of assimilation. It may do so because naming patterns for married women in early modern England and France were sharply opposed. Tracing whether immigrant French women in the 18th century chose to name themselves in the English manner or in French style may give us some index of the extent to which (and pace at which) they assimilated: that is, lost a sense of strong identification not only with their natal family but with their natal community and shifted their sense of identity to the host society.[7]

Laws and customs of marital names

The opposing naming systems for married women are simple to state. In 18th-century France, if Marie Dupont married François Girard, she would for her entire lifetime be called Marie Dupont, femme de François Girard. French women did not name themselves as English women did: upon marriage, they did not assume the names of their husbands, only their titles (if any). As long as French women lived, they would be known by their own birth names. In contemporaneous England, if Mary Smith married Anthony Brown, she would be called Mary Brown.

In early modern France, the persistence of birth surnames for wife as for husband was established in tandem with the use of the family name as the principal identifier, which had replaced the use of patronymic or occupational label, nickname or title of one's farm in all but the most isolated locales.[8] French practice of marital naming long before the Revolution expressed the principle of the immutability of names that would be fully spelled out in the legislation of 6 Fructidor Year II. This law made it illegal to bear any name other than what was on the birth certificate and continues to be the reason why in France today 'it is extremely difficult to discard one's name'.[9] The French practice of marital naming would seem also to relate to a sense, which is still enforced by French courts, that families have a kind of propriety right in their names.[10] On these various grounds, both before and after the Revolution, personal practice, official documents (including wills, whether made by men or by women), and the état-civil all used married women's birth names.[11]

In England, by contrast (though not in Scotland or Wales),[12] the family surname had been established as standard practice by the beginning of the 17th century, and so had the custom of the wife taking her husband's surname.[13] As early as 1632, in the legal treatise entitled *Lawe's Resolution of Women's Rights*, the anonymous author ('T.E'.) stated that 'The Wife must take the name of her husband, Alice Greene becommeth Alice Musgrave; She that in the Morning was faire weather, is at night perhaps Rainebow or Goodwife Foule; Sweet heart going to Church, and Hoistbrick comming home'.[14] The wife's change of name was, however, a 'must' only as a matter of social convention rather than as a legal requirement; even down to this day, English law has had no requirement as to what a married woman calls herself.[15] The old common-law right of a person to change her/his name by simple use (without permission from a court) and to use any name s/he chooses (so long as it was not chosen in order to commit fraud) accorded women, by the same principle, the right to change to their husband's surname upon marriage or not.[16] The uniquely English conventional adoption of the husband's name by the wife and the unmatched legal liberty of self-naming justify one legal historian's conclusion that 'It is not only in geographical position that England is an island'.[17]

So naming practice among early modern French and English women was clearly divergent; we might say the French were realists with respect to marital naming, the English nominalists. And the fact that English law did not force immigrant women to adopt the English naming pattern in order for the marriage to be recognized as legally valid allows us to consider the forms of self-identification used by Huguenot women in England as voluntary expressions of identity – and hence as, in a sense, auto-biographical markers of extent of assimilation.

Findings

How, then, did Huguenot refugee women in 18th-century England identify themselves?

The earliest records on the second Huguenot migration, the records of the French exile churches, where one would anticipate finding the most consistent French practice, are more mixed than we might expect. So, for example, a register containing extracts from wills that left bequests to the French Church in Threadneedle Street attested to receiving donations in 1700 from 'la femme de Jaques denew', in 1704–05 from 'Anne veuve de Simon Noguiere', in 1711 from 'Madame Marie Giuzelin veuve de Monsieur jacques Giuzelin', though also in 1729 from Mme Susanne widow of Etienne Perier'.[18] Similarly, a list of members who asked for *témoignages* so they could go to another church listed in 1709 'Marie Benoist, femme de Charles Brebaut', but in 1710 referred to 'La veuve de Benjamin des Valins' and to 'Simon Joly et Marie sa femme'.[19]

The home-country pattern is more clearly established in the early Threadneedle Street register of abjurations and *reconnaissances*.[20] Here in 1687 we find Jeanne Amyraut, widow of N. Doule professeur en eloquence at Saumur; Jeanne Agere, widow of Pierre Servel of Montpellier; Marie de Guese, wife of Pierre Sanson; Renée de Chievres, wife of Pierre de Royeres, formerly minister at Coutras in Guyenne; and 'Dame Anne Vallée, widow of [monsieur de Chivré] the marquis de La Barre'. This document is of particular utility for our purposes because it applies the French naming pattern in England for Huguenot women in all classes and from all geographical areas of France.[21]

Still, these are not autobiographical sources. The modes of naming used here may well depend upon motives of bureaucratic convenience: more on the logic of the document-maker than on the preferences of the woman concerned. Or more on someone's – e.g., the Church's – prescriptions as to what women should call themselves than on the ways the women wished to identify themselves.

To find truly 'autobiographical' self-identifications, I turned to wills, which, as Jack Goody has said, are 'in effect the written version of the "dying words", the permanent expression of the deathbed wish'.[22] I assembled a dataset of 100 wills proved in London that had been made by Huguenot women in England: ten from each decade 1710–1810.[23] This corpus of wills manifests the mixed and unstable situation in which the individual wills were produced, for the labels (in the margins) according to which the wills are classified shift among the naming formats. Sometimes they designate the case by the woman's married name with a birth name alias: so, for example, Anne Peine alias La Fargue or Susanne Nompar de Caumont alias de Beringhen. At other times they label through the birth name with the husband's name as an alias: so Perside de Lescure alias Badiffe or Marie Fournier alias Puol. And sometimes they use the customary 'formerly': Marianne-Ursule Guise formerly d'Hervart or Jane Margaret Tirel formerly Bistord.

The key portions of the wills for our purposes, however, are the two places where the women testators identify themselves. The opening of the will reads 'I — living in the parish of — ' or 'I — being of sound mind . . . ' And then the will always concludes with the woman testator's own signature.

From those two 'autobiographical' elements in these wills we can identify the following trends in naming patterns. By the end of the 18th century, wives were no longer using the French naming pattern: from 1790 onward I found not a single case of what still prevailed as convention across the Channel in France. Leading up to this end result, the trend across the preceding century had been as follows: In the first third of the period, from 1710–40, 59 per cent of the will-making Huguenot women had declared their own name according to the French pattern. The practice persisted into the second period but much more weakly, with 36 per cent of women in 1740–70 calling themselves in the French fashion. Thereafter, as I said, French naming practice dropped to nil.

Another cultural artifact that disappeared with the same timing was the French-language will, of which I found none after 1770. In the first period (1710–40) 77 per cent of the women's wills had been in French; in the second period 36 per cent. This coincident disappearance of naming pattern and will language leads us to ask whether the naming pattern had been all along just a matter of the language of the will, French naming appearing in French-language wills and English naming being used in English-language wills? That was not, however, the case. French-pattern names were found 68 per cent of the time in French-language wills and 32 per cent of the time in English-language wills. English-pattern names were found 41 per cent of the time in French-language wills. Indeed, this last datum may be among the most significant of the findings. If the disappearance by 1800 of French-language wills and French marital naming is not surprising, given what else we know about the direction and pace of Huguenot integration in England, the early 18th-century experience is a bit more arresting: in particular, the fact that in the 1710s and 1720s 57 per cent of the women using the English naming pattern were doing so in French-language wills. In other words, of the total women testators in my sample who wrote a will before 1730, 21 per cent wrote within their French-language community but went by English-style names.

What does it mean?

Data such as these are not self-interpreting, and as arduous as it is to collect and process them, it is yet more difficult to determine what they may mean. Here are my hypotheses. As my study is as yet incomplete, this should be regarded as only a pre-liminary report on my findings accompanied by a few highly speculative suggestions.

First, *persistence* of the French naming pattern well past mid-century would indi-cate the continuing presence of whatever particular conditions permitted French immigrant women to keep their own names. What might those have been? That marital naming not be something the English felt so strongly about that, in the absence of legal requirement, they enforced it through informal pressures to conform; perhaps that immigrant women maintained strong ties to the home country; perhaps that they did not intermarry with English men; that French immigrant men and/or the French community as a whole validated continuation of the French naming pattern, maybe sensing its importance as a token of the bilateral nature of marriage/kinship.

More significantly, the association between individuals and Huguenot culture was more elastic than I had originally assumed, internal diversity probably more normal. My point of departure had been that *disappearance* of the French marital naming pattern could be taken as a marker of very advanced cultural assimilation. Despite the perennial hopes of host populations, attachments to one's own culture do not erode easily – least easily eroded of all, perhaps, might be attachment to the name one's culture of origin has assigned. So I guessed that the decision to adopt an English-style naming would signal advanced or virtually complete refashioning of oneself in the image of the host: that one who keeps her own French name may be very far assimi-lated in other respects, but one who gives it up has probably already given up the rest of her ethnic identity: lost any sense of strong identification with the natal group and shifted her sense of identity to the core society.

This assumption has been undermined by two of my findings. First, the early variability on naming serves as a reminder that communities – immigrant or native – normally (and I use this word deliberately) exhibit a pluralism of preferences – segmented by class,[24] age, locality, personal idiosyncrasy, time on the ground – not simply when the community's solidarities are 'eroding' but when they are at their most coherent. Indeed, it undercuts the conventional notion that linear movement from coherence to detachment is the shape that best describes the experience of integration/ assimilation.[25]

A second finding lends substance to this revision: the use of the English naming pattern in some families known to be deeply embedded in the Huguenot community. A case in point is Jane Migault, daughter-in-law of the famous memoir-writer Jean Migault, the schoolmaster from Poitou. She, obviously, adopted her husband's surname, and yet the list of friends in her husband's will shows their personal cultural milieu: Du Pont, Loubert, Bilonard, Girard, Delafons, Bornin, Trible, Courtauld, Bonvillieres.

Indeed, the meanings of the women's names will only become fully clear when naming choices can be correlated with other information in the wills (forms of property, family structure, patterns of bequests) and with the principal differences between French inheritance practices and English in the period (greater power of the

English to exheredate, lesser preference for sons and first-borns among the French, more legacies to collaterals and distant kin among the French, and so on). This kind of contextualization can yield fuller meanings of the self-identifications that are the wills' most obvious and obviously significant feature.

Even more broadly read, the wills might allow us to imagine the life stories that lay behind testamentary provisions: the only autobiographies these women ever wrote. To give just one example, many women in their wills placed themselves firmly in a universe of women through the prominence of females among their legatees: often nieces or god-daughters, sometimes back in France (once or twice mentioned as being nuns, once or twice with the proviso that they move to England as Protestants) or in other parts of the Refuge; but mostly their own daughters. And the testators' words sometimes conveyed a certain urgency not only about the arrangements for the bequest but also about the security of the donee. So, for example, the widowed Marie Granger (English-named), living in the parish of St James, London, writing her French-language will in 1712, stipulated that half her estate should go to her daughter Magdalen, which she was to receive 'upon her own acquittances and for her own proper and separate use without the said sieur [Thomas] Champion de Crespigny her husband's intermeddling or intervening' and further stipulated that the other half of the estate should go to the children of her deceased daughter Martha, to be managed by the surviving daughter Magdalen 'without the intermeddling and intervening of the said sieur d'Auteuil their father who shall have no direction or management in the said portion belonging to the children'. The wills themselves, then, may offer us a broad entrée into the lives of the English *réfugiées*.

But like the will itself, it all starts with a name. And 'What's in a Name?', Juliet asked; in 1847 Elizabeth Cady Stanton answered: 'There is a great deal in a name. It often signifies much, and may involve a great principle'.[26]

Appendix

This paper sets aside two issues that merit further discussion: the relationship of naming practices to property laws and to the power dynamics within marriage. The author of *Lawe's Resolution of Women's Rights* (1632) connects the name pattern to the laws of property: 'Because women lose the name of their ancestors, and by marriage usually are transferred into another family, they participate seldom in heirship with males. . . . A wife however gallant soever she be, glittereth but in the riches of her husband, as the moon hath no light but it is the sun's'.[27] The English case is however far more complex than this would suggest. On the one hand, the system of trusts under Equity law made it possible for women's property to be kept separate.[28] But the common law of property also (and this is usually ignored) reserved her real estate to her own control. For this reason, Alan Macfarlane has called the English situation for women 'a strange irony': that English women lost their name even as they kept their real property as well as their individual and civil rights. 'The obliteration of the wife's name and separate identity in kinship was somehow combined with her preserved separateness and individuality as a property-owner and as a citizen'.[29] By contrast, French women, who kept their own name, slipped into lifelong coverture and found their property absorbed into the community, of which their husband was the master.

'La puissance qu'a le mari le rend maître absolu de tous les biens de la communauté et lui donne le droit d'en disposer, même pour la part qu'y a sa femme, sans qu'elle puisse disposer elle-même, sans son mari, en aucune manière, de sa part, pendant que le mariage et la communauté durent'.[30]

Though later feminists have sometimes used marital naming to symbolize loss or maintenance of identity, the assumption that name patterns reflect the lesser or greater autonomy of married women does not work, at least not in the French-English case under discussion here. Property law was too disparate and too complex on both sides of the Channel, and power relations too alike, to allow the contrasting naming patterns to stand for contrasting relationships between husband and wife.[31] At least as much in France as in England was the wife subsumed to 'son mari, son chef, son seigneur et son maître'.[32]

NOTES

1   The inventory I have compiled includes escape accounts by persons with the following surnames: Aigaliers, Allix, Arbaud (2), Aulnis, Babault, Baudouin de la Bruchardière, Brousson, Cabrit, Cabrol, Chalmot, Changuion, Chauffepié (2), Chenu de Chalezac, Collot, Cosne, Dumont de Bostaquet, DuNoyer, Durand, Faisses, Fontaine, Gamond, Giraud, Lacoste, Lambert de Beauregard, La Motte Fouqué, Lamp, Lamy, La Rochefoucauld, Lautere, Massanes, Migault, Minet, Mirmand, Molinier, Montacier, Nissolle, Péchels, Perigal, Pineton de Chambrun, Rebotier, Rival, Robillard de Champagné, Rochegude, Savois, Terrasson, Turquand, Vieusseux-Léger. Two accounts are anonymous.

2   Robin Gwynn, 'Patterns in the study of Huguenot refugees in Britain: past, present and future', in Irene Scouloudi (ed.), *Huguenots in Britain and their French background, 1550–1800* (London, 1987), 222.

3   An exception here would be intermarriage, in which (of course) women are as well represented as men. I am sceptical of what intermarriage between a French immigrant and an English person by itself – apart from the decision on naming taken by the bride – might signify for assimilation, since such pairings had been common for a very long time and were no more cross-cultural (perhaps even less) than, for example, marriage between a Breton and a Provençal. The significant dimension of French bride-English groom pairings would be precisely the consequence for the woman's name.

4   For a basic sociological overview of current approaches to issues of assimilation and group adaptation, see Joe R. Feagin and Clairece Booher Feagin, *Racial and ethnic relations* (6th edn., New Jersey, 1999), esp. ch. 2.

5   Paul John Eakin, *Fictions in autobiography: studies in the art of self-invention* (Princeton, 1985), 214.

6   I could add, in the interest of full disclosure, that this topic has a particular personal interest to me, since I have recently changed my surname – to take back the birth name abrogated at marriage, though my marital status itself has not changed. But then, as is often said, all writing of history is autobiographical.

7   Assimilation is 'the more or less orderly adaptation of a migrating group to the ways and institutions of an established host group' (Feagin and Feagin, 35). It assumes an asymmetry: rather than natives and new arrivals adjusting to each other in their interactions, one gives up its own cultural heritage to conform to the other, which remains steady.

8   Albert Dauzat, *Les noms de personnes: origine et évolution* (Paris, 1925); H. Blaquière, 'Du prénom au surnom', *Revue internationale d'onomastique* 21 (1969): 105–8.

9   Roderick Munday, 'The French law of surnames: a study in rights of property, personality and privacy', *Legal Studies: The Journal of the Society of Public Teachers of Law* 6 (1986), 94.

10   For an excellent discussion of post-Revolutionary applications of the principles of immutability and familial proprietary right, see Munday, 'French law of surnames' and Roderick Munday, 'The girl they named Manhattan: the law of forenames in France and England', *Legal Studies: The Journal of the Society of Public Teachers of Law* 5 (1985), 331–44. In neither article, unfortunately, does Munday apply these principles directly to women's marital naming or suggest how the current practice of adopting the husband's surname at marriage squares with the principle of immutability.

11   There were regional exceptions well into the modern era. Any study of Huguenot assimilation must remember the situation of immense variation that French emigrants came out of: in languages, laws, family patterns. As Fernand Braudel famously remarked: 'France is diverse to the point of absurdity'. See Braudel, *The identity of France*, vol. 1: *History and environment*, trans. Siân Reynolds (New York, 1988), 37. The Huguenot exiles came into the Refuge, then, bearing their local cultures and to a very important extent only became united as 'French' in the Refuge. One of the advantages of tracing assimilation by the marital naming pattern is, however, that it was one of the most uniform practices across French regions even by the time of the Revocation.

12   Scottish law required use on all legal documents of the wife's birth name, along with the husband's surname as a mere alias: Una Stannard, *Mrs Man* (San Francisco, 1977), 114.

13   There were exceptions: in parts of West Cumberland, in Dorset, in the Channel Islands and in the North where kin groups were especially strong, women might use their birth name for their entire life.

14   T.E., *Lawe's Resolution of Women's Rights* (London, 1632), 125.

15   In a 1992 survey, 11 per cent of English married women identified themselves with their birth name. See Stephen Wilson, *The means of naming: a social and cultural history of personal naming in western Europe* (London, 1998), 257.

16   Sir Edward Coke, *Commentaries on Littleton* (1628), 3, a[m]. This was confirmed in 1823 by King vs. Inhabitants of St Faith's, *Dowling and Ryland Report* (9 vols., London, 1822–31), vol. 3, 348. Two excellent discussions by Roderick Munday of these common law principles are in 'Girl they named Manhattan', and 'French law of surnames', 79–95.

17   Courtney Stanhope Kenny, *The history of the law of England as to the effects of marriage on property and on the wife's legal capacity* (London, 1879), 7. The uniqueness of the English naming system was the subject of an extended exchange in the following issues of *Notes and Queries*: 23 December 1865, 13 August 1887, 10 September 1887, 8 October 1887, 25 February 1888, 12 May 1888, 9 June 1888, 8 December 1888, 17 August 1889, 21 September 1889. One stated reason for lamenting the English practice was concern over a man's loss of posthumous fame in a patrilineal system if he had only daughters. Roughly twenty percent of all families would have daughters and no sons, according to G. A. Harrison and J. R. Goody, 'The probability of family distribution', *Comparative Studies in Society and History* 15 (1973), 16–20. Of course in England a daughter's husband did sometimes adopt his wife's family name in such situations or add her surname to his own, with or without a hyphen. Or the wife might take the husband's name but have the second son take her maiden name and her property, so refounding her lineage. See Joan Perkin, *Women and marriage in 19th-century England* (Chicago, 1989), ch. 3.

18   French Protestant Church of London, Soho Square, MS 71A: Collection of wills, 1723–1844.

19   French Protestant Church of London, Soho Square, MS 230: Register of members who asked for *témoignages*, 12 April 1674–23 August 1685.

20   HSQS 22, xv.

21 I cannot, however, establish that the French naming pattern is universal even here, because in a few cases this listing groups families under the husband's first and last name, followed by the first names of his wife and children. I would have to see the signature of the wife to ascertain which practice her self-identification conformed to.

22 Jack Goody, 'Inheritance, property and women: some comparative considerations', in Jack Goody *et al.* (eds.), *Family and inheritance: rural society in western Europe, 1200–1800* (Cambridge, 1976), 15.

23 These were identified with the help of Wagner's notebooks on wills, which are located in the Huguenot Library at University College, London. All the wills themselves are in the Public Record Office at Kew. Of course nothing definitive can be advanced until we have a sample that is representative and that allows us to contrast Huguenot women and English women on more dimensions (particularly with respect to patterns of bequests). For the moment, I offer only a few preliminary observations.

24 The testators in the wills in the PRO all stand above a certain level of property ownership. To test the class bias in these wills, I used the records of the Westminster Charity School, an institution set up to assist the children of poor or indigent Huguenot families. The school's records list the parents of the children admitted on the basis of the baptismal certificate. I took a sample of 100 parent-couples whose child-pupils were baptized from 1786 to 1810, in an effort to see whether the disappearance of the wife's birth name so evident in the wills is equally replicated among a lower class group. This sample shows greater persistence of the mother's birth name: one-third of the mothers' names were listed in the French style. However, these data are not directly comparable to the wills, since these documents are bureaucratic rather than autobiographical. The best predictor of the naming pattern of the mothers in the WCS sample comes from the church in which their children were baptized. When the baptism was at Threadneedle Street or La Patente or Artillery, the mother's birth name was used. Practice at the Savoy Church was mixed. Baptisms in such English parishes as St Anne's Westminster, St Giles, Whitechapel, or Marylebone used English-style naming. Perhaps the main utility of this comparison sample, then, is to suggest the complexity of the relationship of individual immigrants to the French community, for two-thirds of these families associated themselves with the English Church but looked for charity to the French community.

25 Thought-provoking reconceptualizations of immigrant community experiences are discussed in James Clifford, 'Diaspora', *Cultural Anthropology* 9 (1994), 302–38; and in Stuart Hall, 'Cultural identity and diaspora', in Jonathan Rutherford (ed.), *Identity: community, culture, difference* (London, 1990), 222–37.

26 Shakespeare, *Romeo and Juliet*, Act 2, Scene 2; Elizabeth Cady Stanton, 'Letter to Rebecca Eyster', quoted in Stannard, *Mrs Man*, 4.

27 T.E., *Lawe's Resolution of Women's Rights*, 9, 129–30.

28 A remarkably clear and discerning discussion that underlines the limits of women's control over equity property is Susan Moller Okin, 'Patriarchy and married women's property in England: questions on some current views', *Eighteenth Century Studies* 17:2 (1983–4), 121–38: 'Rather than separate estates increasing the power of wives in relation to husbands, then, it seems that the power of husbands over wives was so extensive as to greatly weaken the practical significance of separate estate' (135).

29 Alan Macfarlane, *Marriage and love in England: modes of reproduction, 1300–1840* (New York, 1986), 289–90.

30 Robert Joseph Pothier, *Traité de la puissance du mari* (1774), quoted in Jean Portemer, 'Le statut de la femme en France depuis la réformation des coutumes jusqu'à la rédaction du code civil', in *La femme: recueils de la Société Jean Bodin pour l'histoire comparative des institutions* 12 (1962), 460. See also Pierre Petot, 'Le statut de la femme dans les pays coutumiers français du XIIIe au XVIIe siècle', in *La femme*, 243–54.

31   The spectrum of property systems in France was established by the work of Jean Yver, especially his *Essai de géographie coutumière* (Paris, 1966). See Emmanuel Le Roy Ladurie, 'Family structures and inheritance customs in sixteenth-century France', in Goody, *Family and inheritance*, 37–71. For England, see Jack Goody, 'Inheritance, property and women'.

32   Molière, *L'école des femmes* (1662), Act 3, Scene 2.

Contributors

Dr Julia Marciari Alexander, Paintings and Sculpture, Yale Center for British Art, Box 208280, New Haven, CT 06520-8280

Mrs Eileen Barrett, 26 Rama Crescent, Khandallah, Wellington, New Zealand

Dr Margrit Schulte Beerbühl, Historische Seminar II, Heinrich Heine Universität, Universitätstrasse, 40225 Düsseldorf, Germany

Dr Michael Berkowitz, Department of Hebrew and Jewish Studies, University College, Gower Street, London WC1E 6BT

Dr Pierre Boutin, Centre d'Etudes en Rhétorique, Philosophie et Histoire des Idées, Ecole Normale Supérieure, Lyon, France

Professor Geoffrey Cantor, School of History and Philosophy of Science, University of Leeds LS2 9JT

Dr Paula Wheeler Carlo [*Nassau Community College, State University of New York*], 151 Labau Avenue, Staten Island, NY 10301

Professor Patrick Collinson, The Winnats, Cannon Fields, Hathersage, Hope Valley S32 1AG

Dr Aart de Groot, 12 Boskant, Zeist 3708 BP, The Netherlands

Carrie E. Euler, Department of History, The Johns Hopkins University, 3400 N. Charles Street, Baltimore, MD 21218

Dr Amanda Eurich, Department of History, Western Washington University, Bellingham, WA 98225-9056

Dr Raymond Fagel, Department of History, University of Leiden, Doelensteeg 16, 2300 RA Leiden, The Netherlands

Peter Forsaith, The Wesley and Methodist Studies Centre, Westminster Institute of Education, Oxford Brookes University, Oxford OX2 9AS

Dr Peter D. Fraser, Race and Drugs Project, School of Social Science, University of Middlesex, Queensway, Enfield, Middlesex EW3 4SA

Professor Joyce D. Goodfriend, Department of History, University of Denver, 2000 Asbury Avenue, Denver, CO 80208

Miss Eileen Goodway, P.O. Box 1961, Bradford-on-Avon, Wilts BA15 2YD

Professor Nigel Goose, Department of Humanities, University of Hertfordshire, Wall Hall Campus, Aldenham, Herts WD2 8AT

Dr Robin Gwynn, 23 Clyde Road, Napier, New Zealand

Dr Deborah E. Harkness, Department of History, University of California-Davis, Davis, CA 95616

Dr April Lee Hatfield, Department of History, Texas A & M University, College Station, TX 77843-4236

Ms Karen Hearn, Curator, 16th- and 17th-century British Art, Tate Gallery, Millbank, London SW1P 4RG

John McDonnell Hintermaier, Department of History, 207 Dickinson Hall, Princeton University, Princeton, NJ 08544

Dr Raymond Pierre Hylton, Department of History, Virginia Union University, 1500 N. Lombardy Street, Richmond, VA 23220

Robert G. Ingram, Department of History, Randall Hall, University of Virginia, P.O. Box 400180, Charlottesville, VA 22904-4180

Dr Jeffrey Jaynes, Methodist Theological School in Ohio, 3081 Columbia Pike, Delaware, OH 43221

Graham Jefcoate, Early Printed Collections, The British Library, 96 Euston Road, London NW1 2DB

Dr Yitzchak Kerem, P O Box 10642, Jerusalem 891002, Israel

Dr Vivienne Larminie, New Dictionary of National Biography, Great Clarendon Street, Oxford OX2 6DP

Professor Carolyn Lougee Chappell, Department of History, Stanford University, Stanford, CA 94305-2024

Mme Michelle Magdelaine, CNRS, 3 rue Michel-Ange, 75794, Paris Cedex 16

Dr John Marshall, Department of History, The Johns Hopkins University, Baltimore, MD 21218

Dr Nabil Matar, Humanities and Communication Department, Florida Institute of Technology, Melbourne, FL 32901

Dr Jane McKee, Department of Humanities, University of Ulster, Magee College, Londonderry BT48 7JL

Dr Tessa Murdoch, Department of Furniture and Woodwork, Victoria and Albert Museum, South Kensington, London SW7 2RL

Dr Sugiko Nishikawa, Faculty of Letters, Kobe University, 1-1 Rokkodai-cho, Nada-ku, Kobe 657-8051, Japan

Professor Alison G. Olson, Department of History, University of Maryland, 215 Francis Scott Key Hall, College Park, MD 20742-7315

Professor Jeannine Olson, Rhode Island College, Providence, RI 02908 / 1654 Portola Avenue, Palo Alto, CA 94306

Dr William O'Reilly, Department of History, National University of Ireland, Galway, Ireland

Dr Itamar Raban, Ohalo College, Qatzrin, Golan Heights, Israel

Mrs Dianne Ressinger, 4N900 Greenwood Lane, St Charles, IL 60175

Ms Christine Riding, Tate Gallery, Millbank, London SW1P 4RG

Miss Natalie Rothstein, Avalon, Kiln Road, Prestwood, Bucks HP18 9DH

Edgar Samuel, 4 Garden Court, 63 Holden Road, Woodside Park, London N12 7DH

Dr Claire S. Schen, Department of History, Wake Forest University, P.O. Box 7806, Winston-Salem, NC 27109-7806

Professor Dr Christoph Strohm, Evangelisch-Theoloigische Fakultät, Ruhr-Universität Bochum, Universitätstrasse 150, D-44801 Bochum, Germany

Dr Catherine Swindlehurst, 11107 22A Avenue, Edmonton, Alberta T6J 4V7, Canada

Geoffrey Treasure, Beech Grove House, Kington, Herefordshire   HR5 3RH

Professor Hugh Trevor-Roper (Lord Dacre of Glanton), The Old Rectory, Didcot, Oxon OX1 7EB

D. J. B. Trim, Depatment of Humanities, Newbold College, Binfield, Bracknell, Berks RG42 4AN

Mrs Jean Tsushima, Malmaison, Church Street, Great Bedwyn, Wilts SN8 3PE

Dr Bertrand van Ruymbeke [*University of Toulouse*], 6 rue Jacques Labatut, Toulouse 3100, France

Dr David William Voorhees, Papers of Jacob Leisler Project, New York University, 53 Washington Square South, New York, NY 10012-1098

Dr Joseph P. Ward, Department of History, University of Mississippi, University, MS 38677

Dr Gordon M. Weiner, Department of History, Arizona State University, Tempe, AZ 85261

Professor Ruth Whelan, Department of French, National University of Ireland, Maynooth, Co Kildare, Ireland

Professor Myriam Yardeni, Department of General History, University of Haifa, Mount Carmel, Haifa 31905, Israel

Dr Laura Hunt Yungblut, Department of History, University of Dayton, 300 College Park, Dayton OH 45469-1540

Index
